Fetal Medicine

THE CLINICAL CARE OF THE FETUS AS A PATIENT

Dedication

This book is dedicated to the participants, invited lecturers, and the Board of Directors of the Fetus as a Patient Society.

Fetal
Medicine

THE CLINICAL CARE OF THE FETUS AS A PATIENT

Edited by

Frank A. Chervenak

The New York Hospital – Cornell Medical Center, New York, USA

and

Asim Kurjak

Ultrasonic Institute, University of Zagreb, Croatia

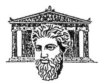

The Parthenon Publishing Group

International Publishers in Medicine, Science & Technology

NEW YORK   LONDON

Library of Congress Cataloging-in-Publication Data
Data available

British Library Cataloguing in Publication Data
Fetal medicine : the clinical care of the fetus as a
    patient
    1. Fetus – Diseases 2. Fetal monitoring
    I. Chervenak, Frank A. II. Kurjak, Asim
618.3'2

ISBN 1-85070-072-9

Published in the USA by
The Parthenon Publishing Group Inc.
One Blue Hill Plaza
PO Box 1564, Pearl River,
New York 10965, USA

Published in the UK and Europe by
The Parthenon Publishing Group Limited
Casterton Hall, Carnforth,
Lancs. LA6 2LA, UK

Copyright © 1999 The Parthenon Publishing Group

Typeset by H&H Graphics, Blackburn, UK
Printed and bound by Butler & Tanner Ltd.
Frome and London, UK

Contents

List of principal contributors ... ix

Color plates ... xiii

Preface ... 1

1   Professional virtues in the clinical care of the fetus as a patient ... 3
F. A. Chervenak, L. B. McCullough and A. Kurjak

Section 1   New developments in ultrasound

2   The embryonic biophysical profile ... 9
C. Comas and J. M. Carrera

3   Advanced sonoembryology by transvaginal three-dimensional ultrasound ... 16
H. Takeuchi

4   The volume and vascularity of the yolk sac ... 24
S. Kupesic and A. Kurjak

5   Clinical importance of evaluation of the intervillous circulation ... 28
A. Kurjak, S. Kupesic, T. Hafner and M. Ivančić-Košuta

6   Screening procedures during the first trimester of pregnancy ... 37
M. L. Brizot, L. M. Lopes, D. A. L. Pedreira, V. Bunduki and M. Zugaib

7   B-mode and Doppler studies of the abnormal fetus in the first trimester ... 46
R. K. Pooh

8   Ultrasound screening for congenital heart defects: routine or selective? ... 52
S. Levi, L. Tecco and G. Faron

9   Fetal pyelectasis: definition, significance and outcome ... 58
G. D'Ottavio, L. Paduano, M. A. Rustico, R. Natale, Y. J. Meir and G. P. Mandruzzato

10   Ultrasonographic morphological assessment of the umbilical cord ... 64
V. D'Addario and E. Di Naro

11   Diagnosis and management of fetal tumors ... 70
C. I. Onyeije and M. Y. Divon

12   Fetal pulmonary arterial and venous flow velocity waveforms during the second half of pregnancy ... 76
J. W. Wladimiroff and J. A. M. Laudy

13   Intrauterine growth restriction and fetal cerebral circulation   81
      G. Clerici and G. C. Di Renzo

14   Human fetal venous return evaluation: a reappraisal   86
      A. Matias, N. Montenegro and J. C. Areias

15   Current perspectives on ultrasonic tissue characterization   93
      K. Maeda, P. E. Kihaile, M. Utsu, N. Yamamoto and M. Serizawa

16   Three-dimensional ultrasonography in prenatal diagnosis   102
      A. Kurjak and M. Kos

Section 2   Advances in fetal diagnosis and therapy

17   New insights into understanding fetomaternal tolerance   111
      S. Hahn, M. R. Bürk, C. Troeger, S. Schatt and W. Holzgreve

18   An update on chorionic villus sampling   117
      Y. H. Yang and J. E. Chung

19   Prenatal diagnosis of hemoglobinopathies   124
      S. T. Chasen

20   Fetal cells in maternal blood: diagnostic aid or disease-causing culprit?   130
      W. Holzgreve, C. Troeger, X. Y. Zhong, S. Schatt, C. van Kaisenberg and S. Hahn

21   Issues in multifetal pregnancy reduction   136
      M. I. Evans, Y. Yaron, L. Littmann, C. Tapin and H. R. Belkin

22   Antepartum testing of fetal well-being   151
      K. B. Lescale and M. Y. Divon

23   Doppler flow studies and fetal heart rate variability   157
      G. P. Mandruzzato, L. Fischer-Tamaro, Y. J. Meir and G. Conoscenti

24   Fetal behavior: integrity of brain stem apparatus   165
      T. Koyanagi, T. Takashima and H. Nakano

25   The development of the senses   171
      B. Arabin, R. van Lingen, W. Baerts and J. van Eyck

26   Fetal hemodynamics and behavioral states   181
      G. Clerici, A. Cutuli and G. C. Di Renzo

27   *In utero* treatment: state of the art   186
      M. I. Evans, A. W. Flake, M. P. Johnson, H. R. Belkin, A. Johnson and M. Harrison

28   Current perspectives on twin-to-twin transfusion syndrome   205
      D. W. Skupski

29   Fetomaternal transfusion: state of the art   211
      I. Szabó and Z. Papp

30   Perinatal cytomegalovirus infection   217
      G. Nigro, M. Mazzocco and E. V. Cosmi

31   Laboratory and clinical diagnosis of intrauterine infection of the fetus   223
      I. Sziller and Z. Papp

32   The assessment of fetal lung maturity   229
      H. H. de Haan, S. Hundertmark, J. van Eyck and B. Arabin

33   Umbilical cord nucleated red cell count as an index of intrauterine hypoxia   238
      F. Saraçoğlu

34   Modern intrapartum surveillance of the fetus – some problems in its evolution   245
      E. Saling

35   New perspectives in fetal surgery: prenatal repair of myelomeningocele   254
      B. Westerburg, R.W. Jennings and M. Harrison

Section 3   Current perspectives in clinical perinatology

36   Discrepancy between gestational age and fetal maturity among ethnic groups   267
      É. Papiernik and G. R. Alexander

37   Intrahepatic cholestasis of pregnancy: physiopathology and fetal outcome   274
      N. Berkane, J. J. Cocheton, P. Merviel, R. Gaudet, D. Brehier and S. Uzan

38   Perinatal Rh hemolytic disease: screening, treatment and personal experience   279
      L. S. Voto and M. Margulies

39   Fetal consequences of maternal inherited hypercoagulable states (thrombophilia) 288
      D. Blickstein and I. Blickstein

40   Pregnancy outcome and obstetric complications following hysteroscopic
      metroplasty   294
      S. Kupesic, A. Kurjak and D. Đulepa

41   Fetal oxygenation and vasoactive agents   301
      E. V. Cosmi and E. Cosmi, Jr

42   Fetal effects of maternally administered hypotensive drugs: fact and fiction?   310
      L. S. Voto, A. Lapidus and M. Margulies

43   Management of HIV in pregnancy   317
      S. R. Inglis

44   Ethical dimensions of HIV infection in pregnancy   331
      F. A. Chervenak, L. B. McCullough and W. J. Ledger

45 Maternal death during pregnancy: management and ethical aspects   336
    E. Gdansky and J. G. Schenker

46 Epidemiology of pre-eclampsia in The Netherlands   343
    J. van Eyck, W. F. de Boer, W. B. Grol and B. Arabin

47 Physiopathology of pre-eclampsia and intrauterine growth restriction   347
    P. Merviel, M. Beaufils, N. Berkane, A. Dumont, J. C. Challier and S. Uzan

48 Induction of labor   355
    K. Vairojanavong

49 Post-term pregnancies: evaluation, management and outcome   362
    Y. J. Meir, G. P. Mandruzzato, G. D'Ottavio, F. Buonomo and G. Conoscenti

50 Cerebral palsy in multifetal pregnancies: facts and hypotheses   368
    I. Blickstein

51 Perinatal asphyxia   374
    D. J. Evans and M. I. Levene

52 Ultrasound screening policies in the newborn period   382
    V. Váradi

53 Computers and fetal medicine   389
    I. E. Zador, L. Chik and R. J. Sokol

Index   397

List of principal contributors

B. Arabin
Department of Perinatology
Isala Clinics
Location Sophia
8025 AB Zwolle
The Netherlands

N. Berkane
Service de Gynécologie-Obstétrique et
    Médicine de la Reproduction
Hôpital Tenon
4 rue de la Chine
75020 Paris
France

D. Blickstein
Division of Hematology
Rabin Medical Center
Beilinson Campus
49100 Petach-Tikva
Israel

I. Blickstein
Department of Obstetrics and Gynecology
Kaplan Medical Center
76100 Rehovot
Israel

M.L. Brizot
Department of Obstetrics and Gynecology
Fetal Medicine Division
São Paulo University
Rua Enéas de Carvalho Aguiar, 255
Instituto Central, 10º Andar
São Paulo - SP CEP: 05406-000
Brazil

S.T. Chasen
Department of Obstetrics and Gynecology
Cornell University Medical College
525 East 68th Street
New York, NY 10021
USA

F.A. Chervenak
The New York Hospital – Cornell Medical Center
Department of Obstetrics and Gynecology
525 East 68th Street
New York, NY 10021
USA

G. Clerici
Institute of Gynecology and Obstetrics
University of Perugia
Policlinico Monteluce
Via A Brunamonti
06122 Perugia
Italy

C. Comas
Department of Obstetrics and Gynecology
Institut Universitari Dexeus
Passcig Bonanova 67
08017 Barcelona
Spain

E.V. Cosmi
Universita Degli Studi Di Roma - 'La Sapienza'
II Istituto di Clinica Ginecologica e Ostetrica
Policlinico Umberto I
Viale Regina Elena 324
00161 Rome
Italy

V. D'Addario
Department of Obstetrics and Gynecology
University of Bari, School of Medicine
Policlinico Hospital
Piazza Giulio Cesare
70100 Bari
Italy

G. D'Ottavio
Department of Obstetrics and Gynecology
Istituto per L'Infanzia
IRCCS, Burlo Garofolo
34100 Trieste
Italy

H.H. de Haan
Department of Obstetrics and Gynecology
Division of Perinatology
Isala Clinics
Location Sophia
PO Box 10400
8000 GK Zwolle
The Netherlands

G.C. Di Renzo
Center of Perinatal Medicine
Institute of Obstetrics and Gynecology
Policlinico Monteluce
Via Brunamonti
University of Perugia
06100 Perugia
Italy

D.J. Evans
Centre for Reproduction, Growth and
    Development
University of Leeds
D Floor, Clarendon Wing
The General Infirmary at Leeds
Leeds LS2 9NS
UK

M.I. Evans
Hutzel Hospital
Department of Obstetrics and Gynecology
Division of Reproductive Genetics
4707 St. Antoine
Detroit, MI 48201
USA

S. Hahn
Laboratory for Prenatal Medicine
Department of Obstetrics and Gynecology
University of Basel
Schanzenstrasse 46
4031 Basel
Switzerland

M. Harrison
The Fetal Treatment Center
University of California, San Francisco
San Francisco, CA 94143-0570
USA

W. Holzgreve
Department of Obstetrics and Gynecology
University of Basel
Schanzenstrasse 46
4031 Basel
Switzerland

S.R. Inglis
Department of Obstetrics and Gynecology
The New York Hospital – Cornell Medical
    Center
525 East 68th Street
New York, NY 10021
USA

T. Koyanagi
Kyushu University, Graduate School of
    Medical Science, Reproductive and
    Developmental Medicine
Reproductive Pathophysiology
Department of Human Development
Maidashi 3-1-1, Higashi-ku
Fukuoka 812-8582
Japan

S. Kupesic
Department of Obstetrics and Gynecology
Medical School, University of Zagreb
Sveti Duh Hospital
Sveti Duh 64
10000 Zagreb
Croatia

A. Kurjak
Department of Obstetrics and Gynecology
Medical School, University of Zagreb
Sveti Duh Hospital
Sveti Duh 64
10000 Zagreb
Croatia

K.B. Lescale
Department of Obstetrics and Gynecology
Lenox Hill Hospital
100 East 77th Street
New York, NY 10021-1883
USA

S. Levi
Ob-Gyn Ultrasound Laboratory
Centre Hospitalier Universitaire Brugmann
1020 Brussels
Belgium

K. Maeda
Department of Obstetrics and Gynecology
Seirei Hamamatsu Hospital
Sumiyoshi 2-12-12
Hamamatsu-Shi
Shizuoka-Ken 430
Japan

G.P. Mandruzzato
Istituto per L'Infanzia
Divisione di Ostetricia
Via dell'Istria 65/1
34137 Trieste
Italy

Y.J. Meir
Department of Obstetrics and Gynecology
'Burlo Garofolo' Hospital
Via dell'Istria 65/1
34137 Trieste
Italy

P. Merviel
Obstetric, Gynecologic and IVF Department
Hôpital Tenon
4 rue de la Chine
75020 Paris
France

N. Montenegro
Department of Obstetrics and Gynecology
Development Unit
Faculty of Medicine of Porto
4200 Porto
Portugal

G. Nigro
2nd Institute of Obstetrics/Gynecology
Viale Regina Elena 324
00161 Rome
Italy

C.I. Onyeije
Department of Obstetrics and Gynecology
Lenox Hill Hospital
100 East 77th Street
New York, NY 10021-1883
USA

É. Papiernik
Service de Gynécologie-Obstétrique I
Maternité Port-Royal
123 Blvd. de Port-Royal
75679 Paris Cedex 14
France

R.K. Pooh
Department of Obstetrics and Gynecology
Clinical Research Institute National Zentsuji
   Hospital
2-1-1, Senyu-cho
Zentsuji City
Kagawa 765-8507
Japan

E. Saling
Institute of Perinatal Medicine
Mariendorfer Weg 28
D-12051 Berlin-Neukoelln
Germany

F. Saraçoğlu
Department of Obstetrics and Gynecology
Ankara Numane Research and Training
   Hospital
Mihatpasa Caddesi No 49/8
Yenisehir
Ankara 06420
Turkey

J.G. Schenker
Department of Obstetrics and Gynecology
Hadassah Medical Center
PO Box 12000
The Hebrew University
91120 Jerusalem
Israel

D.W. Skupski
Director of Maternal–Fetal Medicine
The New York Hospital Medical Center of
    Queens
56-45 Main Street, #4 South
Flushing, NY 11355
USA

I. Szabó
1. Department of Obstetrics and Gynecology
Semmelweis University Medical School
Baross utca. 27
1088 Budapest
Hungary

I. Sziller
Semmelweis University Medical School
Baross utca. 27
1088 Budapest
Hungary

H. Takeuchi
Department of Obstetrics and Gynecology
Juntendo University Urayasu Hospital
2-1-1 Tomioka
Urayasu-shi 279
Japan

J. van Eyck
Isala Clinics
Location Sophia
Department of Perinatal Medicine
Dr. van Heesweg 2
8025 AB Zwolle
The Netherlands

K. Vairojanavong
Department of Obstetrics and Gynecology
Rajavithi Hospital
2 Rajavithi Road
Bangkok 10400
Thailand

V. Váradi
Department of Neonatology
St. Margaret Hospital
1032 Budapest
Bécsi str. 132
Hungary

L.S. Voto
Juncal 2168
1125 Buenos Aires
Argentina

J.W. Wladimiroff
Department of Obstetrics and Gynecology
University Hospital Rotterdam-Dijkzigt
Dr. Molewaterplein 40
3015 GD Rotterdam
The Netherlands

Y.H. Yang
Department of Obstetrics and Gynecology
Division of Reproductive Genetics
Yonsei University College of Medicine
CPO Box 8044
Seoul
Korea

I.E. Zador
Department of Obstetrics and Gynecology
Hutzel Hospital
4707 St. Antoine Blvd.
Detroit, MI 48201
USA

Color plates

Color Plate A Pulsed Doppler signals obtained from the wall of the yolk sac, demonstrating low velocity and absence of diastole

Color Plate B Transvaginal scan demonstrating a 7–8-week gestational sac. Pulsed Doppler signals isolated from the connection of the yolk sac and vitelline duct show absence of diastolic flow (resistance index 1.0)

Color Plate C The same case as in Color Plate B. Subtle Doppler signals are obtained from the umbilical cord. Note the absence of diastolic flow, as in vitelline stalk vessels

Color Plate D Pulsed Doppler signals derived from the yolk sac in a patient with missed abortion. Note the larger diameter (7 mm) of the yolk sac and irregular blood flow signals at its periphery

Color Plate E Transvaginal scan of a gestation lasting 7 weeks, complicated by bleeding. The pulsed Doppler waveform analysis indicates continuous blood flow at the periphery of the yolk sac. A few days after this examination was completed, spontaneous abortion occurred

Color Plate F Venous blood flow signals obtained from the yolk sac at 10 weeks' gestation in a patient with missed abortion

Color Plate G Transvaginal three-dimensional scan of the gestational sac at 8 weeks' gestation. Note the regular volume, shape and surface of the yolk sac

Color Plate H Three-dimensional surface rendering of the yolk sac, demonstrating direct connection between the yolk sac and the embryonic gut

Color Plate I Transvaginal scan demonstrating all the segments of the uterine circulation. Prominent intervillous circulation at the periphery of the gestational sac, measuring 2.0×1.2 cm

Color Plate J Transvaginal color Doppler enables hemodynamic investigation of all the segments of the uterine circulation; uterine, radial and spiral arteries can be studied simultaneously and instantaneously throughout the pregnancy

Color Plate K Transvaginal scan at 10 weeks' gestation. Arterial blood flow velocity waveforms from the intervillous space show low impedance (RI = 0.42)

Color Plate L The same patient as in Color Plate K. Continuous flow of a venous type is another pattern easily obtainable from the intervillous space

Color Plate M Ultrasonic images (a,b, B-mode; c, color Doppler) from normal fetuses at 12–13 weeks of gestation. The posteriorly situated fetal spine and the umbilical vein (UV) serve as landmarks (a, non-ideal plane; b,c, ideal insonation plane). DV, ductus venosus; IVC, inferior vena cava; RA, right atrium

Color Plate N Doppler blood flow waveforms recorded in the umbilical artery (reversed end-diastolic flow (a), middle cerebral artery (b), inferior vena cava (high retrograde flow) (c), ductus venosus (absent flow during atrial contraction) (d) and umbilical vein (dicrotic pulsatile flow) (e), 1 day before death (26 weeks and 6 days)

Color Plate O Transvaginal scan demonstrating a septate uterus. Note two separate endometria in the proliferative phase of the menstrual cycle. Color Doppler exposes small myometrial vessels within the uterine septum

Color Plate P In the same patient as in Color Plate O, color signals explored by pulsed Doppler waveform analysis (right) show moderate-to-high resistance to blood flow (RI = 0.69), typical of radial arteries

Color Plate Q Transvaginal scan demonstrating vascularized septum and two gestational sacs. The patient started bleeding and both pregnancies were aborted

Color Plate R Transvaginal scan of a septate uterus. Note the empty gestational sac on the left and decidually transformed endometrium on the right. Vascular signals are obtained from the septal area and intervillous space of the anembryonic pregnancy

Color Plate S The same patient as in Color Plate R. Blood flow signals isolated from the septal area demonstrate the absence of diastolic flow in radial arteries, indicative of myometrial contractions

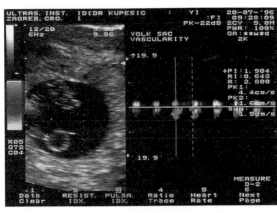

A

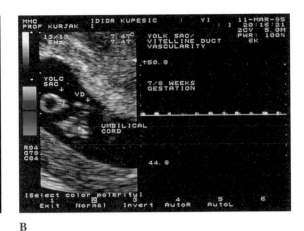

B

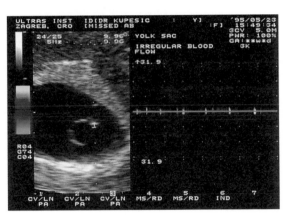

C

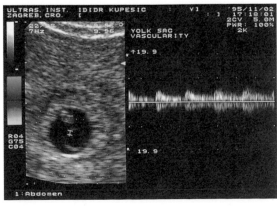

D

E

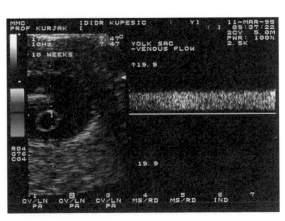

F

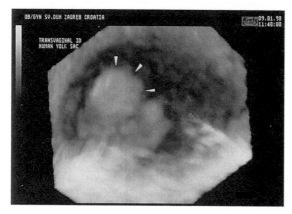

G

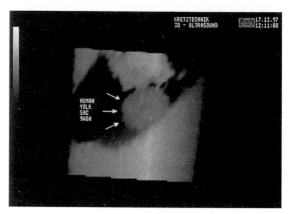

H

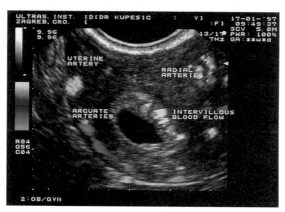

I

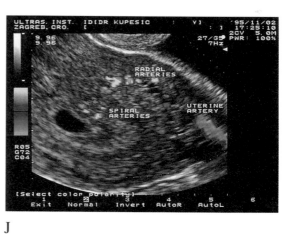

J

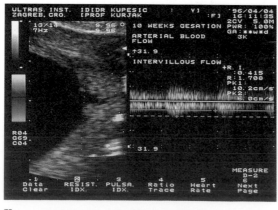

K

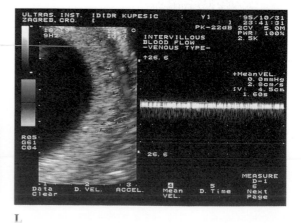

L

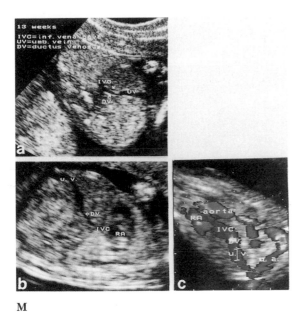

M

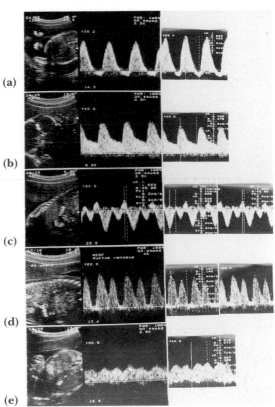

(a)

(b)

(c)

(d)

(e)

N

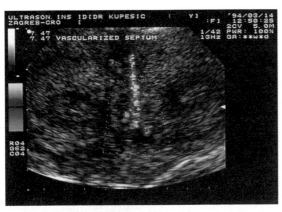

O

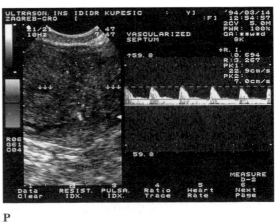

P

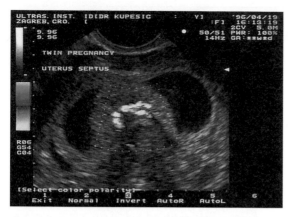

Q

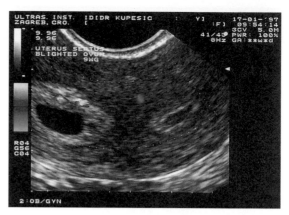

R

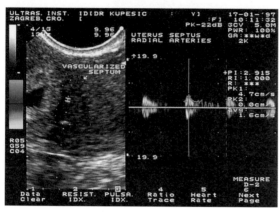

S

Preface

The Fetus as a Patient Society is an international, interdisciplinary group of physicians dedicated to improving all aspects of fetal diagnosis and therapy. This book represents the best current work of the Board of Directors and invited speakers of the Society.

Throughout the world, medicine is challenged to define the nature of the profession. The opening chapter makes explicit the central role of professional virtues in medicine as a fiduciary profession. Now, more than ever, our profession must embody those virtues in the care of pregnant women and fetal patients.

The section on 'New developments in ultrasound' presents the latest breakthroughs in this constantly evolving area. Early ultrasound not only permits evaluation of the intravillous circulation but is an important screen for Down's syndrome and other abnormalities. Later in pregnancy, the ability of ultrasound to define anomalies is constantly improving. Doppler ultrasound and three-dimensional imaging yield amazing *in vivo* information about the structure and function of the fetal patient.

The section on 'Advances in fetal diagnosis and therapy' analyzes new dimensions of genetic diagnosis and fetal assessment. An important historical evolution of intrapartum fetal surveillance is presented. Advances in fetal therapy are detailed with exciting new developments described for prenatal repair of meningomyelocele. 'Current perspectives in clinical perinatology' are presented in the last group of chapters. This section emphasizes new and important clinical dimensions of diagnosing and treating the fetus as a patient. The wide variety of topics reflects the range of modern perinatology.

We are most grateful to the Board of Directors and invited speakers of the Fetus as a Patient Society who have dedicated themselves to the constant improvement of fetal diagnosis and who have made the special effort to present their best work in a concise and readable fashion. Each contribution, while unique, blends together with the rest to reflect the scope of the evolving challenge of fetal medicine and the clinical care of the fetus as a patient.

Frank A. Chervenak, MD
Asim Kurjak, MD

Professional virtues in the clinical care of the fetus as a patient

1

F. A. Chervenak, L. B. McCullough and A. Kurjak

The clinical care of the fetus as a patient involves scientific and technical challenges. These challenges should be met by physicians in a professional manner. Professionalism in medicine is therefore essential to the appropriate application of the science and technology of maternal–fetal medicine.

In the English-speaking world, the concept of medicine as a fiduciary profession was the creation of two physicians in the 18th century: John Gregory (1724–73) in Scotland[1,2] and Thomas Percival (1740–1803) in England[3]. In their seminal works on medical ethics, these two physicians responded to what they regarded as the lack of professionalism in medicine. They were concerned about the excessive competition for patients among physicians and between physicians and surgeons, the unbridled pursuit of reimbursement and prestige, and the lack of scientific rigor in clinical judgement and practice. They believed that there was a need also to define the ethics of a new health-care institution, the infirmary, the forerunner of and model for American hospitals[2].

Gregory and Percival's work in medical ethics was enormously influential. Their books quickly were translated into the major European languages, were widely studied on the Continent, and were brought to the then-young United States by physicians who had studied in Britain, including Benjamin Rush. Published in American editions, these works influenced American medical ethics well into the 19th century. The framers of the first code of medical ethics (1847) of the American Medical Association acknowledged their extensive debt to Gregory and Percival[4].

Because contemporary clinical ethical challenges are strikingly similar to theirs, the importance of Gregory and Percival reaches into our day.

The main concern of Gregory and Percival was the *absence* of professionalism, i.e. the lack of any ethical brake on the physician's pursuit of self-interest and the subsequent inability of the patient to trust the physician to act in the patient's interest. They proposed a solution to this ethical crisis: the physician should blunt self-interest, routinely act to protect the patient's interest and thereby earn the trust of the patient[2].

THE PHYSICIAN AS A FIDUCIARY OF THE PATIENT

Gregory and Percival used the tools of ethics to develop the concept of medicine as a fiduciary profession. In medicine, the physician-fiduciary, as a primary consideration, is expected as a matter of routine and habit to fulfil obligations to protect and promote patients' interests rather than pursue his or her own interests. Virtues are those traits and habits of character that routinely focus the concern and behavior of an individual on the interests of others, and thereby habitually blunt the physician's motivation to act in self-interest as the primary consideration. Four virtues constitute the physician–patient relationship based on the physician as fiduciary[5,6].

The first virtue is self-effacement. This requires the physician not to act on the basis of potential differences between the patient and the physician such as race, religion, national origin, education, gender, manners, socioeconomic status, hygiene, or proficiency in speaking the physician's language. Self-effacement prevents biases and prejudices arising from these differences that could adversely impact on the plan of care for the patient.

The second virtue is self-sacrifice. This requires physicians to accept reasonable risks to themselves. As one example, physicians manifest this virtue in their willingness to care for patients with infectious diseases such as tuberculosis, hepatitis and HIV infection, all of which are a potential threat to the physician's health. In both fee-for-service and managed care, this virtue of self-sacrifice obliges the physician to turn away from economic self-interest and focus on the patient's need for relief when the two are in conflict.

The third virtue, compassion, motivates the physician to recognize and seek to alleviate the stress, discomfort, pain and suffering associated with the patient's disease and illness. Self-effacement, self-sacrifice and compassion provide the basis for a powerful ethical response to the business tool of conflicts of interest by the physician.

This response is strengthened by the fourth virtue, integrity. This virtue imposes an intellectual discipline on the physician's clinical judgements about the patient's problems and how to address them. Integrity prescribes rigor in the formation of clinical judgement. Clinical judgement is rigorous when it is based on the best available scientific information or, when such information is lacking, on consensus and on the careful thought processes of the individual physician that can withstand peer review. In settings that lack such quality control mechanisms, physicians confront a powerful incentive to make the pursuit of remuneration via fee-for-service the primary consideration. Integrity is thus an antidote to the pitfalls of bias, subjective clinical impressions and unexamined clinical 'common sense'. Integrity provides the basis for the physician's ethical response to the business tool of control of clinical judgement and practice.

None of these four virtues is absolute in its ethical demands. The task of medical ethics now, as it was 200 years ago for Gregory and Percival, is to identify both the application and the limits of these four virtues. The concept of legitimate self-interest provides the basis for these limits[5]. Legitimate self-interest includes protecting the conditions for practicing medicine well, fulfilling obligations to persons in the physician's life other than the patient and protecting activities outside the practice of medicine that the physician finds deeply fulfilling.

Percival thought that physicians were entitled as a matter of legitimate self-interest to exceptional levels of compensation, but only when compensation was the side-effect of the steadfast pursuit of excellence in the fiduciary care of patients[2]. We add that physicians have a legitimate interest in repaying their student loans, providing for their families, saving for retirement and other prudent financial concerns. Subordinating the interests of patients to the pursuit of wealth or to personal convenience (as with performing unindicated surgery) obviously violates the virtues of self-effacement and self-sacrifice, deadens compassion and undermines integrity[7].

CONCLUSION

Living the moral life of a fiduciary, we believe along with Gregory and Percival, makes the practice of medicine deeply rewarding and sustains the physician in the face of daily clinical challenges including a decreased number of patients. In other words, being a fiduciary provides, among many other things, a powerful and reliable bulwark against boredom and burnout. Being a fiduciary has benefits for patients, because they can receive care in an environment of trust rather than the ruthless environment of *caveat emptor*. Maintaining such trust is especially important in maternal–fetal medicine, in which increasingly sophisticated scientific and technical challenges arise for the physician.

References

1. Gregory J. *Lectures on the Duties and Qualifications of a Physician.* London: W. Strahan & T. Cadell, 1772

2. McCullough LB. *John Gregory and the Invention of Professional Medical Ethics and the Profession of Medicine.* Dordrecht: Kluwer, 1998

3. Percival T. *Medical Ethics, or a Code of Institutes and Precepts Adapted to the Professional Conduct of Physicians and Surgeons.* Manchester: S. Russell, 1803

4. Baker R, ed. *Anglo-American Medical Ethics and Medical Jurisprudence in the Nineteenth Century.* Vol 2 of *The Codification of Medical Morality: Historical and Philosophical Studies of the Formalization of Western Medical Morality in the Eighteenth and Nineteenth Centuries.* Dordrecht: Kluwer Academic Publishers, 1995

5. McCullough LB, Chervenak FA. *Ethics in Obstetrics and Gynecology.* New York: Oxford University Press, 1994

6. Council on Ethical and Judicial Affairs of the American Medical Association: Ethical issues in managed care. *J Am Med Assoc* 1995;273:330–5

7. Chervenak FA, McCullough LB, Chez R. Responding to the ethical challenges posed by the business of managed care in the practice of obstetrics and gynecology. *Am J Obstet Gynecol* 1996;175:523–7

Section 1

New developments in ultrasound

The embryonic biophysical profile

2

C. Comas and J. M. Carrera

INTRODUCTION

The progressive introduction in clinical practice of biophysical techniques of fetal surveillance over the past two decades has allowed the development of biophysical profiles that include different ultrasound parameters (e.g. fetal corporal and breathing movements, fetal tone, amniotic fluid volume) and cardiotocographic variables (e.g. fetal reactivity). Therefore, it has been possible not only to arrange the information provided by these diagnostic tools into a hierarchical system, but also to establish a comprehensive diagnostic and prognostic approach in relation to the degree of fetal well-being.

The recent introduction of transvaginal ultrasonography and color Doppler, as well as advances in the knowledge of physiopathology of the embryo, have prompted us to design an 'embryonic biophysical profile' with a similar philosophy and perspective to those of the 'fetal biophysical profile'. Our research group, which over the past 20 years has been interested in the ultrasonographic study of the 'habitat' of the embryo and especially of the kinetic characteristics, has focused its attention for the past 5 years on the assessment of different embryonic parameters derived from the use of new technologies. This chapter summarizes our experience in this field in an attempt to develop a profile and, if possible, one or various scores that would allow, on the basis of an ultrasound study, the classification and integration of all data that could be useful for predicting the embryonic condition and the outcome of the fetus.

From a practical point of view, two types of embryonic biophysical profile are distinguished: a biophysical profile of the embryonic condition and an early biophysical profile of chromosome abnormalities.

BIOPHYSICAL PROFILE OF THE EMBRYONIC CONDITION

Attempts to evaluate the embryonic condition by means of ultrasonography developed almost simultaneously with the introduction of this type of examination in obstetrics. In 1980, our group coined the expression 'sonographic signs of ovular warning'[1], which proved popular in the literature of that time; 13 sonographic signs or variables were identified that mostly referred to the aspect of the yolk sac and to the characteristics of the incipient placenta. It is currently considered that such a profile should primarily include data on five basic parameters: embryonic kinetics, embryonic biometry, embryonic heart rate activity, umbilical Doppler and nuchal translucency.

Embryonic kinetics

The recognition of a kinetic pattern of the embryo is a sonographic finding that consistently reflects biopathological condition. The use of transvaginal ultrasonography has increased interest in analysis of this parameter. At present, the two embryonic kinetic patterns classically defined in the literature, i.e. rapid movement and slow movement, can be accurately studied by means of transvaginal ultrasonography; it has been shown that there is a significant correlation between type of pattern and outcome of pregnancy. The interest in these findings merits an in-depth study of this parameter.

Embryonic biometrical measurements

Crown–rump length is a particularly efficient parameter for the prediction of embryonic death and the risk of fetal malformations and chromosome abnormalities (as discussed later in this chapter).

Embryonic heart rate

Anomalies of the embryonic heart rate have been traditionally considered a crucial sign in the evaluation of the embryo's condition, especially when sustained bradycardia is detected. The recent construction of normality curves for the heart rate activity of the embryo and the study of chromosomal defects in the embryo have allowed identification of two types of condition. Abnormally increased heart rate activity is associated with pregnancy loss in chromosomally normal embryos, whereas low heart rate tracings are consistently associated with chromosome abnormalities, particularly in cases of trisomy 21[2].

Umbilical Doppler

The detection of an increased resistance index in the umbilical circulation, usually reported in the second half of pregnancy, is a warning sign related to the appearance of perinatal complications. The utility of this index in the prediction of imminent embryonic death or chromosomal defects in early stages of gestation has been recently reported (results of umbilical resistance indexes are commented on in detail in the next section).

Nuchal translucency

Besides the association between increased nuchal translucency and chromosomal defects – analyzed in the following section – the prognostic value of this finding in the prediction of perinatal outcome (with a significant increase in perinatal morbidity and mortality) and its association with structural defects has been reported. Therefore, in the presence of increased nuchal translucency,

once the karyotype analysis has been performed, close attention should be paid to the obstetric follow-up of the fetus.

EARLY BIOPHYSICAL PROFILE OF CHROMOSOME ABNORMALITIES

The current implications of prenatal diagnosis in our society have been one of the reasons for obstetric techniques to evolve towards earlier and less aggressive methods. In this context, we assess the usefulness of ultrasonography and Doppler studies as markers of chromosomal defects in the first weeks of gestation and, accordingly, their use as an early and non-invasive screening method for chromosome abnormalities in clinical practice. Several forceful arguments in favor of the indication of these procedures include the harmlessness of the method, the optimal cost/benefit ratio, the improved image resolution, better knowledge of embryological development, the chronological advance in the possibility of making a diagnosis and the high percentage of detection of chromosomal defects.

Three main aspects of early sonographic diagnosis of chromosome abnormalities are distinguished. These include indirect sonographic signs, detection of associated malformations and identification of sonographic markers, with maximum attention focused on the possibilities of early antenatal screening. The importance of early ultrasound studies is related to the fact that early sonographic anomalies found in aneuploid fetuses are transient in about 50% of the cases and disappear spontaneously at more advanced gestational ages.

After the ultrasound study it would be helpful to be able to assign to pregnant women an individual theoretical risk of a fetus that is potentially a carrier of chromosomal defects and to establish the need for an invasive procedure according to a previously determined arbitrary value. In the sonographic study of the second trimester of pregnancy, different methods have been proposed in order to make an overall assessment of a number of qualitative and quantitative sonographic parameters. At the present time, however, an ultrasound score for the first trimester of pregnancy is not yet available, although there is considerable research in this field. Nuchal translucency thickness is the most promising ultrasound marker of the first trimester in the early prenatal screening program for aneuploidies, particularly autosomal trisomies. The inclusion of this marker in the protocol of indications of fetal cytogenetic studies in the first trimester of pregnancy has been already suggested, although more extensive studies confirming the effectiveness and reproducibility of this measure in the general population are required.

Finally, combining data of different epidemiological, biochemical and sonographic markers, each of which has been shown to be reliable in recognizing malformations, allows improvement of the results of a screening program for aneuploidies. During the first trimester of pregnancy, it seems advisable to integrate the information provided by maternal age, biochemical markers (maternal serum pregnancy-associated plasma protein A, inhibin, α-fetoprotein, neutrophil alkaline phosphatase) and ultrasound markers. Recent reports have shown promising results of the combined application of these studies at early stages of gestation[3–11]. Although at present they have not yet become a widespread routine practice, future perspectives are directed towards integrating clinical, biochemical and ultrasound variables with the advantages derived from earliness in the diagnosis.

Indirect signs

It has been traditionally considered that the presence of some indirect ultrasonographic signs of chromosomal defects would suggest the need for fetal cytogenetic studies. Although these signs are usually detected during the second half of pregnancy, some of them may be useful for early antenatal screening for aneuploidy.

Placental sonographic findings suggestive of polyploidy are usually found during the second half of gestation, although they have been recently documented at earlier stages. The paternal origin of the extra chromosome is responsible for degeneration of the placenta, with increased thickness and cystic images (from small and multiple sonolucent areas to a single cyst), and a tendency to increase in volume and echogenicity as pregnancy progresses.

The presence of a single umbilical artery is an ultrasound sign associated with a large number of syndromes, perinatal complications, intrauterine growth retardation and fetal malformations, accompanied by chromosomal defects in a variable percentage (between 12 and 47%) of cases. Its detection is facilitated by the use of transvaginal color Doppler. However, early assessment of this parameter is associated with a higher rate of false-positive results, so that it is recommended to confirm the diagnosis during the second half of pregnancy.

An umbilical cord pseudocyst has recently been associated with fetal chromosome abnormalities, particularly trisomies 18 and 13[12–14]. The indication of fetal cytogenetic studies is controversial when this is an early and single finding, since in cases of chromosomal defects it is usually associated with other signs, malformations, or ultrasound markers. Although in the series published in the literature[12–14], umbilical cord pseudocyst is usually diagnosed during the second half of gestation, the use of transvaginal ultrasonography and color Doppler allows diagnosis at earlier stages.

Measurement of an increased resistance index of the umbilical circulation is a warning sign, usually reported in the second half of pregnancy, related to the appearance of perinatal complications and fetal chromosome abnormalities. The applicability of this finding for predicting aneuploidy and/ or imminent fetal death at earlier stages of gestation has recently been reported[6,15–17]. Increased resistance to the umbilical–placental circulation has been suggested as a useful predictor of chromosomal defects, especially of autosomal trisomies in early pregnancy, although the predictive value of this parameter as a screening test in the general population remains to be evaluated.

Early detection of an abnormal embryonic and/or fetal heart rate pattern has been associated with spontaneous pregnancy failure, although in most studies the fetal karyotype was not analyzed. Abnormal heart rate activity has recently been associated with chromosome abnormalities, although the number of cases reported is small and results of the different series are not always consistent[2,7,8].

Malformations

The association of fetal malformations detected in the second trimester of gestation and chromosome abnormalities is well documented. However, the clinical implications of the same congenital defects found in early pregnancy are uncertain and controversial. There are a large number of fetal malformations of which an early ultrasonographic diagnosis is not possible, because of the natural history of embryonic development. Accordingly, anatomical and physiological development of the embryo and the fetus throughout the gestational period should be taken into account in the assessment of fetal malformations, particularly when this evaluation is being performed in the context of the first trimester of pregnancy. Thus, some congenital anomalies are expressed late, because they develop as pregnancy progresses, requiring a certain silent period until detection. This group of malformations, including renal (obstructive uropathy), cardiac (myocardial hypertrophy), intestinal (duodenal atresia) and central nervous system (hydrocephalus) anomalies, constitute an important source of misdiagnoses (false negatives).

Ultrasonographic markers

During past years, different research groups have reported the presence of phenotypic sonographic features suggestive of chromo-some abnormalities, named 'sonographic markers'. Although evidence provide by these findings is not sufficient to make the diagnosis of aneuploidy, they are useful for screening purposes. It has been shown that sonographic markers contribute to precise identification early in pregnancy of a group of high-risk women, independently of maternal age, family or personal history and results of biochemical tests. On the other hand, as a result of the clinical use of transvaginal ultrasonography, new subtle variations from normality are continuously added to the list of anatomical and/or biometrical anomalies indicative of aneuploidy. Since the overall incidence of these markers is high, ranging between 1 and 5%, with a predictive value around 1%, their implications in terms of the couple's anxiety and costs should be re-evaluated.

Biometrical markers

Some embryonic and fetal biometrical abnormalities associated with chromosomal defects are detectable early in the prenatal period. These include anomalies of yolk sac size, increase in the extraembryonic celom, reduction in the length of the umbilical cord and intrauterine growth retardation.

Yolk sac size is a prognostic factor in the assessment of correct evolution of pregnancy, although the effectiveness of this marker is reduced by the large biological variation of its measurement. On the other hand, a decrease in yolk sac size has been suggested as an ultrasound marker of aneuploidy in relation to decreased maternal serum levels of α-fetoprotein in trisomic fetuses, although results are still inconclusive[18,19]. In addition, increase in the extraembryonic celom and reduced length of the umbilical cord have been reported as early screening markers of aneuploidy, but the usefulness of these findings is still controversial and further studies are needed to confirm their accuracy in clinical practice[20].

Severe and symmetrical intrauterine growth retardation in the second trimester of pregnancy is an indication for karyotype analysis due to the incidence of aneuploidy in approximately 25% of fetuses. The aneuploid placenta provides inadequate respiratory and nutritional support, which prevents normal embryo–fetal development. The impact of aneuploidy on fetal growth can be documented at earlier stages of gestation, probably due to the inherent effect of the chromosomal defect on cellular growth and proliferation, which is manifested by a reduction in the parameters defining embryonic growth. Measurement of the crown–rump length as evidence of early intrauterine growth impairment, and proportional to the degree of severity of the chromosomal defect, has been proposed as an early ultrasound sign for the detection of aneuploidies[21-24]. In fact, crown–rump length is a sensitive parameter for the prediction of embryonic death, risk of fetal malformations and chromosome anomalies.

Nuchal markers

Ultrasound markers related to abnormal fluid accumulation in the nuchal fold are very useful in the early prenatal screening of aneuploidies and merit special consideration. Thickening of the nuchal fold in the first trimester of gestation as an early sonographic marker of trisomy 21 was initially suggested by Szabó and Gellén[25] in 1990. The usefulness of this sign was subsequently confirmed by these authors[20,25] and others[26-31], although there is no consensus in the current literature regarding its predictive value. In general, nuchal translucency of ≤ 3 mm between 10 and 14 weeks has a sensitivity of 28–100% and a specificity of 48–99% in the diagnosis of trisomy 21. At present, however, it seems more appropriate to use a variable cut-off value in relation to gestational age, usually the 95th centile of the normal curve, instead of a predetermined fixed cut-off point. The effectiveness of this parameter in the overall screening of common autosomal trisomies (trisomies 18, 21 and 13) and less common disorders (trisomy 10), sex-linked chromosomal defects and polyploidies has been demonstrated[2,5,18,27-32]. The assessment of the nuchal fold offers promising perspectives in the early prenatal screening of aneuploidies as the most sensitive and specific ultrasound marker for the most frequent autosomal trisomies.

Other markers

This group includes a series of ultrasound markers that cannot be classified into the aforementioned categories and that are mostly reported in the second half of pregnancy, although some of them may be useful at earlier stages.

The increase in the echogenicity of the yolk sac has recently been reported as an early ultrasound marker of trisomy 21, although data are still preliminary. Ventricular echogenic foci have been associated with cardiac tumors and chromosomal defects, although in most cases this is a benign sign, detected late and secondary to a variation from normality in the development of papillary muscles and chordae tendineae. Bilateral ectasia of the renal pelvis can be used as an additional sign in the ultrasound screening for trisomy 21. Hyperechogenicity in the hemiabdomen is associated with a significant increase in the risk of aneuploidy, although it can be attributed to other clinical conditions and may be a finding present in euploid fetuses or those of high perinatal risk. The usefulness of this observation has been mostly defined in the second trimester of pregnancy, but recent studies support its value as an early sign of trisomy 21.

References

1. Carrera JM. *Ecografía obstétrica*. Barcelona: Salvat Editores, 1990
2. Martinez JM, Comas C, Ojuel J, Puerto B, Borrell A, Fortuny A. Fetal heart rate patterns in pregnancies with chromosomal disorders or subsequent fetal loss. *Obstet Gynecol* 1996;87:118–21
3. Pandya PP, Brizot ML, Kuhn P, Snijders RJM, Nicolaides KH. First-trimester fetal nuchal translucency thickness and risk for trisomies. *Obstet Gynecol* 1994;84:420–3
4. Nicolaides KH, Brizot ML, Snijders RJM. Fetal nuchal translucency: ultrasound screening for fetal trisomies in the first trimester of pregnancy. *Br J Obstet Gynaecol* 1994;101:782–6
5. Pandya PP, Goldberg H, Walton B, *et al.* The implementation of first-trimester scanning at 10–13 weeks' gestation and the measurement of fetal nuchal translucency thickness in two maternity units. *Ultrasound Obstet Gynecol* 1995;5:20–5
6. Martinez JM, Borrell A, Antolin E, *et al.* Combining nuchal translucency with umbilical Doppler velocimetry for detecting fetal trisomies in the first trimester of pregnancy. *Br J Obstet Gynaecol* 1997;104:11–14
7. Jauniaux E, Gavrill P, Khun P, Kurdi W, Hyett J, Nicolaides KH. Fetal heart rate and umbilico-placental Doppler flow velocity waveforms in early pregnancies with a chromosomal abnormality and/or increased nuchal translucency thickness. *Hum Reprod* 1996;11:435–9
8. Hyett JA, Noble PL, Snijders RJM, Montenegro N, Nicolaides KH. Fetal heart rate in trisomy 21 and other chromosomal abnormalities at 10–14 weeks of gestation. *Ultrasound Obstet Gynecol* 1996;7:239–44
9. Brizot ML, Snijders RJM, Bersinger NA, Kuhn P, Nicolaides KH. Maternal serum pregnancy-associated plasma protein A and fetal nuchal translucency thickness for the prediction of fetal trisomies in early pregnancy. *Obstet Gynecol* 1994;84:918–22
10. Noble PL, Abraha HD, Snijders RJM, Sherwood R, Nicolaides KH. Screening for fetal trisomy 21 in the first trimester of pregnancy: maternal serum free β-hCG and fetal nuchal translucency thickness. *Ultrasound Obstet Gynecol* 1995;6:390–5
11. Brizot ML, Snijders RJM, Butler J, Bersinger NA, Nicolaides KH. Maternal serum hCG and fetal nuchal translucency thickness for the prediction of fetal trisomies in the first trimester of pregnancy. *Br J Obstet Gynaecol* 1995;102:127–32
12. Sepulveda W, Pryde PG, Greb AE, Romero R, Evans MI. Prenatal diagnosis of umbilical cord pseudocyst. *Ultrasound Obstet Gynecol* 1994;4:147–50
13. Jauniaux E, Donner C, Thomas C, Francotte J, Rodesh F, Avni FE. Umbilical cord pseudocyst in trisomy 18. *Prenat Diagn* 1988;8:557–63
14. Rizzo G, Arduini D. Umbilical cord pseudocyst in trisomy 13. *Ultrasound Obstet Gynecol* 1994;4:438
15. Martinez JM, Comas C, Ojuel J, Puerto B, Borrell A, Fortuny A. Umbilical artery pulsatility index in early pregnancies with chromosome anomalies. *Br J Obstet Gynaecol* 1996;103:330–4
16. Montenegro N, Beires J, Pereira Leite L. Reverse end-diastolic umbilical artery blood flow at 11 weeks' gestation. *Ultrasound Obstet Gynecol* 1995;5:141–2
17. Martinez Crespo JM, Comas C, Borrell A, Puerto B, Antolin E, Ojuel J, Fortuny A. Reversed end-diastolic umbilical artery velocity in two cases of trisomy 18 at 10 weeks' gestation. *Ultrasound Obstet Gynecol* 1996;7:447–9
18. Comas C, Martinez JM, Puerto B, *et al.* Estudio ecográfico transvaginal en el primer trimestre de la gestación. Valor predictivo de los marcadores ecográficos en el diagnóstico prenatal de aneuploidías. Resultados preliminares. *Prog Diagn Prenat* 1994;6:225–35
19. Wathen NC, Cass PL, Campbell DJ, Wald N, Chard T. Alpha-fetoprotein levels and yolk sac size in the first trimester of pregnancy. *Prenat Diagn* 1992;12:649–52
20. Szabó J, Gellén J, Szemere G. Nuchal edema as an ultrasonic sign of trisomy 21 during the first trimester of pregnancy [Letter]. *Orv Hetil* 1992;133:3167–8
21. Drugan A, Johnson MP, Isada NB, *et al.* The smaller than expected first-trimester fetus is at increased risk for chromosome anomalies. *Am J Obstet Gynecol* 1992;167:1525–8
22. Benacerraf BR. Intrauterine growth retardation in the first trimester associated with triploidy. *J Ultrasound Med* 1988;7:153–4
23. Pedersen JF, Molsted-Pedersen L. Early fetal growth delay detected by ultrasound marks increased risk of congenital malformation in diabetic pregnancy. *Br Med J* 1981;283:269–71
24. Pedersen JF. Ultrasound studies on fetal crown-rump length in early normal and diabetic pregnancies. *Dan Med Bull* 1986;33:296–304
25. Szabó J, Gellén J. Nuchal fluid accumulation in trisomy-21 detected by vaginosonography in the first trimester. *Lancet* 1990;3:1133
26. Pandya PP, Kondylios A, Hilbert L, Snijders RJM, Nicolaides KH. Chromosomal defects and outcome in 1015 fetuses with increased nuchal translucency. *Ultrasound Obstet Gynecol* 1995;5:15–19

27. Brun JL, Saura R, Horovitz J, *et al.* First trimester diagnosis of fetal nuchal edema. Report of 29 cases. *Fetal Diagn Ther* 1994;9:246–51

28. Comas C, Martinez JM, Ojuel J, *et al.* First-trimester nuchal edema as a marker of aneuploidy. *Ultrasound Obstet Gynecol* 1995;5:26–9

29. Schulte-Vallentin M, Schindler H. Non-echogenic nuchal oedema as a marker in trisomy 21 screening [Letter]. *Lancet* 1992;339:1053

30. Nicolaides KH, Azar G, Byrne D, Mansur C, Marks K. Fetal nuchal translucency: ultrasound screening for chromosomal defects in the first trimester of pregnancy. *Br Med J* 1992;304:867–9

31. Brambati B, Cislaghi C, Tului L, *et al.* First-trimester Down's syndrome screening using nuchal translucency: a prospective study in patients undergoing chorionic villus sampling. *Ultrasound Obstet Gynecol* 1995;5:9–14

32. Savoldelli G, Binkert F, Achermann J, Schmid W. Ultrasound screening for chromosomal anomalies in the first trimester of pregnancy. *Prenat Diagn* 1993;13:513–18

Advanced sonoembryology by transvaginal three-dimensional ultrasound

H. Takeuchi

3

INTRODUCTION

In the first edition of this book, sono-embryology, particularly sonoembryology of the central nervous system and its efficacy for diagnosing anomalies in early pregnancy, was described by the present author[1]. By applying expertise in sonoembryology to the routine transvaginal examination in early pregnancy in our department, to date eight cases of anencephaly have been successfully diagnosed at up to 10 weeks of amenorrhea. However, under the same diagnostic conditions, anencephaly failed to be diagnosed in three cases. In daily clinical practice, it was considered that routine use of sono-embryology was not always feasible.

Recently, the technique of three-dimensional ultrasound has remarkably progressed. Three-dimensional visualization of the embryo and fetus in early pregnancy by the transvaginal method has become possible[2]. Several papers on the usefulness of transvaginal three-dimensional ultrasound in early pregnancy have been published[3-5]. If the embryological characteristics in appearance are discernible, three-dimensional sono-embryology, different from conventional two-dimensional sonoembryology, can be performed. Consequently, we have obtained a new capability for observation of the embryo and fetus. Furthermore, by making use of the refined objectivity of three-dimensional ultrasound, it is considered that fetal anomalies can be detected earlier and more accurately.

By using the newly developed transvaginal probe, we obtained three-dimensional images of embryos and fetuses from 6 to 11 weeks of pregnancy, and studied their morphological appearance. During our study period, we have encountered several cases of a fetus with morphological abnormality. In this chapter, the three-dimensional sonoembryology and diagnosis of morphological abnormalities in early pregnancy is presented.

METHOD OF THREE-DIMENSIONAL ULTRASOUND USED IN THIS STUDY

The equipment used in this study was the three-dimensional ultrasound machine Voluson 530D (Kretztechnik, Zipf, Austria) with a 6.5-MHz transvaginal probe Type S-VDW 5–8,which was developed in 1997 as the second-generation type. As the probe is very light and slim, with a diameter of 24 mm at the tip, and weight of 150 g, it can be manipulated as easily as the conventional two-dimensional transvaginal probe.

After positioning the probe over the region of interest by using the B-mode method, a volume box was positioned on the monitor. Volume scanning was activated by sweeping the transducer automatically with angles of 10–95° within 5 s. During this time the probe is put into the fixed position. By this method, the data set from the pyramid-shaped volume in the uterus is acquired. Storage of acquired data was accomplished on removable hard disk cartridge with 540-Mbit capacity, allowing repeated study of the fetus without re-examination of the patient.

By using software installed in the workstation of the machine, every possible plane in the stored volume box could be accessed. Initially, the fetus was represented in three orthogonal planes in three windows on the monitor. Each of the windows could be selected and its viewing plane could be rotated in all three axes. When changing the axes in one selected window, the planes in the other two windows changed simultaneously, so that each of them might keep a 90° difference between them in the viewing angle. The aim of this procedure was to put the volume box in a well-defined orientation. For achieving a three-dimensional image of the volume, the extent of the region of interest had to be selected in all three axes, permitting the speckle reduction level to be adjusted. Finally, in both surface-rendering and volume-rendering modes, a rotating three-dimensional computer image of the region of interest was calculated. Surface rendering allows visualization of the fetal skin surface, whereas volume rendering provides information about the internal structures, such as bones.

In this study we used only surface rendering for visualization of the appearance of the embryo and fetus. For surface reconstruction, a dimension in which the fetus was directly facing the examiner was selected by adequate rotation of planes. The calculation time for reconstructing each single image was less than 0.3 s. This image could be rotated on the screen to provide a better representation of the fetal appearance.

THREE-DIMENSIONAL SONO-EMBRYOLOGY OF THE EMBRYO AND FETUS

A total of 57 embryos and fetuses from 6 to 11 weeks of pregnancy were used for studying three-dimensional sonoembryology in the early stage of pregnancy. All of the studied embryos and fetuses had their structural normality confirmed postnatally. The sonoembryological information that was obtained by three-dimensional surface mode in every week of 6–11 weeks of pregnancy was as follows.

Six weeks of pregnancy

The head of the embryo at this age is recognizable due to the round prominence of the forebrain (Figure 1). This is easily differentiated from the tail. The heart bulge is barely discernible. The gross form and posture of the embryo can be identified. Limb buds are not large enough to be discerned.

Seven weeks of pregnancy

The embryo flexes sharply into a 'C' shape (Figure 2). The head and chest are almost in contact. On account of this, the region which appears to be the vertex corresponds to the hindbrain (rhombencephalon). By two-dimensional imaging, this part of the vesicles is depicted first as an echo-free space, but no structural appearance can be visualized by three-dimensional imaging. Although the spine winds smoothly from the head to the tail region, the tail cannot be depicted clearly. The heart bulge and limb buds can occasionally be observed.

Eight weeks of pregnancy

When the crown–rump length reaches more than 15 mm, growth and expansion of the lateral ventricle, third ventricle and midbrain ventricle give rise to erection of the head, causing apparent dissociation of the head from the body (Figure 3). The vertex moves to the position of the midbrain. As a result, the neck being inconspicuous, the head can be differentiated from the trunk. The smooth head shape with narrow width in the ventral or dorsal view is an important characteristic at this age of the embryo. Although the nasal process, ears and eyes are developing, the appearance of the face is hardly visualized, owing to its small size and its close position to the body. The rapidly growing intestine is beginning to herniate into the umbilical cord, and a large insertion of the cord occupies the anterior abdominal wall region. The arms curve over the heart bulge, and can be visualized in most cases. The feet are also visualized.

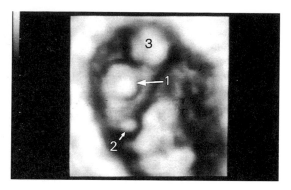

Figure 1 *Transvaginal three-dimensional surface image of an embryo at 6 weeks and 5 days of amenorrhea with crown–rump length of 7 mm. The forebrain (1) is protruded dominantly, but the heart bulge is not so clearly shown. The tail (2) is visualized. The yolk sac (3) with its stalk is seen*

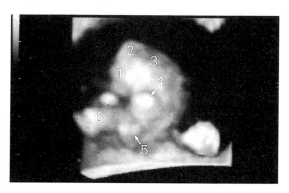

Figure 3 *A lateral view of an embryo at 8 weeks and 5 days of amenorrhea with crown–rump length of 20 mm. The forebrain (1) is still very close to the body, but the midbrain (2) ascends to the vertex, causing the descent of the hindbrain (3). The arm (4) and leg (5) are discernible. A large umbilical cord (6) and yolk sac (7) are noted*

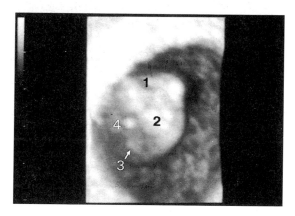

Figure 2 *The embryo at 7 weeks and 2 days of amenorrhea with crown–rump length of 12 mm is discerned diagonally from the upper and lateral side. The dorsal region of the head and trunk are mainly visualized. The hindbrain (1) is at the vertex, and the arm bud (2) and leg bud (3) are inconspicuously seen. The heart bulge is not visualized in this case. The umbilical cord (4) is barely discerned*

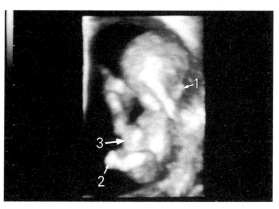

Figure 4 *A fetus at 9 weeks and 6 days of amenorrhea with crown–rump length of 28 mm is discerned three-dimensionally from the left lateral direction. A relatively large spherical head is in an erect position, and the neck is identifiable. As a result, the face can now be visualized. In this image, the external ear (1) is successfully depicted. The elbow and hand in the arm, and the knee and foot (2) in the leg, are also identifiable. The fetus now has a complete human appearance. Physiological midgut herniation (3) is the only abnormal finding in the appearance of the body*

Nine to ten weeks of pregnancy

The cerebral hemispheres expand like two large balloons, and the head as a whole has a round spherical appearance with a size of almost half the fetal length (Figure 4). The head is in a more erect position and therefore the face can now be visualized. Also, the neck is identifiable. The external ear is well advanced in form and occasionally discerned in the three-dimensional surface image. Midgut herniation into the cord is the dominant finding in the abdomen. A smoothly visualized dorsal region from the neck to the tail assures an intact spine. The arms with elbow and hand extended to the front of the body can be discerned. The legs with knee and foot which approach the midline are also seen. The findings show that at this gestational age the embryonic period is complete and the fetal period begins.

Accordingly, when a fetus has a gross anomaly, there is a possiblity of visualizing it by three-dimensional surface imaging at this age of gestation.

Eleven weeks of pregnancy

A well-developed and expanded forehead is still characteristic of the head (Figure 5). As the head extends and the chin is raised from the thorax, the neck develops. The eyes remain closed. The face profile shows the nose and lips, depending on cases. The herniated midgut is beginning to return to the abdominal cavity. The tail disappears by regression, and distinguishing features of the external genitalia appear in this gestational week (Figure 6). The limbs are longer and more differentiated. The size of the body at this age seems to be appropriate for visualization of the whole body appearance of the fetus by transvaginal three-dimensional ultrasound.

The visualization rate of fetal parts in gestational weeks 6–11

The results are shown Table 1. The differentiation of the head from the trunk is possible from 6 weeks of gestation. Recognition of the morphology of the head itself has to be done after 7 weeks. Interpretation of the entire head should be done in and after 10 weeks, when the neck is formed. That is, if there is any anomaly that deforms the appearance of the head, the anomaly is probably detectable

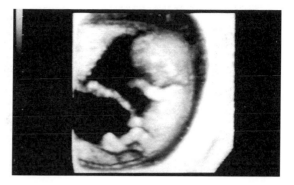

Figure 5 *The size of the head with dominant forehead is seen relatively smaller than the body in a fetus with a crown–rump length of 41 mm at 10 weeks and 5 days of amenorrhea*

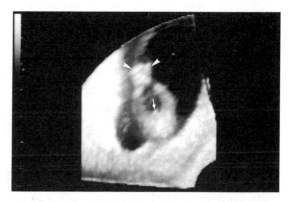

Figure 6 *The three-dimensional surface image of the fetus at 11 weeks and 3 days of pregnancy was rotated on the screen, and the view from the caudal direction was obtained. External genitalia (arrow) are distinguishable between both femurs. The legs are crossed at the ankles. Both feet (arrowheads) are recognizable*

around 7 weeks of pregnancy, but the diagnosis of the anomaly must be performed from 9 or 10 weeks of pregnancy.

Table 1 *Visualization rate (%) of appearance of fetal parts in weeks 6–11 of pregnancy by transvaginal three-dimensional surface imaging (n = 57)*

	Weeks of pregnancy					
	6 (n = 7)	7 (n = 5)	8 (n = 14)	9 (n = 11)	10 (n = 10)	11 (n = 10)
Differentiation of head from trunk	71	100	100	100	100	100
Clear visualization of head shape	14	80	93	91	100	100
Midgut herniation into cord	0	0	71	91	90	80
Intact spine	0	0	71	73	90	90
Existence of extremities (limb buds)	0	60	93	100	90	100
Whole length of extremities	0	0	71	91	90	100
Small parts (e.g. ears, fingers)	0	0	0	18	20	60

It is possible to follow the umbilical hernia from its development to its disappearance by three-dimensional ultrasound, although full observation is not always practicable in every case, owing to the fetal position. It is considered that the extent of herniation can be quantitatively described. The dorsal region, namely the spinal region, can be evaluated in and after 8 weeks. If meningomyelocele develops at such an early stage, early detection is expected.

Among anatomical structures that protrude on the surface, the extremities are the most dominant. At and after 7 weeks of pregnancy, their growth is noted. On account of their size, the fingers are visualized at 11 weeks. Anomaly of the extremities can be seen from around 9 weeks. Although small parts such as the external ears are observed after 9 weeks, it is considered to be difficult to detect their morphological abnormality until 11 weeks of pregnancy.

DIAGNOSIS OF FETAL MORPHOLOGICAL ABNORMALITIES

Two cases of fetal morphological abnormalities that were successfully visualized and were effectively diagnosed by three-dimensional surface imaging during the study period are presented.

Case 1

The first case was anencephaly diagnosed at 9 and 10 weeks of amenorrhea. A primigravid woman who had regular menstrual periods visited our out-patient clinic at 9 weeks and 3 days of amenorrhea. Conventional transvaginal two-dimensional ultrasound scanning was performed to confirm intrauterine pregnancy. A living fetus with crown–rump length of 26 mm was clearly visualized. Cranial vault and brain vesicles, which should be sonoembryologically delineated in this size of fetus, were not seen. These findings indicated that the fetus had a severe anomaly of the head.

Transvaginal three-dimensional ultrasound scanning was performed, and reconstruction of the fetal image by surface mode was immediately carried out. The appearance of the fetal head showed its distinct abnormality. No cranial vault was seen, and a topknot-like mass at the vertex was characteristic of acrania and exencephaly (Figure 7). No other morphological abnormalities were found. We informed the parents of the diagnosis, and they elected to terminate the pregnancy.

Prior to termination at 10 weeks and 2 days of amenorrhea, three-dimensional surface imaging was repeated (Figure 8). Three-dimensional imaging revealed that the deformity of the head had progressed remarkably. The topknot-like mass at the vertex had increased its volume during these 6 days. Acrania and exencephaly were confirmed. In comparison with the view of the delivered fetus, images by three-dimensional surface mode had correctly delineated the appearance of this abnormality *in utero*, as shown in Figure 9.

Case 2

The second case was of fetal hydrops at 9 weeks of pregnancy. Conventional two-dimensional transvaginal ultrasound at the second visit of the patient to our out-patient clinic, without any abnormal symptoms in 11 weeks and 1 day of amenorrhea, revealed a living fetus with 28-mm crown–rump length, which corresponded to 9 weeks and 6 days of pregnancy. Subcutaneous fluid retention was clearly seen.

By using three orthogonal planes in the multiplanar method, the width of nuchal translucency in an appropriately selected sectional plane was measured at 5.5 mm, as shown in Figure 10. Furthermore, the abnormally swollen subcutaneous part of the fetal body was successfully visualized by three-dimensional surface mode, as seen in Figure 11. It was considered that three-dimensional ultrasound was very useful for evaluation of fetal hydrops.

DISCUSSION

Three-dimensional ultrasound has almost 25 years of history[6]. Every effort has been made

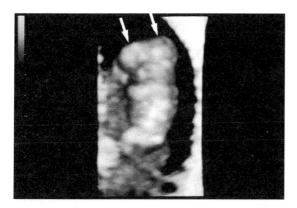

Figure 7 *Anencephalic fetus at 9 weeks and 3 days of amenorrhea with crown–rump length of 26 mm is visualized by three-dimensional surface mode. Left laterally, the dorsal view of the fetus shows the abnormal shape of the head. The topknot-like mass (arrows) at the vertex without the cranium is characteristic of acrania and exencephaly*

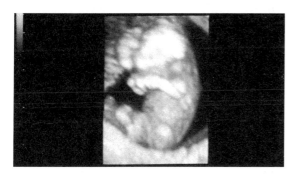

Figure 8 *At 10 weeks and 2 days of amenorrhea, just before termination, a three-dimensional image was repeated. A remarkably increased mass at the vertex was noted*

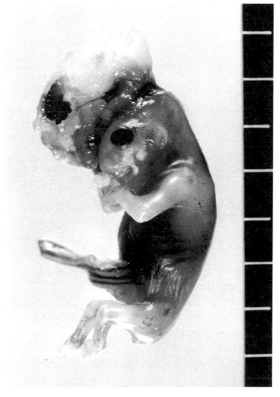

Figure 9 *The fetus delivered at 10 weeks and 2 days of amenorrhea showed the feature of acrania and exencephaly*

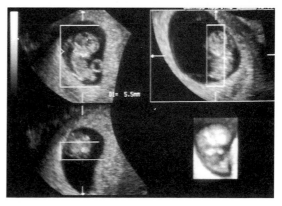

Figure 10 *By using triple orthogonal planes, the thickness of nuchal translucency was measured. Accurate measurement can be achieved by selecting the optimal section for delineation of nuchal translucency*

for technical improvement to provide a practical diagnostic modality. Most of the three-dimensional ultrasound systems developed in the past years required a long time to construct the three-dimensional image, and their image quality was generally inferior to that of two-dimensional images[7–10]. Therefore, these systems were not practical for routine clinical use. Improvements have for the first time enabled the use of three-dimensional ultrasound in routine prenatal examinations, especially in the diagnosis of fetal malformations[11,12]. The transabdominal method is applied for this purpose. When the transvaginal probe was developed, it was immediately introduced into clinical practice[2]. By using simultaneous display of triple orthogonal sections, optimal images from irregular and difficult-to-image objects such as uterine anatomy[13], endometrial

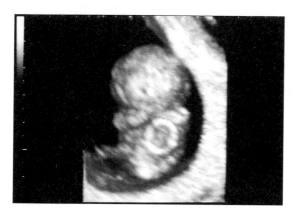

Figure 11 *The same embryo as in Figure 10, visualized three-dimensionally. The round and double-contoured head and trunk show characteristics of fetal hydrops. The circular structure attached to the abdomen is the yolk sac*

thickness[14] or follicular size[15] can be obtained. On the other hand, the surface-rendering method was applied for visualizing the form of the embryo and fetus in early pregnancy[4,16]. Bonilla-Musoles[5] stated that, in 1996, 'we were in the early stages of the development of three-dimensional imaging, but this method heralded a new era in the provision of early and reliable recognition of fetal abnormalities'. Later, the machine and transducer used by his group were much improved, and the time for acquisition and reconstruction were remarkably reduced. The quality of the surface-mode image has also been improved. Therefore, the capability of transvaginal three-dimensional surface imaging for visualizing the form or appearance of the embryo and fetus in early pregnancy was studied, to add new information to sonoembryology.

For assessing and evaluating the morphological progress of the embryo and fetus, a description of the external form, namely the shape of the body, is used. The chief methods used in embryology are the study of serial histological sections and of the reconstructions made from them[17]. In conventional sonoembryology, several temporarily obtainable sections were used, but since correct reconstruction of sectional images was difficult to perform, the external form or appearance of the embryo and fetus

could not be described. By using three-dimensional ultrasound, serial sections and reconstructed images of the embryo and fetus can be obtained. Blaas and colleagues[3] reported that they could successfully obtain three-dimensional images of brain ventricles of 7–10-week embryos by their own transvaginal equipment with a special computer graphic system. Although their result was excellent, the method they used was complicated and experimental. We aimed to obtain three-dimensional sonoembryology that was acceptable in daily clinical practice.

In this study, the embryo and fetus from 6 to 11 weeks of pregnancy were used, as the whole body of these could be visualized by the transvaginal method. It was confirmed that their external morphology, according to the embryological description, could be barely visualized. Therefore, the gestational age of an embryo or fetus can be estimated, and its normality or abnormality of development can be recognized by interpretation of transvaginal three-dimensional surface imaging. It is possible to diagnose anomalies at an early stage. Bonilla-Musoles[5] described a case of myelomeningocele which was visualized at 9 weeks of pregnancy by transvaginal three-dimensional surface mode. We had cases of anencepaly and hydrops diagnosed at 9 or 10 weeks of pregnancy.

We were able to conclude that transvaginal three-dimensional ultrasound by surface mode offers quite new but basic information in sonoembryology. This modality is capable of diagnosing morphological abnormalities of the fetus in early stages of pregnancy.

In terms of the technical procedure in obtaining three-dimensional surface image, the information acquired by volume scanning is first stored in a removable hard disk. Stored image information is reconstructed into a three-dimensional surface image through the built-in work station, as occasion arises. Therefore, it takes time to finish the procedures, and this is considered to be the disadvantage of this modality. However, the off-line procedure between acquisition and reconstruction of image information is an advantage, and improves the quality of the examination. The shortened acquisition time by automatic rapid scanning of the transducer achieves a safer examination for the fetus and offers more stable echo information to the examiner. Short examination time and less operator dependancy are important requirements for daily examinations. Furthermore, reconstruction and interpretation of both three-dimensional and two-dimensional images by the expertise of skilled sonographers can be performed with centralization. Separation between acquisition and reconstruction of image information shows the possibility of constructing a system for screening fetal abnormalities at 9–11 weeks of pregnancy. In this ultrasound screening system, every pregnant woman could be given the opportunity to be screened for fetal aneuploidy and anomaly without visiting a specialized center. The technique of telemedicine will bring more effective application of this screening system.

In conclusion, transvaginal three-dimensional ultrasound by surface mode adds new and basic information to sonoembryology, and makes sonoembryology applicable daily for expert detection of abnormalities of the embryo and fetus in early stages of pregnancy. Moreover, when the appropriate system using this modality is constructed, screening of fetal aneuploidy and anomaly at 9–11 weeks of pregnancy will be conducted reliably and effectively.

References

1. Takeuchi H. Sonoembryology in the central nervous system. In Kurjak A, Chervenak FA, eds. *The Fetus as a Patient*. Carnforth, UK: Parthenon Publishing, 1994:141–50
2. Feichtinger W. Transvaginal three-dimensional imaging. *Ultrasound Obstet Gynecol* 1993;3:375–8
3. Blaas H-G, Eik-Nes T, Kiserud T, Berg S, Angelsen B, Olstad B. Three-dimensional imaging of the brain cavities in human embryos. *Ultrasound Obstet Gynecol* 1995;5:228–32
4. Bonilla-Musoles F, Raga F, Osbome NG, Blanes J. Use of three dimensional ultrasonography for the study of normal and pathologic morphology of the human embryo and fetus: preliminary report. *J Ultrasound Med* 1995;14:757–65
5. Bonilla-Musoles F. Three-dimensional visualization of the human embryo: a potential revolution in prenatal diagnosis. *Ultrasound Obstet Gynecol* 1996;17:393–7
6. Szilard J. An improved three-dimensional display system. *Ultrasonics* 1974;76:273–6
7. Brinkley JF, Muramatsu SK, McCallum WD, Popp RL. *In vitro* evaluation of ultrasonic three dimensional imaging and volume system. *Ultrasonic Imaging* 1982;14:126–39
8. Fredfelt KE, Holm HH, Pedersen JF. Three dimensional ultrasonic scanning. *Acta Radiol Diagn* 1984;125:237–41
9. Sohn C, Grotepass J, Schneider W, Funk A, Jung H. Erste Untersuchungen zur dreidimensionalen Darstellung mittels Ultraschall. *Z Geburtsh Perinat* 1988;192:241–8
10. Baba K, Satoh K, Sakamoto S, Ishii S. Development of an ultrasonic system for three-dimensional reconstruction of the fetus. *J Perinat Med* 1989; 17:19–24
11. Merz E, Bahlmann F, Weber G. Volume (3-D)-scanning in the evaluation of fetal malformations – a new dimension in prenatal diagnosis. *Ultrasound Obstet Gynecol* 1995;5:222-7
12. Merz E, Bahlmann F, Weber G, Machiella D. Three-dimensional ultrasonography in prenatal diagnosis. *J Perinat Med* 1995;23:213–22
13. Jurkovic D, Geipel A, Gruboeck D, Jauniaux E, Natucci M, Campbell S. Three-dimensional ultrasound for the assessment of uterine anatomy and detection of uterine anomalies: a comparison with hysterosalpingography and two-dimensional sonography. *Ultrasound Obstet Gynecol* 1995;5:233–7
14. Gruboeck K, Jurkovic D, Lawton F, Sawas M, Tailor A, Campbell S. The diagnostic value of endometrial thickness and volume measurements by three-dimensional ultrasound in patients with postmenopausal bleeding. *Ultrasound Obstet Gynecol* 1996;8:272–6
15. Brunner M, Obruca A, Bauer P, Feichtinger W. Clinical application of volume estimation based on three-dimensional ultrasonography. *Ultrasound Obstet Gynecol* 1995;6:358–61
16. Maymon R, Halperin R, Weinraub Z, Herman A, Schneider D. Three-dimensional transvaginal sonography of conjoined twins at 10 weeks: a case report. *Ultrasound Obstet Gynecol* 1998;11:292–4
17. O'Rahilly R, Muller F. *Human Embryology and Teratology*. New York: Wiley-Liss, 1992

The volume and vascularity of the yolk sac

4

S. Kupesic and A. Kurjak

The yolk sac appears sonographically as a round, translucent, cyst-like structure, often located near the periphery of the gestational sac[1]. Furthermore, this fragile structure is the first to be observed by ultrasound imaging within the gestational sac, even before the embryo itself. By transvaginal high-resolution ultrasound, the yolk sac should be detected in all pregnancies over 5 weeks when the gestational sac exceeds 8 mm in diameter[2]. In normal pregnancies, its diameter increases gradually from 5 to 11 weeks of gestation and then decreases[3]. However, the evaluation of the biological function of the yolk sac by B-mode ultrasound is limited, since the diameter cannot be related to the metabolic activity of its constitutive cell layers[4]. The ability to detect blood flow velocity waveforms by sensitive color Doppler units, even in minor structures such as the yolk sac, has aroused enthusiasm in clinicians interested in the physiology and pathophysiology of early pregnancy.

COLOR DOPPLER STUDIES OF THE YOLK SAC IN NORMAL PREGNANCY

Little is known about transitory organs such as the yolk sac, which is active during only the first few weeks of embryonic life. The description of the human yolk sac has proven surprisingly controversial over the years. Recently, interesting results have been published on the assessment of yolk sac vascularization in normal pregnancy. Kurjak and colleagues[5] performed a transvaginal color Doppler study on 105 patients whose gestational age ranged from 6 to 10 weeks from the last menstrual period. Transvaginal

Table 1 *Visualization rate of yolk sac vascularity between 6 and 10 weeks of gestation*

Gestational age (weeks)	n	Visualization rate		PI ± SD
		n	%	
6	15	5	33.33	3.42 ± 0.58
7	21	18	85.71	3.14 ± 0.82
8	28	24	85.71	3.10 ± 0.94
9	23	18	78.26	3.12 ± 0.85
10	18	11	61.11	3.45 ± 0.72
Total	105	76	72.38	3.24 ± 0.94

color and pulsed Doppler examination was performed before the termination of pregnancy for psychosocial reasons.

The first color and pulsed signals from the yolk sac were obtained between 5 and 6 weeks of gestation. The visualization rate of the yolk sac vessels in the 6th week of gestation was 33.33%, and this increased to a value of 85.71% during the 7th and 8th weeks of gestation (Table 1). As the functional activity of the yolk sac progressively declined, the visualization rate of 78.26% for 9 weeks' gestation and 61.11% for 10 weeks' gestation paralleled this process. The overall visualization rate for yolk sac vessels was 72.38%. The highest visualization rates (85.71%) were obtained in the 7th and 8th weeks of gestation. A characteristic waveform profile included: low velocity (5.8 ± 1.7 cm/s) and absence of diastolic flow (Color Plate A). The pulsatility index (PI) showed a mean value of 3.24 ± 0.94 without significant changes between subgroups ($p > 0.05$). The distribution of mean PI values for yolk sac vascularity is shown in Table 1.

Vitelline stalk vessels showed similar peak systolic velocity (PSV) (5.4 ± 1.8 cm/s) and PI values (3.14 ± 0.91) ($p > 0.05$) to those obtained from the yolk sac. The distribution of the vitelline artery PI values is shown in Table 2. Transvaginal color Doppler ultrasound and spectral analysis of the vitelline artery at 7–8 weeks' gestation are shown in Color Plate B. At the same time one can detect blood flow signals in the umbilical circulation (Color Plate C) characterized by similar Doppler features. The overall visualization rate for vitelline arteries was 66.67%. Color and pulsed Doppler signals could be obtained from the vitelline duct during the 7th week of gestation in 85.71% of patients. The peak of visualization (89.28%) occurred during the 8th week of gestation (Table 2). The process of the elongation of the vitelline duct together with the removal of the yolk sac from the body wall is paralleled by a decreased rate of vitelline duct visualization during the 9th (73.91%) and 10th (55.55%) weeks of gestation. Although the reports on yolk sac and vitelline circulation are very exciting, one should realize that such studies are not ethically feasible in ongoing human pregnancies, since the secondary yolk sac is the source of primary germ cells and blood stem cells[6].

VASCULARIZATION OF THE YOLK SAC IN ABNORMAL PREGNANCIES

Kurjak and associates[7,8] recently performed research analyzing the vascularization of the yolk sac in abnormal pregnancies. They obtained three types of signal from the yolk sac in patients with missed abortion: irregular blood flow (Color Plate D), permanent diastolic flow (Color Plate E) and venous blood flow signals (Color Plate F). The prognostic significance of analyzing the secondary yolk sac circulation is not clearly established, since these vessels persist inside the wall of the yolk sac up to 1 month after the cellular death of the other components[9]. It seems that changes in both yolk sac appearance (size, shape and echogenicity) and vascularization are probably a

Table 2 *Visualization rate of the vitelline stalk vascularity between 6 and 10 weeks of gestation*

Gestational age (weeks)	n	Visualization rate		
		n	%	PI ± SD
6	15	—	—	—
7	21	18	85.71	3.02 ± 0.92
8	28	25	89.28	3.05 ± 0.89
9	23	17	73.91	3.08 ± 0.91
10	18	10	55.55	3.38 ± 0.82
Total	105	70	66.67	3.14 ± 0.92

consequence of poor embryonic development or even embryonic death, rather than being the primary cause of early pregnancy failure.

VOLUME OF THE YOLK SAC IN NORMAL PREGNANCY

It is well known that the prognostic significance of the yolk sac diameter as determined by ultrasound is not clearly established. Most abnormal pregnancies have been demonstrated to have normal yolk sac measurements[10–12], with only a minority of abnormal early pregnancies presenting yolk sac dimensions that either 'too small' or 'too large'[3,13]. Increased echogenicity of the yolk sac walls has been reported as a sign of dystrophic changes that occur in non-viable cellular material, indicating early pregnancy loss[14].

Recently, we performed a study on 80 women with uncomplicated singleton pregnancy (between 5 and 12 weeks' gestation)[15]. The volumes of the gestational and yolk sacs were measured by three-dimensional ultrasound (Voluson 530, Kretztechnik, Austria). Regression analysis revealed exponential growth of the gestational sac volume (Figure 1). The yolk sac volume was found to increase gradually from 5 to 10 weeks of gestation. However, when the yolk sac reaches its maximum size and volume at around 10 weeks, it has already started to degenerate (Figure 2), which can be proved by a significant reduction in visualization rates

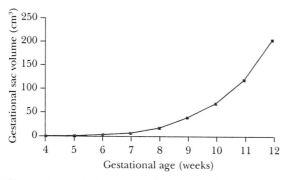

Figure 1 *Gestational sac volume determined by three-dimensional ultrasound*

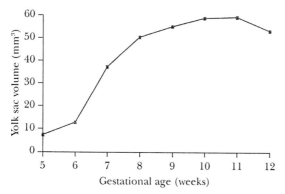

Figure 2 *Yolk sac volume determined by three-dimensional ultrasound*

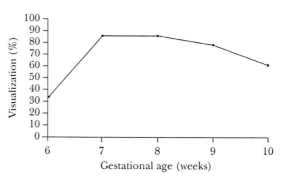

Figure 3 *Yolk sac vascularity determined by transvaginal color Doppler*

of the yolk sac vascularity (Table 1, Figure 3). This suggests that the evaluation of the biological function of the yolk sac by measurement of the diameter and/or the volume is limited (Color Plate G). Therefore, the combination of functional and volumetric studies is necessary, to illuminate some of the important moments during early pregnancy:

(1) Simultaneous beginning of yolk sac angiogenesis and vascular development of the embryo[5];

(2) Non-invasive evaluation of the functional capacity of the yolk sac[5];

(3) Definition of the shift from embryo-vitelline to embryo–placental circulation[8];

(4) Three-dimensional ultrasound studies of the direct connection between the yolk sac and the embryonic gut (Color Plate H);

(5) Evaluation of yolk sac degeneration and location by three-dimensional ultrasound at the end of the first trimester.

References

1. Mantoni F, Pedersen JF. Ultrasound visualization of the human yolk sac. *J Clin Ultrasound* 1979;7:459–61
2. Bree RL, Marn CS. Transvaginal sonography in the first trimester: embryology, anatomy, and hCG correlation. *Semin Ultrasound CT MR* 1990;11:12–21
3. Jauniaux E, Jurkovic D, Henriet Y, Rodesch F, Hustin J. Development of the secondary human yolk sac. Correlation of sonographic and anatomical features. *Hum Reprod* 1991;6:1160–6
4. Jauniaux E, Gulbis B, Jurkovic D, Campbell S, Collins WP, Ooms HA. Relationship between protein concentrations in embryological fluids and maternal serum and yolk sac size during human early pregnancy. *Hum Reprod* 1994;9:161–6
5. Kurjak A, Kupesic S, Kostovic L. Vascularization of yolk sac and vitelline duct in normal pregnancies studied by transvaginal color and pulsed Doppler. *J Perinat Med* 1994;22:433–40
6. Witschi E. Migration of the germ cells of human embryos from the yolk sac to the primitive gonadal folds. *Contrib Embryol Carnegie Inst* 1948;32:67–80
7. Kurjak A, Kupesic S, Kos M, Latin V, Zudenigo

D. Early hemodynamics studied by transvaginal color Doppler. *Prenat Neonat Med* 1996;1:38–49

8. Kurjak A, Kupesic S. Parallel Doppler assessment of yolk sac and intervillous circulation in normal pregnancy and missed abortion. *Placenta* 1998;19:619–23

9. Hustin J, Jauniaux E. Implantation and the yolk sac. In Kurjak A, ed. *Textbook of Perinatal Medicine.*Carnforth, UK: Parthenon Publishing, 1998:960–9

10. Crooij MJ, Westhuis M, Schoemaker J, Exalto N. Ultrasonographic measurements of the yolk sac. *Br J Obstet Gynaecol* 1982;89:931–4

11. Reece EA, Sciosca AL, Pinter E, *et al.* Prognostic significance of the human yolk sac assessed by ultrasonography. *Am J Obstet Gynecol* 1988;159:1191–4

12. Goldstein SR, Kerenyi T, Scher J, Papp C. Correlation between karyotype and ultrasound findings in patients with failed early pregnancy. *Ultrasound Obstet Gynecol* 1996;8:314–17

13. Lindsay DJ, Lyons EA, Levi CS, Zheng XH. Endovaginal appearance of the yolk sac in early pregnancy: normal growth and usefulness as a predictor of abnormal pregnancy outcome. *Radiology* 1992;83:115–22

14. Harris RD, Vincent LM, Askin FB. Yolk sac calcification: a sonographic finding associated with intrauterine embryonic demise in the first trimester. *Radiology* 1988;166:109–16

15. Kupesic S, Kurjak A. Volume and vascularity of the yolk sac. *J Perinat Med* 1998; in press

Clinical importance of evaluation of the intervillous circulation

5

A. Kurjak, S. Kupesic, T. Hafner and M. Ivančić-Košuta

Many investigations are currently directed at the intervillous space, probing in particular its size and form, its source of blood supply and the mechanism of circulation within it. However, a good deal of information is already available, especially as the result of recent Doppler demonstration of the continuous blood flow in the intervillous space.

COLOR DOPPLER AND THE INTERVILLOUS CIRCULATION

Color Doppler has been a potent tool for research into the development and hemodynamics of the intervillous circulation (Color Plate I). This technique has had a great impact on resolving some controversies on the intervillous circulation in early pregnancy.

The classical embryological postulation was that the formation of the intervillous space, and the circulation of maternal blood within it, commenced within a few days after implantation. This concept was was challenged in 1987 and 1988 by the experiments of Hustin and colleagues[1,2]. They examined slice radiographs of hysterectomy specimens with pregnancy *in situ* collected at 7, 8 and 9 weeks of gestation and found no contrast medium in the intervillous space. When the examination was performed at 13 weeks of gestation, the placenta was rapidly filled with contrast medium. Histological examination of these hysterectomy specimens showed occlusion of the uteroplacental arteries by trophoblastic cells up to 12 weeks of gestation. Reconstruction of serial spiral arterial sections was also suggestive of the absence of the intervillous circulation before 12 weeks of gestation. At 13 weeks, on the other hand, the uteroplacental arteries were free of trophoblastic plugs, and contrast medium was found in the intervillous space, encircling the chorionic villi. This was partially confirmed *in vivo* by means of hysteroscopy, examination of chorionic villous sampling material and transvaginal sonography. These results suggest that the early placenta is bathed predominantly by fluid derived from maternal plasma and uterine gland secretions. The authors believed that blood flow in the intervillous space was absent or incompletely developed before 12 weeks of gestation. Transformation of spiral arteries continues during the first trimester, when they widen progressively. Around 12 weeks of gestation, all trophoblastic plugs are eventually loosened and dislocated. This allows free entry of maternal blood to the intervillous space and the establishment of a fully developed placental circulation.

Further support has been supplied by a more recent study[3] using a polarographic oxygen electrode inserted under ultrasound guidance. This demonsrated that, between 8 and 10 weeks of gestation, placental po_2 levels were significantly lower than endometrial po_2 levels, whereas between 12 and 13 weeks, the levels were similar. Intraplacental po_2 levels increased significantly from 8–10 to 12–13 weeks of gestation. These results suggest that the increase of placental po_2 may be related to the establishment of continuous maternal blood flow in the intervillous space at the end of the first trimester.

The advent and development of transvaginal color Doppler has enabled *in vivo* hemodynamic investigation of almost all segments of the embryonic/fetal and uteroplacental circulation[3–10] (Color Plate J). In 1991 and 1992 Jauniaux and co-workers[11,12] and Jaffe and Warsoff[13] were unable to detect 'intraplacental' flow before 12 weeks of gestation using transvaginal color Doppler. They found the appearance of intraplacental flow at around 14 weeks of gestation to coincide with the appearance of pandiastolic flow in the umbilical artery and with an abrupt increase in uterine artery peak systolic velocity[14,15]. In agreement with the theories of Hustin and colleagues[1,2], they hypothesized that the simultaneous appearance of intraplacental flow, pandiastolic umbilical artery flow and abrupt increase in uterine artery blood flow velocity was to be explained by sudden loosening and disappearance of the trophoblastic plugs in the spiral arteries. At this time Kurjak and associates[15] were unable to demonstrate an abrupt change in the uteroplacental circulation between 12 and 14 weeks of gestation.

It must be emphasized that color Doppler measurements in the studies mentioned above were performed on devices of relatively moderate capability in detection of low velocities. After the introduction of the new generation of far more sensitive color Doppler devices in the past few years, several authors have reported a positive finding of intervillous circulation during the first trimester of pregnancy.

In 1995 Kurjak and colleagues[16] presented the first report on a combined Doppler and morphopathological study of the intervillous circulation. Using transvaginal color Doppler, they detected continuous intervillous flow of two types in all examined patients: pulsatile artery-like (Color Plate K) and continuous vein-like flow (Color Plate L). Parallel histological study has shown that the lumen of spiral arteries was never completely obstructed by the trophoblastic plugs. These data indicate that establishment of the intervillous circulation is a continuous process rather than an abrupt event at the end of the first trimester.

Shortly after, several other groups reported similar findings. Valentin and colleagues[17] performed a combined study of

uteroplacental and luteal flow with pathomorphologic analysis. Color Doppler measurements revealed a positive finding of intervillous circulation from the 6th week of normal pregnancy onward. The same two types of Doppler signal, the pulsatile and the continuous, were detected and measured with a visualization rate of more than 90% on 64 pregnancies from 5 to 11 weeks of gestation. The authors stated that the high blood velocities recorded from the subchorionic arteries were not compatible with these arteries being completely occluded by trophoblastic plugs. At the pathomorphological analysis, trophoblast plugging of the spiral arteries was incomplete, allowing the passage of red blood cells. The authors concluded that the intervillous circulation was present as early as the first trimester.

Merce and co-workers[18] reported similar results in the group of 108 normal singleton pregnancies of 4 to 15 gestational weeks. They were able to detect intervillous flow from 5 weeks 6 days of gestation. They obtained a slightly undulating vein-like signal with a tendency towards increasing velocity throughout the first trimester. They also recorded arterial signals in retrochorionic segments of the uteroplacental vasculature. The conclusion was that their results were in accordance with the classical embryological concept of establishment of intervillous flow from the 4th to the 7th weeks of gestation. According to Merce and colleagues[18], the uteroplacental circulation is the earliest to be effected in pregnancy, with pronounced changes from week 4 onwards. The intervillous circulation and primitive umbilical blood flow were identified from week 5 onwards.

In more recent publications, Kurjak and colleagues[19,20] studied a group of 60 normal pregnancies of gestational age from 6 to 12 weeks and, for the first time, a group of 34 pathological early pregnancies (22 cases of missed abortion and 12 cases of anembryonic pregnancy) between 7 and 12 weeks of gestation. The same Doppler features were detected in the intervillous space of all

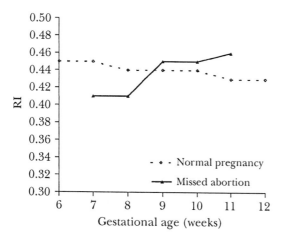

Figure 1 *Spiral artery resistance index (RI) in normal pregnancy and missed abortion*

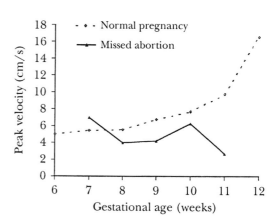

Figure 3 *Peak velocity of the continuous intervillous flow in normal pregnancy and missed abortion*

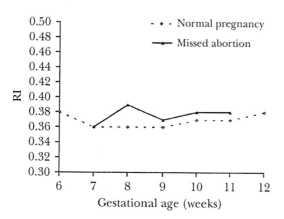

Figure 2 *Resistance index (RI) of arterial intervillous flow in normal pregnancy and missed abortion*

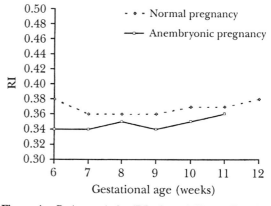

Figure 4 *Resistance index (RI) of arterial intervillous flow in normal and anembryonic pregnancy*

pregnancies; pulsatile artery-like signals with a characteristic spiky outline, and vein-like continuous signals. There was no difference in Doppler parameters between the group with missed abortion and the group with normal pregnancy (Figures 1–3). However, lower impedance (measured as resistance index (RI) and pulsatility index (PI)) was detected in most of the patients with anembryonic pregnancies (Figures 4 and 5). These results are significantly different from those published by Jauniaux and co-workers[21], who found increased intervillous blood flow in 70% of abnormal pregnancies before 12

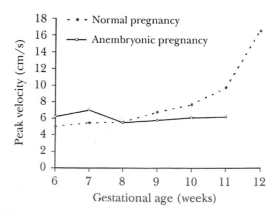

Figure 5 *Peak velocity of the continuous intervillous flow in normal and anembryonic pregnancy*

weeks of gestation. In these cases a histopathological examination showed that the trophoblastic shell was discontinuous and thinner, and that the intervillous space had been massively infiltrated by maternal blood. The authors hypothesized that trophoblast plugs in the spiral arteries restricted the flow of maternal blood in the intervillous space, protecting vulnerable villi from the high pressure of arterial blood. According to this concept, the premature entry of maternal blood in the intervillous space could disrupt the maternoembryonic interface, causing the separation of the early placenta and, eventually, abortion. In the research into placental development and formation of the uteroplacental circulation, of crucial importance was experimental work with animal models, particularly non-human primates, mostly *Macaca* species. The classical work by Ramsey and co-workers on the circulation in the intervillous space of the primate placenta is the base for all contemporary research in this field[22]. Recently, Nimrod and colleagues[23,24] reported the assessment of early uteroplacental circulation in cynomolgus monkeys (*Macaca fascicularis*) by the color Doppler technique. They were able to detect the intervillous circulation from day 18 after conception. Regardless of the the known differences in the depth of trophoblastic invasion of the spiral arteries between human and monkey, this finding can be considered as additional evidence of early establishment of the intervillous circulation in all primate placentas, although the 'argument by analogy' must be used with caution.

Jauniaux and associates speculated that the finding of focal intervillous flow in the first trimester was a sign of consecutive formation of echo-poor areas as an early sign of pregnancy complications[21,25]. If this were true, how could one explain the high rate of visualization of these signals in normal pregnancies reported by our group[26,27] and the Malmö group[17]? It is hard to believe that all these pregnancies were destined to fail. According to Jauniaux and colleagues[21], continuous flow in the intervillous space

during the first trimester is a highly pathological event, causing the disruption of the maternoembryonic interface by high-pressure blood flow and consequent spontaneous abortion. In the opinion of Jauniaux[28], this fact is the most striking evidence in favor of Hustin's concept. In fact, we also believe that the high pressure of arterial blood can disrupt the maternoembryonic interface and cause spontaneous abortion. However, this fact is not incompatible with the finding of continuous intervillous flow during the first trimester of pregnancy. This can be explained by there being some areas where trophoblastic plugs in spiral arteries are loosened, allowing the intervillous circulation of blood. In the beginning, there are only a few areas of such flow, giving enough oxygen and nutrients for the progression of pregnancy. At this stage the intervillous space is not undisrupted, as in the mature placenta. There are parts with active continuous intervillous flow and parts in which such flow has not yet been established, and nutrients and oxygen diffuse through the intercellular fluid. The number of areas with established intervillous flow increases with embryonic and placental growth, in order to maintain a state of metabolic balance. This process ends with a fully formed intervillous space under the mature placenta. Such a hypothesis can be in concordance with findings of lower oxygen levels in the placental tissue than in the endometrium between 8 and 10 weeks of pregnancy[28]. Also, it can be in concordance with the fact that in cases of inappropriate trophoblastic plugging of spiral arteries the uncontrolled pressure of arterial blood can mechanically disrupt the maternoembryonic interface.

Merce and colleagues[18] recently reported that the abnormal Doppler patterns, such as the increase of retrochorial vascular resistance and the presence of intervillous flow in pregnancies with a gestational sac measuring less than 12 mm, were found with a greater incidence of miscarriage. However, intervillous flow was also detectable in pregnancies with normal outcome, but in a smaller proportion than in those ending with miscarriage (11 vs. 53 %). This finding confirms that intervillous circulation exists throughout early pregnancy, but at the same time the limitation of the amount and pressure of incoming maternal blood seems to be essential for normal pregnancy development.

STUDIES IN LATE PREGNANCY

The intervillous circulation in the second and third trimesters can effectively be assessed by color Doppler. Many authors have researched the hemodynamics of development of the uteroplacental circulation[1-29]. This vascular system undergoes dramatic adaptation during pregnancy with the main aim of adequately supplementing the intervillous space under the placenta with maternal blood. Doppler assessment of the uteroplacental circulation is the topic of another chapter in this book and, therefore, we elaborate just the intervillous flow.

First-trimester pregnancies should be assessed by the transvaginal route and second- and third-trimester pregnancies by the transabdominal route. During the B-mode examination, the placental site must be located (chorion frondosum in pregnancies less than 9–10 weeks). The color flow imaging technique is then used to locate color-coded areas of flow inside the placental tissue and under the decidual plate. In first-trimester pregnancies, color-coded areas are visualized inside the chorion frondosum or early placenta. The pulsed Doppler sample volume (gate) should then be positioned on the color-coded areas and the flow velocity waveform obtained.

The sample volume size should be selected between 1 and 2 mm and carefully positioned on the site from which the most regular and sharpest signal can be obtained. This is not an easy task. Turbulent flow results in an irregular, ill-defined Doppler signal. For proper measurement, the Doppler velocity waveform must be as clear as possible. Also, it is helpful if the patient stabilizes and slows down her breathing. In the same area, especially in advanced pregnancies, blood flow inside the fetal placental vessels can also be detected. Distinction between the maternal intervillous circulation and the fetal intravillous circulation is easily achieved by heart rate analysis.

The following data are results of our new, yet unpublished, study. If the pulsed Doppler signal is sampled from such a color-coded area, two types of flow pattern can be detected: a pulsatile, artery-like signal and a continuous vein-like signal. The same two types of Doppler waveform pattern can be followed throughout the pregnancy. The pulsatile, artery-like waveform should match the fountain-like blood spurts coming from the openings of the spiral arteries on the decidual plate. As previously mentioned there are between 100 and 200 spiral arteries under the insertion of the term placenta.

The velocities of blood (peak systolic, end diastolic and temporal maximum averaged) progressively rise up to approximately 20–22 weeks, when they reach a plateau and remain stable to term (Table 1). Near and after term there is a slight, statistically non-significant, decrease of blood flow velocities. Possibly, the reduced velocity of blood flow in the intervillous space after term could be responsible for the increased degenerative processes in the placenta in this period. This still remains the object of further investigations. It is interesting that Burchell[30] has observed blood stasis in the intervillous space in late pregnancy. His impressive research was based on radiographic scanning of the human placenta *in vivo*, from the 7th week to the 41st week of pregnancy. The diffusion and disappearance of the contrast dye in the intervillous space were much slower in late pregnancy.

Because of the impossibility of defining the angle of insonation during Doppler measurements, absolute values of blood flow velocities must be considered carefully. One must be aware of the fact that this causes great variability in the results. When a large number of measurements are taken, an approximate range of values can be obtained. Peak systolic velocity in early pregnancy (7–9 weeks) is around 29 cm/s; it rises to around 37 cm/s at

Table 1 *Resistance index (RI), pulsatility index (PI), peak systolic velocity (PSV), end-diastolic velocity (EDV) and temporal averaged maximum velocity (TAMV) obtained from the intervillous space and in the spiral arteries in different gestational age groups*

Gestational age (weeks)	Intervillous blood flow					Spiral artery blood flow				
	RI (SD)	PI (SD)	PSV (SD)	EDV (SD)	TAMV (SD)	RI (SD)	PI (SD)	PSV (SD)	EDV (SD)	TAMV (SD)
7–9	0.48 (0.05)	0.71 (0.09)	28 (10)	18 (7)	25 (9)	0.58 (0.06)	0.88 (0.11)	31 (16)	22 (12)	26 (15)
10–12	0.41 (0.06)	0.61 (0.11)	28 (12)	21 (9)	26 (10)	0.51 (0.07)	0.73 (0.09)	36 (14)	20 (16)	31 (15)
13–15	0.34 (0.07)	0.43 (0.08)	35 (14)	22 (10)	30 (15)	0.43 (0.05)	0.55 (0.11)	41 (21)	26 (15)	37 (15)
16–22	0.29* (0.06)	0.34* (0.09)	40 (19)	35 (17)	37 (19)	0.41* (0.06)	0.55* (0.12)	37 (16)	23 (15)	32 (15)
23–28	0.30 (0.07)	0.36 (0.10)	36 (20)	30 (14)	32 (16)	0.40 (0.06)	0.52 (0.11)	42 (15)	26 (11)	34 (13)
29–36	0.25 (0.06)	0.29 (0.08)	36 (12)	26 (9)	32 (10)	0.34 (0.07)	0.42 (0.10)	31 (9)	21 (6)	26 (7)
37–42	0.27 (0.06)	0.31 (0.09)	32[†] (14)	23** (10)	27[†] (12)	0.37 (0.09)	0.48 (0.15)	30[†] (12)	19** (9)	25[†] (11)

SD, standard deviation; *, $p < 0.01$; **, $p < 0.05$; [†], $p < 0.07$

mid-pregnancy (16–22 weeks). The velocity remains stable thereafter. The slight, non-significant decrease at term is noted.

The impedance to flow in the intervillous space, measured in terms of the RI and PI, is low. It is characterized by a slight decrease to mid-pregnancy, and afterwards it remains constant. From an RI of 0.48 (PI = 0.71) at 7–9 weeks of gestation, the impedance decreases to an RI of 0.29 (PI = 0.34) at 16–22 weeks of gestation. There is no significant change until term. At term, RI = 0.27 (PI = 0.31). Low resistance is in concordance with the fact that the intervillous space is a voluminous vascular pool, which enables the blood to flow around the villi that are freely floating inside it. The mechanisms of regulation of the blood circulation through the intervillous space, if any, are still obscure to our knowledge. Karimu and Burton[31] suggest an interesting hypothesis. They found that the fetal vasculature provides hydraulic support to the villous tree, and that changes in the umbilical perfusion pressure

could therefore alter the disposition of the villi inside the intervillous space. As fetal blood pressure rises, for example during acute hypoxic episodes, the villi move apart. The enlargements and the clefts between adjacent villi have a secondary effect upon the maternal circulation, promoting more even perfusion of the intervillous space at higher overall flow rates. Their work was carried out *in vitro* in laboratory conditions. We still do not have any *in vivo* color and pulsed Doppler evidence of this effect. However, this topic remains open to interesting research work.

The continuous, vein-like Doppler blood flow pattern represents circulation in veins that are draining blood out of the intervillous space. Venous orifices are randomly dispersed on the decidual plate. The Doppler signal shows turbulent, continuous flow. It is well known that the inadequate development of the uteroplacental circulation can lead to placental insufficiency and fetal growth restriction. The impaired adaptation of the uteroplacental vasculature, which is often seen in pre-eclamptic, gestotic patients, results in reduced placental perfusion with maternal blood and an increased rate of placental degenerative processes and subnormal development of the villous tree[32-35].

INTERVILLOUS CIRCULATION IN HYPERTENSIVE PREGNANCY

It has been more than 25 years since Brosens and co-workers[36] demonstrated that in cases of pre-eclampsia there is a failure of physiological invasion of the trophoblast into the myometrial parts of the spiral arteries. A highly significant correlation between depth of trophoblast invasion of spiral arteries in pregnancy-induced hypertension (PIH) and arcuate artery impedance has been reported[14]. We hypothesized that the intervillous circulation was impaired in patients with PIH, owing to the maladaptation of the uteroplacental vasculature. The results of our study are still unpublished. In a group of 31 women with PIH in the gestational age range from 29 to 36 weeks, we found significantly higher RI and PI of Doppler signals from the intervillous space and spiral arteries than in those measured in a group of normal pregnancies. Impaired adaptation of the uteroplacental vasculature in patients with PIH has been reported in various histopathological studies[36-38]. Color Doppler studies have also shown that the uteroplacental vasculature of those patients is characterized by higher vascular impedance[39]. The results of our study were not surprising, because of the fact that the pulsatile circulation in the intervillous space is caused by transmitted pressure over a fountain-like sprout of blood coming from the spiral artery orifice on the decidual plate of the placenta[36].

Analysis of blood flow velocities in the intervillous space and spiral arteries between the two groups yielded interesting results. Blood flow velocity in the intervillous space was lower in the group with PIH, although the difference was significant at the end of diastole only. We speculate that blood stasis, i.e. a slower exchange rate of blood in the intervillous space, could be responsible for a higher incidence of cases with lower total placental volume, lower parenchymal volume and villous area, with increased areas of infarction in patients with hypertensive disease[38]. Contrary to this, the velocity of blood flow in the spiral arteries in PIH was higher than in normal pregnancy. The impaired trophoblast invasion in PIH resulted in a smaller diameter of spiral arteries. A smaller diameter of the vessel would result in a higher velocity of fluid running within it, and this could be the explanation for the noted phenomenon. In spite of the increased velocities, the amount of blood flow would be decreased in a system with a reduced diameter of the vessel. This could produce a state of placental and fetal hypo-oxygenation and malnutrition.

Color Doppler is a valuable tool for *in vivo* investigation of the uteroplacental and intervillous circulation. Its use can increase our knowledge of the physiology of the intervillous circulation and our knowledge of the intervillous space.

References

1. Hustin J, Shaaps JP. Echographic and anatomic studies of the maternotrophoblastic border during the first trimester of pregnancy. *Am J Obstet Gynecol* 1987;157:162–8
2. Hustin J, Shaaps JP, Lambotte R. Anatomical studies of the uteroplacental vascularization in the first trimester of pregnancy. *Troph Res* 1988; 3:49–60
3. Kurjak A, Zudenigo D, Predanic M, Kupesic S, Funduk-Kurjak B. Transvaginal color Doppler study of fetomaternal circulation in threatened abortion. *Fetal Diagn Ther* 1994;9:341–7

4. Kurjak A, Zalud I, Salihagic A, Crvenkovic G, Matijevic R. Transvaginal color Doppler in the assessment of abnormal early pregnancy. *J Perinat Med* 1991;19:155–65

5. Kurjak A, Predanic M, Kupesic S, Zudenigo D, Matijevic R, Salihagic A. Transvaginal color Doppler in the study of early normal pregnancies and pregnancies associated with uterine fibroids. *J Matern Fetal Invest* 1992;3:81–5

6. Kurjak A, Kupesic S, Predanic M, Salihagic A. Transvaginal color Doppler assessment of the uteroplacental circulation in normal and abnormal early pregnancy. *Early Hum Dev* 1992;29:385–9

7. Kurjak A, Predanic M, Kupesic S, Funduk-Kurjak B, Demarin V, Salihagic A. Transvaginal color Doppler study of middle cerebral artery blood flow in early normal and abnormal pregnancy. *Ultrasound Obstet Gynecol* 1992;2:424–8

8. Kurjak A, Zudenigo D, Funduk-Kurjak B, Shalan H, Predanick M, Sosic A. Transvaginal color Doppler in the assessment of the uteroplacental circulation in normal early pregnancy. *J Perinat Med* 1993;21:25–34

9. Kurjak A, Zudenigo D, Predanic M, Kupesic S. Recent advances in the Doppler study of early fetomaternal circulation. *J Perinat Med* 1994; 22:419–39

10. Kurjak A, Kupesic S, Kostovic LJ. Vascularization of yolk sac and vitelline duct in normal pregnancies studied by transvaginal color Doppler. *J Perinat Med* 1994;22:433–40

11. Jauniaux E, Jurkovic D, Campbell S. *In vivo* investigations of anatomy and physiology of early human placental circulations. *Ultrasound Obstet Gynecol* 1991;1:435–45

12. Jauniaux E, Jurkovic D, Campbell S, Hustin J. Doppler ultrasonographic features of the developing placental circulation: correlation with anatomic findings. *Am J Obstet Gynecol* 1992;166: 585–7

13. Jaffe R, Warsof SL. Transvaginal color Doppler imaging in the assessment of uteroplacental blood flow in the normal first-trimester pregnancy. *Am J Obstet Gynecol* 1991;164:781–5

14. Khong TY, Pearce JM. Development and investigation of the placenta and its blood supply. In Lavery JP, ed. *The Human Placenta. Clinical Perspectives.* Rockville: Aspen Publishers, 1987:25–45

15. Kurjak A, Predanic M, Kupesic-Urek S. Transvaginal color Doppler in the assessment of placental blood flow. *Eur J Obstet Gynecol Reprod Biol* 1993;49:29–32

16. Kurjak A, Laurini R, Kupesic S, Kos M, Latin V, Bulic K. A combined Doppler and morphopathological study of intervillous circulation. Presented at *The Fifth World Congress of Ultrasound in Obstetrics and Gynecology. Ultrasound Obstet Gynecol* 1995;6(Suppl 2):116

17. Valentin L, Sladkevicius P, Laurini R, Sodeberg H, Marsal K. Uteroplacental and luteal circulation in normal first trimester pregnancies: Doppler ultrasonographic and morphologic study. *Am J Obstet Gynecol* 1996;174:768–75

18. Merce LT, Barco MJ, Bau S. Color Doppler sonographic assessment of placental circulation in the first trimester of normal pregnancy. *J Ultrasound Med* 1996;15:135–42

19. Kurjak A, Kupesic S. Doppler assessment of the intervillous blood flow in normal and abnormal early pregnancy. *Obstet Gynecol* 1997;89:252–6

20. Kurjak A, Dudenhausen JW, Hafner T, Kupesic S, Latin V, Kos M. Intervillous circulation in all three trimesters of normal pregnancy assessed by color Doppler. *J Perinat Med* 1997;25:373–80

21. Jauniaux E, Zaidi J, Jurkovic D, Campbell S, Hustin J. Comparison of color Doppler features and pathohistological finding in complicated early pregnancy. *Hum Reprod* 1994;9:2432–7

22. Ramsey EM, Chez RA, Doppman JL. Radioangiographic measurement of the internal diameters of the uteroplacental arteries in Rhesus monkeys and man. *Carnegie Inst Contrib Embryol* 1979;38:59–70

23. Nimrod C, Simpson N, De Vermette R, Fournier J. Placental and early fetal haemodynamics: the suitability of the monkey model. Presented at *The Fetus as a Patient*, May 1996, Grado, Italy

24. Nimrod C, Simpson N, Hafner T, *et al.* Assessment of early placental development in the cynomolgus monkey (*Macaca fascicularis*) using colour and pulsed wave Doppler sonography. *J Med Primatol* 1996;25:106–11

25. Jauniaux E, Nicolaides KH. Placental lakes, absent umbilical artery diastolic flow and poor fetal growth in early pregnancy. *Ultrasound Obstet Gynecol* 1996;7:141–4

26. Kurjak A, Kupesic S. Doppler proof of the presence of intervillous circulation [Letter]. *Ultrasound Obstet Gynecol* 1996;7:463–4

27. Kurjak A, Kupesic S, Hafner T, Latin V, Kos M, Harris RD. Intervillous blood flow in patients with missed abortion. *Croatian Med J* 1998;39:41–4

28. Jauniaux E. Intervillous circulation in the first trimester: the phantom of the color Doppler obstetric opera [Editorial]. *Ultrasound Obstet Gynecol* 1996;8:73–6

29. Rodesch F, Simon P, Donner C, Jauniaux E. Oxygen measurements in endometrial and trophoblastic tissues during early pregnancy. *Obstet Gynecol* 1992;80:283–5

30. Burchell RC. Arterial blood flow into the human intervillous space. *Am J Obstet Gynecol* 1967;98: 303–11

31. Karimu AL, Burton GJ. Star volume estimates of the intervillous clefts in the human placenta: how changes in umbilical arterial pressure might influence the maternal placental circulation. *J Dev Physiol* 1993;19:137–42

32. Salafia CM, Minor VK, Pezzullo JC, Popek EJ, Rosenkrantz TS, Vintzileos AM. Intrauterine growth restriction in infants of less than thirty two weeks gestation: associated placental pathologic features. *Am J Obstet Gynecol* 1995;173: 1049–57

33. Jackson MR, Walsh AJ, Morrow RJ, Mullen JB, Lye SJ, Ritchie JW. Reduced placental villous tree elaboration in small-for-gestational-age pregnancies: relationship with umbilical artery Doppler waveforms. *Am J Obstet Gynecol* 1995;172: 518–25

34. Arabin B, Jimenez E, Vogel M, Weitzel HK. Relationship of utero- and fetoplacental blood flow velocity waveforms with pathomorphological placental findings. *Fetal Diagn Ther* 1992;7:173–9

35. Harris JWS, Ramsey EM. The morphology of human uteroplacental vasculature. *Contrib Embryol* 1996;38:43–58

36. Brosens I, Robertson WB, Dixon HG. The role of the spiral arteries in the pathogenesis of pre-eclampsia. *Obstet Gynecol Annu* 1972;1:177–91

37. Khong TY, DeWolf F, Robertson WB, Brossens I. Inadequate maternal vascular response to placentation in pregnancies complicated by pre-eclampsia and small-for-gestational-age infants. *Br J Obstet Gynaecol* 1986;93:1049–59

38. Boyd PA, Scott A. Quantitative structural studies on human placentas associated with pre-eclampsia, essential hypertension and intrauterine growth retardation. *Br J Obstet Gynaecol* 1985;92:714–21

39. Fleischer A, Schulman H, Farmakides G, *et al.* Uterine artery Doppler velocimetry in pregnant women with hypertension. *Am J Obstet Gynecol* 1986;154:806–13

Screening procedures during the first trimester of pregnancy

6

M. L. Brizot, L. M. Lopes, D. A. L. Pedreira, V. Bunduki and M. Zugaib

INTRODUCTION

In recent years the interest in screening for fetal abnormalities has shifted to the first trimester of pregnancy, owing to technical improvements in early diagnosis (chorionic villous sampling) and also to the introduction of transvaginal ultrasound scans and new laboratory tests. Special attention has been given to screening for chromosomal abnormalities, multiple pregnancy complications, cardiac defects and fetal infection.

Several of the new procedures discussed below are being routinely introduced in prenatal care. The degree of confidence of early screening tests has already been ascertained for many of them.

SCREENING FOR CHROMOSOMAL ABNORMALITIES

Prevalence

The prevalence of chromosomal abnormalities depends on maternal age and gestational age. The older the mother the higher the risk for trisomies, and the earlier the gestation the higher the risk. This is because fetuses with chromosomal defects are more likely to die *in utero* than normal fetuses[1,2].

Pregnancy dating

Very early intrauterine growth restriction has been associated with some fetal chromosomal abnormalities[3-5]. The first important issue for analysis of first-trimester growth restriction is correct pregnancy dating. Pregnancy dating errors are expected to occur in as much as 40% of cases at the first prenatal visit, when assignment of gestational age derives only from menstrual history.

Once the estimated date is confirmed we can then make the diagnosis of early growth restriction and analyze its correlation with aneuploidy and other fetal complications. The impact of aneuploidy on fetal growth has been investigated by some authors. In trisomy 18 fetuses, the crown–rump length measurement (CRL) is significantly smaller than that observed in normal fetuses, in which CRL is derived from menstrual history. This difference does not seems to occur in trisomies 21 and 13 or other aneuploidies[3,4].

The larger the size discrepancy, the higher the possibility of chromosomal abnormality[3]. For routine clinical use the predictive values for fetal aneuploidies have to be calculated on the basis of the sensitivity and specificity of the CRL discrepancies, taking into account the prevalence of aneuploidy in the population.

Another issue of CRL measurement and early growth restriction is that if CRL is smaller than expected for gestational age in aneuploid fetuses and if it is used alone for dating, this could interfere with biochemical screening results[5].

Nuchal translucency

In the first trimester a common feature of chromosomal abnormality is an abnormal nuchal fluid collection called increased nuchal translucency (NT) thickness by some authors and nuchal edema, cystic hygroma, or nuchal thickening by others[6,7].

The first screening study that involved measurement of NT thickness was in 1273 women with singleton pregnancies, undergoing fetal karyotyping at 10–14 weeks, and reported that in 84% of fetuses with trisomy 21 and in 4.5% of chromosomally normal fetuses the NT was ≥ 2.5 mm, or ≥ 3 mm when using machines that give measurements to the nearest millimeter[6]. Additionally, the study showed that the risks for fetal trisomies can be calculated by combining data from maternal age and fetal NT thickness and formed the basis for the introduction of a new method of screening. Subsequent studies have confirmed that this method of screening not only gives the option of first-trimester diagnosis, but is the most sensitive method for the detection of trisomies; in a multicenter study of more than 100 000 pregnancies the sensitivity for trisomy 21 was 77% for a false-positive rate of 5% and a cut-off value of 1 in 300[8].

An essential issue on screening using NT measurement is that the same criteria should be used to achieve uniformity of results from different operators. The technique proposed by the multicenter study[8] was as follows:

(1) Transabdominal or transvaginal sonography;

(2) Good sagittal section of the fetus, as for measurement of fetal crown–rump length;

(3) Magnification such that the fetus occupies at least 75% of the image;

(4) Care taken to distinguish between fetal skin and amnion;

(5) Maximum thickness measured of the subcutaneous translucency between the skin and the soft tissue overlying the cervical spine;

(6) Calipers placed on the lines (just limiting the black space) as shown in Figure 1;

(7) More than one measurement taken during the scan, and the maximum recorded.

From October 1995 screening for chromo-

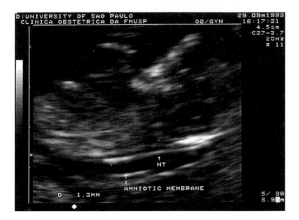

Figure 1 *Ultrasound image of a nuchal translucency thickness measurement, showing the correct parameters for measurement: fetal position, image size, caliper placement and visualization of the amniotic membrane*

somal and fetal abnormalities by ultrasound scan between 10 and 14 weeks has been offered to all women attending our antenatal clinic at São Paulo University. Information leaflets explaining the risk for trisomies based on their age and how this risk may be altered by the fetal NT thickness are given to the women[6,9]. The same leaflet provides information on the difference between screening and diagnosis and we offer the option of invasive testing for women with maternal age of 35 years or over, or for those whose adjusted risk is considered to be high after the NT thickness measurement. To calculate the risk for trisomies we use the software provided by the Fetal Medicine Foundation (International Multi-centre Study)[8].

During a period of 3 years (October 1995 to September 1998), ultrasound examination was performed in 2169 singleton pregnancies with a live fetus and a fetal CRL of 38–84 mm. The median CRL was 62 mm, which corresponds to the gestational age of 12^{+3} weeks. The fetal NT was successfully measured in all cases. From those with an expected date of delivery up to 31 August, we have complete follow-up on 1224 (87%) pregnancies. The maternal age was ≥ 35 years in 23%, and we observed 1.47% (18/1224) of chromosomal abnormalities (Table 1). The cut-off risk of ≥ 1/100 was observed in 3.8% of the normal

Table 1 *Fetal chromosomal abnormalities observed in 2169 pregnancies (1224 completed follow-up) screened by fetal nuchal translucency (NT) thickness measurement at 10–14 weeks' gestation at the University of São Paulo, Brazil, between October 1995 and August 1998*

Case	Maternal age (years)	NT (mm)	Background risk	Adjusted risk	Prenatal karyotype	Outcome
1	42	2.3	1 in 25	1 in 49	NP	alive, trisomy 21
2	39	3.2	1 in 72	1 in 36	failure	alive, trisomy 21
3	38	5.0	1 in 91	1 in 2	trisomy 21	alive
4	39	3.9	1 in 72	1 in 2	trisomy 21	NND
5	32	4.4	1 in 390	1 in 15	trisomy 21	IUD (37 weeks)
6	37	3.8	1 in 137	1 in 7	trisomy 21	IUD (32 weeks)
7	30	2.9	1 in 518	1 in 87	trisomy 21	IUD (16 weeks)
8	31	2.1	1 in 469	1 in 1069	trisomy 21	TOP
9	33	4.3	1 in 330	1 in 5	trisomy 21	TOP
10	42	2.5	1 in 31	1 in 13	trisomy 21	TOP
11	40	2.2	1 in 20*	1 in 31	trisomy 21[†]	TOP
12	35	6.0	1 in 209	1 in 3	trisomy 13	IUD (14 weeks)
13	25	13.0	1 in 853	1 in 12	trisomy 18	IUD (15 weeks)
14	27	1.4	1 in 660	1 in 3881	47, XXY[‡]	TOP (16 weeks)
15	39	3.0	1 in 72	1 in 7	der 18/21**	TOP (19 weeks)
16	43	4.3	1 in 25	1 in 2	trisomy 20	SA (13 weeks)
17	23	21.5	1 in 926	1 in 13	45,X	ongoing 34 weeks
18	25	6.5	1 in 759	1 in 10	45,X	ongoing 32 weeks

NP, not performed; IUD, intrauterine death; TOP, termination of pregnancy; NND, neonatal death; SA, spontaneous abortion; *, previous chromosomally abnormal child with trisomy 21; [†], karyotype: 46,XY-21,+t(21,21); [‡], holoprosencephaly and facial cleft, karyotype by amniocentesis and confirmed by skin fibroblast culture after TOP; **, karyotype: 46,XX der(18,21) (q11,q11)+18 (confirmed by chorionic villous sampling and amniocentesis)

pregnancies, in 91% with trisomy 21 and in 85.7% with other chromosomal defects. In this study population 18.6% (82/441) of the women with maternal age ≥ 35 years opted for an invasive test, and the uptake for adjusted risk of ≥ 1 in 100 after the NT scan was 58% (43/74). Additionally, about half of the patients with abnormal fetal karyotype diagnosed during the prenatal period opted to continue with the pregnancy (Table 1). These aspects are different from reports by other studies, in which the uptake for invasive tests in advanced maternal age was approximately 50%[10] and the choice of continuing the pregnancy after prenatal diagnosis of a chromosomal abnormality was found to be around 5.0%[11]. Our patients' choices may have been influenced by several factors. First, abortion is illegal unless it is for a lethal condition; therefore, patients do not have this option available and most of them cannot afford an abortion at illegal clinics. Second,

this study involves patients with limited educational levels, and a considerable percentage of them do not have a clear understanding of the consequences of the chromosomal abnormality; despite genetic counselling and psychological interviews, they have difficulty in appreciating the severity of the fetal condition. Third, we cannot forget the religious and cultural aspects involved in decision making.

Increased NT thickness is not just a marker of chromosomal abnormality but is also associated with an increased risk of other fetal defects, mainly cardiac, diaphragmatic, renal, abdominal wall and several genetic syndromes[12,13]. Therefore, it is necessary to perform further detailed ultrasound scans and fetal echocardiography to diagnose such defects.

Apart from NT screening, several other benefits of the ultrasound scan between 10 and 14 weeks of gestation are now well recognized. These include accurate dating of the pregnancy, detection of major malformations and missed abortion and early diagnosis of multiple pregnancy with the possibility of determining chorionicity.

Maternal serum biochemistry

Several studies have shown that fetal chromosomal abnormalities are associated with abnormal levels of maternal serum biochemical markers, not only in the second but also in the first trimester of pregnancy[14–16].

During the first trimester in pregnancies with trisomy 21 fetuses, the maternal serum concentration of free β-human chorionic gonadotropin (free β-hCG) is increased, pregnancy-associated plasma protein A (PAPP-A) is decreased but α-fetoprotein (AFP), inhibin-A and pregnancy-specific β-1 glycoprotein (SP1) are not significantly different from normal. In trisomy 18 pregnancies, free β-hCG, PAPP-A, SP1 and AFP are significantly decreased[14–16].

The efficacy of the individual parameters was assessed by comparing sensitivity for a 5% false positive rate. Screening by first-trimester maternal serum free β-hCG or PAPP-A, which have respectively a 33% and 44% sensitivity rate, would not offer a dramatic improvement over screening based only on maternal age (sensitivity of 25–30% for the same false-positive rate). However, studies have demonstrated that there is no significant association between the maternal serum biochemistry and fetal NT thickness and therefore the data could be combined in the calculation of risks for trisomies. The association between maternal age, ultrasound (NT thickness) and biochemical parameters (free β-hCG and PAPP-A) in the first trimester can improve the detection rate to more than 90%[16]. The cost benefit of this association is still being evaluated. At this time, only a few centers in the world offer it in routine practice.

MULTIPLE PREGNANCY

The first-trimester scan (10–14 weeks) has brought the opportunity of better management of multiple pregnancy, especially owing to the following aspects.

(1) In multiple pregnancies the outcome is mainly related to the number of fetuses and chorionicity. The higher the number of fetuses the higher the risk of premature delivery, perinatal death and handicap.

(2) This is the best time to determine chorionicity. In dichorionic twin pregnancies there are two placentas and they can either be adjacent to each other or on opposite sides of the uterus. When they are next to each other the inter-twin membrane is thick and at the junction with the placenta there is a placental extension called the lambda sign or 'twin peak'. In monochorionic pregnancies the inter-twin membrane is thin and there is no lambda sign at the junction with the placenta. Monochorionic pregnancies have a higher risk of spontaneous abortion, prematurity and handicap, mainly due to complications related to the twin-to-twin transfusion syndrome. Chorionicity will also influence the management of a twin pregnancy when one of the fetuses is severely compromised, increasing the risk for the co-twin because of the vascular communications.

(3) Screening by NT thickness has proven to be the most effective method of screening for chromosomal abnormalities in multiple pregnancies; this has approximately the same detection rate as for single pregnancies. However, a small increase in the false-positive rate is expected[17], due to the fact that an increased NT in one of the fetuses or a discordance in NT by more than 1 mm can be an early marker for a higher risk of subsequent development of severe twin-to-twin transfusion syndrome.

SCREENING FOR CARDIAC DEFECTS

Congenital malformations of the fetal heart have been diagnosed by transabdominal fetal

Table 2 *Indications for early fetal echocardiography*

Indication	Number of cases	Congenital heart disease
Increased nuchal translucency (≥ 2.5 mm)	63	11 (13.2%)
Family history of congenital heart disease	11	
Pregestational diabetes	4	1 (25%)
Arrhythmias	3	
Fetal abnormalities by ultrasound	1	
Risk for chromosomal abnormalities	1	
Total	83	12 (14.4%)

echocardiography, which is a well-established technique[18]. However, precise diagnosis before 17 weeks' gestation has been difficult. With the development of high-frequency transducers, it has become possible to detect heart diseases earlier in pregnancy[18,19]. With the use of two-dimensional echocardiography enhanced by color-coded Doppler imaging, it has been possible to define small structures and vessels of the fetal heart between 12 and 16 weeks' gestation and thus improve diagnosis as well as sensitivity. However, the sensitivity of early fetal echocardiography is only 64% compared to 78% for transabdominal examination at 20–22 weeks' gestation[19]. The lesser resolution, more time-consuming examination and need for high-level training of the examiner are the most important disadvantages of this technique. It is therefore unjustified to use early fetal echocardiography for screening, despite its great potential[18].

Knowing that increased NT thickness is seen in about 70–80% of fetuses with chromosomal abnormalities, and a high proportion of such fetuses have abnormalities of the heart and great vessels[12], we believe that detailed early fetal echocardiography performed by a specialist should be offered to all fetuses with increased NT; this group of fetuses has become the most recent indication for early fetal echocardiography.

In the past 2 years, we have performed early fetal echocardiography according to the indications shown in Table 2. The criteria for considering the examination complete were the adequate visualization of the four-chamber view, outflow tracts with measurement and double-crossing of the aorta and the pulmonary trunk, ductus and aortic arch. The atrioventricular and semilunar valves were carefully analyzed not only by real-time cross-sectional imaging but also by Doppler and color flow imaging. Because at this early gestational age the resolution within the fetal heart may be poor, when we could not achieve the criteria described, we rescheduled the patient for weekly scans until all views were obtained. In all cases, a further transabdominal echocardiographic examination was performed at 24–28 weeks' gestation and after birth. Any suspicions of murmur or heart disease were an indication for neonatal echocardiography.

As indicated in Table 3, increased NT is strongly associated with very severe forms of congenital heart disease. Fetal echocardiography at this stage in our experience seems to be a very sensitive technique (Figure 2).

The pathophysiology of increased NT thickness is still unclear; a few studies have suggested possible mechanisms[12,20]. However, it is accepted that measurement of NT is a useful tool for screening for aneuploidies. In our series it was strongly associated with congenital heart disease (14.4%). Increased NT thickness seems to be the most important indication for early transvaginal echocardiography performed by a specialist.

SCREENING FOR FETAL INFECTIONS

Our current knowledge on prenatal diagnosis and treatment of some congenital infections leads us to re-evaluate the diseases that should be screened in early pregnancy. We believe

Table 3 *Nuchal translucency (NT) thickness and fetal cardiac defects detected by early transvaginal fetal echocardiography*

Case no.	Gestational age (weeks)	Cardiac defect	NT (mm)	Karyotype	Outcome
1	13	hypoplastic LV	13.9	trisomy 18	FD
2	15	DORV	3.4	trisomy 21	TOP
3	16	hypoplastic LV	cystic hygroma	45,X	FD
4	15	VSD	4.4	trisomy 21	ND
5	12	AVSD, A-V block	7	normal	TOP
6	14	TV atresia, A-V block	3.5	normal	FD
7	11	TV insufficiency, PS	3.7	trisomy 21	ND
8	14	hypoplastic LV	7.0	normal	ND
9	15	hypoplastic LV	cystic hygroma	45,X	ongoing
10	15	TOF	5.0	normal	ongoing
11	13	VSD	6.2	normal	TOP

LV, left ventricle; FD, fetal death; DORV, double outflow right ventricle; TOF, tetralogy of Fallot; TOP, termination of pregnancy; VSD, ventricular septal defect; ND, neonatal death; AVSD, atrioventricular septal defect; A-V, atrioventricular; TV, tricuspid valve; PS, pulmonary stenosis

(a)   (b)

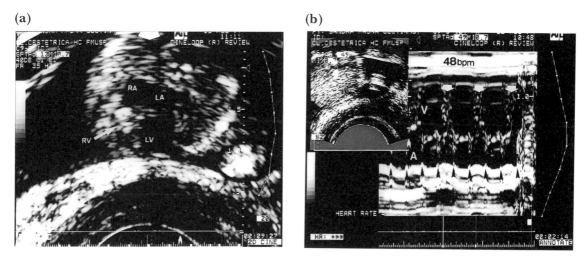

Figure 2 *Tricuspid atresia associated with complete heart block at 14 weeks. (a) Four-chamber view and hypoplastic right ventricle clearly seen (white arrow). (b) M-mode showing complete atrioventricular block. Atrial wall at atrial rate of 137 bpm (black arrow heads) and ventricular wall at ventricular rate of 48 bpm (white arrows)*

that the first step is to establish which are the most common congenital infections occurring in a given geographic area (incidence). In general, around 90% of the babies congenitally infected with cytomegalovirus (CMV) and toxoplasma are asymptomatic in the neonatal period[21] (Figure 3). Detection of these infections are best accomplished by serological screening of the neonate.

The second step is to include in the screening the diseases with known effective prenatal treatment; these are considered to be syphilis and toxoplasmosis. However, fetal toxoplasmosis can be considered treatable only if early diagnosis is made. Much controversy has occurred in the past 10 years about using screening for toxoplasmosis in low-incidence areas. We agree with Desmonts[22] that, in these areas, it is difficult to explain to the mother of a congenitally infected baby (Figure 3) how much we could have done to avoid the outcome if we had diagnosed her infection early. What could have been done was:

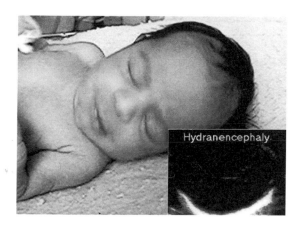

Figure 3 *Congenital toxoplasmosis in a baby at birth. Note that it looks perfectly normal. The ultrasound scan shows hydranencephaly diagnosed at 34 weeks (lower right). The mother started prenatal care susceptible for toxoplasmosis and early in pregnancy she acquired the infection (no clinical symptoms) and transmitted it to the unborn baby*

(1) Spiramycin, introduced soon after maternal diagnosis of acute infection, could have prevented vertical transmission in 60%;

(2) If fetal infection was present, it could have treated[21];

(3) If fetal treatment was not considered (there are those who do not believe in the efficacy of this treatment), at least early termination of the pregnancy could have been offered, even though termination would be accomplished only after invasive diagnosis of fetal infection. This would avoid termination of a non-infected fetus, since vertical transmission in the first trimester reaches a maximum of 15%.

The third step is to establish what can be done during, or immediately after, pregnancy for preventing the infection. If maternal serological status is known in early pregnancy, HIV, hepatitis B and rubella are included. For the HIV-positive pregnant women, the use of zidovudine during pregnancy and delivery, and for the neonate, seems to reduce vertical transmission; there is contraindication for invasive procedures, breast feeding and invasive maneuvers during delivery[23]. If the patient is a chronic AgHBS carrier, care must be taken to avoid contact of the neonate with maternal blood during delivery, and immunoglobulin as well as vaccination must be given very soon after birth; breast feeding is controvertial in these cases[24]. Rubella vaccine is contraindicated during pregnancy. The best moment for vaccination can be soon after birth if the mother starts the pregnancy susceptible for the infection, because around 50% of congenital rubella cases are born from multiparous women[25]. In our population routine infection screening includes: toxoplasmosis, rubella, HIV, syphilis and hepatitis B. It is equally important to give advice on how to avoid these infections (Table 4).

For the prevention of toxoplasmosis, the results with our proposed program (Table 4) that started in 1992 showed that only 8.7% of all susceptible women were sent to receive information on how to prevent the infection and were asked to repeat the serology. Among these, 45.8% completed the proposed systematic serological screening. After this first experience, our laboratory started to send a notice to the patient's doctor, with information that the patient was susceptible for the disease and should be sent to the program. This simple measure increased the referred number of patients up to 16.2% and, in this second stage, the percentage of patients who underwent the total number of serology screenings requested increased to 67.8%. Although these results are far from the ideal 100% coverage, the increasing number of referrals because of maternal seroconversion shows that obstetricians are increasingly considering prevention.

After 6 years of working on prevention, we have experienced our first three cases of seroconversion during pregnancy. So far, a total of ten cases of congenital toxoplasmosis have been diagnosed prenatally. These patients were referred because of positive maternal screening in early pregnancy ($n = 5$), diagnosis of fetal hydrocephaly ($n = 4$) and maternal seroconversion ($n = 1$). This last fetus was the only one for whom we could improve the prognosis; all nine others died either *in utero* or between 3 and 6 months after birth, or are alive but seriously handicapped.

Table 4 *Initial serological screening in pregnancy and preventive measures to avoid infection*

Disease	Immune status	Preventive measures
Toxoplasmosis	susceptible	avoid eating raw or undercooked meat or eggs
		avoid contact of raw meat with mucus of mouth and eyes
		avoid contact with soil
		wash fruits and vegetables before eating
		avoid contact with cat's feces; if not possible, throw away its feces daily and feed the cat well-cooked meat
		repeat serology at 20 and 30 weeks
Rubella	susceptible	avoid contact with persons with suspicious infection
		vaccinate after delivery
HIV	infected	prescribe zidovudine
		avoid invasive procedures and breast feeding
		take care in delivery
Hepatitis B	AgHBS carrier	avoid invasive procedures and breast feeding
		vaccinate the neonate
Syphilis	negative	if high risk, test again in the third trimester
		if unknown status during labor, test after delivery

References

1. Snijders RJM, Holzgreve W, Cuckle H, Nicolaides KH. Maternal age specific risk for trisomies at 9–14 weeks gestation. *Prenat Diagn* 1994;14:543–52
2. Snijders RJM, Sebire NJ, Nicolaides KH. Maternal age and gestational age specific risk for chromosomal defects. *Fetal Diagn Ther* 1995;10:356–67
3. Drugan A, Johnson MP, Isada NB, *et al.* The smaller than expected first-trimester fetus is at increased risk for chromosome anomalies. *Am J Obstet Gynecol* 1992;167:1525–8
4. Kuhn P, Brizot M, Pandya PP, Snijders RJ, Nicolaides KH. Crown–rump length in chromosomally abnormal fetuses at 10 to 13 weeks' gestation. *Am J Obstet Gynecol* 1995;172:23–5
5. Macintosh MCA, Brambati B, Chard T, Grudzinskas JG. Crown–rump length in aneuploid fetuses: implications for first trimester biochemical screening for aneuploidies. *Prenat Diagn* 1995;15:691–5
6. Nicolaides KH, Brizot ML, Snijders RJM. Fetal nuchal translucency thickness: ultrasound screening for fetal trisomy in the first trimester of pregnancy. *Br J Obstet Gynaecol* 1994;101:782–6
7. Shulman LP, Emerson D, Felker R, Phillips O, Simpson J, Elias S. High frequency of cytogenetic abnormalities with cystic hygroma diagnosed in the first trimester. *Obstet Gynecol* 1992;80:80–2
8. Snijders RJM, Noble P, Sebire NJ, Souka A, Nicolaides KH. UK multicentre project on assessment of risk of trisomy 21 by maternal age and fetal nuchal-translucency thickness at 10–14 weeks of gestation. *Lancet* 1998;351:343–6
9. Pandya PP, Snijders RJM, Johnson SJ, Brizot M, Nicolaides KH. Screening for fetal trisomies by maternal age and fetal nuchal translucency thickness at 10 to 14 weeks of gestation. *Br J Obstet Gynaecol* 1995;102:957–62
10. Youings S, Gregson N, Jones P. The efficacy of maternal age screening for Down's syndrome in Wessex. *Prenat Diagn* 1991;11:419–25
11. Pandya PP, Snijders RJM, Johnson SJ, Nicolaides KH. Natural history of trisomy 21 fetuses with increased nuchal translucency thickness. *Ultrasound Obstet Gynecol* 1995;5:381–3
12. Hyett JA, Perdu M, Sharland GK, Snijders RJM, Nicolaides KH. Increased nuchal translucency at 10–14 weeks of gestation as a marker for major cardiac defects. *Ultrasound Obstet Gynecol* 1997;10:242–6

13. Souka A, Snijders RJM, Novakov A, Soares W, Nicolaides KH. Defects and syndromes in chromosomally normal fetuses with increased nuchal translucency thickness at 10–14 weeks gestation. *Ultrasound Obstet Gynecol* 1998;11:391–400

14. Brizot ML, Snijders RJM, Bersinger NA, Kuhn P, Nicolaides KH. Maternal serum pregnancy associated placental protein A and fetal nuchal translucency thickness for the prediction of fetal trisomies in early pregnancy. *Obstet Gynecol* 1994;84:918–22

15. Brizot ML, Snijders RJM, Butler J, Bersinger NA, Nicolaides KH. Maternal serum hCG and fetal nuchal translucency thickness for the prediction of fetal trisomies in the first trimester of pregnancy. *Br J Obstet Gynaecol* 1995;102:127–32

16. Noble PL, Abraha HD, Snijders RJM, Sherwood R, Nicolaides KH. Screening for fetal trisomy 21 in the first trimester of pregnancy: maternal serum free β-hCG and fetal nuchal translucency thickness. *Ultrasound Obstet Gynecol* 1996;6:390–5

17. Sebire NJ, Snijders RJM, Hughes K, Scpulveda W, Nicolaides KH. Screening for trisomy 21 in twin pregnancies by maternal age and fetal nuchal translucency thickness at 10–14 weeks of gestation. *Br J Obstet Gynaecol* 1996;103:999–1003

18. Gembruch U. Prenatal diagnosis of congenital heart disease. *Prenat Diagn* 1997;17:1283–98

19. Yagel S, Weissman A, Rotstein Z, *et al.* Congenital heart defects: natural course and *in utero* development. *Circulation* 1997;96:550–5

20. Montenegro N, Matias A, Areias JC, Castedo S, Barros H. Increases in fetal nuchal translucency: possible involvement of early cardiac failure. *Ultrasound Obstet Gynecol* 1997;10:265–8

21. Remington JS, McLeod R, Desmonts G. Toxoplasmosis. In Remington JS, Klein JO, eds. *Infectious Diseases of the Fetus and Newborn Infant.* 4th edn. Philadelphia: WB Saunders, 1995:140–267

22. Desmonts G. Preventing congenital toxoplasmosis. *Lancet* 1990;20:1017–18

23. Henderson JL, Weiner CP. Congenital infection. *Curr Opin Obstet Gynecol* 1995;7:130–4

24. Crumpacker CS, Zeldis JB. Hepatitis. In Remington JS, Klein JO, eds. *Infectious Diseases of the Fetus and Newborn Infant,* 4th edn. Philadelphia: WB Saunders, 1995:805–34

25. Grangeot-Keros L. Rubella and pregnancy. *Pathol Biol* 1992;40:706–10

B-mode and Doppler studies of the abnormal fetus in the first trimester

7

R. K. Pooh

INTRODUCTION

After the introduction of the high-frequency transvaginal transducer, sonographic assessment of embryos and fetuses in the early stage has rapidly advanced. Clear visualization of embryonal and fetal morphology has established sonoembryology[1] and malformation assessment in early pregnancy. Advanced transvaginal color Doppler studies of the fetomaternal circulation[2] have enabled clear visualization of the intrauterine circulation and evaluation of fetal function in early pregnancy.

B-MODE STUDIES IN THE FIRST TRIMESTER

Early sonographic detection of congenital anomalies

For the past decade, many reports have been published on early sonographic detection of fetal congenital anomalies. Major anomalies of individual structure that have been detected by the end of 13 weeks of gestation are shown in Table 1.

Anomalies of the central nervous system

Congenital anomalies of the central nervous system are common, with the birth prevalence being approximately 3 per 1000. Calvarial ossification starts at 10 weeks of gestation and the hyperechogenic skull appears in the sonographic image by 11 weeks in normal pregnancy. Acrania, exencephaly and anencephaly are not independent anomalies. It is considered that dysraphia (absent cranial vault, acrania) occurs at a very early stage, and

Table 1 *Major congenital anomalies detected by the end of 13 weeks' gestation*

Anomalies of the central nervous system
Acrania, exencephaly, anencephaly
Encephalocele, iniencephaly
Spina bifida
Holoprosencephaly
Dandy–Walker malformation

Cardiac defects
Atrioventricular septal defect
Ventricular septal defect
Coarctation of the aorta

Abdominal wall defects
Omphalocele
Gastroschisis
Body stalk anomaly

Urinary tract defects
Bilateral renal agenesis
Multicystic dysplastic kidney disease
Megacystis

Skeletal anomalies
Achondrogenesis type II
Thanatophoric dwarfism
Osteogenesis imperfecta type II
Congenital lethal arthrogryposis

Others
Diaphragmatic hernia
Conjoined twin

disintegration of the exposed brain (exencephaly) during the fetal period results in anencephaly. Bronshtein and Ornoy[3] reported a case which showed the progression from acrania to anencephaly. Encephalocele, iniencephaly and spina bifida also result from open neural tube defects. Encephalocele is a condition with a cranial defect with protrusion of the brain; the lesion is occipital in most cases. It is detectable from 11 weeks by close observation of the skull shape. The skull deformity with bilateral indentation, often seen in a fetus with myelomeningocele, is called the lemon sign. Sonographic detection of this sign is possible from 12 weeks. Early detection of meningocele at 10 weeks has been reported[4]. Holoprosencephaly, caused by a disorder of prosencephalic development, is often associated with a chromosomal abnormality such as trisomy 13. Alobar-type holoprosencephaly is detectable from 10 weeks' gestation by depicting a single ventricle and accompanying facial anomalies[5]. Dandy–Walker malformation is characterized by the presence of cystic dilatation of the fourth ventricle and a defect of the cerebellar vermis. Achiron and colleagues[6] demonstrated the hypoechoic lesion in the posterior fossa of an 11-week fetus with this malformation.

Cardiac defects

Cardiac defects are the most common congenital abnormalities, with a birth prevalence of 4–10 per 1000. However, the sonographic detection rate of the major cardiac defects is still low, even at the mid-gestation scan. Although the four-chamber view of the heart can be visualized at 13–14 weeks' gestation in normal fetuses[7], other cardiac anatomical surveys cannot be completed during the first trimester. There are several reports on the early detection of major cardiac defects such as atrioventricular septal defect and ventricular septal defect in the first trimester; more than 80% of the cases were associated with increased nuchal translucency[8]. Although there is a limitation on demonstrating heart structure in the first trimester in practice, a detection of increased nuchal translucency should be followed by detailed observation of cardiac structure.

Abdominal wall defects

In normal fetuses, physiological midgut herniation is visualized at 8–10 weeks of gestation, and the return of the intestinal loops into the abdominal cavity is completed by the end of 11 weeks. Therefore, a pathological situation such as omphalocele can be clearly detectable from 12 weeks. However, if the omphalocele contains the liver, it can be detected as a pathological condition even at 10 weeks[9]. Gastroschisis is a rare anomaly with right-sided abdominal wall defect, protruding and free-floating intestinal loop and an intact umbilical cord. The differentiation between omphalocele and gastroschisis may be simplified by using color Doppler. The body stalk anomaly is rare, characterized by a major abdominal wall defect, severe kyphoscoliosis and short umbilical cord. In cases detected in the first trimester, the protruding part of the fetal structure in the extra-amniotic (celomic) cavity was demonstrated by ultrasound[10].

Urinary tract defects

The fetal kidneys can be visualized from 12 weeks' gestation and the bladder is recognizable in most normal fetuses at 12 weeks' gestation. Bronshtein and colleagues[11] detected several cases of bilateral renal agenesis (Potter syndrome) in the first and early second trimesters and described the diagnostic criteria for renal agenesis in the early fetus. These differed from those used in the second half of gestation, because in cases of bilateral renal agenesis the amniotic fluid was of normal volume until the 17th week and in some cases a cystic structure compatible with the urinary bladder was detected in the pelvis. Multicystic dysplastic kidney disease may be caused by an early injury to the mesonephros or early obstructive uropathy, and early detection of this disease is difficult. However, there have been some reported cases with unilateral multicystic dysplastic kidney disease detected from 12 weeks' gestation. Megacystis is caused by urethral atresia and several cases have been detected from 11 weeks.

Skeletal anomalies

Limb buds are visualized at 8 weeks' gestation and long bones of the upper and lower extremities are recognizable from 11 weeks by sonography. Limb movements are normally visualized by 11 weeks' gestation. Skeletal dysplasia is classified into lethal and non-lethal groups. Some cases of lethal skeletal dysplasia have been detected in the first trimester[12]: achondrogenesis type II, thanatophoric dwarfism and osteogenesis imperfecta type II. Extremity contractures rarely occur in conjunction with musculoskeletal or neurological disorders. Congenital lethal arthrogryposis is a condition with multiple joint contractures including bilateral talipes and fixed flexion or extension deformities of the limb joints. In families with a previous history of this sequence, a few cases have been detected in the first trimester[13].

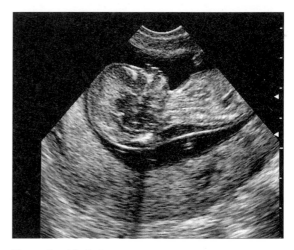

Figure 1 *Nuchal translucency at 12 weeks' gestation*

Increased nuchal translucency

It has been well established that increased nuchal translucency (Figure 1) is an early marker for fetal chromosomopathies. However, even if chromosomal abnormalities are excluded, structural abnormalities are occasionally found in chromosomally normal fetuses with increased nuchal translucency. Hyett and colleagues[14] reported that the prevalence of major cardiac defects in chromosomally normal fetuses with increased nuchal translucency was 17 per 1000, ranging from 5.4 per 1000 (translucency of 2.5–3.4 mm) to 233 per 1000 (translucency of 5.5 mm or more). They suggested that measurement of nuchal translucency thickness may prove to be a useful method of screening for abnormalities of the heart and great arteries. Souka and colleagues[8] studied the pregnancy outcome in chromosomally normal fetuses with increased nuchal translucency, and reported that the rates of miscarriage and perinatal death increased with fetal nuchal translucency thickness. They also combined the data from 15 studies providing data on fetal defects in chromosomally normal pregnancies with increased nuchal translucency thickness, and reported that 16% of fetuses experienced a wide range of structural abnormalities, and that the prevalence of major cardiac defects,

diaphragmatic hernia, exomphalos, body stalk anomaly and fetal akinesia deformation sequence appeared to be substantially higher than in the general population[8]. Therefore, sonographic detection of increased nuchal translucency should be followed by careful observation of the fetal morphology and by a follow-up scan thereafter. Counselling parents is an important task in clinical practice when increased nuchal translucency is detected. About 90% (nuchal translucency below 4.5 mm), 80% (translucency of 4.5–6.4 mm) and 45% (translucency of 6.5 mm or more) of chromosomally normal pregnancies resulted in healthy live births[8]. In addition, nuchal translucency is one of the sonographic markers for detecting fetal chromosomopathy or structural abnormalities such as cardiac defects, but does not constitute a fetal structural abnormality in itself. These data and facts should be given to parents with affected pregnancies.

First-trimester screening for structural and chromosomal abnormalities

It is still controversial when a sonographic screening for fetal anomalies should start during pregnancy. Detailed sonographic visualization of the fetal anatomy is obtained in most fetuses at 12–13 weeks' gestation, and sonographic examination at this age depicts detailed structures of individual organs. It was reported that 81% of chromosomally abnormal fetuses were diagnosed in the first-trimester sonographic examination[15] and 64.7% of major structural abnormalities were diagnosed at the 12–13-week scan[16]. A higher detection rate of major structural abnormalities may be obtained in the second trimester than in the first trimester. In contrast, the detection rate of trisomy 21 becomes lower after 16 weeks than before this age. As a screening protocol for both structural and chromosomal abnormalities, the first scan at 12–13 weeks and the second scan at about 18–20 weeks are recommended.

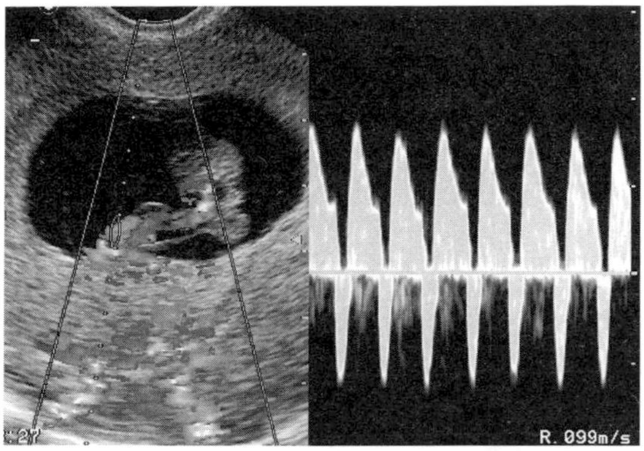

Figure 2 *Reversed end-diastolic flow in the umbilical artery at 9 weeks' gestation, seen in a fetus with hydrops*

DOPPLER ASSESSMENT IN THE FIRST TRIMESTER

Color or power Doppler assessment often simplifies the diagnosis of morphological abnormalities detected by B-mode. In addition, Doppler assessment of the fetal circulation in early pregnancy may be helpful for evaluation of cardiac function and prediction of the outcome of pregnancy.

Doppler assessment of arterial circulation in the abnormal fetus

In normal early pregnancy, the blood flow velocity waveform of the umbilical artery has absent end-diastolic flow; this is a physiological phenomenon until 12 weeks.

A few studies have been reported on the relationship between an abnormal fetus and Doppler evaluation of arterial flow in the first trimester. Martinez and colleagues[17] examined both the umbilical artery pulsatility index and nuchal translucency measurements in the first trimester and suggested that the presence of chromosomal anomalies may be strongly suspected when an increased nuchal translucency thickening is associated with an abnormally high pulsatility index of the umbilical artery. Jauniaux and colleagues[18] compared some parameters including fetal heart rate and umbilical artery pulsatility index of each trisomy group with a control

group, and concluded that fetuses with trisomy 21 showed a significantly increased heart rate, but no significant differences of the Doppler features were found between the groups. The authors also reported that, in some fetuses with trisomy 18 or triploidy, an increased resistance to blood flow in the umbilical artery could be found in early pregnancy, probably due to an abnormal development of the villous vascularization[18].

It is well known that absent and reversed end-diastolic blood flow of the umbilical artery is a sign of fetal adverse outcome in the late second and third trimesters. Although it is rare to detect reversed end-diastolic flow of the umbilical artery in early pregnancy (Figure 2), five cases with reversed flow between 9 and 13 weeks' gestation have been reported[19–22]. Increased nuchal translucency, hydrops or cystic hygroma was observed in all cases. Four out of five had chromosomal anomalies of trisomy 18 ($n = 2$), trisomy 13 ($n = 1$) and 45,X ($n = 1$) and one case had normal chromosome. Although pregnancies were terminated in two cases, intrauterine fetal death was confirmed between 1.5 days and 5 weeks after the detection of reversed end-diastolic flow in the remaining three cases. Even in the first trimester, reversed end-diastolic flow of the umbilical artery may be a sign indicating fetal cardiac insufficiency and may predict fetal demise thereafter.

Doppler assessment of venous circulation in the abnormal fetus

Many reports have been published in the 1990s on the venous Doppler assessment of the fetal circulation in the second and third trimesters. In the fetal venous circulation, the ductus venosus is an important vessel, which communicates between the oxygenated bloodstream from the umbilical vein and the central venous system. Kiserud and colleagues[23] reported a reduced minimum velocity or reversed blood flow in the ductus venosus during atrial contraction in growth-retarded fetuses or fetuses with cardiac diseases. Figure 3 shows a reversed blood flow in the ductus venosus during atrial contraction, seen in an abnormal fetus in the early second trimester. Recently, venous Doppler studies in the first trimester have been published. Montenegro and colleagues[24] carried out the nuchal translucency measurement and Doppler assessment of the ductus venosus at 10–13 weeks' gestation, and the results showed that the forward velocity in the ductus venosus during atrial contraction was consistently less than 2 cm/s in five chromosomally abnormal fetuses with increased nuchal translucency thickness ($p < 0.001$), compared with chromosomally normal fetuses with increased nuchal translucency. Matias and colleagues[25] reported three trisomic fetuses with congenital heart diseases or increased

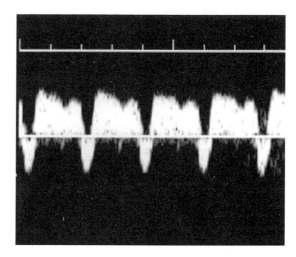

Figure 3 *Reversed flow in the ductus venosus during atrial contraction in an abnormal fetus at 16 weeks' gestation. A similar flow pattern was reported in the first trimester[25]*

endocardial thickness. In all three cases, increased nuchal translucency and abnormal venous return, such as a high retrograde flow in the inferior vena cava, a decreased or reversed flow in the ductus venosus and a dicrotic pulsatile flow in the umbilical vein, were observed at 12–13 weeks' gestation[25]. It is of interest that all cases had a normal umbilical artery blood flow pattern. Venous Doppler assessment in the first trimester may have value in clinical practice for the evaluation of fetal compromise.

References

1. Timor-Tritsch IE, Peisner DB, Raju S. Sonoembryology: an organ oriented approach using a high-frequency vaginal probe. *J Clin Ultrasound* 1990;18:286–98
2. Kurjak A, Zudenigo D, Predanic M, Kupesic S. Recent advances in the Doppler study of early fetomaternal circulation. *J Perinat Med* 1993;21:419–39
3. Bronshtein M, Ornoy A. Acrania: anencephaly resulting from secondary degeneration of a closed neural tube: two cases in the same family. *J Clin Ultrasound* 1991;19:230–4
4. Bernard JP, Suarez B, Rambaud C, Muller F, Ville Y. Prenatal diagnosis of neural tube defect before 12 weeks' gestation: direct and indirect ultrasonographic semeiology. *Ultrasound Obstet Gynecol* 1997;10:406–9
5. Weissman A, Achiron R. Ultrasound diagnosis of congenital anomalies in early pregnancy. In Jurkovic D, Jauniaux E, eds. *Ultrasound and Early Pregnancy.* Carnforth, UK: Parthenon Publishing, 1996:95–119
6. Achiron R, Achiron A, Yagel S. First trimester transvaginal sonographic diagnosis of Dandy–

Walker malformation. *J Clin Ultrasound* 1993;21: 62–4

7. Gembruch U, Knopfle G, Bald R, Hansmann M. Early diagnosis of fetal congenital heart disease by transvaginal echocardiography. *Ultrasound Obstet Gynecol* 1993;3:310–17

8. Souka AP, Snijders RJM, Navakov A, Soares W, Nicolaides KH. Defects and syndromes in chromosomally normal fetuses with increased nuchal translucency thickness at 10–14 weeks of gestation. *Ultrasound Obstet Gynecol* 1998;11: 391–400

9. Pagliano M, Mossetti M, Ragno P. Echographic diagnosis of omphalocele in the first trimester of pregnancy. *J Clin Ultrasound* 1990;18:658–60

10. Ginsberg NE, Cadkin A, Strom C. Prenatal diagnosis of body stalk anomaly in the first trimester of pregnancy. *Ultrasound Obstet Gynecol* 1997;10:419–21

11. Bronshtein M, Amit A, Achiron R, Noy I, Blumenfeld Z. The early prenatal sonographic diagnosis of renal agenesis: techniques and possible pitfalls. *Prenat Diagn* 1994;14:291–7

12. Souka AP, Nicolaides KH. Diagnosis of fetal abnormalities at the 10–14-week scan. *Ultrasound Obstet Gynecol* 1997;10:429–42

13. Hyett J, Noble P, Sebire NJ, Snijders R, Nicolaides KH. Lethal congenital arthrogryposis presents with increased nuchal translucency at 10–14 weeks of gestation. *Ultrasound Obstet Gynecol* 1997; 9:310–13

14. Hyett JA, Perdu M, Sharland GK, Snijders RSM, Nicolaides KH. Increased nuchal translucency at 10–14 weeks of gestation as a marker for major cardiac defects. *Ultrasound Obstet Gynecol* 1997;10: 242–6

15. Economides DL, Whitlow BJ, Kadir R, Lazanakis M, Verdin SM. First trimester sonographic detection of chromosomal abnormalities in an unselected population. *Br J Obstet Gynaecol* 1998; 105:58–62

16. Economides DL, Braithwaite JM. First trimester ultrasonographic diagnosis of fetal structural abnormalities in a low risk population. *Br J Obstet Gynaecol* 1998;105:53–7

17. Martinez JM, Borrell A, Antolin E, *et al.* Combining nuchal translucency with umbilical Doppler velocimetry for detecting fetal trisomies in the first trimester of pregnancy. *Br J Obstet Gynaecol* 1997;104:11–14

18. Jauniaux E, Gavrill P, Khun P, Kurdi W, Hyett J, Nicolaides KH. Fetal heart rate and umbilico-placental Doppler flow velocity waveforms in early pregnancies with a chromosomal abnormality and/or an increased nuchal translucency thickness. *Hum Reprod* 1996;11: 435–9

19. Martinez Crespo JM, Comas C, Borrell A, *et al.* Reversed end-diastolic umbilical artery velocity in two cases of trisomy 18 at 10 weeks' gestation. *Ultrasound Obstet Gynecol* 1996;7:447–9

20. Montenegro N, Beires J, Leite LP. Reverse end-diastolic umbilical artery blood flow at 11 weeks' gestation. *Ultrasound Obstet Gynecol* 1995;5:141–2

21. Comas C, Carrera M, Devesa R, *et al.* Early detection of reversed diastolic umbilical flow: should we offer karyotyping? *Ultrasound Obstet Gynecol* 1997;10:400–2

22. Pooh RK, Nakagawa Y, Nagamachi N. Interesting findings in early sonographic detection. *Adv Obstet Perinatol* 1998;9:59–73

23. Kiserud T, Eik-Nes SH, Blaas H-G, Hellevik LR, Simensen B. Ductus venosus blood velocity and the umbilical circulation in the seriously growth-retarded fetus. *Ultrasound Obstet Gynecol* 1994;4: 109–14

24. Montenegro N, Matias A, Areias JC, Castedo S, Barros H. Increased fetal nuchal translucency: possible involvement of early cardiac failure. *Ultrasound Obstet Gynecol* 1997;10:265–8

25. Matias A, Montenegro N, Areias JC, Brandão O. Anomalous fetal venous return associated with major chromosomopathies in the late first trimester of pregnancy. *Ultrasound Obstet Gynecol* 1998;11:209–13

Ultrasound screening for congenital heart defects: routine or selective?

8

S. Levi, L. Tecco and G. Faron

INTRODUCTION

Congenital heart defects (CHD) are among the most frequent congenital anomalies and the most threatening to patient life. Specific care is possible, from surgery and drug therapy to termination of pregnancy (TOP). Prenatal diagnosis is particularly helpful in the case of severe anomalies, allowing the parents to choose among various available solutions, including complete fetal examination, karyotyping, maternal transport to a specialized tertiary unit before birth, or TOP.

Six to ten per 1000 births and terminations are complicated by CHD[1-3]. The range is broad and the incidence depends very much on the method of recording and diagnosing birth defects[4] and on the duration of the follow-up. Eight per 1000 is the most commonly quoted incidence, and this includes about 50% of ventricular septal defects (VSD). CHD represented 21% of 4615 congenital anomalies collected in the Eurofetus study[5].

Depending on the type of CHD, and on the combination with other structural or chromosome anomalies, death is the outcome of major undiagnosed defects in more than 75% for some CHD, and nearly 30% of the average CHD[5].

The diagnosis of CHD can be made by fetal echocardiography at various stages of pregnancy, depending on the defect and the examination conditions, such as maternal obesity. Fetal echocardiography is a specialized examination generally reserved for particular cases. The selection of cases for expert echocardiography is based on the presence of high-risk factors for CHD, including history and signs. Among the signs,

previous abnormal or suspicious sonograms have a prominent role. Accordingly, routine ultrasound screening may play an important role in finding relevant signs of CHD. Prenatal diagnosis of congenital anomalies, and of CHD in particular, should be followed by karyotyping, since the risk of chromosome anomaly is significantly higher and its diagnosis has an important impact on therapy options. Parental choice of therapy options is possible only if the diagnosis is made in time and is sufficiently precise to allow effective counselling. Counselling is based on the possible outcome of the CHD at stake, and encompasses the entire spectrum of the possible attitudes towards the particular anomaly. Parents' wishes, available effective treatment, subsequent severe handicaps and postnatal costs can be considered only when prenatal diagnosis is made.

We have performed a systematic overview of the data published in the specialized literature and analyzed the studies on prenatal CHD diagnosis from 1980.

OBJECTIVES OF THE STUDY

We aimed first to find rational arguments to show the usefulness of prenatal diagnosis of CHD for alleviating the weight of CHD on patients and public health, by reducing morbidity and mortality through cost-effective measures. Second, we wished to select the best method for prenatal detection and diagnosis of CHD: examination of high-risk patients only or routine check-up of pregnant women as a part of obstetric care.

STUDY DESIGN

Papers published before 1980 were not expected to be useful, although prenatal diagnostic ultrasound has been used from 1958 onwards[6], and ultrasound fetal cardiology from 1972[7]. Emphasis was given to papers

(1) Concerned with examination of high-risk pregnancies, or of low-risk pregnancies when significant data were reported on whether CHD was diagnosed or not;

(2) On chromosome anomalies detected following CHD diagnosis;

(3) Reporting on outcome;

(4) Describing the method used for CHD screening and its sensitivity.

When the data seemed to have been collected in a sufficiently homogeneous way, we adopted a qualitative analysis to enhance the significance of the results.

RESULTS

Frequency of CHD

As underlined in the introduction, the published frequency of CHD varies widely. It is important to consider the method used for counting CHD before accepting any given number. One of the main criteria for the completeness of CHD recording is the competence of the professional examining the newborn babies: pediatric cardiologists diagnose 20% more cases that do non-specialists[4]. A second criterion is the duration of time considered for anomaly recording: from the usual few days after birth to a 12-month survey. For example, 30% more CHD can be discovered between these limits[8]. However, severe anomalies will not remain ignored for many days, even when searched for by less expert examiners. The majority among late diagnosed CHD are medium and small VSD, and their proportion among all CHD may be considered as a marker of the completeness of CHD registration[4]. For example, an incidence of nearly 1% CHD is

coupled with more than 0.6% VSD[4]. We counted a total of 421 CHD in samples including 58 352 pregnant women at low risk of congenital anomalies (0.7%)[8–15]. On the basis of a single paper, it was possible to compare the recording of CHD made soon after birth and an additional recording made 12 months later in the same population. The comparison shows an increase from 47 to 65 CHD in 7024 cases, corresponding to incidences of 0.67% and 0.93%, respectively[8]. Considering that the difference is mostly due to missed VSD, 18 VSD were probably missed at postnatal examination and the total contribution of VSD to CHD should be 0.6%, similar to the proportion shown above[4].

Severity

Severity depends on several factors, e.g. the type of anomaly, the health of the patient with CHD, the association with other congenital anomalies, chromosome anomalies and other genetic conditions, and also, from the patient's point of view, the ability to take care of the affected newborn baby. Association with a chromosome anomaly occurred, in our readings, in 163 of 1215 CHD (13%) (Figure 1); 56 were trisomy 21, 46 trisomy 18 and 15 trisomy 13[5,9,12,14,16]. Association with congenital anomalies, including other CHD, occurred in 43%[5]. Among 160 CHD, 67 led to perinatal

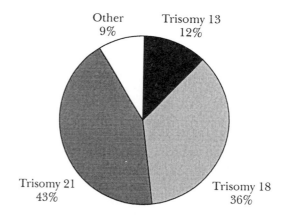

Figure 1 *Distribution of chromosome anomalies* (n = 163) *among congenital heart defects* (n = 1215) (13%): *trisomies 13, 18, 21 and miscellaneous*

death or TOP[8,11,12,15,17]. In a series of 15 types of major anomalies affecting 452 CHD cases, 28% of patients with a defect not diagnosed died perinatally, against 61% including TOP in detected cases[5].

Prenatal diagnosis

Diagnosis of CHD is frequently the result of expert echocardiography; patients are usually selected for echocardiography because of existing high-risk factors for CHD. The main indications are positive family history, maternal diseases including diabetes, infections and metabolic diseases, teratogens, aneuploidy and other genetic non-chromosomal conditions, and, finally, abnormal sonograms. The prominent role of abnormal or suspicious previous sonograms has been shown by several studies. The most significant signs collected during ultrasound examination are suspected CHD, extracardiac malformation, abnormal obstetric features such as polyhydramnios, non-immune hydrops, intrauterine fetal growth retardation and fetal arrhythmia (also detectable by fetal auscultation). The proportions of the various indications for echocardiography are 58% for clinical signs and 42% for previous abnormal ultrasound scans[9,15–19]. On the other hand, the relative contribution of ultrasound and of clinical signs to CHD diagnosis is, respectively, 85% and 15%[16,19–22] (Figures 2–4). The method used for ultrasound examination is relevant to the detection of CHD. Although the use of complete echocardiography including color Doppler is indispensable for CHD diagnosis[23], it cannot be included in routine obstetric ultrasound examination or even in routine ultrasound scanning targeted on malformation screening. Echocardiography is a complex examination that requires special qualification and high-tech equipment.

The sensitivity of CHD detection and diagnosis depends first on the design of the study. Examining low-risk pregnancies or high-risk pregnancies does not generate the same reported sensitivity. The same is true

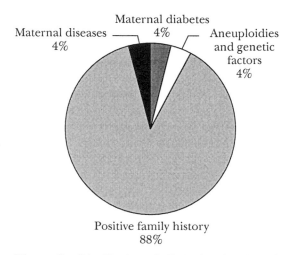

Figure 2 *Distribution of clinical indications for echocardiography: positive family history, maternal diseases excluding diabetes, maternal diabetes, aneuploidies and genetic factors*

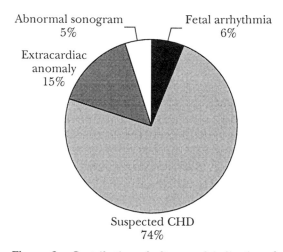

Figure 3 *Contribution of ultrasound indications for echocardiography to diagnosis of congenital heart defects (CHD): suspected CHD on previous sonograms, suspected or diagnosed extracardiac malformations on previous sonograms, abnormal basic obstetric ultrasound scan, fetal arrythmia detected by any means (sonogram, Doppler, etc.)*

when a specific screening method is considered. Similar detection rates for CHD would not be yielded by superficial overview of the cardiac area, as practised some years ago; looking at the four-chamber view – as advocated in 1986[24] – or the five-chamber view[15]; and examining, in addition, the outlet of the great arteries. Therefore, figures on sensitivity should be given along with the

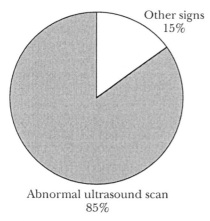

Figure 4 *Contribution of indications for echocardiography to diagnosis of congenital heart defects: all the indications listed in Figure 3 (abnormal ultrasound scan) and those listed in Figure 2 (other signs)*

method used for heart scanning. Series on mid-trimester routine ultrasound examination for low-risk pregnancies, with no particular method described, disclose sensitivities ranging from 7 to 47% (average 21%)[12-14]. The CHD prevalences corresponding to the examples quoted above are as different as 1% and 0.4% (average 0.7%). This particular inverse relationship between sensitivity and prevalence is in agreement with our opinion that published prevalence has an influence on the corresponding sensitivity[25].

The four-chamber view, applied in low-risk pregnancies, led also to very different sensitivities, ranging from 5 to 81% (average 27%), coupled with prevalences ranging from 1 to 0.4% (average 0.8%)[10-14]. In two studies comparing a simple obstetric scan with the four-chamber view, the sensitivity was 47% and 81%, respectively, in one[12] and 7% against 11% in another in which less good results were obtained[14]. Complete echo-cardiography, performed in low-risk pregnancies, was able to detect 26–88% (average 53%)[8,9,11]. The four-chamber view in high-risk pregnancies was capable of displaying a broad range of sensitivities: 31%[26] to 92%[16]; comprehensive echo-cardiography in high-risk pregnancies led to the highest sensitivities, ranging from 50%[27] to 96%[19] (average 78%)[9,17,18,20,28].

COMMENTS

Considering that the choice of a policy aiming at detection of CHD is the most relevant issue for studies like the present one, it is clear that performing echocardiography on a selection of pregnant women at high risk for CHD will lead to a high detection rate and precise diagnosis. However, such a policy will deceive by misdiagnosing more than 90% of the CHD existing in a standard population of pregnant women. Therefore, an increase of CHD detection could be obtained through a primary scan – routine second-trimester obstetric ultrasound examination or, better, targeted ultrasound scanning for congenital anomalies – and the patients with suspicious sonograms then referred for expert echocardiography (Figure 4). Suspicious sonograms include a large variety of signs, such as any congenital anomaly, including CHD, any anomaly of amniotic fluid volume, excessive nuchal thickness or nuchal translucency, fluid collections in the fetus, fetal arrhythmia or abnormal fetal heart axis. Enhancing the quality of basic ultrasound scanning and of anomaly screening should strongly improve the rate of CHD diagnosis[13,25]. Therefore, we can conclude that there is no conflict between strategies favoring examination of high-risk pregnancies only and those suggesting routine obstetric and targeted ultrasound for congenital anomalies. Indeed, since previous abnormal sonograms provide 85% of diagnosed CHD in indicated echocardiography programs, any routine ultrasound program significantly influences CHD screening, being of the utmost importance in showing signs indicating specialized echocardiography, as evidenced in our study. Routine ultrasound examination should necessarily include the four-chamber view to detect 50% and more significant CHD, almost ignoring the large number of small and medium VSD. Evaluation of screening programs for low-risk pregnancies is possible only when the incidence of CHD is similar to those found in low-risk populations, i.e. a minimum of 0.6% where CHD are recorded after birth, and nearly 1% where CHD are recorded for a longer period of 6–12 months. In high-risk pregnancies, the precise distribution of the various indications, and their relative contribution to CHD diagnosis, should be mentioned.

ACKNOWLEDGEMENTS

We are grateful to the team of consultants, residents and fellows of the Ultrasound Gynecology and Obstetrics laboratory for their help in reading the abundant literature on ultrasound and CHD, and for selecting the papers in which useful information was found in accordance with our study scheme, namely Rosine Lejeune MD, Theresa Cos MD, Philippe Charles MD, Fatna Amhai MD, Kawakeb El Mourabi MD, Catherine Van Pachterbeke MD and Berthe Zinga MD, and to Mrs Monique Van Noten for the efficacious management of the references.

References

1. Boughman JA, Neill CA, Ferencz C, Loffredo CA. The genetics of congenital heart disease. *Prenat Diagn* 1997;17:1283–98
2. Eurocat Working Group. *15 Years of Surveillance of Congenital Anomalies in Europe 1980–1994* (report 7). *European Union Project*. Brussels: Scienfic Institute of Public Health – Louis Pasteur, 1997
3. Grandjean H, Larroque D, Levi S, the Eurofetus team. Sensitivity of routine ultrasound screening of pregnancies in the Eurofetus database. In Levi S, Chervenak F, eds. *Ultrasound Screening for Fetal Anomalies: Is It Worth It? Ann NY Acad Sci* 1998; 847:118–24
4. Pexieder T, Bloch D, Eurocat Working Party on Congenital Heart Disease. Eurocat subproject on epidemiology of congenital heart disease – first analysis of the completed study. In Clark EB, Markwald RR, Takao A, eds. *Developmental Mechanisms of Heart Disease*. New York: Futura Publishing, 1995:655–68
5. Levi S. *Cost-effectiveness of Antenatal Screening for Fetal Malformation by Ultrasound*. An evaluation of antenatal mass screening by ultrasound for the diagnosis of birth defects (1990–1993). Contract MR4*-0225-B. Brussels: European Commission, 1995
6. Donald I, MacVicar J, Brown TG. Investigation of abdominal masses by pulsed ultrasound. *Lancet* 1958;1:1188–94
7. Winsberg F. Echocardiography of the fetal and newborn heart. *Invest Radiol* 1972;7:152
8. Rustico MA, Benettoni A, D'Ottavio G, Maieron A, *et al.* Fetal heart screening in low-risk pregnancies. *Ultrasound Obstet Gynecol* 1995;6:313–19
9. Stumpflen I, Stumpflen A, Wimmer M, Bernaschek G. Effect of detailed fetal echocardiography as part of routine prenatal ultrasonographic screening on detection of congenital heart disease. *Lancet* 1996;348:854–7
10. Buskens E, Grobbee DE, Frohn-Mulder IME, *et al.* Efficacy of routine fetal ultrasound screening for congenital heart disease in normal pregnancy. *Circulation* 1996;94:67–72
11. Achiron R, Glaser J, Gelernter I, Hegesh J, Yagel S. Extended fetal echocardiographic examination for detecting cardiac malformations in low-risk pregnancies. *Br Med J* 1992;304:671–4
12. Vergani P, Mariani S, Ghidini A, *et al.* Screening for congenital heart disease with the four-chamber view of the fetal heart. *Am J Obstet Gynecol* 1992;167:1000–3
13. Levi S, Schaaps JP, Dehavay P, Defoort P, Coulon R. End-result of routine ultrasound screening for congenital anomalies: the Belgian multicentric study 1984–92. *Ultrasound Obstet Gynecol* 1995;5:366–71
14. Tegnander E, Eik-Nes SH, Johansen OJ, Linker DT. Prenatal detection of heart defects at the routine fetal examination at 18 weeks in a non-selected population. *Ultrasound Obstet Gynecol* 1995;5:372–80
15. Ott WJ. The accuracy of antenatal fetal echocardiography screening in high- and low-risk patients. *Am J Obstet Gynecol* 1995;172:1741–9
16. Copel JA, Pilu G, Green J, Hobbins JC, Kleinman CS. Fetal echocardiography screening for congenital heart-disease. The importance of the 4-chamber view. *Am J Obstet Gynecol* 1987;157:648–55
17. Giancotti A, Torcia F, Giampa G, *et al.* Prenatal evaluation of congenital heart disease in high-risk pregnancies. *Clin Exp Obstet Gynecol* 1995;22:225–9
18. Cooper MJ, Enderlein MA, Dyson DC, Roge CL, Tarnoff H. Fetal echocardiography: retro-

spective review of clinical experience and an evaluation of indications. *Obstet Gynecol* 1995; 86:577–82

19. Wheller JJ, Reiss R, Allen HD. Clinical experience with fetal echocardiography. *Am J Dis Child* 1990;144:49–53

20. Parness IA, Yeager SB, Sanders SP, *et al.* Echocardiographic diagnosis of fetal heart defects in mid trimester. *Arch Dis Child* 1988;63: 1137–45

21. Allan LD, Sharland GK, Milburn A, *et al.* Prospective diagnosis of 1006 consecutive cases of congenital heart disease in the fetus. *J Am Coll Cardiol* 1992;23:1452–8

22. Fermont L, Batisse A, Piechaud JF, Lebidois J. Détection prénatale des cardiopathies congénitales. *Rev Pediat* 1989;6:17–28

23. Sharland GK, Chita SK, Allan LD. The use of colour Doppler in fetal echocardiography. *Int J Cardiol* 1990;28:229–36

24. Allan LD, Crawford DC, Chita SK, Tynan MT. Prenatal screening for congenital heart disease. *Br Med J* 1986;292:1717–19

25. Levi S. Screening for congenital malformations by ultrasound. In Kurjak A, ed. *Textbook of Perinatal Medicine.* Carnforth, UK: Parthenon Publishing, 1998:587–609

26. Wigton TR, Sabbagha RE, Tamura RK, Cohen L, *et al.* Sonographic diagnosis of congenital heart disease: comparison between the four-chamber view and multiple cardiac views. *Obstet Gynecol* 1993;82:219–24

27. Hata T, Takamori H, Hata K, *et al.* Antenatal diagnosis of congenital heart disease and fetal arrhythmia by ultrasound. *Gynecol Obstet Invest* 1988;26:118–25

28. Buskens E, Grobbee DE, Hess J, Wladimiroff JW. Prenatal diagnosis of congenital heart disease: prospects and problems. *Eur J Obstet Gynecol Reprod Biol* 1995;50:5–11

Fetal pyelectasis: definition, significance and outcome

9

G. D'Ottavio, L. Paduano, M. A. Rustico, R. Natale, Y. J. Meir and G. P. Mandruzzato

DEFINITION

Mild dilatation of the fetal pelvis or pyelectasis is a common sonographic finding. Its incidence depends, amongst other things, on the different definitions of pyelectasis by different authors. The distinction between physiological and pathological pyelectasis is still under debate, and there is not a uniform definition of this condition. Although, according to Blakiston's *Gould Medical Dictionary*, pyelectasis is a 'dilation of a renal pelvis' presumably without involvement of calyces, several authors still include in their series also pelvicalyceal mild dilatations. Moreover, the threshold of significance of fetal pyelectasis that results in relevant postnatal disease has been controversial.

In the early 1980s, Grignon and colleagues[1] reported a grading classification for prenatal pelvis dilatation: they stated that mild pyelectasis of < 10 mm should be considered normal. This grading system was further modified by Homsy and co-workers[2], who introduced the grades 'mild' (a renal pelvis size of < 15 mm with normal calyces), 'moderate' (a renal pelvis size of > 15 mm with slight calyceal dilatation) and 'severe' pelvis dilatation (a renal pelvis size of > 15 mm and moderate to severe calyceal dilatation with or without cortical involvement). According to these authors, moderate to severe renal pelvis dilatation requires further diagnostic workup.

More recently, the Society for Fetal Urology have proposed a classification of hydronephrosis independent of measurements, based on a grading from 0 to 4 of different degrees of dilatation (grade 0 = no hydronephrosis; grade I = only renal pelvis visualized; grade II = renal pelvis and few calyces seen; grade III = renal pelvis and almost all calyces seen; grade IV = hydronephrosis and parenchymal thinning[3].

Anatomical variations and environmental influences such as maternal state of hydration have recently been suggested for the ultrasonographic observation of minimal pelvic dilatations[4]. Pyelectasis has been thought to result from an overproduction of urine, a transient reflux and also a possible genetic predisposition[5]. However, recent studies involving the long-term prenatal and postnatal follow-up of fetuses with pyelectasis have concluded that there are clinically significant associations with fetal aneuploidy, obstructive uropathy and vesicoureteral reflux (VUR).

REVIEW OF THE LITERATURE

Although varying degrees of pyelectasis have been reported to be significant, there are no consistent guidelines in the literature that relate severity of pyelectasis to appropriate perinatal management (Table 1). Corteville and co-workers[7] recommended postnatal follow-up for renal pevis dilatation of > 4 mm before 33 weeks and > 7 mm after 33 weeks. Mandell and associates[8] found no good correlation between the degree of dilatation *in utero* and after birth. They therefore suggested as thresholds for significant pyelectasis 5 mm between 15 and 20 weeks, ≥ 8 mm between 20 and 30 weeks and ≥ 10 mm after 30 weeks. Anderson and colleagues[9] proposed a cut-off level of 6 mm between 24

Table 1 *Literature and present study criteria: upper limit of fetal renal pelvis (anteroposterior diameter) to define fetal pyelectasis*

Authors	Year	No. of fetuses	Pelvis size and gestational age
Corteville et al.[7]	1991	63	≥ 4 mm before 33 weeks; > 7 mm after 33 weeks
Mandell et al.[8]	1991	154	≥ 5 mm at 15–20 weeks; > 8 mm at 20–30 weeks; ≤ 10 mm after 30 weeks
Adra et al.[16]	1995	68	≥ 8 mm after 28 weeks
Ouzounian et al.[10]	1996	84	≥ 5 mm at any gestational age
Wilson et al.[17]	1997	65	≥ 6 mm at 19 weeks or after
Persutte et al.[11]	1997	294	≥ 4 mm and < 10 mm at any gestational age
Present study	1999	58	≥ 5 mm at 21 weeks

and 30 weeks; therefore they suggested postnatal renal sonography and voiding cystourethrography (VCUG) for all babies with antenatal pyelectasis of 4 mm or more.

Ouzounian and associates[10] evaluated 84 patients for a total of 98 fetal kidneys with pyelectasis, which was more common in the left kidney and in males. Using a receiver-operating characteristic curve, they found that fetal pyelectasis of 8 mm was 91% sensitive and 72% specific in predicting subsequent hydronephrosis. Use of a threshold of 5 mm showed a sensitivity of 100% and a specificity of 24%. They concluded that antenatal detection of a pelvic diameter of 5 mm at any gestational age should have follow-up ultrasound examination and detailed postnatal evaluation.

Persutte and co-workers[11], who considered isolated dilatations measuring between 4 and 10 mm, found a prevalence of this phenomenon of 5.5% (i.e. finding the condition would require the assessment and postnatal surveillance of about 5% of all fetuses). Their results confirmed another important point: as a rule, dilatation that corresponds to a real pathology gradually increases in size over the period of pregnancy. However, in their experience, the major problem of screening for urinary tract malformations was linked to the antenatal detection of VUR.

The early recognition of congenital reflux seems to be important for several reasons. Reflux nephropathy is among the most frequent causes of hypertension and chronic renal failure in children and young adults.

Furthermore, it represents the fourth most frequent cause of pediatric renal transplantation in the USA[12], while recent data from the Italian registry on chronic renal insufficiency in children (ITALKID) indicate that males with primary VUR are the predominant group of patients with renal insufficiency at age 1–15 years[13]. The difficulties of detection depend above all on the fact that *in utero* VUR is a condition frequently associated with less severe degrees of dilatation; moreover, the postnatal sonogram is of no practical value in determining whether primary VUR is present or not: its value lies in excluding urinary tract obstruction[14].

VCUG is the gold standard for the postnatal detection of VUR. However, VCUG should not be used routinely in all patients with persistent pyelectasis, because the procedure is expensive and exposes babies to radiation and occasionally induces urinary tract infection via catheterization[15].

In the study of Adra and co-workers, approximately two-thirds of fetuses with persistent pyelectasis beyond 28 weeks were found to have pathological urinary features at birth: ureteropelvic junction obstruction (37%) and VUR (3.3%) with a higher incidence of VUR in boys[16]. The majority of these infants were managed conservatively with spontaneous resolution of the renal pathologies in the first several years of life.

The various pathological urinary tract features identified at birth reflect the difficulty in predicting postnatal renal pathologies on the basis of the finding of mild dilatation of the fetal renal pelvis on prenatal ultrasound examination. However, the presence of unilateral versus bilateral pyelectasis may be considered as a potential prognostic indicator of postnatal renal pathological processes[17].

PYELECTASIS AS A MARKER OF CHROMOSOMAL ABNORMALITIES

The association between isolated fetal pyelectasis and Down's syndrome is also controversial. Benacerraf and colleagues[18] included fetal pyelectasis (> 4 mm at 14–20 weeks) in their sonographic scoring system for prenatal detection of chromosomal abnormalities, giving this feature the score of 1. They indicated pyelectasis as a weak marker of chromosomal abnormalities not requiring, as an isolated feature, fetal karyotyping.

Nicolaides and co-workers[19] showed that isolated pyelectasis was associated with a 1.6-fold increase in chromosomal abnormalities over the maternal age-related risk. On the other hand, Corteville and colleagues[20] indicated that the risk for Down's syndrome in fetuses with isolated pyelectasis was only 1 : 340, a risk that does not warrant amniocentesis for assessment of the fetal karyotype. Out of 11 340 fetuses evaluated before birth, 82 (0.72%) showed isolated pyelectasis that was associated with trisomy 21 in three of these 82 fetuses[20].

Wickstrom and colleagues[21] showed that the risk for Down's syndrome in cases of isolated pyelectasis was related to the estimated prevalence of trisomy 21 relative to both maternal age and gestational age. Specifically, the risk for Down's syndrome was increased (beyond the traditional risk of 1 : 250) in women 31 or 32 years old, during weeks 16–20. Furthermore, the risk was increased at all gestational intervals in women 33 years of age or older.

OUR EXPERIENCE

During a period of 5 years, from March 1991 to June 1996, 4048 fetuses from an unselected population of pregnant women underwent sonographic investigation of the genito-urinary tract. These sonograms, as a part of a routine maternal–fetal health-care program, were obtained at 21 and 30 weeks' gestation with a 3.5- or 5.0-MHz sector-array transducer (Acuson, Mountain View, CA). Pyelectasis was defined as a pelvic fluid-filled space with anteroposterior diameter of ≥ 4 mm and < 10 mm, without involvement of calyces. When pyelectasis was identified, a detailed evaluation of bilateral fetal kidneys was undertaken and all the patients had two or more examinations until term.

Of fetuses evaluated in our center during the study period, 58 (1.43%) were found to have pyelectasis on prenatal sonographic examination at 21 weeks' gestation, as an isolated ultrasonographic finding. In 23 cases the pyelectasis was unilateral, whereas in the remaining 35 cases the dilatation was bilateral, for a total of 93 fetal kidneys involved. The size of dilatation and the number of dilated pelves was found to be similar in the right and left kidneys. Of the 58 patients in the present study, 42 were male and 16 female, yelding a male to female predilection of 2.5 : 1.

According to the laterality of the prenatal sonographic findings, we found after birth in case of a unilateral lesion: two cases of ureteropelvic junction obstruction, both treated with pyeloplasty; a case of urinary tract infection and 11 spontaneous resolutions in a variable period of time. In case of bilateral prenatal lesions, we found after birth: one non-obstructive ureter, three urinary tract infections, 30 cases of spontaneous resolution (of which only one required about 2 years), a case of Down's syndrome (associated *in utero* with an increased thickness of the nuchal fold) and no cases of mechanical obstruction requiring surgical repair (Table 2). In all cases, either unilateral or bilateral, in which the renal pelvis was ≤ 4 mm there was no urological problem after birth.

For pelvic dilatation ranging between 5 and 6 mm in case of increasing size during pregnancy, we found three cases of persistent urinary tract infection (VCUG negative in all of them) and one case of non-obstructive megaureter that measured 10 mm before

Table 2 *Outcome of cases of prenatally detected pyelectasis according to the laterality of the findings*

Laterality	No. of cases	Outcome
Unilateral pyelectasis	23	
	left kidney	1 urinary infection 1 UPJ obstruction – surgery 11 spontaneous resolutions
	right kidney	1 UPJ obstruction – surgery 9 spontaneous resolutions
Bilateral pyelectasis	35	3 urinary infections 1 non-obstructive megaureter 1 slow resolution (2 years of life) 1 Down's syndrome 29 spontaneous resolutions

UPJ, ureteropelvic junction

Table 3 *Outcome of cases of prenatally detected pyelectasis according to the dilatation found at 21 weeks*

Laterality	Dilatation of 4 mm		Dilatation of 5–6 mm		Dilatation of 7–9 mm	
Unilateral (23 cases)	11	all negative	10	1 urinary tract infection 9 spontaneous resolutions	2	2 UPJ obstruction – surgery
Bilateral (70 kidneys; 35 cases)	36	all negative	27	1 non-obstructive megaureter 2 urinary tract infections 1 slow resolution (2 years) 1 Down's syndrome 22 spontaneous resolutions	7	1 hypospadias 6 spontaneous resolutions

UPJ, ureteropelvic junction

birth. The remaining cases, which showed stable or reducing measurements before birth, resolved spontaneously in a period of time varying between 2 months and 3 years of life. These included a case of Down's syndrome.

In case of pelvic dilatation of 7 mm or more, we had two cases of hydronephrosis due to ureteropelvic junction obstruction with rapid increase during pregnancy, a case of associated hypospadias and six spontaneous resolutions in a period of time lasting from 6 months to 2 years of life (Table 3).

Table 4 shows the intrauterine evolution of fetal pyelectasis detected at 21 weeks' gestation. Only in case of ureteropelvic junction obstruction was a significant worsening *in utero* observed, associated in both cases with an increasing involvement of calyces.

Our data suggested that:

(1) Isolated fetal pyelectasis of 4 mm or less, detected within 20–22 weeks, should be considered 'physiological'. In fact, 62% of such dilatations resolved *in utero*; although 28% of these cases showed a worsening during the rest of pregnancy, none of them has reached 10 mm in width at term, and neither have they been associated with calycectasy. None of these infants showed urological pathology after birth, with the exception of a baby who developed a urinary tract infection in the presence of a contralateral greater pelvic dilatation.

(2) A dilatation of 5 mm should be kept under observation. Of these cases, 36% showed a regression *in utero* whereas 27% resulted in worsening of the dilatation; among these cases one developed a non-obstructive megaureter.

Table 4 Sonographic evolution of the cases of fetal pyelectasis complicated by renal pathologies

Case no.	Duration of follow-up (years)	21 weeks		30 weeks		Before delivery		Outcome
		Right (mm)	Left (mm)	Right (mm)	Left (mm)	Right (mm)	Left (mm)	
1	1	–	6	4	7	11	13	UTI (1 month); VCUG negative; resolution
2	5	4	5	7	7	7	10	left non-obstructive megaureter; scintigraphy negative
3	6	5	5	8	8	normal	normal	UTI (1 year); VCUG negative; resolution
4	3	4	5	4	11	11	12	UTI; VCUG negative; resolution
5	6	5	5	9	5	14	7	18 mm after birth; VCUG negative; resolution (2 years)
6	5	5	6	3	3	3	4	Down's syndrome
7	2	7	–	12	–	17	–	UPJ obstruction; surgery (1 year)
8	6	–	8	–	15	–	28	UPJ obstruction; surgery (18 months)
9	5	7	4	9	3	9	3	hypospadias

UTI, urinary tract infection; VCUG, voiding cystourethrography; UPJ, ureteropelvic junction

(3) The vast majority of babies with a prenatal pelvic dilatation of 6 mm required postnatal investigation; nevertheless, no pathological cases were detected in this group. Only 21% of fetuses had a complete resolution of the sonographic finding during pregnancy.

(4) A value of 7 mm or more should be considered 'on guard'. Among the fetuses of this group, 67% showed a worsening of the dilatation *in utero* and two developed a ureteropelvic junction obstruction.

(5) Such classification is valid also for the examination at 30 weeks' gestation, since five out of the six calyceal dilatations detected at that time were in the group showing an early dilatation of 6 mm or greater.

(6) Furthermore, other critical prognostic factors in the evaluation of a pelvic dilatation are the unilaterality (all cases of obstruction and megaureter were unilateral) and the sonographic finding of calycectasy at 30 weeks' gestation.

(7) The absence of VUR in our study group may have depended on the highly selected nature of the cases (only mild pyelectasis without calycectasy). In fact, this type of dilatation unfavorably correlates with the sonographic feature of massive VUR, while a mild to moderate reflux has a high rate of spontaneous resolution *in utero*. Therefore, VUR could not have been highlighted during our postnatal investigations.

(8) Minimal isolated pyelectasis (4 mm within 21 weeks) should be considered a sonographic feature of morphological evolution depending on functional maturation. Such maturation will occur *in utero* in the vast majority of fetal kidneys. However, in about one-third of cases, the evolution will be completed after birth (even after 2 or 3 years of life) without the evidence of any pathological feature.

Our data suggested that most fetuses with sonographically detected renal pelvis of < 7 mm (isolated pyelectasis without dilated calyces), within 20–22 weeks' gestation, did not have significant postnatal sequelae. However, a sonographic examination at approximately 30 weeks should be recommended in order to differentiate the cases that will not require further surveillance (stable dilatation or lack of calyceal involvement) from those that should be followed after birth for an early detection of any urinary tract pathology or until complete regression of the antenatal sonographic anomalous renal findings.

As far as the problem of fetal pyelectasis as a marker of chromosomal aberration is concerned, only one case was present in our study population; although it was associated with nuchal fold thickening, we are not able to draw any conclusion. Review of the literature supports the opinion that isolated pyelectasis without any other abnormal ultrasound finding does not increase the risk for fetal aneuploidy to a degree justifying amniocentesis.

References

1. Grignon A, Filion R, Filiatrault D, *et al.* Urinary tract dilatation *in utero*: classification and clinical application. *Radiology* 1986;160:645-7
2. Homsy YL, Williot P, Danais S. Transitional neonatal hydronephrosis: fact or fantasy? *J Urol* 1986;136:339-41
3. Fernbach SK, Maizels M, Conway JJ. Ultrasound grading of hydronephrosis: introduction to the system used by the Society for Fetal Urology. *Pediatr Radiol* 1993;23:478-80
4. Robinson JN, Tice K, Kolm P, Abuhamad AZ. Effect of maternal hydration on fetal renal pyelectasis. *Obstet Gynecol* 1998;92:137-41
5. Degani S, Leibovitz Z, Shapiro I, *et al.* Fetal pyelectasis in consecutive pregnancies: a possible genetic predisposition. *Ultrasound Obstet Gynecol* 1997;10:19-21
6. Larger B, Simeoni U, Montoya Y, *et al.* Antenatal diagnosis of upper urinary tract dilatation by ultrasound. *Fetal Diagn Ther* 1996;11:191-8
7. Corteville JE, Gray DL, Crane JP. Congenital hydronephrosis: correlation of fetal ultrasonographic findings with infant outcome. *Am J Obstet Gynecol* 1991;165:384-8
8. Mandell J, Blyth BR, Peters CA. Structural genitourinary defects detected *in utero*. *Radiology* 1991;178:193-6
9. Anderson NG, Abbott GD, Mogridge N, *et al.* Vesicoureteric reflux in the newborn: relationship to renal pelvic diameter. *Pediatr Nephrol* 1997;11:610-16
10. Ouzounian JG, Castro MA, Fresquez M, *et al.* Prognostic significance of antenatally detected fetal pyelectasis. *Ultrasound Obstet Gynecol* 1996;7:424-8
11. Persutte WH, Koyle M, Lenke RR, *et al.* Mild pyelectasis ascertained with prenatal ultrasonography is pediatrically significant. *Ultrasound Obstet Gynecol* 1997;10:12-18
12. Kohaut EC, Tejani A. The 1994 annual report of the North American Pediatric Renal Transplantation Cooperative Study. *Pediatr Nephrol* 1996;10:422-34
13. Ardissino GL, Bonaudo R, Daccò V for the Italian Registry of Childhood Chronic Renal Insufficiency in Conservative Treatment. *Pediatr Nephrol* 1995;9:abstr C69
14. Clauntice-Engle T, Anderson NG, Allan RB, *et al.* Diagnosis of obstructive hydronephrosis in infants: comparison sonograms performed 6 days and 6 weeks after birth. *Am J Roentgenol* 1995;164:963-7
15. Assael BM, Guez S, Marra G, *et al.* Congenital reflux nephropathy: a follow up of 108 cases diagnosed perinatally. *Br J Urol* 1998;82:252-7
16. Adra AM, Mejides AA, Dennaoui MS, *et al.* Fetal pyelectasis: is it always 'physiologic'? *Am J Obstet Gynecol* 1995;173:1263-6
17. Wilson RD, Lynch S, Lessoway VA. Fetal pyelectasis: comparison of postnatal renal pathology with unilateral and bilateral pyelectasis. *Prenat Diagn* 1997;17:451-5
18. Benacerraf BR, Nadel A, Bromley B. Identification of second-trimester fetuses with autosomal trisomy by use of a sonographic scoring index. *Radiology* 1994;193:135-40
19. Nicolaides KH, Shawwa L, Brizot M, *et al.* Ultrasonographically detectable markers of fetal chromosomal defects. *Ultrasound Obstet Gynecol* 1993;3:56-69
20. Corteville JE, Gray DL, Crane JP. Fetal pyelectasis and Down syndrome: is genetic amniocentesis warranted? *Obstet Gynecol* 1992;79:770-2
21. Wickstrom E, Maizels M, Sabbagha RE, *et al.* Isolated fetal pyelectasis: assessment of risk for postnatal uropathy and Down syndrome. *Ultrasound Obstet Gynecol* 1996;8:236-40

Ultrasonographic morphological assessment of the umbilical cord

10

V. D'Addario and E. Di Naro

INTRODUCTION

Currently, the ultrasonographic assessment of the umbilical cord during pregnancy is usually limited to the investigation of Doppler flow velocimetry of the umbilical vessels and to the evaluation of vessel number. There have been only a few pathological studies and case reports concerning whether there is a correlation between prenatal morphometry of the umbilical cord (i.e. umbilical cord diameter or area) and perinatal outcome or duration of pregnancy. Little is known about the amount of Wharton's jelly and its role in several conditions during pregnancy (e.g. pre-eclampsia, dysmaturity, intrauterine growth restriction (IUGR), fetal distress and perinatal mortality)[1,2].

It has been demonstrated by computerized microscope morphometry that the amount of Wharton's jelly at birth is lower in cases of fetuses with IUGR than in normal newborns[3], and Weissman and Jakobi showed that the umbilical cord in cases of diabetic patients was larger than in uncomplicated pregnancies[4]. Silver and colleagues reported that, in post-term pregnancies, antepartum variable decelerations were more frequent in fetuses with a lower mean umbilical cord diameter, and a 'lean' umbilical cord was frequently associated with a severe reduction of amniotic fluid volume and with fetal distress[5]. In addition, our group recently demonstrated that in cases of 'lean' umbilical cord, the risk for the fetus of being small for gestational age at birth with fetal distress at the time of delivery was increased in comparison to those with normal umbilical cord size[6].

The aim of this chapter is to evaluate the role of the ultrasonic morphological assessment of the umbilical cord in the monitoring of the fetal condition.

ULTRASONOGRAPHIC MEASUREMENT OF THE UMBILICAL CORD

Weissmann and co-workers[7] were the first to establish nomograms of the umbilical cord, vein and artery diameters. Using data from 368 uncomplicated pregnancies, they reported a progressive increase of the cord diameter up to 36 weeks of gestation. The diameter of the cord rises from 0.5 mm at 8–9 weeks' gestation to 17.4 mm at 36 weeks and then remains unchanged until term.

Raio and colleagues[8] recently published the first nomogram for the sonographic assessment of the umbilical cord area (Figure 1) from data generated in 557 patients with uncomplicated pregnancy. They reported an increase of the cross-sectional area and diameter of the umbilical cord up to 32 weeks with a subsequent progressive reduction. The mean cross-sectional area at 10 weeks was 8.11 mm^2; this rose to 187.95 mm^2 at 32 weeks. These modifications of the umbilical cord during pregnancy can be explained by the consideration that there is, towards the end of pregnancy, a documented progressive reduction of the amount of Wharton's jelly. It is possible to hypothesize an active metabolic role for the umbilical cord, as was suggested by Vizza and co-workers[9]. These authors demonstrated that the structure of Wharton's jelly is a communicating system of cavities that could represent a way to store the ground substance of the jelly and might play a fundamental role in the passage through

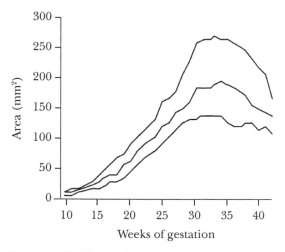

Figure 1 *Umbilical cord area according to gestational age. The curves represent the 10th, 50th and 90th centiles. Reprinted with permission from reference 8*

this structure of water and metabolites from and to the amniotic fluid and umbilical vascular structures. In fact, Weissman and Jakobi found in patients with gestational diabetes that the umbilical cord was larger than in non-diabetic patients. There was a different amount of Wharton's jelly, with an increased content of fluid and plasma proteins within the empty spaces of the Wharton's jelly fibers[4]. Silver and colleagues[5] observed, in post-term pregnancies, a reduction of the cord size and amniotic fluid, due to a different content of water in the amniotic fluid and umbilical cord. This showed a significant correlation with increased peripartum morbidity.

Experimental studies suggest that the amount of Wharton's jelly is also important because it has a contractile function similar to that of smooth muscle cells, with a direct influence on umbilical blood flow[10]; a reduction of the content of Wharton's jelly could therefore be responsible for some cases of fetal growth retardation. This concept has been recently confirmed by Raio and co-workers[6], who reported an association between a 'lean' umbilical cord and small-for-gestational-age infants at birth. It has also been reported that fetuses with IUGR have a total reduction of the umbilical cord area with a cord smaller than normal fetuses, owing to a different amount of jelly and the size of the

umbilical vein not correlated with a pathological umbilical artery Doppler flow[3]. A possible explanation for this observation could be dehydration or a reduction of the extracellular matrix component often present in cases of IUGR.

It is now clear that there is a strong correlation between the amount of Wharton's jelly and fetal growth, with a direct action on the umbilical cord vessel. In conclusion, the ultrasonographic measurement of the cross-sectional area could be considered a fundamental parameter to look for during routine examination; in case of detection of a 'lean' umbilical cord, careful monitoring of the fetal condition is suggested.

DISCORDANT UMBILICAL ARTERIES

Discordant umbilical arteries are one of the umbilical vessel anomalies detectable during a prenatal ultrasound examination. Little is known about the clinical significance of their antenatal detection. Dolkart and co-workers[11] were the first to report cases of discordant umbilical arteries and associated discrepancy in Doppler velocimetry between the two vessels. They reported six cases. Raio and associates[12], in the largest study in this field, reported that morphological placental alterations and anomalous placental insertion of the umbilical cord are often present in cases of discordant umbilical arteries (Table 1). These findings are also common in cases of single umbilical artery (SUA): a high incidence of marginal insertion (18% of cases) and of velamentous insertion (9%) as well as an increased rate of placental anomalies (i.e. chorioangiomas and infarction) are reported[13].

Raio and colleagues[12] noted, in three of their 14 cases, the presence of bipartite and succenturiate placenta and, in agreement with Abuhamad and co-workers[14], they found that the left vessel was often the smaller, thus confirming the analogy with the single artery. Raio and co-workers suggested that, at the origin of the SUA, there is probably a secondary atresia or atrophy of one vessel in a normally developed cord.

Table 1 *Placental and cord characteristics in 14 cases of discordant umbilical arteries. Reprinted with permission from reference 12*

Patient number	Umbilical cord insertion	Placental weight (g)	Placental findings
1	central	200	infarcts
2	velamentous	440	chorangiosis
3	central	500	
4	marginal	400	
5	central	520	
6	central	480	absence of Hyrtl anastomosis
7	eccentric	480	infarcts
8	velamentous	670	
9	marginal	700	
10	eccentric	510	bipartite
11	marginal	700	bipartite
12	central	400	
13	marginal	400	succenturiate
14	central	450	infarcts, chorangiosis

In the current opinion the discordant umbilical arteries are considered to be simply a morphological defect. However, Raio and colleagues demonstrated that there is also a different downstream resistance to blood flow in the two arteries. Such a difference was observed in cases of placental infarction when the infarcted area was supplied by one of the two arteries and in cases of eccentric and marginal umbilical cord insertion frequently associated with the absence of Hyrtl anastomosis.

This absence of interarterial anastomosis between the two umbilical arteries and associated different impedance to flow has also been reported in a case of discordant umbilical arteries[15]. The different blood pressures in the umbilical arteries could be responsible for their secondary atrophy or atresia.

A different downstream resistance to blood flow is also connected with a reduced vascularization of stem villi[15] and with placental abnormalities in the area supplied by the smaller artery.

In conclusion, the clinical significance of discordant umbilical arteries is connected with their association with placental anomalies, responsible for an increased risk of small-for-gestational-age infants, low Apgar score and preterm delivery. Furthermore, the difference in Doppler velocimetry between the two arteries, with a high resistance pattern in the smaller one, should be considered as the expression of a benign condition.

SINGLE UMBILICAL ARTERY

The incidence of SUA is reported to be 0.5–2.5% in uncomplicated neonates, but is higher in aborted (1.5–7%) and aneuploid fetuses (9–11%). Of cases of SUA, 5–11% occur in multiple pregnancies, and multiple gestations have a 3–7-fold increased risk of SUA[16]. Three theories are accepted about the pathogenesis of SUA:

(1) Primary agenesis of one artery;

(2) Secondary atrophy of a previously normal artery;

(3) Persistence of the original allantoic artery of the body stalk.

The second theory seems to be the most reliable.

Ultrasonography has made the prenatal diagnosis of SUA possible, by the recognition of only two vessels in the transverse section of the cord; in the longitudinal section, a loss of the typical helicoidal appearance of the cord can be recognized (Figure 2). Most cases of SUA are diagnosed in the late second trimester. Color Doppler imaging should allow earlier and more confident diagnosis of SUA, but its apparent efficacy has to be confirmed[17]. The sonographic demonstration of the umbilical arteries in the fetal pelvis has been suggested as supportive evidence of SUA. Furthermore, the patent artery is usually larger than normal and it may approximate to the vein diameter[18]. Despite the apparently easy recognition of SUA, a low sensitivity of ultrasound is reported (65%)[19]. In a series of 87 cases of suspected SUA, five false-positive diagnoses were reported[20].

The most important clinical implication of SUA is its possible association with prenatal

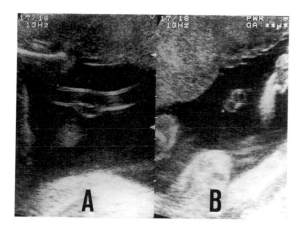

Figure 2 *Single umbilical artery: (A) longitudinal scan; (B) transverse scan*

complications, such as fetal anomalies, aneuploidies, IUGR and placental abnormalities. It has been estimated that the risk of anomalies is seven times greater than in infants with two arteries[13]. The list of anomalies identified as being associated with SUA is long. After an accurate review of the literature, Persutte and Hobbins divided the reported abnormalities into three groups: those believed to be identifiable by prenatal ultrasonography; those believed to be difficult to identify; and those believed to be not identifiable. Using these criteria they concluded that prenatal ultrasonography can consistently identify only 37% of fetal anomalies associated with SUA[21]. This low accuracy becomes an important observation to be kept in mind when counselling a patient with a fetus affected by SUA. The percentage of aneuploidy in fetuses with SUA is reported to be 5–12%[20,22]. However, after reviewing 30 cases of SUA, Nyberg and co-workers[23] showed that 50% (6/12) of fetuses with major congenital anomalies had a fetal aneuploidy. Of the remaining 18 fetuses with either minor or non-identifiable abnormality, none had aneuploidy. Following this observation they concluded that fetal karyotyping should be offered only if concomitant anomalies are seen with prenatal ultrasound. Considering that only 37% of fetal anomalies associated with SUA are prenatally identifiable, however,

is that conclusion acceptable? The answer to this question still remains unclear.

Intrauterine growth restriction complicates 28% of all cases of SUA and 15–20% of cases with associated anomaly[16]. Low birth weight, prematurity, low placental weight and other placental abnormalities are frequently associated with SUA[13] and, together with the associated anomalies, are responsible for the high perinatal mortality rate (mean 20%). It is well known that during fetal development an adaptive mechanism such as dilatation of the umbilical and fetal vessels warrants an adequate blood supply to the fetus, reducing the resistance to blood flow. This mechanism, in case of SUA, could be in part limited and in theory lead to a 'lean' umbilical cord by reducing the amount of Wharton's jelly. In fact the 'lean' umbilical cord is known to be associated with fetal and neonatal death, oligohydramnios, fetal distress and a small-for-gestational-age infant. Raio and colleagues[24] found that, in 22 patients who delivered an infant with only an SUA and without other congenital anomalies, the umbilical artery and vein areas were above 2 standard deviations from the mean in 13 cases (59.1%). The amount of Wharton's jelly was below 2 standard deviations in all cases. This finding suggests that the increased perinatal morbidity and mortality observed in case of SUA, even in the absence of congenital or chromosomal anomalies, could be in part a consequence of the reduced content of Wharton's jelly.

Considering the frequent association of SUA with the previously reported compli-cations, the obstetric management of the fetuses affected by this cord anomaly should be different from routine management. First of all, a careful, detailed ultrasonographic examination, including fetal echocardio-graphy, should be performed to rule out associated anomalies. Fetal karyotyping is indicated when associated anomalies are found; when no associated abnormality can be identified, it is prudent to offer fetal karyo-typing when parents wish it. Serial sonography to assess fetal growth and enhanced fetal monitoring are required. Finally, pediatricians should be alerted in order to search for subtle anomalies by accurate physical examination and non-invasive techniques.

CYSTIC LESIONS OF THE UMBILICAL CORD

Cystic lesions of the umbilical cord are represented by the omphalomesenteric duct cyst and the allantoid cyst. The former is due to persistence and dilatation of a segment of the omphalomesenteric duct; the latter is a cystic dilatation of the allantoid remnant. Both are generally located close to the fetal insertion of the umbilical cord and may vary widely in size. The differentiation between the two types of cyst relies on the different lining epithelium: the omphalo-mesenteric cyst is lined by epithelium of gastrointestinal origin, the allantoid cyst by a flattened or occasionally transitional epithelium.

The prenatal ultrasonographic diagnosis of these cysts has been reported[25]. They appear as a cystic structure of the umbilical cord close to the fetal abdomen (Figure 3). The differential diagnosis between the two

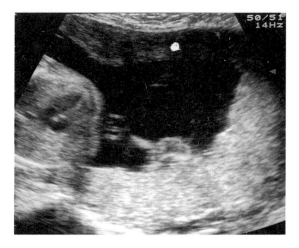

Figure 3 *Cyst of the umbilical cord*

types of cyst is not possible, even though the allantoid cyst is sometimes associated with a dilatation of a patent urachus in the fetal abdomen.

The prognosis is good in both cases; the only theoretical risk is the development of a vascular compression by an expanding cyst.

References

1. Bankowski E, Sobolewski K, Romanowicz L, Chyczewski L, Jawosrski S. Collagen and glycosaminoglycans of Wharton's jelly and their alterations in EPH-gestosis. *Eur J Obstet Gynecol Reprod Biol* 1996;66:109–17
2. Goodlin RC. Fetal dysmaturity, 'lean cord', and fetal distress. *Am J Obstet Gynecol* 1987;156:716
3. Bruch JF, Sibony O, Benali K, Challer C, Blot P, Nessmann C. Computerized microscope morphometry of umbilical vessels from pregnancies with intrauterine growth retardation and abnormal umbilical artery Doppler. *Hum Pathol* 1997;28:1139–45
4. Weissman A, Jakobi P. Sonographic measurements of the umbilical cord in pregnancies complicated by gestational diabetes. *J Ultrasound Med* 1997;16:691–4
5. Silver RK, Dooley SL, Tamura RK, Depp R. Umbilical cord size and amniotic fluid volume in prolonged pregnancy. *Am J Obstet Gynecol* 1987;157:716–20
6. Raio L, Ghezzi F, Di Naro E, Gomez R, Maymon E, Mueller M. Prenatal diagnosis of a 'lean' umbilical cord:an early and simple marker for the fetus at risk for SGA at birth. *Am J Obstet Gynecol* 1998;178:164, abstr. 54
7. Weissman A, Jakobi P, Bronshtein M, Goldstein I. Sonographic measurements of the umbilical cord and vessels during normal pregnancies. *J Ultrasound Med* 1994;13:11–14
8. Raio L, Ghezzi F, Di Naro E, Gomez R, Mueller M, Maymon E, Mazor M. Umbilical cord area and fetal anthropometric parameters. *Am J Obstet Gynecol* 1998;178:164, abstr. 578
9. Vizza E, Correr S, Goranova V, *et al.* The collagen skeleton of the human umbilical cord at term. A scanning electron microscopy study after 2N-NaOH maceration. *Reprod Fertil Dev* 1996;8:885–94
10. Gebrane-Younes J, Minh HN, Orcel L. Ultrastructure of human umbilical vessels: a possible role in amniotic fluid formation? *Placenta* 1986;7:173–85

11. Dolkart LA, Reimers FT, Kuonen CA. Discordant umbilical arteries: ultrasonographic and Doppler analysis. *Obstet Gynecol* 1992;79:59–63

12. Raio L, Ghezzi F, Di Naro E, Gomez R, Saile G, Bruhwiler H. The clinical significance of antenatal detection of discordant umbilical arteries. *Obstet Gynecol* 1998;91:86–91

13. Heifetz SA. Single umbilical artery: a statistical analysis of 237 autopsy cases and review of the literature. *Perspect Pediatr Pathol* 1994;8:345–78

14. Abuhamad AZ, Shaffer W, Mari G, Copel JA, Hobbins JC, Evans AT. Single umbilical artery: does it matter which artery is missing? *Am J Obstet Gynecol* 1995;173:728–32

15. Hitschold T, Braun S, Weiss E, Berle P, Beck T, Muntefering H. A case of discordant flow velocity waveforms in nonanastomosing umbilical arteries: a morphometric analysis. *J Matern Fetal Invest* 1992;2:215–19

16. Leung AKG, Robson WLM. Single umbilical artery. *Am J Dis Child* 1989;143:108–11

17. Jauniaux E, Campbell S, Vyas S. The use of color Doppler imaging for prenatal diagnosis of umbilical cord abnormalities: report of three cases. *Am J Obstet Gynecol* 1989;161:1195–6

18. Persutte WH, Lenke RR. Transverse umbilical arterial diameter: a new technique for the prenatal diagnosis of single umbilical artery. *J Ultrasound Med* 1994;13:763–6

19. Jones TB, Sorokin Y, Bhatia R, Zador I, Bottoms SF. Single umbilical artery: accurate diagnosis? *Am J Obstet Gynecol* 1993;169:358–60

20. Catanzarite VA, Hendricks SK, Maida C, Westbrook C, Cousins L, Schrimmer D. Prenatal diagnosis of the two-vessel cord: implications for patient counselling and obstetric management. *Ultrasound Obstet Gynecol* 1995;5:98–105

21. Persutte WH, Hobbins J. Single umbilical artery: a clinical enigma in modern prenatal diagnosis. *Ultrasound Obstet Gynecol* 1995;6:216–29

22. Saller DN, Keene CL, Sun CY, Schwartz A. The association of single umbilical artery with cytogenetically abnormal pregnancies. *Am J Obstet Gynecol* 1990;163:922–7

23. Nyberg DA, Mahony BS, Luthy D, Kapur R. Single umbilical artery: prenatal detection of concurrent anomalies. *J Ultrasound Med* 1991;10:247–51

24. Raio L, Ghezzi F, Di Naro E, Balestreri D, Ferronato R, Lusher KP. Amount of Wharton's jelly in the umbilical cord with single artery. *Ultrasound Obstet Gynecol* 1998;12(Suppl 1):171

25. Rosemberg JC, Chervenak FA, Walker BA. Antenatal sonographic appearance of omphalomesenteric duct cyst. *J Ultrasound Med* 1986;5:719

Diagnosis and management of fetal tumors 11

C. I. Onyeije and M. Y. Divon

INTRODUCTION

The term fetal tumor is utilized to describe a tumor that arises in the prenatal period. As with neoplastic lesions in the adult, fetal tumors may arise in a wide variety of tissues and hence may present with any of a number of pathophysiological findings.

Fetal tumors are distinctly uncommon, but are often severe entities which present challenging diagnostic and treatment dilemmas when present. Recent advances in prenatal ultrasound imaging have increased the ability to detect and follow the natural history of several fetal tumors.

Timely and accurate detection of fetal tumors is important in order to determine prognosis as well as to determine management options. These tumors can be associated with such complications as hydrops fetalis[1], mechanical obstruction of the birth canal[2] and polyhydramnios[3].

On occasion, when a fetal tumor is suspected on the basis of ultrasound findings, additional diagnostic tests such as biochemical markers, color flow Doppler velocimetry, magnetic resonance imaging (MRI) and computed tomography may be useful. The science of prenatal therapeutic interventions for fetal tumors is in its infancy. This review describes the characteristic findings of fetal tumors. Where applicable, we have commented on the role of ultrasound and additional diagnostic modalities.

We chose to categorize fetal tumors by site of occurrence, similar to the system utilized by Wienk and colleagues[4], who divided the body into three regions: the head and neck, the thorax and the abdomen/pelvis.

FETAL HEAD AND NECK TUMORS

Fetal tumors of the head and neck region may involve the cranial, cervical, or oronaso-pharyngeal regions (Table 1).

Intracranial tumors

Intracranial fetal tumors are often diagnosed on ultrasound scanning during routine sonographic assessment of size/date discrepancy, or in the course of the evaluation of an abnormal maternal serum marker[5]. Although a variety of tumors have been described, intracranial teratomas appear to be the most frequently detected. More than 50% of these tumors are associated with polyhydramnios[6], and hydrocephalus is also frequently noted. In many cases, the growth of an intracranial teratoma is aggressive, and it may completely replace the normal intracranial structures.

A specific diagnosis is impossible with most intracranial tumors until brain biopsy is performed. In the case of sarcomas, lipomas, oligodendromas or craniopharyngiomas, the tumor has been noted to be echogenic on sonography with varying degrees of distortion of intracranial anatomy. Recently, some authors have recommended fetal MRI for evaluation of intracranial tumors in fetuses at risk for the tuberous sclerosis complex (TSC) since the intracranial lesions associated with TSC are generally isoechoic and less visible by ultrasonography[7].

Neuronal migration disorders are often inherited in an autosomal dominant or X-linked manner[8] and are associated with neonatal seizures. We have recently reported

Table 1 *Selected tumors of the fetal head and neck region*

Region	Tumor	Sonographic findings	Associated findings
Intracranial	teratoma	mixed echogenic and transonic multilocular complex structure; varying echodensity	polyhydramnios, hydrocephalus, macrocephaly
	sarcoma	bizarre echogenic and transonic regions with distortion of surrounding structures	hydrocephaly
	lipoma	echogenic mass adjacent to corpus callosum	
	oligodendroma	varying echodensity, both echogenic and transonic	polyhydramnios
	craniopharyngioma	peripherally located transonic areas with distorted fetal brain	polyhydramnios
	heterotopia	supratentorial, isoechoic mass causing marked shift of midline structures	none
Cervical	teratoma	mixed echogenic and transonic multilocular complex structure; varying echodensity	polyhydramnios
	goiter	echoic mass	extension of the fetal head
Oronasopharyngeal	myoblastoma	echogenic mass	
	epignathus	large, oddly shaped mass in facial region demonstrated on sagittal section	polyhydramnios

a case of prenatally diagnosed congenital heterotopia[5] (Figure 1). The ability to diagnose such lesions *in utero* could provide affected parents with additional information regarding fetal involvement.

Cervical tumors

The fetal neck is the site of a number of neoplastic and non-neoplastic conditions which may result in tumors. The differential diagnosis of these tumors is broad and encompasses disorders with markedly different prognostic implications.

Cervical teratomas are composed of tissues from all three germ layers but foreign to the site in which the tumor is located. These tumors are often large and bulky, and may be larger than the size of the fetal head[9]. On ultrasound examination, cervical teratomas are generally unilateral, asymmetric, mobile and well delineated. Polyhydramnios occurs in 20 to 40% of cases, and is more common with larger tumors[10]. An empty stomach may

be the first sonographic evidence of esophageal obstruction due to a cervical teratoma[11]. Generally, cervical teratomas are isolated anomalies; however, cases have been reported in association with trisomy 13[12] and hypoplastic left ventricle[13].

Once detected or suspected, cervical teratomas should prompt serial ultrasound examinations of fetal growth, amniotic fluid volume and fetal well-being[9]. Obstetric complications include preterm labor (due to polyhydramnios) and malpresentation or dystocia due to hyperextension of the fetal head.

Since mortality rates for untreated infants approach 100% regardless of tumor size[14], delivery should be planned in a tertiary center where access to a multidisciplinary team including neonatology and pediatric surgical staff is available[15]. Delayed surgical intervention can result in a number of serious neonatal complications including airway obstruction[13], pneumonia[14] and atelectasis[16]. Some authors have recommended *in utero*

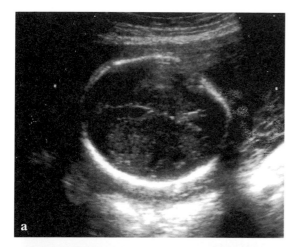

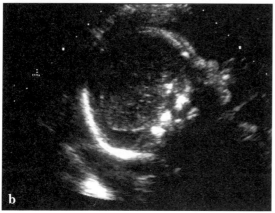

Figure 1 *Prenatal cranial ultrasonography in axial (a) and sagittal (b) views at 23 weeks' gestation. Note isoechoic left hemispheric mass displacing midline structures*

intubation[17] or tracheostomy[18] prior to clamping of the umbilical cord, to facilitate neonatal assessment and preoperative planning. With surgery, the neonatal mortality rates drop to less than 17%[9]. However, parents should be informed that these infants will be most likely to require multiple surgical procedures to complete the removal of the tumor and achieve acceptable cosmetic results.

A fetal goiter is another notable tumor of the fetal cervical region. This tumor is most commonly seen in areas of the world where iodine deficiency is common, and is caused by maternal ingestion of iodide. Although a large goiter may cause hyperextension of the fetal head and preclude vaginal delivery[19], these tumors have been noted to decrease in size (*in utero*) with adequate maternal treatment[20].

Oronasopharyngeal tumors

The most commonly diagnosed tumor of the fetal oronasopharyngeal region is the epignathus (i.e. the nasopharyngeal teratoma)[4]. As with other teratomas, this tumor represents a collection of tissue derived from various germ layers. In this case, the teratoma originates from the fetal facial bones. These tumors may be detected in sagittal section of the fetal head, as they often protrude from the fetal mouth, lip, nose or hard palate. Polyhydramnios is often seen as a consequence of the inability of the fetus to swallow[4].

Myoblastomas are very rare tumors under the control of intrauterine estrogens derived from the fetal ovaries. These tumors, which are found only in females, may arise in a variety of locations; however, the oral cavity is the most common site[21].

TUMORS OF THE FETAL THORACIC REGION

Tumors of the thoracic region may arise in the heart, lungs or mediastinal region.

The heart

Congenital rhabdomyomas are the most common primary cardiac tumor of the fetus, neonate, or young child[4]. When intracardiac tumors are noted in a fetus, the majority of cases will be associated with a family history of TSC[7]. TSC is an autosomal dominant condition in which there is a defect in tumor suppression. As a result, these individuals develop multiple (usually benign) tumors at a variety of locations including the skin, brain, kidneys and heart.

Fetal complications of rhabdomyomas include hydrops fetalis and high-output cardiac failure. Both the tumor and its complications can be diagnosed prenatally with the use of sonography. Since affected mothers will have a 50% risk of transmitting

TSC to their neonates, these mothers should be offered fetal echocardiography to rule out rhabdomyoma[22]. When the tumor is detected, these fetuses should undergo serial evaluations to detect hydrops. Interestingly, most cases of rhabdomyoma noted at birth (without hydrops) can be treated medically and the tumors eventually resolve[23].

The prognosis for TSC at birth includes a 60–70% risk of seizures, and a 50% risk of mental retardation or learning difficulties[7]. Mothers at risk for delivering an infant with TSC should be counselled appropriately by skilled genetic counsellors.

The lungs and mediastinum

There have been no documented cases of true neoplasms originating from the lungs prenatally. On occasion, masses in the fetal lung are detected and these congenital malformations include bronchogenic cysts, extralobular pulmonary sequestration and congenital cystic adenomatoid malformations[24].

Mediastinal tumors in the neonate generally consist of cystic enlargement of the thymus gland anteriorly or neurogenic tumors in the posterior mediastinal regions. Compression of surrounding structures by mediastinal tumors may cause hydrops fetalis, polyhydramnios or hypoplasia of the lungs.

TUMORS OF THE FETAL ABDOMINOPELVIC REGION

Tumors of the abdomen, pelvis and sacrococcygeal area are numerous but uncommon. Owing to the generally poor prognosis of these tumors and their association with obstetric complications, early identification of these tumors can assist in making decisions regarding pregnancy management (i.e., termination of pregnancy) and delivery.

The abdomen

Prenatally detected tumors of the fetal liver are uncommon. The most commonly described tumor of the fetal or neonatal liver is the hemangioendothelioma[25]. Previous descriptions of prenatally described hepatic tumors have concentrated on adverse, and often catastrophic, fetal outcomes. Oligo-hydramnios, growth restriction, preterm labor and intrapartum fetal hepatic rupture have been described in association with liver tumors[26].

Gastric teratomas are rare and have been noted in association with polyhydramnios due to gastrointestinal tract obstruction[27].

The differential diagnosis of tumors of the fetal kidney includes hydronephrosis, multicystic kidneys, polycystic kidneys, Wilms' tumor (nephroblastoma) and renal hamartomas. When a tumor with solid and cystic components is noted by ultrasound, the focus of diagnostic possibilities shifts from predominantly cystic lesions to Wilms' tumor or renal hamartomas. Descriptions of these masses may be found in the literature[2]. As with many other fetal tumors, definitive diagnosis may not be possible until biopsy is performed after birth.

Sacrococcygeal tumors

The sacrococcygeal region is the most common location for a teratoma in the fetus and newborn[4]. The appearance of these tumors on prenatal ultrasound examination is one of a solid and cystic lesion with varying echodensity. These tumors may become quite large and result in dystocia, or abnormal presentation.

Prenatal aspiration of cystic components of sacrococcygeal teratomas in order to avoid soft tissue dystocia has been described by Mintz and colleagues[28]. Assessment of maternal serum α-fetoprotein may assist in the differentiation of these lesions from meningomyeolocele.

OTHER TUMORS

Chorioangiomas of the placenta are highly vascular, benign lesions composed of blood vessels and connective tissue which arise from the chorion. Sonographically these lesions appear as well circumscribed, complex masses which often protrude into the amniotic cavity. As a result of arteriovenous shunt mechanisms, these pregnancies are often complicated by fetal cardiac enlargement, congestive heart failure, hydrops, polyhydramnios and low birth weight[29]. Preterm labor often ensues, owing to polyhydramnios; therefore, recent reports have proposed serial amnioreduction to lower this risk[30].

CONCLUSION

Fetal tumors are uncommonly encountered events with serious implications for maternal and fetal well-being. Because of the heterogeneous nature of these events, an individualized approach is important in developing a management plan for any given pregnancy. Serial ultrasonographic assessment appears to be the best means of determining the risk of obstetric complications and route of delivery. When a tumor is detected, genetic and pediatric surgical consultation may be helpful prior to delivery, in order to provide patients with adequate information. In addition, termination of pregnancy should be considered when lethal or severe entities are detected early in pregnancy.

References

1. Walton JM, Rubin SZ, Soucy P, *et al.* Fetal tumors associated with hydrops: the role of the pediatric surgeon. *J Pediatr Surg* 1993;28:1151–3
2. Apuzzio JJ, Unwin W, Adhate A, *et al.* Prenatal diagnosis of fetal renal mesoblastic nephroma. *Am J Obstet Gynecol* 1986;154:636–7
3. Fung TY, Fung YM, Ng PC, *et al.* Polyhydramnios and hypercalcemia associated with congenital mesoblastic nephroma: case report and a new appraisal. *Obstet Gynecol* 1995;85:815–17
4. Wienk MA, Geijn HP, Copray FJS, *et al.* Prenatal diagnosis of fetal tumors by ultrasonography. *Obstet Gynecol Surv* 1990;45:639–53
5. Onyeije CI, Sherer DM, Jarosz CJ, *et al.* Prenatal sonographic findings associated with sporadic subcortical heterotopia. *Obstet Gynecol* 1998;91:799–801
6. Lipman SP, Pretorius DH, Rumack CM, *et al.* Fetal intracranial teratoma: US diagnosis of three cases and a review of the literature. *Radiology* 1985;157:491–4
7. Webb DW, Osborne JP. Tuberous sclerosis. *Arch Dis Child* 1995;72:471–4
8. Pellicer A, Cabanas F, Perex-Higueras A, *et al.* Neural migration disorders studied by cerebral ultrasound and colour Doppler flow imaging. *Arch Dis Child* 1995;73:F55–61
9. Garmel SH, Crombleholme TM, Semple JP, *et al.* Prenatal diagnosis and management of fetal tumors. *Semin Perinatol* 1994;18:350–65
10. Langer JC, Tabb T, Thompson P, *et al.* Management of prenatally diagnosed tracheal obstruction: access to the airway *in utero* prior to delivery. *Fetal Diagn Ther* 1992;7:12–16
11. Suita S, Ikeda K, Nakano H, *et al.* Teratoma of the neck in a newborn infant – a case report. *Z Kinderchir* 1982;35:9–11
12. Dische MR, Gardner HA. Mixed teratoid tumors of the liver and neck in trisomy 13. *Am Soc Clin Pathol* 1978;69:631–7
13. Grundy SR, Wesley JR, Klein MD, *et al.* Cervical teratomas in the newborn. *J Pediatr Surg* 1983;18:382–6
14. Hurlbut HJ, Webb HW, Moseley T. Cervical teratoma in infant siblings. *J Pediatr Surg* 1967;2:424–6
15. Zerella JT, Finberg FJ. Obstruction of the neonatal airway from teratomas. *Surg Gynecol Obstet* 1990;170:126–31
16. Gonzalez-Crussi F. *Extragonadal Teratomas, Atlas of Tumor Pathology*, second series, fascicle 18. Bethesda MD: Armed Forces Institute of Pathology, 1982:118–27
17. Kelly MF, Berenholz L, Rizzo KA, *et al.* Approach for oxygenation of the newborn with airway obstruction due to a cervical mass. *Ann Otol Rhinol Larnygol* 1990;99:179–82
18. Levine AB, Alvarez M, Wedgewood J, *et al.* Contemporary management of a potentially lethal fetal anomaly: a successful perinatal approach to epignathus. *Obstet Gynecol* 1990;76:962–6
19. Abuhamad AZ, Fisher DA, Warsof SL, *et al.* Antenatal diagnosis and treatment of fetal goiterous hypothyroidism: case report and review of the literature. *Ultrasound Obstet Gynecol* 1995;6:368–71
20. Weiner S, Scharf JI, Bolognese RJ, *et al.* Antenatal

diagnosis and treatment of a fetal goiter. *J Reprod Med* 1980;24:39–42

21. Gergely RZ, Eden R, Schifrin BS, *et al.* Antenatal diagnosis of congenital sacral teratoma. *J Reprod Med* 1980;24:229–31

22. Holley DG, Martin GR, Brenner JI, *et al.* Diagnosis and management of fetal cardiac tumors: a multicenter experience and review of published reports. *J Am Coll Cardiol* 1995;26:516–20

23. Smythe JF, Dyck JD, Smallhorn JF, *et al.* Natural history of cardiac rhabdomyomas in infancy and childhood. *Am J Cardiol* 1990;66:1247–9

24. Mayden KL, Tortora M, Chevernak FA. The antenatal sonographic detection of lung masses. *Am J Obstet Gynecol* 1984;148:349–51

25. Foucar E, Williamson RA, Yiu-Chiu V, *et al.* Mesenchymal hamartoma of the liver identified by fetal sonography. *Am J Radiol* 1983;140:970–2

26. Van de Bor M, Verwey RA, van Pel R. Acute polyhydramnios associated with fetal hepatoblastoma. *Eur J Obstet Gynecol Reprod Biol* 1985; 20:65–9

27. Esposito G, Cigliano B, Paludetto R. Abdominothoracic gastric teratoma in a female newborn infant. *J Pediatr Surg* 1983;18:304–5

28. Mintz MC, Mennuti M, Fishman M. Prenatal aspiration of sacrococcygeal teratoma. *Am J Roentgenol* 1983;141:367–8

29. Hadi HA, Finley J, Strickland D. Placental chorioangioma: prenatal diagnosis and clinical significance. *Am J Perinatol* 1993;10:146–9

30. Guzman ER, Vintzileos A, Benito C, *et al.* Effects of therapeutic amniocentesis on uterine and umbilical artery velocimetry in cases of severe symptomatic polyhydramnios. *J Matern Fetal Med* 1996;5:299–304

Fetal pulmonary arterial and venous flow velocity waveforms during the second half of pregnancy

12

J. W. Wladimiroff and J. A. M. Laudy

Owing to recent improvement in color-coded Doppler techniques and the introduction of power angiography it has now become possible to study lung flow during fetal life. It should be emphasized that flow velocity waveforms rather than volume flow is the subject of current Doppler investigations, putting restrictions on the interpretation of Doppler hemodynamic data during normal and abnormal lung development. An additional limitation is the lack of pressure measurements inherent to non-invasive Doppler techniques. Nevertheless, a number of centers have reported on flow velocity waveform characteristics, providing us for the first time with relevant information on arterial and venous pulmonary flow velocity characteristics during the second half of gestation.

As obstetricians we would consider the availability of an accurate prenatal test for detecting pulmonary hypoplasia as highly desirable. Fetal two-dimensional biometric indices have been shown to have a sensitivity and specificity that are insufficient for clinical management. Recent reports have indicated the possible value of fetal lung volume measurements using echo-planar magnetic resonance[1] or three-dimensional ultrasonography[2-4] in predicting lung hypoplasia. The latter technique, although having a high patient acceptability, provides only indirect determinations of lung volume, which are calculated by subtracting the fetal heart volume from the fetal thoracic volume. Fetal lung volume demonstrates a close association with gestational age[2-4]. In a recent study from our own center, an approximately seven-fold rise in fetal lung volume during the second half of pregnancy was established[4].

THE NORMAL FETAL LUNG CIRCULATION

Intrapulmonary arteries and veins connect to the developing main pulmonary artery and proximal pulmonary vein at 32–50 days of gestation. The definite branching pattern of the major intrapulmonary arteries is achieved by 16 weeks of gestation[5]. This is followed by a massive rise in small intrapulmonary arteries during the remainder of pregnancy[6]. Growth of the pulmonary veins coincides with growth of the pulmonary arteries[7]. The pulmonary circulation represents a high-resistance, high-pressure, low-flow system *in utero*. Regulation of fetal pulmonary flow depends on the high resistance of the pulmonary vasculature[5]. The marked increase in small intrapulmonary arteries is parallelled by an increase in the cross-sectional area of the pulmonary arterial bed, producing a lower total resistance, as well as an increase in total amount of vascular wall muscular tissue, providing a more widespread mechanism for controlling resistance[5,6,8].

PULMONARY ARTERY FLOW VELOCITY WAVEFORMS

Most Doppler studies of the human fetal pulmonary circulation have been performed in the proximal branch pulmonary arteries[9-13]. Agreement exists regarding the nature of the systolic component of the proximal branch pulmonary artery waveform, which is characterized by a rapid initial flow acceleration

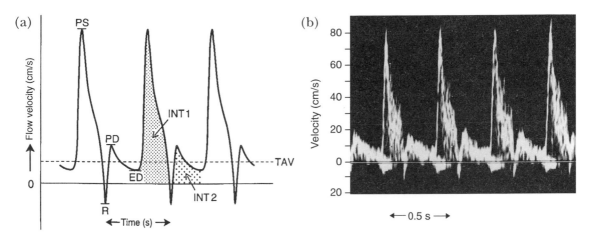

Figure 1 *(a) Schematic presentation of three Doppler flow velocity waveforms from the branch pulmonary artery. INT1, systolic integral; INT2, diastolic integral; PS, peak systolic; PD, peak diastolic; ED, end-diastolic; TAV, time-averaged velocity; R, reverse. (b) Doppler ultrasound recording of four consecutive left branch pulmonary artery velocity waveforms at 34 weeks of gestation. Reproduced with permission from reference 10*

phase followed by an equally rapid deceleration phase (Figure 1). Opinions differ regarding the end-diastolic component, which has been reported as forward flow being absent[5], present[10,11,13], or a combination of present and absent[9]. Moreover, discrepancies are reported on the gestational age-dependency of peak systolic velocities, which vary from significant increase[9,13] to gestational age independency[10,11]. Also, in the proximal branch pulmonary artery, the pulsatility index as well as the resistance index[12] have been described as remaining constant[5,10,11] or as depicting a gestational age-related decrease[9,13]. We believe that sample site and equipment-related differences alone do not explain these discrepancies. However, a standardization of recording techniques would be a helpful first step.

More problematic is our understanding of the possible underlying mechanisms responsible for the arterial waveform pattern described earlier. Several factors, such as vascular pressure, resistance, impedance, vessel compliance and ventricular contractility may play a role[5]. This creates a problem regarding the accurate hemodynamic interpretation of separate Doppler indices in the fetal pulmonary circulation. We have questioned the significance of the pulsatility index as a measure of downstream impedance in fetal pulmonary hemodynamics[10]. Measurement of peak diastolic velocity and diastolic integral rather than the pulsatility index has been suggested by us as being more useful in detecting gestational age-related changes in fetal pulmonary vascular resistance[10]. Several studies have appeared on peripheral arterial lung flow velocity patterns[9,13,14]. Also here, methodological differences appear to be at the root of discrepancies in waveform description. Rasanen and colleagues[9] examined the fetal distal branch pulmonary arterial vascular impedance and analyzed the relationships between proximal (after the bifurcation of the main pulmonary artery) and distal (beyond the first bifurcation of the branch pulmonary artery) pulmonary arterial blood velocity waveforms. Data in the studies by Mitchell and colleagues[12] were collected in the midportion of the fetal lung and by Rizzo and colleagues[14] and Laudy and colleagues (unpublished data) in the most distal area of the fetal lung. Nevertheless, Rasanen and co-workers[9] and Laudy and co-workers (unpublished data) observed a significant change in pulsatility index (or resistance index) with advancing gestational age. Again, standardization of defining measurement techniques should be persued.

(a) 21 weeks (b) 32 weeks

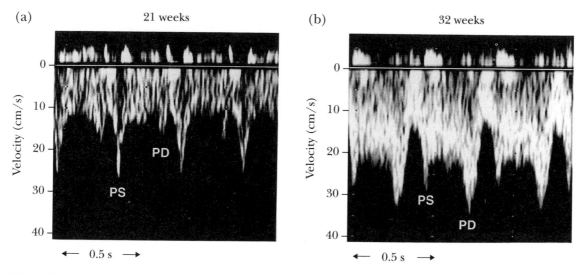

Figure 2 *Pulmonary venous flow velocity waveform, consisting of biphasic forward components, with examples at 21 weeks (a) and 32 weeks (b) of gestation. Note the higher peak diastolic (PD) velocity at 32 weeks in relation to the peak systolic (PS) velocity. Reproduced with permission from reference 16*

PULMONARY VENOUS FLOW VELOCITY WAVEFORMS

Fetal pulmonary venous blood flow was first identified by color-coded Doppler[15]. The pulmonary venous blood flow velocity waveform just proximal to the entrance into the left atrium shows a pulsatile forward flow velocity pattern[16] (Figure 2), equal to that established postnatally in sheep and humans[17,18]. In the adult, the pulmonary venous flow velocity waveform mirrors the atrial pressure wave, resulting in an almost exact correspondence between the pulmonary venous velocity waveform and the inverse of the left atrial pressure waveform[17]. If we assume a similar relationship in the human fetus, then the systolic component of the pulmonary venous flow velocity waveform coincides with a drop in atrial pressure, whilst the diastolic component coincides with rapid emptying of the left atrium during ventricular relaxation. This would suggest that pulmonary venous blood flow is determined by suction of blood from the pulmonary veins into the left atrium and left ventricle[18]. A 1.5–2.5-fold increase has been shown for the systolic and diastolic component of the pulmonary venous flow velocity waveform during the second half of pregnancy[16]. Increase in volume flow and a rise in pressure gradient between the pulmonary venous system and the left atrium may play a role[19]. The S/D ratio shows a decline which is determined by the more pronounced rise in peak diastolic velocity relative to peak systolic velocity[16]. This may suggest a further reduction in atrial pressure after the rapid filling wave across the mitral valve during diastole with advancing gestational age.

LUNG HYPOPLASIA

Here, we should raise the question as to the validity of fetal pulmonary artery Doppler velocimetry in the prediction of pulmonary hypoplasia. Can hemodynamic changes be expected in the presence of lung hypoplasia? If so, will hemodynamic changes be reflected in pulmonary artery Doppler flow velocity waveform recordings, in the presence of pulmonary hypoplasia? The answer regarding the first part of the question should be positive. Several postmortem studies have demonstrated increased pulmonary vascular muscularization in hypoplastic lungs[20,21]. This may result in raised pulmonary vascular

(a)   Normal

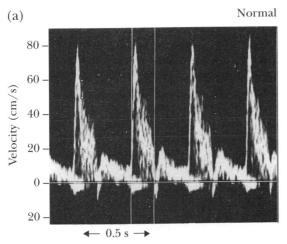

← 0.5 s →

(b)   Pulmonary hypoplasia

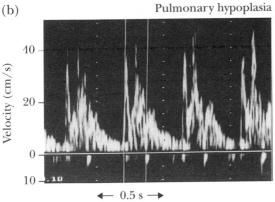

← 0.5 s →

Figure 3 *Doppler flow velocity waveforms from the left branch of the fetal pulmonary artery in a normally developing fetus (a) and a fetus with lung hypoplasia (b) at 34 weeks of gestation. Note the difference in velocity scale (cm/s) used in both figures. Reproduced with permission from reference 22*

resistance and reduced pulmonary arterial compliance. To answer the second part of the question, hemodynamic changes in the pulmonary vascular bed should have a bearing on pulmonary blood flow and may, therefore, result in changes in pulmonary artery Doppler flow velocity waveforms. So far, only a few papers have dealt with this issue[12,22,23], in every case representing lung hypoplasia associated with lethal renal pathology or diaphragmatic hernia rather than the more common pathological state of premature rupture of the membranes. We observed a significant reduction in

pulmonary artery systolic and diastolic velocities (Figure 3). A decreased total size of the pulmonary vascular bed, reduced to vessel count per unit of lung tissue and increased pulmonary vascular muscularization was established in lung hypoplasia at postmortem examination. Reduced volume flow and/or raised downstream impedance may have been responsible for these Doppler velocity changes. The presence of raised downstream impedance is further supported by marked changes in the shape of the pulmonary arterial waveform, characterized by a second needle-shaped peak occurring during mid-systole, even higher than the first systolic peak[22]. Mitchell and co-workers[12], studying peripheral pulmonary arteries, observed a high resistance pattern quite different from that of normal fetuses. In the third report, a significant reduction in pulsatility index was found[23]. It should be realized that so far we are dealing with merely anecdotal data; larger series are needed to obtain a more realistic view as to the clinical significance of Doppler velocimetry in the detection of lethal lung hypoplasia. In further studies attention should be focused on severe oligohydramnios due to premature rupture of the membranes as to the most common cause of pulmonary hypoplasia. Serial Doppler recordings should be performed to pick up any initial change in Doppler indices. Detailed clinical or postmortem examination should confirm or refute the diagnosis of pulmonary hypoplasia after birth.

CONCLUSIONS

Normal proximal pulmonary artery and venous waveforms depict characteristic flow patterns which may change with gestational age. The underlying mechanisms responsible for these waveforms still need to be elucidated, particularly for the arterial waveforms. Abnormal Doppler flow velocity waveforms have been documented in the presence of lung hypoplasia. However, data so far are anecdotal; prospective serial studies are needed.

References

1. Baker PN, Johnson IR, Gowland PA, Freeman A, Adams V, Mansfield P. Estimation of fetal lung volume using echoplanar magnetic resonance imaging. *Obstet Gynecol* 1994;83:961–4

2. D'Arcy TJ, Hughes SW, Chiu WSC, *et al.* Estimation of fetal lung volume using enhanced 3-dimensional ultrasound: a new method and first result. *Br J Obstet Gynaecol* 1996;103:1015–20

3. Lee A, Kratochwil A, Stümpflen L, Deutinger J, Bernaschek G. Fetal lung volume determination by three-dimensional ultrasonography. *Am J Obstet Gynecol* 1996;175:588–92

4. Laudy JAM, Janssen MMM, Struijk PC, Stijnen T, Wladimiroff JW. Three-dimensional ultrasonography of normal fetal lung volume: a preliminary study. *Ultrasound Obstet Gynecol* 1998;11:13–16

5. Emerson DS, Cartier MS. The fetal pulmonary circulation. In Copel JA, Reed KL, eds. *Doppler Ultrasound in Obstetrics and Gynecology.* New York: Raven Press, 1995:307–23

6. Levin D, Rudolph A, Heymann M, Phibbs R. Morphological development of the pulmonary vascular bed in fetal lambs. *Circulation* 1976;53:144–51

7. Hislop A, Reid L. Fetal and childhood development of intrapulmonary veins in man: branching pattern and structure. *Thorax* 1973;28:313–19

8. Morin FC, Egan EA. Pulmonary hemodynamics in fetal lambs during development at normal and increased oxygen tension. *J Appl Physiol* 1992;21:163–84

9. Rasanen J, Huhta JC, Weiner S, Wood DC, Ludomirski A. Fetal branch pulmonary arterial vascular impedance during the second half of pregnancy. *Am J Obstet Gynecol* 1996;174:1441–9

10. Laudy JAM, De Ridder MAJ, Wladimiroff JW. Doppler velocimetry in branch pulmonary arteries of normal human fetuses during the second half of gestation. *Pediatr Res* 1997;41:897–901

11. Stanley JR, Veille JC, Zaccaro D. Description of right pulmonary artery blood flow by Doppler echocardiography in the normal human fetus 17 to 40 weeks gestation. *J Matern Fetal Invest* 1994;4:S14

12. Mitchell JH, Roberts AB, Lee A. Doppler waveforms from the pulmonary arterial system in normal fetuses and those with pulmonary hypoplasia. *Ultrasound Obstet Gynecol* 1998;11:167–72

13. Chaoui R, Taddei F, Rizzo G, Bast C, Lenz F, Bollmann R. Doppler echocardiography of the main stems of the pulmonary arteries in the normal human fetus. *Ultrasound Obstet Gynecol* 1998;11:173–9

14. Rizzo G, Capponi A, Chaoui R, Taddei F, Arduini D, Romanini C. Blood flow velocity waveforms from peripheral pulmonary arteries in normally grown and growth-retarded fetuses. *Ultrasound Obstet Gynecol* 1996;8:87–92

15. Caruso G, Serio R, Pece A, Botticella A, De Luca I. Anomalies of the venous flow during fetal life. Presented at the *4th Bilthoven Symposium of the European Society of Cardiology.* Bilthoven, December 1994:18

16. Laudy JAM, Huisman TWA, De Ridder MAJ, Wladimiroff JW. Normal fetal pulmonary venous blood flow velocity. *Ultrasound Obstet Gynecol* 1995;6:277–81

17. Ramjagopalan B, Friend JA, Stallard T, Lee G. Blood flow in pulmonary veins: I Studies in dog and man. *Cardiovasc Res* 1979;13:667–76

18. Keren G, Sherez J, Megidish R, Levitt B, Laniado S. Pulmonary venous flow pattern – its relationship to cardiac dynamics. A pulsed Doppler echocardiographic study. *Circulation* 1985;71:1105–12

19. Levin DL, Rudolph AM, Heymann MA, Phibbs RH. Morphological development of the pulmonary vascular bed in fetal lambs. *Circulation* 1976;53:144–51

20. Barth PJ, Rüschoff J. Morphometric study on pulmonary arterial thickness in pulmonary hypoplasia. *Pediatr Pathol* 1992;12:653–63

21. Levin DL. Morphologic analysis of the pulmonary vascular bed in congenital left sided diaphragmatic hernia. *J Pediatr* 1978;92:805–9

22. Laudy JAM, Gaillard JLJ, Van den Anker JN, Tibboel D, Wladimiroff JW. Doppler ultrasound imaging: a new technique to detect lung hypoplasia before birth? *Ultrasound Obstet Gynecol* 1996;7:189–92

23. Twining P. The value of fetal pulmonary artery flow as a predictor of pulmonary hypoplasia in congenital diaphragmatic hernia. *Ultrasound Med Biol* 1997;23:S106

Intrauterine growth restriction and fetal cerebral circulation

13

G. Clerici and G. C. Di Renzo

INTRODUCTION

Intrauterine growth restriction (IUGR) is a common symptom of many possible maternal–fetal conditions and/or the expression of a genetic alteration; the most common etiology is related to chronic fetal hypoxemia. Sonography and, particularly, Doppler ultrasound technologies can help the obstetrician in the evaluation of fetal well-being, by studying fetal hemodynamic adaptations to different maternal and fetal pathophysiological conditions, which are correlated with hypoxemia. Fetal hypoxemia may be the result of fetomaternal pathophysiological processes that can produce completely different fetal hemodynamic modifications, not only in relation to the quality but particularly in relation to the chronology of the hemodynamic events. However, fetal hypoxia is mostly due to placental vascular insufficiency and it is important to point out that fetal hypoxemia–acidemia is part of the terminal pathway starting from placental functional and structural alterations, through fetal IUGR and leading to intrauterine fetal death.

PATHOPHYSIOLOGICAL BASIS

Several mechanisms are involved in the beginning of the process that leads the fetus to the hemodynamic changes, from the adaptation to the decompensation, during hypoxemia. These include fetomaternal immunological tolerance alterations; failure of endothelial vasodilator tone control (possibly alterations of the nitric oxide system); reduction of maternal plasma expansion; increased maternal blood viscosity at low shear rate; inappropriate trophoblastic invasions with histological, morphological and functional placental alterations; and others. All these processes are involved in the hemodynamic alterations of both uterine and umbilical arteries which characterize the IUGR fetus[1-7].

When the structural and functional placental alterations appear and/or increase, the fetus adapts itself to this situation with decreased growth, alterations in behavior (i.e. decrease in the episodes of body movements) and hemodynamic changes, in order to maintain the supply of oxygen and substrates for tissues with active metabolism such as the brain, heart and adrenals[8]. Only when the obstruction of placental vessels is over 60% is there a detectable and clear alteration in the umbilical artery velocity waveform profile[7]. Thus, when a particular level of po_2 is reached, there is a redistribution of the fetal blood flow. These hemodynamic modifications, known as the 'brain-sparing effect', which produce a 'fetal hemodynamic centralization', are thought to be protective against hypoxic insult and consist of vasodilatation with an increase of blood flow in the fetal structures that are most sensitive to hypoxemia (such as the brain, adrenals and coronary arteries) and a decrease of blood supply in the peripheral vascular districts such as the pulmonary, intestinal, cutaneous, renal and skeletal vessels[8-16].

These changes in arterial perfusion are mediated by neuronal stimulation, either directly through stimulation of the vagal center or through chemoreceptors in the aorta and in the carotid arteries. If the uteroplacental vascular bed alterations persist, this produces a further increase of the impedance to flow in the umbilical artery and in the fetal aorta and, mainly as a result of the hypoxemia, in the renal artery. Moreover, these factors cause a further increase of the hypoxemic fetal status balanced by a more pronounced fetal blood flow redistribution with lowest impedance to flow values in the cerebral vessels. The centralization of blood flow influences cardiac hemodynamics with a decrease in the left ventricle afterload due to the cerebral vasodilatation and an increase in the right ventricle afterload due to the systemic vasoconstriction. This phase is characterized by the extreme response of the fetus to hypoxemia which leads, after a time, to the decompensatory phase.

The last phase is characterized by the impairment of fetal cardiac function which is unable to balance all the factors mentioned above. Due to the persistent severe hypoxemia and to the consequent polycythemia and increased blood viscosity, there is impairment of fetal cardiac contractility which is the most important factor leading to the terminal decompensatory phase. The impairment of the cardiac function causes a decrease in the cardiac afterload and an increase in the cardiac preload, leading to an increase of the atrioventricular gradient, abnormal ventricular filling with increase of the venous pressure beyond the inferior vena cava, i.e. the hepatic and ductus venosus circulation. Moreover, during this stage, the reduced cardiac output and the high blood viscosity also cause a reduction in cerebral perfusion, leading to the disappearance of the so-called brain-sparing effect. The disappearance of the latter may also be caused by a mechanical mechanism induced by the edema produced by the brain damage of the hypoxic insult[11].

FETAL HEMODYNAMIC ADAPTATION AND ITS CHRONOLOGY

Doppler silent stage

Although instead of considering the processes that lead to the uteroplacental vascular insufficiency are present, the fetal hemodynamic profile might remain 'normal' for even a long period of time. The umbilical artery velocity waveform shows a positive blood flow pattern throughout the cardiac cycle, and the impedance to flow values expressed as pulsatility index (PI) are normal with a non-significant slight increase. Doppler velocimetry of the remaining main fetal vessels and districts (particularly the aorta, renal artery, femoral artery and cerebral vessels) are also normal. Under these 'normal' conditions the mean PI of the middle cerebral arteries is found to be higher than that of either the internal carotid or the anterior cerebral arteries, while that of the posterior cerebral artery is usually found to be lower than that of the middle and anterior cerebral arteries, and higher than that of the umbilical artery. The middle cerebral artery, because of its relatively great dimension and the simplicity of its sampling, has been one of the most investigated cerebral vessels and appears to be one of the most sensitive to initial hypoxemia[9]. In particular, it seems that its subcortical segment (M_2) modifies earlier than the proximal part of the vessel (M_1). The ratio between the flow indices of the two parts of the vessel (M_2/M_1) became lower than two standard deviations in the presence of initial fetal hypoxemia[10].

In conclusion, the alteration in the uteroplacental vascular bed and the alterations in the placental metabolites and gas exchange, in this initial stage, produce only small and non-significant fetal hemodynamic modifications (slight increase of the impedance to flow in the umbilical artery and the fetal peripheral vessels and a slight decrease in the cerebral vessels). The main hemodynamic change that it is possible to detect with Doppler technology is the decrease in the impedance to flow values characterizing the subtcortical segment of the middle cerebral artery (M_2), but this event is of doubtful clinical application.

Early stage of fetal blood flow redistribution

Fetal Doppler velocimetry shows an increase in the impedance to flow values (PI) of the umbilical artery but also of the aorta and the renal artery. The increase of the vascular resistance of the aorta is probably related to different factors such as the increase in vascular impedance in the umbilicoplacental vessels and arterial vasoconstriction of the peripheral vessels due to progressive hypoxemia.

During this phase it is possible to observe some hemodynamic modifications that involve the whole fetal organism. These modifications are related to the substantial redistribution of the cardiac output in the direction of the tissues that are important for fetal life. The inversion of the cerebro-placental ratio, the brain-sparing effect, is the most evident hemodynamic change. At this stage, a statistically significant increase of the blood flow and a decrease of the resistance in all the cerebral vessels examined can be noted. Furthermore, owing to the hemodynamic redistribution, a decrease of the peripheral flow in the umbilical artery, abdominal aorta, renal artery, femoral artery and other vessels can be observed, with high impedance to flow values[8-15].

The ratio between the PI of the middle cerebral artery and the PI of the umbilical artery (cerebroplacental ratio) can be considered as the Doppler flow expression of the brain-sparing effect; the decrease of this ratio below two standard deviations is a sign of the incipient severe hypoxemia and, in its presence, it is possible to observe anomalies of the fetal biophysical profile, reduction of fetal heart rate variability and reduction of amniotic fluid volume[13] (Figure 1).

During this stage, the PI of the umbilical artery and of the fetal aorta is elevated, but Doppler velocimetry frequency values continue to be positive throughout the cardiac cycle, even in the end-diastolic phase. However, it is possible to find high-velocity frequencies during diastole in all cerebral vessels, suggesting an increase of the fetal cerebral blood flow.

Advanced stage of fetal hemodynamic redistribution

This phase is essentially characterized by a further increase in the impedance to flow in

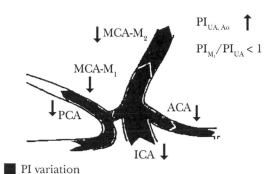

Figure 1 *Fetal blood flow redistribution during hypoxemia due to uteroplacental vascular insufficiency: the 'brain-sparing effect'. PI, pulsatility index; UA, umbilical artery; Ao, fetal aorta; MCA-M$_1$, -M$_2$, segments of the middle cerebral artery; ACA, anterior cerebral artery; PCA, posterior cerebral artery; ICA, internal carotid artery. Modified from reference 11*

the umbilical artery, the fetal aorta and the renal artery. In the umbilical artery flow velocity profile, a decrease of the diastolic frequencies is observed, moving progressively to the absence of diastolic flow. The end-diastolic frequency disappears first, but subsequently the lack of blood flow is evident in the whole of diastole. This occurs, usually, when 80% of villus arterioles are occluded[7]. Aortic velocity waveforms exhibit a similar pattern, with absence of diastolic frequencies, usually preceding that observed in the umbilical artery. At the same time the impedance to flow values in the cerebral vessels shows a further decrease, leading to the lowest PI values in this district, as a result of concurrent maximal vasodilatation of the cerebral vessels[11]. Moreover, during this phase, it is possible to find a relative decrease of the right cardiac output and an increased left cardiac output characterized by increased time to peak velocity in the aorta and by a decrease of the same parameter in the pulmonary arteries, suggesting a preferential shift of cardiac output in favor of the left ventricle, leading to improved perfusion to the brain.

Decompensatory phase

During this phase, the cardiac output and the peak velocity of the main arterial trunks gradually decline and, as a consequence, cardiac filling is impaired, suggesting a progressive deterioration of cardiac function. These factors cause changes that induce hemodynamic alterations in all cardiovascular districts (intracardiac and arteriovenous). The incipient heart failure produces a decreased cardiac output, which causes a decrease in the peak velocity of the outflow tracts, leading to reversed flow in the aorta, in the umbilical artery and, as a terminal sign, in other arteries such as the cerebral vessels[16]. However, during this phase, the increased viscosity of the fetal blood, the decrease of the cardiac output and, probably, the cerebral edema, produce a decrease in brain perfusion, shown by the decrease of blood velocity, especially during diastole. This is thus the disappearance of the brain-sparing effect[11,16] (Figure 2).

At the same time, the impairment of the cardiac contractility causes an increased atrioventricular gradient, abnormal ventricular filling underlined by a decrease in the E/A ratio (E, peak due to ventricular diastole; A, peak due to atrial systole) of the atrioventricular blood flow velocity waveforms. The increased pressure gradient in the right atrium leads, during atrial contractions, to evidence of the reversed flow

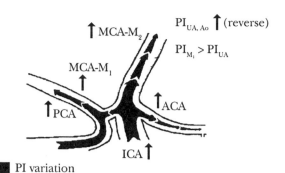

Figure 2 *Fetal cerebral artery velocity waveform profiles during the 'decompensatory phase'. PI, pulsatility index; UA, umbilical artery; Ao, fetal aorta; MCA-M$_1$, -M$_2$, segments of the middle cerebral artery; ACA, anterior cerebral artery; PCA, posterior cerebral artery; ICA, internal carotid artery. Modified from reference 11*

in the ductus venosus and to a high percentage of abnormal reversed flow in the inferior vena cava. The next step is the extension of the abnormal reversal of blood flow from the inferior vena cava beyond the ductus venosus and the hepatic circulation into the umbilical vein, causing typical end-diastolic pulsations in this vessel. It has been observed that this hemodynamic pattern is associated with the onset of severe fetal heart rate anomalies and with severe acidemia at birth[13].

References

1. Jauniaux E, Jurkovic D, Campbell S, Hustin J. Doppler ultrasonographic features of the developing placental circulation: correlation with anatomic findings. *Am J Obstet Gynecol* 1992;166: 585–7
2. Warwick BG, Trudinger BJ, Baird PJ. Fetal umbilical artery flow velocity waveforms and placental resistance: pathological correlation. *Br J Obstet Gynaecol* 1985;92:31–8
3. Nordenvall M, Ullberg U, Laurin J, Lingman G, Sandstedt B, Ulmsten U. Placental morphology in relation to umbilical artery blood velocity waveforms. *Eur J Obstet Gynecol Reprod Biol* 1991;40: 179–90
4. Trudinger BJ, Warwick BG, Colleen MC. Utero-placental blood flow velocity–time waveforms in normal and complicated pregnancy. *Br J Obstet Gynaecol* 1985;92:39–45
5. Trudinger BJ, Warwick BG, Colleen MC. Flow velocity waveforms in maternal uteroplacental and fetal umbilical placental circulations. *Am J Obstet Gynecol* 1985;152:155–63
6. Trudinger BJ, Warwick BG, Colleen MC, Bombardieri J, Collins L. Fetal umbilical artery flow velocity waveforms and placental resistance: clinical significance. *Br J Obstet Gynaecol* 1985;92: 23–30
7. Trudinger BJ, Stevens D, Connelly A, *et al.* Umbilical artery flow velocity waveforms and placental resistance: the effects of the embolization of the umbilical circulation. *Am J Obstet Gynecol* 1987;157:1443–8

8. Mari G, Deter RL. Middle cerebral artery flow velocity waveforms in normal and small-for-gestational-age fetuses. *Am J Obstet Gynecol* 1992; 166:1262–70

9. Veille JC, Penry M. Effect of maternal administration of 3% carbon dioxide on umbilical artery and fetal renal and middle cerebral artery Doppler waveforms. *Am J Obstet Gynecol* 1992;167:1668–71

10. Luzi G, Coata G, Caserta G, Cosmi EV, Di Renzo GC. Doppler velocimetry of different sections of the fetal umbilcal artery in relation to perinatal outcome. *J Perinat Med* 1996;24:327–34

11. Clerici G, Luzi G, Di Renzo GC. Cerebral circulation from healthy to IUGR and distressed fetus: what happens and how we can explain it? In Kurjak A, Di Renzo GC, eds. *Modern Methods of the Assessment of Fetal and Neonatal Brain.* Rome: CIC International, 1996:36–50

12. Bilardo CM, Snijders RM, Campbell S, Nicolaides KH. Doppler study of fetal circulation during long-term maternal hyperoxygenation for severe early onset intrauterine growth retardation. *Ultrasound Obstet Gynecol* 1991;1:250–7

13. Scherjon SA, Smolders-DeHaas H, Kok JH, Zonderwan HA. The 'brain sparing' effect: antenatal cerebral Doppler findings in relation to neurologic outcome in very preterm infants. *Am J Obstet Gynecol* 1993;169:169–75

14. Weiner Z, Farmakides G, Schulman H, Penny B. Central peripheral hemodynamic changes in fetuses with absent end-diastolic velocity in umbilical artery: correlation with computerized fetal heart rate pattern. *Am J Obstet Gynecol* 1994; 170:509–15

15. Van Den Wijngaard JAGW, Groenenberg IAL, Wladimiroff JW, Hop WCJ. Cerebral Doppler ultrasound of the human fetus. *Br J Obstet Gynaecol* 1989;96:845–9

16. Sepulveda W, Shennan AH, Peek MJ. Reverse end-diastolic flow in the middle cerebral artery: an agonal pattern in the human fetus. *Am J Obstet Gynecol* 1996;174:1645–7

Human fetal venous return evaluation: a reappraisal

14

A. Matias, N. Montenegro and J. C. Areias

INTRODUCTION

The introduction of the Doppler ultrasound technique has allowed the non-invasive study of blood flow velocity in the human fetus *in utero*[1,2]. The widespread use of Doppler clinical studies has successfully demonstrated afterload and cardiac contractility in the fetal circulation[3]. More recently, the preload and hemodynamics of the fetal venous compartment have been extensively studied in depth as an indirect tool for assessing cardiac function[4]. During recent years, a step forward in ultrasound technology has enabled researchers to study the venous circulation early in gestation. This is a promising tool to be used in clinical obstetric practice for fetal surveillance[5–7].

THE ANATOMY AND PHYSIOLOGY OF HUMAN FETAL VENOUS RETURN

Developmental anatomy

The presence of three shunts (foramen ovale, ductus arteriosus and ductus venosus) and the placenta are unique to the fetal circulation. Blood flow from the yolk sac is transported in an embryo of 7 weeks of gestation through the hepatic sinusoids via the paired vitelline vessels into the sinus venosus, whereas blood from the chorionic villi bypasses the liver to empty into the sinus via the umbilical veins. The right umbilical vein and the proximal portion of the left umbilical vein degenerate. The rest of the left umbilical vein anastomoses with the hepatic sinusoids to create a new sphincter-like channel, the ductus venosus[8].

The umbilical vein enters the abdomen to follow the inferior edge of the liver. As it approaches the liver hilus, it gives off branches to the left and medial portions of the liver until it finally communicates with the portal sinus.

The ductus venosus is a branchless structure that connects the ventral side of the umbilical sinus to the hepatic veins and inferior vena cava below the atrial inlet. It courses from caudal to cranial, from ventral to dorsal, and slightly oblique to the left side (Color Plate M)[6]. Its outlet, however, has been reported to be more variable, but mostly related to the left and medial hepatic veins[9].

The inferior vena cava (IVC) widens at the level of the confluence, where it receives the right hepatic vein and the ductus venosus shortly before entering the fetal heart (subdiaphragmatic vestibulum)[7]. The Eustachian valve (belonging to the IVC) contributes to this functional unit by forming the right anterior wall of the interatrial tube.

Physiological behavior

The ductus venosus is a blood vessel that functions mostly in fetal life as a regulatory shunt of the umbilical venous flow to the heart. Well-oxygenated blood from the umbilical vein will stream preferentially through the ductus venosus towards the left atrium through the foramen ovale. However, the proportion of the umbilical blood to be shunted through the ductus venosus depends on the umbilicocaval pressure gradient, blood viscosity and cross-sectional area of the inlet of the ductus venosus. Ductus venosus blood flow velocities are the highest venous velocities, because the blood is accelerated towards the heart through a narrow isthmus. The time-averaged flow velocity in the ductus venosus is 2.7 and 3.2 times higher than that in the IVC and umbilical vein, respectively, in early pregnancy[6].

Angiographic studies in fetal sheep and pre-viable human fetuses have demonstrated that the inferior caval blood flow is divided into a high-velocity blood flow to the foramen ovale (left pathway), and a right flow, with lower velocities, directed to the tricuspid valve[10]. During induced hypoxemia, hemorrhage or partial clamping of the cord in animal preparations, the proportion of umbilical blood directed through the ductus venosus increases to secure optimal oxygen delivery to the coronary and cerebral arteries[11].

DOPPLER EVALUATION OF FETAL VENOUS RETURN IN THE FIRST TRIMESTER

The transvaginal Doppler technique allows the characterization of fetal hemodynamics as early as 6 weeks of gestation, while using higher emission frequencies and more directly focused beams. However, both transvaginal and transabdominal approaches are feasible and use energy output levels clearly situated in the lower regions for acoustic power output of diagnostic ultrasound equipment. The energy exposure on the surface of the fetus (intensity spatial peak temporal average (Ispta) = 1.2–1.9 mW/cm^2) is well within the Food and Drug Administration guidelines (94 mW/cm^2).

Normal fetuses

Methodological concern and technical issues about obtaining reproducible and reliable blood flow waveforms in the ductus venosus were recently addressed by our group[7]. Once again one should stress the importance of a standardized technique: in the late first trimester of pregnancy only a ventral mid-sagittal plane enables the record of the highest velocities in the ductus venosus.

Another difficulty appeared when trying to distinguish the proximal (near the IVC) and distal (near the umbilical vein) end of the ductus venosus to avoid 'contamination' from neighboring vessels. The sample volume should be placed in the isthmic portion.

Flow velocity waveforms in the ductus venosus are characterized by a pulsatile pattern, which consists of a systolic and diastolic component with a continuously forward flow even during atrial contraction. The absence of reverse flow in the ductus venosus may be the result of the placental pressure gradient over the ductus venosus and umbilical vein[12]. Diastolic reversal of ductus venosus flow was observed late in pregnancy but as a sign of unfavorable prognosis in cases of congestive heart failure[13,14].

Concerning the IVC velocity tracings, the sample volume should be placed close to the right atrium, but not too close. If it is placed too proximally turbulence should be expected and other blood flow waveforms might be recorded. In this way, the so-called subdiaphragmatic vestibulum[12] will gather information on changes in general venous return, since the IVC, ductus venosus and right hepatic vein are confluent at this site.

IVC velocity profiles are usually triphasic. One blood flow peak velocity occurs during ventricular systole and a second one during early diastole, when the atrioventricular (AV) valves open. A third wave occurs during atrial contraction, in the reverse direction; it is more striking in the first trimester of pregnancy, probably owing to lower cardiac compliance.

Blood flow waveforms in the umbilical vein should be acquired in its mid-hepatic portion, in the absence of fetal respiratory movements. Umbilical venous velocities usually have a non-pulsatile forward pattern. However, early in gestation, waveforms can be sporadically 'slightly undulatory' until 13 weeks of gestation[15], probably reflecting a high placental resistance.

Abnormal venous return and increased nuchal translucency

Although the underlying mechanism of increased nuchal translucency thickness (NT) remains to be clarified, it has been hypothesized that temporary heart failure could be a contributing factor[16,17]. An increase in mRNA expression of atrial natriuretic peptide and brain natriuretic peptide was found in the fetuses with increased NT, supporting evidence for heart strain[18].

In order to investigate cardiac failure in fetuses with increased NT, our group studied the characteristics of the late diastolic trough in the ductus venosus in those fetuses. As the blood velocity in the ductus venosus mirrors the pressure gradient between the umbilical vein and the right atrium, it may provide indirect information on compromised cardiac function.

None of the hemodynamic parameters of the ductus venosus, with the exception of the velocity during atrial contraction, showed any variation in the chromosomally abnormal fetuses with increased NT[19,20]. More recently, other reports appeared in the literature describing similar alterations in the ductus venosus blood flow in fetuses with trisomies[21]. Although the decrease or inversion of flow during atrial contraction in such fetuses may imply compromised atrial function (Figures 1 and 2), the unaltered peak systolic and diastolic velocities support the preferential streaming of blood through the ductus venosus and its capacity of enduring severe hemodynamic stress[14,22].

If this proves to be true in larger-scale studies, the systematic assessment of velocity during atrial contraction in the ductus venosus, whenever nuchal translucency thickness is increased, would dramatically reduce the need for invasive testing, despite a slight decrease in sensitivity[18].

Abnormal venous return and the early detection of cardiac defects

Cardiac defects are the most prevalent congenital anomalies, affecting around

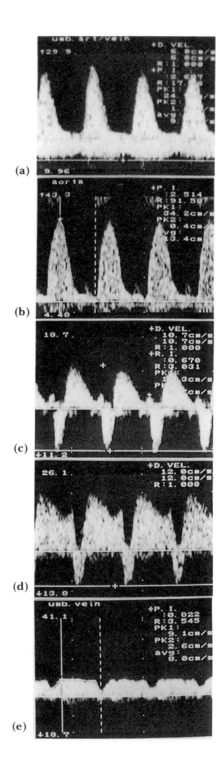

Figure 1 *Doppler blood flow waveforms in the umbilical artery (a), aorta (b), inferior vena cava (c), ductus venosus (d) and umbilical vein (e) at 13 weeks of gestation in a case of trisomy 13. Fetal heart rate = 165 beats/min; nuchal translucency = 4 mm*

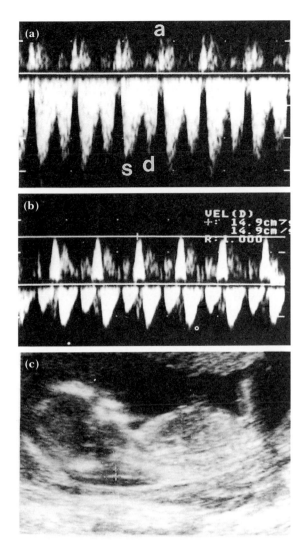

Figure 2 *Doppler blood flow waveforms in the ductus venosus (a) (reversed flow during atrial contraction) and in the inferior vena cava (b) (high retrograde flow) at 13 weeks of gestation in a case of trisomy 21 with a complete atrioventricular septal defect (nuchal translucency = 4 mm) (c)*

Therefore, efforts in fetal cardiology are focusing on an earlier diagnosis of cardiac malformations to the better understanding of their natural history, to optimize management earlier in pregnancy and to minimize emotional trauma to the parents by earlier counselling or earlier termination of pregnancy.

We recently described alterations in the ductus venosus during atrial contraction in aneuploidic fetuses with cardiac defects (Figure 2)[19]. No relevant changes were recorded, either in the umbilical artery or the descending thoracic aorta.

It is well known that fetal systemic vascular resistance may influence venous return and the filling patterns of the right heart. Increased placental resistance, peripheral vasoconstriction or cardiac impairment eventually increases end-diastolic ventricular pressure. Thus, more prominent changes were expected and identified in the venous return: dicrotic pulsatile flow in the umbilical vein with notches synchronous with atrial contraction, a high retrograde flow in the IVC and a decreased or reversed flow in the ductus venosus during atrial contraction (Figures 1 and 2)[19].

DOPPLER EVALUATION OF FETAL VENOUS RETURN IN THE SECOND AND THIRD TRIMESTERS

In the past two decades, Doppler assessment of umbilical artery blood flow has become a routine procedure in high-risk pregnancies. Absence or reversal of end-diastolic blood flow (ARED flow) in the umbilical artery and aorta, accepted as signs of ominous prognosis, have been used as a guide for obstetric management[24], but both seem of limited value in determining the optimal time for delivery.

Since systemic venous blood velocity is a direct reflection of variations in central venous pressure, conditions of decreased right ventricular output or contractility can be traced by venous hemodynamic evaluation. As changes in the venous compartment seem to follow the establishment of arterial redistribution, the sequential evaluation of

4/1000 live births. Current screening policies adopted the 18–22 week ultrasound scan, while first-trimester echocardiography is merely anecdotal in the literature[23].

Nuchal translucency has been proposed as a sensitive marker for major cardiac defects[16,19] and an indication for specialist echocardiography. Indeed, pathological studies have demonstrated a high prevalence of cardiac defects and abnormalities of the great arteries in fetuses with increased NT[16].

venous return might help to monitor and categorize the progressive worsening of fetal condition in hemodynamically compromised preterm fetuses[25,26].

We carried out a longitudinal study, on a nearly daily basis, of the Doppler arterial and venous blood flow patterns in intrauterine growth-restricted fetuses with ARED flow in the late second and early third trimesters of pregnancy[25]. Changes in the venous return were found to be discriminatory: presence of dicrotic pulsations in the umbilical vein, increase in the retrograde flow in the IVC and reduction or inversion in end-diastolic blood velocity in the ductus venosus (Color Plate N).

The increase in downstream vascular impedance in cases of high afterload extends beyond the ductus venosus, transmitting pressure waves in the umbilical venous circulation. The appearance of end-diastolic venous pulsations corresponding to heart atrial contraction was found in human fetuses with non-immune hydrops, and in hypoxic lambs during cord compression and maternal aortic occlusion[4,13]. Blood flow waveforms in the umbilical vein just before fetal death can have similar characteristics to those in the IVC, which might suggest a maximally open ductus venosus.

The reversed flow during atrial contraction in the IVC, higher than 15% of forward flow, was already described in fetuses with severely increased placental resistance, arrhythmia and non-immune hydrops, and correlated with increased perinatal mortality[4,13].

Worsening changes in the fetal heart performance could be further transmitted through the IVC to the ductus venosus. Peak systolic and diastolic velocities remained within the normal range, probably owing to the redistribution of umbilical flow preferentially through the ductus venosus. The decrease in end-diastolic venous blood velocity during atrial contraction appears as a warning sign in fetuses with intrauterine growth restriction or cardiac defects[14,22], reflecting severe heart strain and increased central venous pressure.

The progressive deterioration of right ventricular filling caused an increased flow velocity in early diastole (E-wave) and a steep abrupt acceleration and deceleration in the transtricuspid flow. This 'restricted' ventricular filling pattern is most probably the result of a decrease in ventricular compliance. Myocardial hypoxemia may result in a stiffness of the myocardium and thus increase the pressure in the right atrium.

Neither the arterial vessels nor the heart seem to offer the possibility of reliable categorization of chronic fetal deterioration[25,26]. In addition, Rizzo and co-workers[27] demonstrated that Doppler indices from the venous vessels correlated better with fetal acidosis than did indices from peripheral vessels. These preliminary results suggest that the evaluation of the venous compartment in hemodynamically disturbed preterm fetuses along with the assessment of right ventricular filling appears to be a useful model for investigating the physiopathology of fetal deterioration and to establish the sequence of events in case of fetal compromise.

CONCLUSIONS

Doppler evaluation of fetal venous flow may yield relevant information on cardiac function, central venous hemodynamics and alterations due to the reduced umbilical venous return from the placenta, from early phases of pregnancy. Alterations in the ductus venosus blood flow waveform were found in fetuses with increased nuchal translucency (with chromosomopathy and/or cardiac defects). In the second half of pregnancy, changes in the venous return recorded in cases of intrauterine growth restriction, cardiac defects, monochorionic twin pregnancy, arrythmia, anemia or hypoxemia, suggest that they may be used as discriminatory signs of fetal compromise. The most sensitive vessel to reflect central dysfunction appears to be the ductus venosus, since it is the main distributor of oxygenated blood during a major period of intrauterine life.

In conclusion, Doppler blood evaluation of the venous return to the heart, although still an investigational tool for demonstrating cardiac failure, seems promising in the evaluation of fetal compromise and should be further assessed for use in fetal medicine.

ACKNOWLEDGEMENTS

We would like to acknowledge our colleagues Jura Wladimiroff, Torvid Kiserud, Kypros Nicolaides and Kurt Hecher, for inestimably contributing to the clinical significance of Doppler fetal venous return evaluation.

References

1. Campbell S. The prediction of fetal maturity by ultrasonic measurements of the biparietal diameter. *J Obstet Gynecol Br Commonwealth* 1969;76:603–9

2. Fitzgerald DE, Drumm JE. Non-invasive measurement of the fetal circulation using ultrasound: a new method. *Br Med J* 1977;2:1450–1

3. Marsal K, Eik-Nes SH, Lindblad A, Lingman G. Blood flow in the fetal descending aorta, intrinsic factors affecting fetal blood flow, ie, fetal breathing movements and cardiac arrhythmia. *Ultrasound Med Biol* 1984;10:339–48

4. Reed KL, Appleton CP, Anderson CF, Shenker L, Sahn DJ. Doppler studies of vena cava flows in human fetuses, insights into normal and abnormal cardiac physiology. *Circulation* 1991;81:498–505

5. Wladimiroff JW, Huisman TWA, Stewart PA. Fetal cardiac flow velocities in the late first trimester of pregnancy: a transvaginal Doppler study. *J Am Coll Cardiol* 1991;17:1357–9

6. Huisman TWA, Stewart PA, Wladimiroff JW, Stijnen T. Flow velocity waveforms in the ductus venosus, umbilical vein and inferior vena cava in normal human fetuses at 12–15 weeks of gestation. *Ultrasound Med Biol* 1993;19:441–5

7. Montenegro N, Matias A, Areias JC, Barros H. Ductus venosus revisited: a Doppler blood flow evaluation in the first trimester of pregnancy. *Ultrasound Med Biol* 1997;23:171–6

8. Moore KL. The cardiovascular system. In Moore KL, ed. *The Developing Human*. Philadelphia: WB Saunders, 1997:279–83

9. Balique JG, Regairaz C, Lemeur P, Espalien P, Hugonnier G, Cuilleret J. Anatomical and experimental study of the ductus venosus. *Anat Clin* 1984;6:311–16

10. Franklin KJ, Barclay AE, Prichard MML. Some observations on the cardiovascular system in the viable foetal lamb. *J Anat* 1940;75:75–87

11. Behrman RE, Lees MH, Peterson EN, de Lannoy CW, Seeds AE. Distribution of the circulation in the normal and asphyxiated fetal primate. *Am J Obstet Gynecol* 1970;108:956–69

12. Wladimiroff JW, Huisman TWA. Venous return in the human fetus. In Kurjak A, Chervenak FA, eds. *The Fetus as a Patient: Advances in Diagnosis and Therapy*. Carnforth, UK: Parthenon Publishing, 1994:425–34

13. Gudmundsson S, Huhta JC, Wood DC, Tulzer G, Cohen AW, Weiner S. Venous Doppler ultrasonography in the fetus with non-immune hydrops. *Am J Obstet Gynecol* 1991;164:33–7

14. Kiserud T, Eik-Nes SH, Hellevik LR, Blaas HG. Ductus venosus blood velocity changes in fetal cardiac diseases. *J Matern Fetal Invest* 1993;3:15–20

15. Rizzo G, Arduini D, Romanini C. Umbilical vein pulsations: a physiological finding in early gestation. *Am J Obstet Gynecol* 1992;167:675–7

16. Hyett JA, Moscoso G, Papapanagiotu G, Perdu M, Nicolaides KH. Abnormalities of the heart and the great arteries, in chromosomally normal fetuses with increased nuchal translucency thickness at 11–13 weeks of gestation. *Ultrasound Obstet Gynecol* 1996;7:245–50

17. Montenegro N, Matias A, Areias JC, Castedo S, Barros H. Increased fetal nuchal translucency: possible involvement of early cardiac failure. *Ultrasound Obstet Gynecol* 1997;10:265–8

18. Hyett JA, Brizot ML, Von Kaisenburg C, McKie AT, Farzaneh F, Nicolaides KH. Cardiac gene expression of atrial natriuretic peptide and brain natriuretic peptide in trisomic fetuses. *Obstet Gynecol* 1996;87:506–10

19. Matias A, Montenegro N, Areias JC, Brandão O. Anomalous venous return associated with major chromosomopathies in the late first trimester of pregnancy. *Ultrasound Obstet Gynecol* 1998;10:209–13

20. Matias A, Gomes C, Flack N, Montenegro N, Nicolaides K. Screening for chromosomal abnormalities at 11–14 weeks: the role of ductus venosus blood flow. *Ultrasound Obstet Gynecol* 1998;12:380–4

21. Huisman TWA, Bilardo CM. Transient increase in nuchal translucency thickness and reversed end-diastolic ductus venosus flow in a fetus with trisomy 18. *Ultrasound Obstet Gynecol* 1998;10:397–9

22. Kiserud T, Eik-Nes SH, Blaas HG, Hellevik LR, Simensen B. Ductus venosus blood velocity and the umbilical circulation in the seriously growth-

retarded fetuses. *Ultrasound Obstet Gynecol* 1994;4: 109–14

23. Carvalho JS, Moscoso G, Ville Y. First trimester transabdominal fetal echocardiography. *Lancet* 1998;351:1023–7

24. Karsdorp VHM, van Vugt JMG, van Geijn HP, *et al.* Clinical significance of absent or reverse end-diastolic velocity waveform in the umbilical artery. *Lancet* 1994;344:1664–8

25. Areias JC, Matias A, Montenegro N. Venous return and right ventricular diastolic function in ARED flow fetuses. *J Perinatal Med* 1998;26: 157–67

26. Hecher K, Campbell S, Doyle P, Harrington K, Nicolaides K. Assessment of fetal compromise by Doppler ultrasound investigation of the fetal circulation. Arterial, intracardiac and venous blood flow velocity studies. *Circulation* 1995; 91:129–38

27. Rizzo G, Capponi A, Talone PE, Arduini D, Romanini C. Doppler indices from inferior vena cava and ductus venosus in predicting pH and oxygen tension in umbilical blood at cordocentesis in growth-retarded fetuses. *Ultrasound Obstet Gynecol* 1996;7:401–10

Current perspectives on ultrasonic tissue characterization

15

K. Maeda, P. E. Kihaile, M. Utsu, N. Yamamoto and M. Serizawa

INTRODUCTION

A real-time ultrasound image is expressed by the pixel echogenicity from which the nature of the subject tissue is estimated. The visual impression, however, is insufficient for exact determination. Many academic investigations have focused on ultrasonic tissue characterization; the changes of ultrasonic frequency, velocity, attenuation, non-linearity, backscatter, echodensity and texture analysis of B-mode have been reported. Akaiwa[1], our colleague, reported objective results in the frequency-dependent attenuation values in various tissues, but the method needed a special computer system and great efforts by the investigator. Such a special investigative system could not be used generally in hospitals.

More detailed and quantitative evaluation was needed in placental studies than the four-grade classification of the images reported by Grannum and colleagues[2]. Various studies on placental tissue characterization have been reported[3–5]. We have attempted to establish a new objective parameter[4–7].

Fetal lung maturity has usually been estimated by tests on the amniotic fluid obtained by uterine puncture. Non-invasive analyses of ultrasonic images of the fetal lung have been reported[8–12]. However, the visual image evaluation was subjective, the mean gray levels were altered by the change of device gain and other controls, and therefore, we needed new, simple but objective methods.

THE NEW ECHOGENICITY PARAMETER: GRAY-LEVEL HISTOGRAM WIDTH

Ultrasound devices and ultrasonic phantom

The ultrasonic imaging devices used in this study[7] were the UIP-100 computer system, SSD-258, SSD-650, SSD-680 (Aloka, Tokyo, Japan), SSA-270A (Toshiba, Tokyo, Japan), and U-Sonic RT-8000 (Yokogawa Medical System, Tokyo, Japan). The UIP-100 system was composed of the Aloka SSD-270, DEC PDP 11 computer, special obstetric programs, frequency-dependent attenuation and displays of the gray-level histogram and its parameters. Other commercial equipment included common obstetric programs and the histogram function. The ultrasound frequency was 3.5 MHz in Aloka machines, and 3.75 MHz in Toshiba and Yokogawa machines. The transducers were usually of the convex transabdominal type, and a linear transducer was compared to the convex transducer in SSD-650. The region of interest (ROI) shape was usually square, but there were circular or traced ones. The fetal lung and liver were studied mainly by the SSD-2000 machine (Aloka, Tokyo, Japan). Its convex transducer frequency was 3.5 MHz. The ultrasonic phantom, used in the tests of the various imaging devices, was RMI-412 (Radiation Measurement Inc., Middleton, WI). The transabdominal transducers were tested by the phantom after being attached to the top of the phantom via ultrasound jelly.

Determination of gray-level histogram width

Pixel brightness was expressed by gray scales in a sonographic device in which the full scale was 64 when 6-bit memories were used. We analyzed the most primitive parameter, the range of the distribution of pixel gray levels, which was expressed as the base width of the gray-level histogram. The pixel numbers at each gray scale were counted in a ROI, and a distribution histogram was composed that was 100% at the gray scale of the highest pixel number (n), and the other gray-scale bars were expressed by the percentages of n (Figure 1). In addition to the histogram, the pixel numbers in the ROI, the gray scale of the highest pixel number and some of the histogram parameters were displayed on the screen. The base width of the histogram was the distance between the highest and lowest gray scales, and the number of the histogram bars contained in the histogram was divided by 64 when the memory was 6 bits, or the histogram base length was divided by the full gray-scale span on the permanent record of the screen image. The result, expressed as a percentage, was called the gray-level histogram width (GLHW) (Figure 1). The GLHW was directly determined by the UIP-100 computer system (Aloka, Tokyo, Japan). Manually determined GLHW with common sonographs were used in this study at the same time as those obtained by the UIP-100 computer system.

Studies on the influence of the device gain, contrast and image depths on GLHW values

GLHW values were measured in the ROIs placed at the homogeneous image of the RMI-412 phantom, using various device gains, contrasts and the depths from the surface of the phantom, by using the SSD-680 with an abdominal convex 3.5-MHz transducer. The gray-level histogram and its parameters were displayed on the screen. The ROIs were set at various parts of phantom images. In the studies on the influence of the gain control, the ROI was set at the center of the phantom image, about 5 cm from the phantom surface.

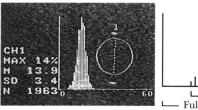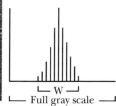

Figure 1 *Gray-level histogram of ultrasonic phantom (RMI-412) displayed on the screen of the SSA-270A machine (left), and the manual determination of gray-level histogram width (GLHW) (right). The histogram bars (W) are counted and divided by full gray scales (64), or the histogram base length is divided by the full gray scale length, and GLHW (%) is obtained*

The GLHW of the ultrasound phantom, obtained by 52–90-dB gains, showed uniform values in each step of the contrast (Figure 2).

The influence of device contrast control from steps 1–6 on the GLHW was studied by the 70-dB gain. The GLHW values of the RMI-412 phantom showed a linear increase when the contrast control was set at higher steps (Figure 2): $y = 5.386 x + 30.33$; $n = 6$; $r = 0.989$; $p < 0.05$, where x = contrast scale and y = GLHW.

The influence of sonographic image depths on the GLHW was tested by the setting of the ROIs at various depths from the surface of the phantom. The gain was 70 dB. The GLHW values of the phantom showed no particular difference at the depths of the ROIs ranging from 2 to 10 cm from the surface (Figure 2).

Comparisons of GLHW values in various sonographic devices

The GLHW values of the RMI-412 phantom were compared among the Aloka UIP-100, SSD-650 and SSD-680, Toshiba SSA-270A and Yokogawa RT-8000. The abdominal transducers were placed on the top of the phantom. The ROIs were set at various parts of the homogeneous images of the phantom. The device gain was arbitrarily changed so as to obtain suitable image quality. Device contrast was, however, set at the lowest step in

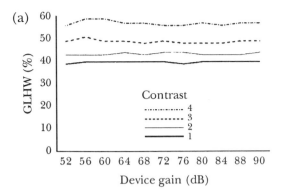

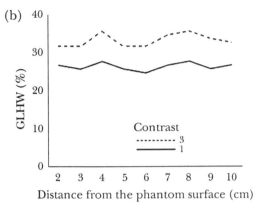

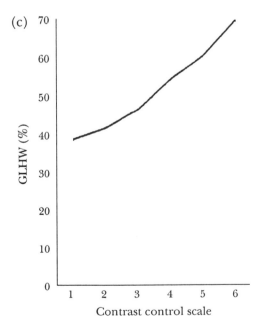

Figure 2 *The influence of device gain (a), image depth (b) and contrast (c), on the gray-level histogram width (GLHW) values in studies on the phantom images. No significant change of GLHW was noted with the control of device gain or image depth, but the value changed linearly when the device contrast increased*

SSD-650 and -680, and the dynamic range was 50–65 dB in the UIP-100, SSA-270A and RT-8000. ROI size was set so as to include more than 500 pixels in a ROI. The GLHW values and the mode of gray levels obtained by manual calculations in common sonographs were compared to the values obtained by the UIP-100 computer system. There was no statistically significant difference of GLHW values of the RMI-412 phantom images among the UIP-100 computer system, Aloka SSD-680 and Toshiba SSA-270A. The Aloka SSD-650 and Yokogawa RT-8000 showed significant, but mild, differences of GLHW values from those of the UIP-100. The values did not change by on–off sensitivity time control (STC) in SSD-650 and -680. However, the mode of pixel gray levels obtained at the peak of the gray-level histogram showed moderate to large and significant differences among tested sonographic devices. Linear and convex transducers of the SSD-650 showed no difference in GLHW values. The GLHW obtained by circular ROI of the SSA-270A showed no difference from the square ROIs of other devices.

Automatic measurement of the base length of the gray-level histogram

The gray-level histogram base length was automatically measured with the ROM programmed by K. Irie and the Aloka technical department. The automatic menu was installed in our SSD-650 and -680 machines. Automatically obtained GLHW values of various tissues were compared to the values of manual measurement of the same subjects. The manually measured GLHW (mean ± SD) was 39.7 ± 13.93%, and the automatic measurement was 42.33 ± 15.93%. There was no significant difference between the two groups. The regression equation was: $y = 1.09\ x - 0.63$; $r = 0.954$; $p < 0.01$; $n = 44$, where y was the automatic and x was the manual measure-ment. From the results, automated and manual methods did not differ in the determination of the histogram, and both results were used in our studies on the GLHW values.

CLINICAL STUDIES ON THE PLACENTA WITH THE GLHW MEASUREMENTS

Gray-level histograms were measured by the UIP-100 and other old scanners in the 222 normal placentas at 20–41 weeks of pregnancy[7]. Grannum[2] grades were 0–1. The placentas were determined by the UIP-100 combined with the SSD-270, -258 and -650 in our early study[4]. An abdominal scan was used in all cases. The measurements were taken on anteriorly located placentas, but not on the placenta located posteriorly beyond the fetal body. Normal ranges of the placental GLHW were determined by the mean ±1.5 SD of normalized GLHW values of every 2 weeks in 20–41 weeks of gestation. Upper and lower ranges and the mean of normal intrauterine prenatal placentas showed a gradual increase during pregnancy (Figure 3).

In the next step, placental GLHW values were freshly measured by the SSD-650, -680 and SSA-270A in 37 normal placentas and in seven highly echogenic placentas of Grannum[2] grade III, and these were compared to the normal ranges obtained by the old machines. Device contrast was the lowest, and the gain, STC and the ROI shape were set deliberately. The GLHW of normal homogeneous placentas, determined by new sonographs, were found almost between the normal ranges of GLHW which were obtained by using the old scanners. The Grannum[2] grade III placentas of very echogenic images showed GLHW values larger than the upper normal range (Figure 3).

The placental GLHW was longitudinally determined in a pregnancy with intrauterine growth restriction (IUGR), which showed a large GLHW in the second trimester. Estimated fetal weight was 294 g, and mean – 3.5 SD at 22 weeks. The patient was hospitalized and received treatments with heparin and corticosteroid, because of positive anticardiolipin antibody and a history of IUGR followed by fetal death in a previous pregnancy. The placental GLHW values showed the decrease, and fetal growth was promoted during hospitalization. The GLHW, estimated fetal weight, fetal heart rate and

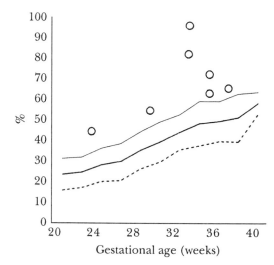

Figure 3 *Normal ranges of placental gray-level histogram width (mean ± 1.5 SD). The circles show the values obtained in the placentas of Grannum grade III, which were generally larger than the upper normal range*

pulsed Doppler flow waveform of the fetal aorta were within normal ranges in the third trimester. A 2660-g normal female baby was born at 38 weeks of gestation by Cesarean section.

STUDIES ON THE GLHW VALUES OF THE FETAL LUNG AND LIVER

The Aloka SSD-2000 device used in the studies on fetal lung and liver

Since the SSD-2000 was a new model not evaluated in the studies on various devices, it was calibrated by using the RMI-412 phantom before its use in the studies on fetal lung and liver[13]. Although the device gain did not influence the GLHW value in the phantom studies, the gain was set at 70 dB in order to study pixel gray levels displayed on the screen. The mean ± SD of GLHW values of the RMI-412 phantom image was 30.47 ± 2.08 (%) at a 65–90-dB gain when the contrast was the lowest, and there was no significant difference of the GLHW values in the gain settings. The phantom GLHW measured by UIP-100 was 36.5 (%), and therefore, the correction factor of the SSD-2000 was $36.5/30.47 = 1.20$. A measured GLHW value was multiplied by 1.2 in the normalization. On the other hand, GLHW values were divided by 1.14, 1.29, 1.43, 1.57 and 1.72, respectively, when the image contrast control scale was 2 to 6, according to the measurement of RMI-412. The GLHW values of the normal placenta measured by the machine were lower than the upper normal range of the placenta.

The GLHW measurements of fetal lung and liver

Pregnant women were normal when they visited our clinic, and the perinatal outcomes were normal in these cases. The sonographic findings of the fetus, its growth, amniotic fluid, umbilical cord and the placenta were normal. There was no abnormal blood flow velocity waveform in the uterine, fetal or umbilical vessels in the cases. Fetal heart rate records were normal. The full bladder technique was applied in early pregnancy. The sonographic images of fetal lung and liver were recorded in 52 fetuses at 24–38 weeks of pregnancy, including 11 at 27–29 weeks, eight at 30–32 weeks, 11 at 33–35 weeks and 11 at 36–38 weeks (Tables 1 and 2). The fetal chest and abdomen were placed on the anterior side of

the fetal trunk, i.e. the interference of the fetal rib shadow was reduced to a minimum. The histographic bars were counted on the permanent record, because automated measurement was not yet installed in the equipment. The number of counted histogram bars was divided by 64, calibrated by the device factor and the contrast scale, and the GLHW values (%) were obtained. Mean and the standard deviation (SD) of the gray level were also displayed on the screen. The measurements were the GLHW, the mean and SD of the gray levels displayed on the screen and the coefficient of variation (CV) of gray levels, in fetal lung and liver. The CV was obtained by dividing the SD by the mean gray level (%). Also, the ratios of GLHW values, mean gray level, gray level SD and gray level CV of fetal lung and liver, were studied.

GLHW values of fetal lung and liver

The GLHW values of the fetal lung were significantly lower at 24–29 weeks of pregnancy than at 30–38 weeks (Table 1, Figure 4). In more detailed analysis, in every 3 weeks of pregnancy, there were significant differences at 24–26 vs. 27–29 weeks and 36–38 weeks (Table 2).

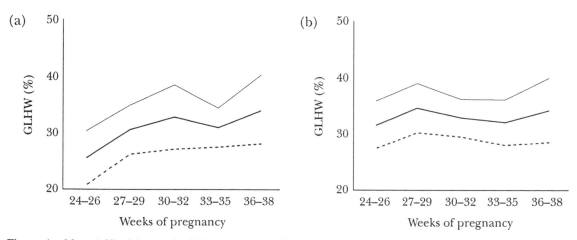

Figure 4 *Mean ± SD of the gray-level histogram width (GLHW) values of the fetal lung (a) and liver (b) determined at 24–38 weeks of pregnancy. The lung GLHW values increased during weeks 24–29, and reached a level of no significant difference at 30–38 weeks. The GLHW values were significantly different between 24–29 and 30–38 weeks. Fetal liver GLHW values, however, showed no significant change during pregnancy*

Table 1 Echogenicity values of the fetal lung and liver at 20–29 and 30–38 weeks of pregnancy. Ranges are shown in parentheses. Modified from reference 13

Weeks of pregnancy	n	Single parameters (mean/SD)				Ratio of fetal lung and liver (mean/SD)			
		GLHW	MGL	GLSD	GLCV	GLHW	MGL	GLSD	GLCV
Lung									
20–29	22	28.18/5.18 (15–37)	20.31/7.09 (10.1–35.9)	4.08/0.82 (2.6–5.6)	21.90/6.94 (15–37)	0.83/0.18 (0.50–1.13)	0.97/0.23 (0.57–1.33)	0.83/0.22 (0.59–1.98)	0.91/0.28 (0.65–1.34)
30–38	30	32.73/5.18 (25–47)	26.89/7.34 (13.0–50.0)	3.80/0.85 (3.1–5.6)	15.23/5.37 (9–26)	1.00/0.16 (0.74–1.22)	1.00/0.22 (0.6–1.61)	0.97/0.17 (0.71–1.22)	0.99/0.26 (0.73–1.63)
Liver									
20–29	22	33.45/4.53 (25–45)	20.39/5.44 (10.9–29.7)	4.90/1.01 (3.2–6.6)	25.45/7.83 (13–42)				
30–38	30	32.86/5.40 (23–47)	27.09/6.40 (14.8–49.8)	3.94/0.77 (4.0–5.2)	15.33/4.60 (9–28)				

GLHW, gray-level histogram width; MGL, mean gray level, displayed on the screen; GLSD, gray-level standard deviation (SD), displayed on the screen; GLCV, gray-level coefficient of variation, GLSD/MGL multiplied by 100; S, significant difference

Table 2 Echogenicity values of the fetal lung and liver in every 3-week period of pregnancy (mean/SD). Modified from reference 13

Weeks of pregnancy	n	Fetal lung				Fetal liver			
		GLHW (%)	Gray levels displayed on the screen			GLHW (%)	Gray levels displayed on the screen		
			Mean	SD	CV(%)		Mean	SD	CV(%)
24–26	11	25.63/4.87 ⌉S	17.56/5.67	3.82/0.68	23.63/7.71	31.90/4.25	17.85/5.42 ⌉S	4.49/0.83	27.45/9.70 ⌉S
27–29	11	30.72/4.39 ⌋	23.07/7.51	4.34/0.89	20.18/5.88	35.00/4.44	22.93/4.30 ⌋	5.30/1.09 ⌉S	23.45/5.08 ⌋
30–32	8	33.00/5.78	22.81/6.26	4.16/1.01	18.87/4.51	33.25/3.32	25.06/6.01	3.81/1.47 ⌋	18.00/4.72 ⌉S
33–35	11	31.09/3.54	27.60/8.33	3.70/0.87	14.36/4.97	30.72/5.90	27.68/8.68	3.75/0.82	14.45/4.47
36–38	11	34.18/6.00	29.15/6.31	3.63/0.76	13.45/5.45	34.72/5.74	27.97/3.75	3.86/0.73	14.27/4.50 ⌋
Difference from 36–38 weeks									
24–26		S	S		S		S		S
27–29			S		S		S	S	S
30–32			S		S				

GLHW, gray-level histogram width; SD, standard deviation; CV, coefficient of variation; S, significant difference

The GLHW values of the fetal liver showed no significant difference between 24–29 weeks and 30–38 weeks of pregnancy (Table 1, Figure 4), and also no difference among the groups examined every 3 weeks of pregnancy (Table 2), i.e. there was no change in fetal liver GLHW during weeks 24–38 of pregnancy.

The fetal lung GLHW was significantly smaller than that of the fetal liver at 24–29 weeks. However, at 30–38 weeks, the lung GLHW showed no significant difference from that of the liver (Table 1). The ratios of fetal lung and liver GLHW values showed a significant increase at 30–38 weeks. The ratios of fetal lung and liver mean gray level showed no significant change. The ratios of fetal lung and liver gray-level SD significantly increased at 30–38 weeks. The ratios of fetal lung and liver gray-level CV showed no significant change (Table 1).

Other echogenicity parameters of fetal lung and liver

Mean gray levels of the fetal lung were significantly larger at 30–38 weeks of pregnancy than at 24–29 weeks. The mean gray level of the fetal liver was significantly larger at 30–38 weeks than at 24–29 weeks. However, there was no difference between fetal lung and liver either at 24–29 weeks or at 30–38 weeks. Gray-level SD of the fetal lung showed no significant difference between the groups at 24–29 weeks and 30–38 weeks of pregnancy, but the values tended to decrease towards the end of pregnancy. The gray-level SD of the fetal liver decreased significantly at 30–38 weeks of pregnancy. The gray-level CV of the fetal lung and liver showed significant decreases at 30–38 weeks of pregnancy (Table 1).

Correlation analysis of the echogenicity parameters

The correlation of the fetal lung GLHW with the weeks of pregnancy was significant but moderate, but the correlation of fetal liver GLHW was low and insignificant. Both mean gray-level values of the fetal lung and liver showed moderate and significant correlation with the weeks of pregnancy. The correlations of the gray-level SD and the gray-level CV of the fetal lung and liver with the weeks of pregnancy were also significant but moderate, except for the lung gray-level SD. A significant correlation was noted in the pregnancy weeks and the ratio of GLHW values of the fetal lung and the liver. The ratios of mean gray level, gray-level SD and gray-level CV of the fetal lung and liver showed no significant correlation with the pregnancy weeks. The GLHW, mean gray level, gray-level SD and gray-level CV values of fetal lung and liver showed various sig-nificant correlations among each parameter.

DISCUSSION

The GLHW, which represents pixel gray-level distribution in the ROI, was uniformly measurable by using various commercial ultrasonic imaging devices. The clinical needs of the gain control are fulfilled in the use of GLHW because the gain change did not influence the GLHW values of the RMI phantom. This might be explained by the fact that the device gain was controlled by the direct current offset of the preamplifier output. It is also a useful feature that the GLHW was not influenced by the image depth within the range of clinical use. The influence of the device contrast control can be corrected by a simple equation.

The placental study in this report confirmed the usefulness of GLHW as a clinical tissue characterization parameter, because we could produce normal GLHW ranges of the placenta which were applicable in both old and new imaging devices. The prolonged observation of GLHW in an IUGR case also showed the utility in longitudinal studies. The echogenicity of the fetal lung has been repeatedly discussed[6,8–11]. Sohn and colleagues[12] reported that the ratio of the frequency component of ultrasound A-mode in the fetal lung and liver was useful in the suspicion of lung immaturity. In our present paper, among the echogenicity parameters, the fetal lung GLHW showed a particular changing pattern as the pregnancy progressed, i.e. the fetal lung GLHW was larger at 30–38 weeks than at 24–29 weeks. The fetal liver GLHW showed uniform values during pregnancy; therefore, the fetal liver is a good reference for the echogenicity of the fetal lung. Although both the GLHW and gray-level SD are related to the distribution of the pixel echogenicity, their characters were different, i.e. the SD showed a decreasing tendency. The gray-level CV of the fetal lung significantly decreased as the pregnancy progressed. The change may indicate the increasing uniformity of tissue echogenicity.

Immaturity of the fetal lung may be estimated by the low echogenicity of the lung in the antepartum stage, particularly with the ultrasonic GLHW measurement. Comparison of the fetal lung GLHW to that of the liver can also be useful in late pregnancy. Hypoplastic lung and other fetal lung abnormalities should be studied by GLHW.

The gray-level histogram was applied in other subjects, e.g. in the analysis of ultrasonic images of ovarian masses[14], and in the examination of periventricular echodensity of the fetal brain[15]. We[7] measured GLHW values of the adult liver. We believe it has usefulness in other general medical fields.

References

1. Akaiwa A. Ultrasonic attenuation character estimated from back scattered radiofrequency signals in obstetrics and gynecology. *Yonago Acta Med* 1989;32:1–10
2. Grannum PT, Berkowitz RL, Hobbins JC. The ultrasonic changes in maturing placenta and the relation to fetal pulmonic maturity. *Am J Obstet Gynecol* 1979;133:915–22
3. Crawford DC, Fenton DW, Price WI. Ultrasonic tissue characterization of the placenta: is it of clinical value? *J Clin Ultrasound* 1985;13:533–7
4. Kihaile PE. Ultrasonic grey-level histograms of prenatal placenta and its relation to fetal well-being. *Yonago Acta Med* 1988;31:139–46
5. Maeda K, Akaiwa A, Kihaile PE, Mio Y, Toda T. Fetal and placental tissue characterization with ultrasound. *Rech Gynecol* 1989;1:301–2
6. Maeda K, Akaiwa A, Kihaile PE. Ultrasound tissue characterization. In Chervenak FA, Isaacson GC, Campbell S eds. *Ultrasound in Obstetrics and Gynecology*. Boston: Little Brown, 1993:55–9
7. Maeda K, Utsu M, Kihaile PE. Quantification of sonographic echogenicity with grey-level histogram width: a clinical tissue characterization. *Ultrasound Med Biol* 1998;24:225–34
8. Reeves GS, Garrett WJ, Warren PS, Fischer CC. Observation of fetal lung reflectivity using real-time ultrasound. *Aust NZ J Obstet Gynaecol* 1984;24:91–4
9. Cayea PD, Grant DC, Doubilet PM, Johns TB. Prediction of fetal lung maturity: inaccuracy of study using conventional ultrasound instruments. *Radiology* 1985;155:473–5
10. Feingold M, Scollins J, Cerrulo CL, Koza D. Fetal lung to liver reflectivity ratio and lung maturity. *J Clin Ultrasound* 1987;15:384–7
11. Fried AM, Loh FK, Umer MA, Dillon KP, Kryscio R. Echogenicity of fetal lung: relation to fetal age and maturity. *Am J Radiol* 1985;145:591–4
12. Sohn C, Stolz W, Gast AS, Bastert G. Die sonographische Diagnostik der fetalen Lungenreife. *Z Geburtshilfe Perinatol* 1992;196:55–60
13. Maeda K, Utsu M, Yamamoto N, Serizawa M. Echogenicity of fetal lung and liver quantified by the grey-level histogram width. *Ultrasound Med Biol* 1999;25; in press
14. Kihaile PE. Ultrasonic tissue characterization of ovarian tumors by the scanning of grey-level histograms. *Yonago Acta Medica* 1989;32:251–60
15. Yamamoto N, Serizawa M, Yamasaki T, Ooi Y, Utsu M, Maeda K. Fetal periventricular ultrasonic echodensity detected in 3 cases of uneventful pregnancy. *48th Congress of Japan Society of Obstetrics and Gynecology. Acta Obstet Gynaecol Jpn* 1996;48(Suppl): 463 (abstr)

Three-dimensional ultrasonography in prenatal diagnosis

16

A. Kurjak and M. Kos

Prenatal two-dimensional ultrasonography enables detailed visualization of fetal anatomy, but also detection of fetal growth and structural abnormalities. The improved two-dimensional technique offers high resolution images, but the fact remains that three-dimensional structures are imaged and analyzed in two-dimensional planes. It is up to the sonographer to construct a three-dimensional mental picture and spatial orientation from a few two-dimensional images. Although some have predicted that ultrasound technology has already reached its theoretical limits, the recent introduction of three-dimensional ultrasonography may lead to the development of entirely new clinical applications. Three-dimensional ultrasonography is still a relatively new diagnostic imaging technique undergoing rapid advances in recent years, particularly in the field of obstetrics and prenatal diagnosis.

The first generation of three-dimensional technology, during the early 1980s, provided a pseudo-three-dimensional image by the simultaneous display of the three orthogonal planes; this offered some advantages over conventional two-dimensional imaging[1,2]. Modern three-dimensional systems are capable of generating surface and transparent views depicting the sculpture-like reconstruction of fetal surface structures or the X-ray-like images of fetal skeletal anatomy. These are the most impressive products within modern three-dimensional ultrasound imaging. The main advantages of three-dimensional techology in perinatal medicine and antenatal diagnosis include scanning in the coronal plane, improved assessment of complex anatomic structures, surface scanning analysis of minor defects, volumetric measuring of organs, 'plastic' transparent imaging of the fetal skeleton, spatial presentation of blood flow arborization and, finally, storage of scanned volumes and images[3–8]. With arbitrary sectional display in three-dimensional ultrasonography, the orientation of tomograms is unlimited, despite the limited manipulation of the probe or inadequate position of fetal structures. These facts are extremely important in the first trimester of pregnancy when the manipulation of the vaginal probe is restricted and limited ultrasound sections are obtainable[9]. During transabdominal scanning, coronal or frontal planes parallel to the fetal abdominal wall are also visible. These views are not available with conventional ultrasound. Additional progress is achieved, owing to the permanent possibility of repeated analysis of previously saved three-dimensional volumes and Cartesian elimination of surrounding structures and artifacts[3,10,11]. Three-dimensional reconstruction of stored images (surface and volume rendering) is the most impressive benefit of three-dimensional scanning. The region of interest is first identified and manually delineated; this is followed by an automatic process of echo extraction. In this way, the surface of the organ of interest is displayed in three dimensions. This enables a detailed morphological analysis to be made of structures such as the fetal face or minor defects. A transparency mode is another way of showing ultrasound images in three dimensions. In this mode, only the strongest and lowest signals are displayed, so that the internal structure of the organ of interest can be analyzed[12].

Although various systems have the capacity for three-dimensional ultrasound data acquisition and three-dimensional image generation, the best three-dimensional images are obtained using special three-dimensional, automatically driven, trans-abdominal and transvaginal transducers. These transducers have to be connected to a two-dimensional high-resolution machine with an integrated three-dimensional control processor and storage unit.

We like to emphasize that the three-dimensional technique is complementary, not alternative technology to the conventional two-dimensional technique in the field of prenatal diagnosis. However, three-dimensional imaging is superior for some specific diagnostic problems. A comparison of two-dimensional and three-dimensional techniques shows that the three-dimensional method provides a diagnostic gain in a large percentage of cases owing to the possibility of surface and transparent mode imaging. The accurate topographic depiction of the desired image plane is then much easier[3,13,14].

FIRST-TRIMESTER APPLICATIONS

Three-dimensional scanning offers advantages in assessing embryonic morphology in the first trimester, owing to the ability to obtain multiplanar images through endovaginal volume acquisition. Limitations of transducer movements prohibit obtaining many images on conventional two-dimensional scanning. The three-dimensional possibility of rotation of the scanned embryo and close analysis of the scanned volume have allowed more systematic review of embryonic and extraembryonic anatomy.

Our experience confirms that transvaginal three-dimensional ultrasonography during the first trimester is related to significant visualization benefit, particularly because of an additional possibility for three-dimensional morphological analysis of extraembryonic 'static' structures such as the gestational sac and yolk sac. Volumetry of the gestational sac and morphological analysis of the yolk sac are easier then ever before (Figure 1). Impressive three-dimensional scanning of embryonic structures might sometimes be impossible, because of intensive embryonic movements.

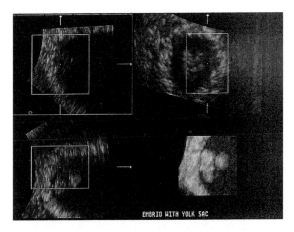

Figure 1 *Human embryo with yolk sac, in the first trimester: three-dimensional rendering mode*

Embryonic developmental disorders related to chromosomal abnormalities are of great interest within modern sonography. During the first trimester, three-dimensional 'surface and sculpture-like imaging' includes excellent morphological follow-up of the physiological midgut herniation process and abdominal anterior wall visualization. Three-dimensional depiction of the retarded resolution of umbilical herniation and the development of omphalocele is possible during weeks 11 and 12 of gestation (Figure 2). Following the possibilites of three-dimensional transparent mode imaging, the morphology related to nuchal translucency and cystic hygroma could be recognizable earlier than biometrically detectable nuchal thickening. Moreover, case reports such as that by Liang and colleagues[15], identifying ectopia cordis at 10 weeks' gestational age, are very encouraging.

SECOND- AND THIRD-TRIMESTER EVALUATION

Besides impressive demonstration of normal fetal structures, three-dimensional ultrasonography is adding a new 'window' to the diagnosis of structural defects. The fetal face is an essential part of routine sonographic examination[10]. Even under optimal conditions, the curvature of the fetal face makes it difficult to obtain adequate images with two-

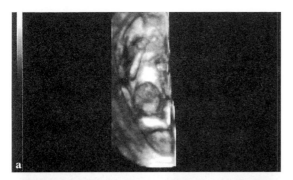

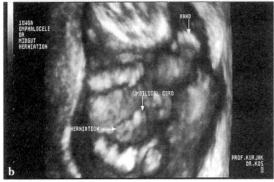

Figure 2 *(a) Embryo at 12 weeks' gestation, showing omphalocele. (b) Embryo at 10 weeks' gestation, showing physiological midgut herniation*

dimensional ultrasonography, and many cross-sectional images are required to produce a complete impression of normality. Volume-rendered three-dimensional images of the fetal face are easily recognizable by both families and physicians. One of the most important aspects of assessing the fetal face with three-dimensional imaging is that the face can be rotated into various anatomic orientations. This allows evaluation of different projections of the face in a rapid and reproducible fashion from the earliest stage of prgenancy[13].

Some defects, such as cleft lip, dysplastic ear, facial dysmorphia, anophthalmia and proboscis are easier to depict with three-dimensional surface mode[10,16-19]. Facial deformities are one marker of chromosomal abnormalities, and three-dimensional technology may be useful for increasing the selectivity of ultrasound screening and confirming normalcy.

Moreover, volumetric data offer a substantial benefit for analysis of some 'subsurface' facial structures. It is possible to obtain three orthogonal slices of fetal orbits, palate, pharynx and soft tissues regardless of the intrauterine head position. On the other hand, surface structures of the face and head become visible despite significant shadowings or malpresentation from overlying structures. The dysmorphic appearance of fetal anencephaly and acrania can be understood much better by presenting the fetal head and neck in three-dimensional volume scanning. The variety of morphological appearance related to development of the cerebrovascular area seems to be much easier to differentiate using a three-dimensional depiction compared to standard two-dimensional imaging (Figure 3).

It is generally agreed that anomalous shape or size of the fetal ears is associated with a number of known morphological and chromosomal syndromes. To recognize a congenital anomaly of the fetal ear *in utero* is generally difficult, possibly owing to the complex shape of the ear and the inherent characteristics of conventional two-dimensional ultrasound. Three-dimensional surface imaging of the fetal ear offers complete analysis of the details related to phenotypic expression of some inherited syndromes. Through the clues of the anomalous ear obtained from three-dimensional imaging, we can diagnose some other, more subtle, fetal anomaly that may be overlooked in simple two-dimensional ultrasound scanning[20,21] (Figure 4).

Many congenital heart defects go undetected in fetuses because the heart is too challenging a moving structure to evaluate. Although some images will be obtained, suggesting adequate cardiac evaluation, false-positive and false-negative results are still significant[22-24].

Similarly, the three-dimensional surface mode enables sculpture-like reconstructions of abdominal defects such as omphalocele or gastroschisis. By use of this modality, the size and extension of the defect are precisely demonstrated. Surface rendering in three-dimensional ultrasonography gives a clear display of normal extremities (Figure 5). Clubfoot, reversible or irreversible patho-

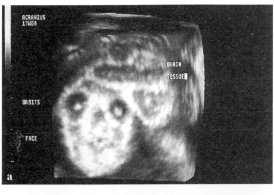

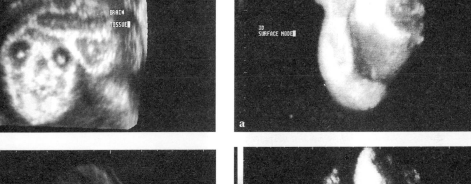

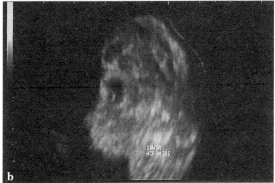

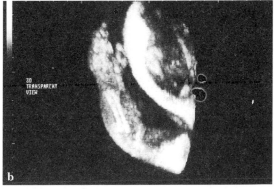

Figure 3 *(a) and (b) Fetus at 17 weeks' gestation, showing acrania. The cerebrovascularization is visible covering the dysmorphic head*

Figure 5 *Normal fetal arm, by (a) surface rendering; and (b) transparent mode*

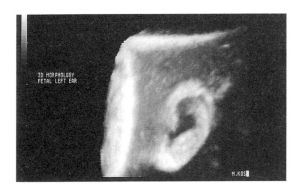

Figure 4 *Normal fetal ear*

logical angulation of the normal anatomical axis and other limb abnormalities are easy to define using three-dimensional orientation[25,26] (Figure 6).

Three-dimensional imaging is also helpful in assessing the precise relationship of the wrist, hand and fingers (Figure 7). Ploeckinger-Ulm and co-workers[27] noted that fetal digits were optimally visualized between 20 and 23 weeks of gestation and that at least one hand was visualized with two-dimensional sonography in 93% of patients, and with three-dimensional sonography in 100% of patients. They reported a study of 72 fetuses examined with the three-dimensional technique, which allowed a complete examination of all digits of the hand in significantly more fetuses from low-risk pregnancies than did two-dimensional ultrasonography (74.3% vs. 52.9%). It is important to note that there will be some fetuses in which it is not possible to obtain adequate volumes of the hands and feet, owing to rapid movements of the extremities.

Transparent mode three-dimensional ultrasonography allows imaging of internal structures, such as the fetal skeleton, depicting its malformation in spatial orientation. Congenital malformations of the fetal spine and ribs can be identified easier by three-

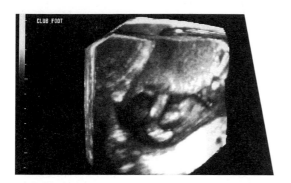

Figure 6 *Fetal leg, showing clubfoot: medial deviation the foot*

dimensional transparent mode reconstruction. This imaging technique allows the sonogram of the spine and thorax to be rotated into a standard anatomic orientation for rapid recognition of abnormalities. Three-dimensional sonography provides several advatages in evaluating neural tube defects. The level and the extent of the defect can be more accurately determined by using the simultaneous display of three orthogonal planes combined with the volume-rendered image. The spine may be evaluated along a curved line in order to evaluate the vertebral bodies in a transverse or axial plane. A specific vertebral body level may be accurately identified by simultaneously evaluating the axial planes of the spine with a volume-rendered image or with the coronal plane[28,29]. It is often difficult to acquire the entire spine in a single volume and thus multiple volumes are often necessary for complete evaluation of the spine.

Using three-dimensional imaging, an experienced ultrasonographer may also depict even subtle malformations such as mild pyelectasis, ambiguous genitalia, clubfoot or single umbilical artery (Figure 8).

Determining chorionicity and amnionicity of multifetal pregnancy is very important, because monochorionic and/or mono-amniotic multifetal pregnancies can be associated with an increased incidence of structural and hemodynamic complications such as twin-to-twin transfusion syndrome, discordant growth, severe malformations, or cord entanglement. Determining chorionicity

and amnionicity during the early second trimester may be much easier by means of three-dimensional sonography, respecting all of the relevant criteria such as counting the number of placentas, determining whether each fetus is within its own amniotic sac, describing the appearance of the dividing membrane and looking for the presence of a triangular projection of placental tissue beyond the chorionic surfaces (lambda or twin peak sign) (Figure 9).

Finally, a three-dimensional surface view reassures the parents with a normal fetus, encouraging a positive fetomaternal relationship[30]. Those with malformed fetuses are provided with clear 'photographic' images of the baby; the sonographer can evaluate the malformation at different angles, giving a clear 'plastic' impression of the shape and severity of the defect to the parents.

Multicenter studies have shown some limitations of three-dimensional ultrasound scanning[3,31]. Fetal and maternal movements during the scanning process lead to motion

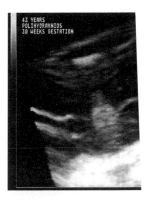

Figure 8   *Single umbilical*

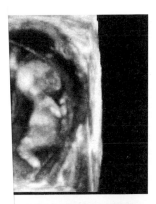

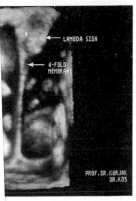

artifacts that can degi
image. Fetal surface
depends on a sufficien
in front of the regio
cases, oligohydramni
structures prevent su
Finally, three-dimensi
stored volumes is a h
operation. Beginners v
and assisted education
with data acquisitio
manipulation, all of wh
three-dimensional ultrasound imaging.

*nancy, with dichorionic/
amniotic twins. (a) Membranes are clearly visible; (b)
chorionicity and amnionicity*

The main advantages of three-dimensional sonography in prenatal diagnosis are:

(1) Improved visualization and diagnosis: evaluation of image planes that cannot be obtained with conventional two-dimensional imaging, owing to anatomic constraints and/or fetal position;

(2) Easy demonstration of the coronal plane: this is the third plane, which cannot be displayed by conventional two-dimensional ultrasonography;

(3) Better recognition of the surface, minor defects related to fetal chromosomal disorders and realistic depiction of fetal surface anatomy;

(4) Transparent mode: new dynamic imaging of fetal skeletal elements;

(5) Improved orientation in the anatomic relationship by interactive rotation of volume-rendered images, particularly in cases of multiple and severe fetal malformations;

(6) Retrospective analysis, consultation and education.

References

1. Baba K, Satch K, Sakamoto S, Okal T, Shiego I. Development of an ultrasonic system for three dimensional reconstruction of the fetus. *J Perinat Med* 1989;17:19–24

2. Fredfelt KE, Holm HH, Pedersen JF. Three dimensional ultrasonic scanning. *Acta Radiol Diagn* 1984;25:237–40

3. Merz E, Bahlaman F, Weber G, Macchiella D.

Three dimensional ultrasonography in prenatal diagnosis. *J Perinat Med* 1995;23:213–22

4. Gregg A, Steiner H, Staudach A, Weiner CP. Accuracy of 3D sonographic volume measurements. *Am J Obstet Gynecol* 1993;168:348–55

5. Kossof G, Griffiths KA, Warren PS, *et al.* Three dimensional volume imaging in obstetrics. *Ultrasound Obstet Gynecol* 1994;4(Suppl 1) abstr 339

6. Kou HC, Chang FM, Wu CH, Yao BL, Liu CH. The primary application of three dimensional ultrasonography in obstetrics. *Am J Obstet Gynecol* 1992;166:880–6

7. Merz A, Macchiela D, Bahlamann F, Weber G. Three dimensional ultrasound for the diagnosis of fetal malformations. *Ultrasound Obstet Gynecol* 1992;2:137–45

8. Chiba Y, Hayashi K, Yamazaki S, Takamizawa K, Sasaki H. New techniques of ultrasound, thick slicing 3D imaging and the clinical aspects in the perinatal field. *Ultrasound Obstet Gynecol* 1994;4:(Suppl 1):abstr 337

9. Feichtinger W. Transvaginal three-dimensional imaging [Editorial]. *Ultrasound Obstet Gynecol* 1993;3:375–8

10. Baba K, Okai T. Clinical applications of three dimensional ultrasound in obstetrics. In Baba K, Jurkovic D, eds. *Three Dimensional Ultrasound in Obstetrics and Gynecology.* Carnforth, UK: Parthenon Publishing, 1997:29–44

11. Kirbach D, Whittingham TA. 3D ultrasound – the Kretz Voluson approach. *Eur J Ultrasound* 1994;1:85–9

12. Jurkovic D, Jauniaux E, Campbell S. Three dimensional ultrasound in obstetrics and gynecology. In Kurjak A, Chervenak F, eds. *The Fetus as a Patient.* Carnforth, UK: Parthenon Publishing, 1994:135–40

13. Merz E, Weber G, Bahlmann F, Mirić-Tešanić D. Application of transvaginal and transvaginal three dimensional ultrasound for the detection or exclusion of malformations of the fetal face. *Ultrasound Obstet Gynecol* 1997;9:237–43

14. Merz E, Bahlmann F, Weber G. Volume scanning in the evaluation of fetal malformations – a new dimension in prenatal diagnosis. *Ultrasound Obstet Gynecol* 1995;5:222–7

15. Liang RI, Huang SE, Chang FM. Prenatal diagnosis of ectopia cordis at 10 weeks of gestation using two-dimensional and three-dimensional ultrasonography. *Ultrasound Obstet Gynecol* 1997;10:137–9

16. Pretorius DH, Nelson RT. Fetal face visualisation using three dimensional ultrasonography. *J Ultrasound Med* 1995;14:349–56

17. Pretorius DH, House M, Nelson TR, *et al.* Evaluation of normal and abnormal lips in fetuses: comparison between three- and two-dimensional sonography. *Am J Roentgenol* 1995;165:1233–7

18. Pretorius DH, Nelson TR. Three dimensional ultrasound of fetal surface features. *Ultrasound Obstet Gynecol* 1992;2:166

19. Lee A, Deutinger J, Bernaschek G. Three dimensional ultrasound: abnormalities of the fetal face in surface and volume rendering mode. *Br J Obstet Gynaecol* 1995;102:40

20. Shih JC, Shy MK, Lee CN, Wu CH, Lin GJ, Hseih FJ. Antenatal depiction of the fetal ear with three dimensional ultrasound. *Obstet Gynecol* 1998;91:500–5

21. Shimizu T, Salvador L, Hughes-Benziee R, Dawson L, Nimrod C, Allanson J. The role of reduced ear size in the prenatal detection of chromosomal abnormalities. *Prenat Diagn* 1997;17:545–9

22. Sklansky MS, Nelson TR, Pretorius DH. Usefulness of gated three-dimensional fetal echocardiography to reconstruct and display structures not visualized with two-dimensional imaging. *Am J Cardiol* 1997;80:665–8

23. Leventhal M, Pretorius DH, Sklansky MS, Budorick NE, Nelson TR, Lou K. Three-dimensional ultrasound of the normal fetal heart: a comparison with two dimensional imaging. *J Ultrasound Med* 1998;17:341–8

24. Nelson TR, Pretorius DH, Sklansky M, Hagen-Ansert S. Three dimensional echocardiographic evaluation of fetal heart anatomy and function: acquisition, analysis and display. *J Ultrasound Med* 1996;15:1–9

25. Lee A, Deutinger J, Bernaschek G. Voluvision: three dimensional ultrasonography of fetal malformations. *Am J Obstet Gynecol* 1994;170:1312–14

26. Lee A, Kratochwil A, Deutinger J, Bernaschek G. Three-dimensional ultrasound in diagnosing phocomelia. *Ultrasound Obstet Gynecol* 1995;5:238–40

27. Ploeckinger-Ulm B, Ulm MR, Lee A, Kratochwil A, Bernaschek G. Antenatal depiction of fetal digits with three dimensional ultrasonography. *Am J Obstet Gynecol* 1996;175:571–4

28. Johnson DD, Pretorius DH, Riccabona M, Budirock NE, Nelson TR. Three dimensional ultrasound of fetal spine. *Obstet Gynecol* 1997;89:434–8

29. Riccabona M, Johnson D, Pretorius DH, Nelson TR. Three dimensional ultrasound: display modalities in the fetal spine and thorax. *Eur J Radiol* 1996;22:141–5

30. Maier B, Steiner H, Weinerroither F, Standach A. The psychological impact of three dimensional fetal imaging on the fetomaternal relationship. In Baba K, Jurkovic D, eds. *Three-dimensional Ultrasound in Obstetrics and Gynecology.* Carnforth, UK: Parthenon Publishing, 1997:67–73

31. Pretorius DH, Nelson TR. Three dimensional ultrasound [Opinion]. *Ultrasound Obstet Gynecol* 1995;5:219–21

Section 2

Advances in fetal diagnosis
and therapy

New insights into understanding fetomaternal tolerance

17

S. Hahn, M. R. Bürk, C. Troeger, S. Schatt and W. Holzgreve

INTRODUCTION

It is now close to 50 years since Sir Peter Medawar alluded to the 'immunological problem of pregnancy[1], and although the riddle of why the mother tolerates and nurtures an allogeneic body within her remains to be resolved, several aspects have been the subject of intense research of late. In this overview we focus on recent developments elucidating key facets of this complex issue and how they have helped to shape current thinking.

By pointing out the anatomical separation of maternal and fetal blood systems, Medawar helped to initiate a concept of immune privilege, a phenomenon whereby tissues grafted into certain sites were protected from rejection by lack of an immunological response. He proposed that the immune system remained ignorant of such antigens by being physically excluded from them. The nature of this shield, however, turned out to be more sophisticated than a simple blood–tissue barrier.

The fact that tissues from different individuals are 'not compatible' results mainly from the ability of T cells to discern self from non-self on the basis of the varying combinations of a large repertoire of different alleles of the major histocompatibility complex (MHC) expressed in an individual. MHC molecules that are recognized as non-self induce a potent immune response, leading to rejection of engrafted tissue.

As a first and simple protection of the fetus from maternal rejection, trophoblasts do not express classic MHC molecules (HLA-A or B), the major markers for 'foreign'. This is further backed up by mechanisms shared with two other classically immune privileged sites, the anterior chamber of the eye[2] and the testis[3]. Here it was demonstrated that the surface molecule, FasL, is constitutively expressed on the surface of parenchymal cells in the eye and Sertoli cells in the testis and induces apoptosis in potentially dangerous cells, such as activated T cells, expressing the Fas receptor.

FasL AND THE QUESTION OF IMMUNE PRIVILEGE

Fas (also termed Apo-1 or CD95) and its ligand, FasL, are important immune regulatory molecules. The apoptotic properties of Fas were independently discovered by the groups of Krammer and Yonehara, when they observed the lysis of certain tumors treated with antibodies to this antigen[4]. Fas was determined to be expressed on a variety of hemopoietic cells, in particular on activated B and T lymphocytes, whereas the cytolytic activity of CD4 and to a lesser extent of CD8 cytotoxic T cells was shown to be attributable to expression of the Fas ligand[5,6].

That Fas–FasL interactions play an important role in immunomodulation was underscored by the cloning of the murine counterparts by the laboratory of Nagata, where debilitating mutations in both the receptor and the ligand were found in the lymphoproliferative and autoimmune prone *lpr* and *gld* mice, respectively[7]. The functional importance of such ligand–receptor interactions in the normal immune response was illustrated by their participation in the elimination of unrequired antigen-presenting cells (B cells and macrophages)[6], the prevention of overt T-cell responses, either directly or by the phenomenon of activation-induced cell death[5,8], and in the induction of peripheral tolerance[4]. That this cytocidal system can be subverted in tumorigenic processes is evident from the detection of aberrant FasL expression in several tumors, including melanomas, colon carcinoma and experimentally derived mastocytomas[9,10], where it is hypothesized to enable the evasion and destruction of these malignant cells by killing tumor-specific immune effector cells.

Since both the placenta and the pregnant uterus have long being viewed as being immune privileged, the recent reports of FasL expression in these tissues is not entirely surprising[11,12]. In human placenta, FasL has been detected by Uckan and colleagues on both syncytiotrophoblast and extravillous trophoblast[12].

Although the most ready interpretation of placental FasL expression is that it prevents the trafficking of activated maternal or fetal lymphocytes across this barrier, it is likely that it has an additional more important function in the induction of maternal–fetal tolerance. Evidence supporting the operating of such a mechanism is provided by mice transgenic for a T-cell receptor specific for the male H-Y antigen[13]. A very strong antigen-specific decrease in these T cells was noted in mice pregnant with male fetuses, which was still evident postpartum, in a pattern strongly paralleling that observed in FasL-mediated elimination of superantigen-stimulated T cells.

This induction of peripheral tolerance is not restricted to FasL and pregnancy, but has also been observed following implants into the testis and by FasL-expressing tumors[14]. In the latter, an additional reduction of the anti-tumor B-cell response was found to occur, indicating the regulatory power of this mechanism.

Several lines of evidence, however, indicate that maternal tolerance of the developing fetus is more than the result of the elimination of maternal lymphocytes specific for fetal or paternal antigens by placental FasL expression: FasL is not an absolute requirement,

since FasL-impaired *gld* mice are fertile, albeit with a reduced litter size. FasL interactions are incapable of explaining the anti-fetal antigen-specific unresponsiveness exhibited by the peripheral T cells of pregnant animals[13], whereby allografts expressing fetal antigens are tolerated during pregnancy but rejected if implanted after parturition. It hence remains open to what extent this phenomenon is attributable to other mechanisms, such as the IDO system recently described by Munn and colleagues[15], discussed below, or the down-modulation of CD8 coreceptors, as observed by Tafuri and colleagues[16].

HLA-G, NK CELLS AND THE ABILITY OF FOREIGN TO BE RECOGNIZED AS SELF

Owing to the central importance of the MHC molecules for discerning self from non-self, it is not surprising that their expression is tightly regulated and controlled. The lytic activity of natural killer (NK) cells is activated when a lack of expression of MHC class 1 molecules is detected on a target cell[17]. This can occur either in virus-infected cells or in tumor cells, the classic target cells for NK cells, where HLA molecules are frequently down-regulated. In this model of 'missing self', NK recognition and activation via MHC class 1 is mediated via inhibitory receptors, termed killer cell inhibitory receptors (KIRs)[17]. Lack of occupation of such a receptor, by the absence of its HLA ligand, would trigger the cytolytic potential of these cells. An enigma that has been puzzling scientists in the field recently is how the HLA-negative trophoblast cells escape destruction by maternal NK cells.

Extravillous trophoblast cells have previously been determined not to express any of the classic MHC class 1 molecules, presumably to protect them from recognition and subsequent attack by maternal T lymphocytes as they invade the endometrium and later the decidua. Granted the activation of NK cells by lack of HLA expression, it was unclear how these fetal cells could evade attack by the numerous uterine NK cells (uNK, previously termed large granular

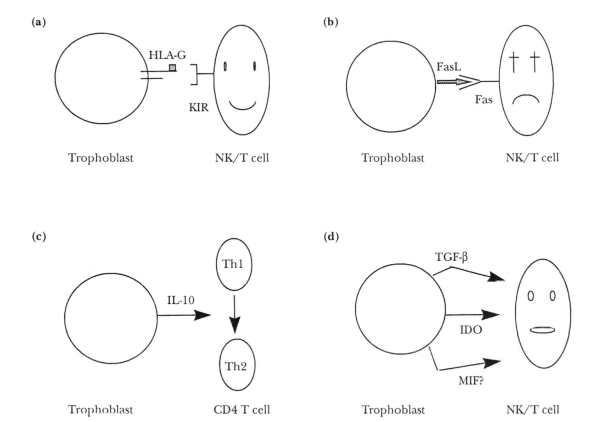

Figure 1 *Means by which fetal–maternal tolerance can be maintained. (a) Expression of non-polymorphic HLA-G by trophoblast cells suppresses the cytolytic activity of natural killer (NK) cells, which would normally kill these classically HLA-negative cells. (b) Expression of FasL by trophoblast cells eliminates activated immune effector cells by induction of apoptosis. (c) Trophoblast expression of Th1-suppressive cytokines, e.g. IL-10, promotes a shift to a Th2 phenotype. (d) T and NK cell activity is directly suppressed either by action of cytokines or by biochemical means*

lymphocytes, LGLs) present in the decidua. This issue has been resolved somewhat by the recent discovery that extra villous trophoblasts express HLA-G, a non-polymorphic HLA-A2-like (MHC) class 1B molecule[18]. First, the tightly regulated pattern of HLA-G expression, which is restricted to the HLA-A and -B negative extravillous trophoblasts and the thymus (discussed below), is highly suggestive that this molecule plays a role in maternal tolerance to the fetal semiallograft. Second, and more conclusively, NK target cells devoid of HLA expression were found to inhibit NK cytolytic activity when expressing a transfected HLA-G construct[19]. Additional attributes of this molecule include its non-polymorphic nature, which implies that it is recognized by a common KIR or KIR-like receptor. This

molecule would be presumed to be highly expressed on the uNK in the endometrium and decidua. Furthermore, HLA-G expression in the thymus means that T lymphocytes are tolerant to it, thereby ensuring that maternal T effector cells will not react against the placental barrier separating mother and fetus.

THE Th1–Th2 PARADIGM AND ITS INFLUENCE ON PREGNANCY OUTCOME

Perhaps the most controversial of the recent hypotheses proposed to account for feto-maternal tolerance is that put forward by the late Wegmann, where a shift in the immune response to a Th2 phenotype is required for successful pregnancy outcome[20]. It is likely that the close proximity to Mossman, a co-discoverer of the CD4 T helper subset phenotypes, was instrumental in the germination of this postulate.

CD4 T helper 1 (Th1) cells were initially characterized by the production of interleukin 2 (IL-2), interferon γ (IFN-γ) and tumor necrosis factor α (TNFα), which would activate a cell-mediated immune response, whereas CD4 T helper 2 (Th2) cells would promote a humoral immune response by the synthesis of interleukins 4, 5 and 10. Additionally, Th1 CD4 T cells have been shown to possess FasL-mediated cytolytic activity, which is lacking in their Th2 counterparts[5,8]. CD8 T cells tend to be mainly of a Th1 phenotype, which correlates well with their chiefly cytolytic activity, although the appearance of non-lytic IL-4-producing subtypes has been reported[5].

Controversial as it may be, several characteristic features of pregnancy can be explained by a shift in the immune response towards a Th2 phenotype, such as the diminished, even suppressed cell-mediated immune response discussed above, which contrasts strongly with the normal to vigorous humoral response[20]. Furthermore, prodigious production of the Th2-promoting cytokines, IL-4 and -5, and the Th1-suppressing cytokine IL-10, by the fetoplacental tissues is likely to tip the scales of the normal Th1–Th2 balance in the direction of Th2.

Since it has been difficult to demonstrate such a phenotypic shift during pregnancy *in vivo*, perhaps the most conclusive evidence is the apparent incompatibility of Th1-like activity with successful pregnancy outcome, as has been observed in both mice and humans. In the former, the injection of or the inflammatory induction of Th1 cytokines, IL-2, IFN-γ or TNFα in pregnant mice results in fetal loss[21]. In humans, the presence of IFN-γ or TNFα in the placenta has recently been observed in malarial infection during pregnancy, thereby strongly associating them with the poor pregnancy outcome, including fetal growth retardation, which occurs following this parasitic infection[21]. *In vitro* experiments suggest that a mechanism by which these cytokines negatively influence pregnancy may be by inhibiting trophoblast development and proliferation[22].

Taken together, these results suggest that inflammatory Th1 cytokines could be deleterious for implantation and fetal development, or, under extreme instances, even be pro-abortive.

INDOLEAMINE 2,3-DIOXYGENASE

Certainly no recent observation in this field has met with more media attention than the recent publication by Munn and colleagues[15], in which the entire question of maternal tolerance to fetal antigens was ascribed to the rudimentary biochemical requirement for an essential amino acid. The initial observation made by this group was that macrophages could induce T-cell tolerance by an indirect biochemical mechanism. By the release of the enzyme indoleamine 2,3-dioxygenase (IDO) which catabolizes tryptophan, macrophages deplete their surroundings of the essential amino acid, thereby starving attacking T cells rather than neutralizing them via a receptor-mediated signal transducing pathway. Since the enzyme is also reportedly expressed in human syncytiotrophoblast cells, the authors pursued this intriguing finding to examine the role of such catabolizing immune repression in pregnancy. In mice they made the stunning observation that the inhibition of this enzyme by a pharmacological inhibitor had an exceptionally strong abortive effect, leading to the reproducible loss of the entire litter when applied early during gestation. Closer examination revealed that the immune-suppressive effect of IDO appeared extensively to down-modulate CD8 T-cell activity. This was demonstrated by showing that fetal reduction mediated by the IDO inhibitor occurred only under conditions of MHC class 1 disparity, which would activate this class of T cells, leading to abortion, or when using adoptively transferred anti-fetal antigen-specific CD8 T cells. No effect was seen when using syngeneic mice or T-cell knock-out mice. Although these data again demonstrate the ability of the maternal immune system to recognize and react to a foreign fetal allogen, the mechanism whereby tolerance is achieved is indeed novel.

ARE THERE OTHER MODES OF TOLERANCE INDUCTION AT PLAY?

The placental barrier that separates mother and fetus is certainly one of the most complex biological systems, particularly from an immunological viewpoint. Recent research has indicated that several systems are involved in maintaining a truce between the maternal and fetal immune effector cells. These have also shown that these immune mediatory systems complement each other. Not expressing HLA-A or -B should make invading trophoblasts invisible to anti-allogeneic T cells, whereas FasL would function in eliminating such activated effector cells, should they arise. HLA-G may function to keep maternal NK cells in a non-cytolytic state. It is very likely that other systems play supplementary roles: for instance, in a shift from a mainly cytolytic Th1 to a mainly humoral Th2 immune response or by other means, such as the production of transforming growth factor β (TGF-β) by trophoblast cells, which has been shown to suppress NK cell activity.

It is also probable that many features may be shared between the various immune-privileged sites such as the testis, eye and placenta, and indeed tumors, which often subvert these mechanisms as means of immune evasion. In this manner, it is highly likely that the recent report that macrophage migration inhibitory factor (MIF) in the anterior chamber of the eye inhibits NK cell activity[23] may also function in the placenta.

ACKNOWLEDGEMENTS

This work was supported in part by Swiss National Science Foundation Grant Number 3200–047112.96, a Roche Research Fellowship (98–79) to M.R.B. and a grant of the German Foundation to C.T. (Tr 452/1–1).

References

1. Medawar P. Some immunological and endocrinological problems raised by the evolution of viviparity in vertebrates. *Symp Soc Exp Biol* 1953; 7:320–38
2. Griffith TS, Brunner T, Fletcher SM, Green DR, Ferguson TA. Fas ligand-induced apoptosis as a mechanism of immune privilege. *Science* 1995; 270:1189–92
3. Bellgrau D, Gold D, Selawry H, Moore J, Franzusoff A, Duke RC. A role for CD95 ligand in preventing graft rejection. *Nature (London)* 1995;377:630–2
4. Nagata S. Apoptosis by death factor. *Cell* 1997;88:355–65
5. Hahn S, Gehri R, Erb P. Mechanism and biological significance of CD4-mediated cytotoxicity. *Immunol Rev* 1995;146:57–79
6. Stalder T, Hahn S, Erb P. Fas antigen is the major target molecule for CD4+ T cell-mediated cytotoxicity. *J Immunol* 1994;152:1127–33
7. Nagata S, Suda T. Fas and Fas ligand: lpr and gld mutations. *Immunol Today* 1995;16:39–43
8. Hahn S, Stalder T, Wernli M, *et al.* Down-modulation of CD4+ T helper type 2 and type 0 cells by T helper type 1 cells via Fas/Fas-ligand interaction. *Eur J Immunol* 1995;25:2679–85
9. Hahne M, Rimoldi D, Schroter M, *et al.* Melanoma cell expression of Fas(Apo-1/CD95) ligand: implications for tumor immune escape. *Science* 1996;274:1363–6
10. Hahn S, Erb P. The immunomodulatory role of CD4-positive cytotoxic T-lymphocytes in health and disease. *Int Rev Immunol* 1999; in press
11. Hunt JS, Vassmer D, Ferguson TA, Miller L. Fas ligand is positioned in mouse uterus and placenta to prevent trafficking of activated leukocytes between the mother and the conceptus. *J Immunol* 1997;158:4122–8
12. Uckan D, Steel A, Cherry A, *et al.* Trophoblasts express Fas ligand: a proposed mechanism for immune privilege in placenta and maternal invasion. *Mol Hum Reprod* 1997;3:655–62
13. Jiang SP, Vacchio MS. Multiple mechanisms of peripheral T cell tolerance to the fetal 'allograft'. *J Immunol* 1998;160:3086–90
14. Griffith TS, Yu X, Herndon JM, Green DR, Ferguson TA. CD95-induced apoptosis of lymphocytes in an immune privileged site

induces immunological tolerance. *Immunity* 1996;5:7–16

15. Munn DH, Zhou M, Attwood JT, *et al.* Prevention of allogeneic fetal rejection by tryptophan catabolism. *Science* 1998;281:1191–3

16. Tafuri A, Alferink J, Möller P, Hämmerling G, Arnold B. T cell awareness of paternal allo-antigens during pregnancy. *Science* 1995;270:630–3

17. Ljunggren H, Kärre K. In search of 'missing self': MHC molecules and NK cell recognition. *Immunol Today* 1990;11:237–44

18. Kovats S, Main EK, Librach C, Stubbelbibe M, Fisher SJ, DeMars R. A class 1 antigen, HLA-G, expressed in human trophoblasts. *Science* 1990;248:220–3

19. Pazmany L, Mandelboim O, Vales Gomez M, Davis DM, Reyburn HT, Strominger JL. Protection from natural killer cell-mediated lysis by HLA-G expression on target cells. *Science* 1996;274:792–5

20. Wegmann TG, Lin H, Guilbert L, Mosmann TR. Bidirectional cytokine interactions in the maternal–fetal relationship: is successful pregnancy a TH2 phenomenon? *Immunol Today* 1993;14:353–6

21. Fried M, Muga RO, Misore AO, Duffy PE. Malaria elicits type 1 cytokines in the human placenta: IFN-gamma and TNF-alpha associated with pregnancy outcome. *J Immunol* 1998:160:2523–30

22. Raghupathy R. Th1-type immunity is incompatible with successful pregnancy. *Immunol Today* 1997;18:478–82

23. Apte R, Sinha D, Mayhew E, Wistow G, Niederkorn J. Role of macrophage migration inhibitory factor in inhibiting NK cell activity and preserving immune privilege. *J Immunol* 1998;160:5693–6

An update on chorionic villus sampling   18

Y. H. Yang and J. E. Chung

INTRODUCTION

Mid-trimester amniocentesis remains the most common technique for prenatal diagnosis, but, because of a growing awareness of the psychological effects and medical risks of second-trimester termination, the interest in chorionic villus sampling (CVS) as a rapid prenatal diagnostic technique has been renewed. Mohr[1] was the first to attain chorionic tissue via endoscopic biopsy; a tubular knife was inserted and used to cut off the tissue drawn in by suction. Using a modified endoscope, Hahnemann[2] reported a further series of transcervical biopsies. Without optical guidance, a group of Chinese investigators (Department of Obstetrics and Gynaecology, Tieutung Hospital, 1975) inserted a blunt metal cannula and aspirated chorionic villus for fetal sex determination. Researchers in the Soviet Union were the first to report success in placental biopsies using ultrasound guidance[3], and in 1983, Ward and colleagues[4] obtained chorionic villus under the guidance of real-time ultrasound with a plastic catheter, and reported a 90% sampling success rate. Simoni and co-workers[5] developed a process for the rapid and direct preparation of karyotypes. It was the recent development of ultrasonography and direct preparation of karyotypes from chorionic villus that enabled CVS to be used as a means of rapid prenatal diagnosis in early pregnancy. With the development of recombinant DNA technology and human gene mapping, CVS is also currently used for the prenatal diagnosis of Mendelian diseases and congenital metabolic disorders.

EMBRYOLOGY AND ANATOMY OF THE CHORIONIC VILLUS

The inner cell mass (ICM) and outer cell mass (OCM) can be distinguished, on day 4 following conception, in the late morula 32-cell stage. The ICM is composed of eight cells, and the OCM is composed of 24 cells. Two cells from the ICM are destined to be the embryo, and the remaining six cells are destined to be the extraembryonic tissue such as the yolk sac, chorion, amnion and the mesodermal core of the chorionic villus. The embryonic disc from the ICM is apparent by day 7 and it is composed of two layers: the epiblast and the hypoblast. The epiblast differentiates caudally into chorion and the mesodermal core of the chorionic villus. The OCM differentiates into trophoblasts, which are composed of an outer layer of syncytiotrophoblast and an inner layer of cytotrophoblast that overlies the mesodermal core. Four weeks after conception, chorionic villi have an outer layer of hormonally active and invasive syncytiotrophoblast, a middle layer of cytotrophoblast, from which syncytio-trophoblast is derived, and an inner mesodermal core containing blood capillaries for oxygen and nutrient exchange[6]. Nine weeks after conception, the chorionic villus actively differentiates to form the chorion frondosum, which is 1–1.5 cm thick, and this is destined to be the placenta. The mitotically active cytotrophoblast, which undergoes rapid differentiation, is taken for direct chromosome preparations[5], and the mesodermal core is used as the source of chromosomes derived by tissue culture[6–8]. The developing gestational sac in the period of 10–12 weeks' gestation only partially fills the uterine cavity, allowing safe transcervical passage of instruments into the chorion frondosum.

TECHNIQUES

Time

The ideal period for CVS is between 10 and 12 weeks after the last menstrual period, when the hyperechoic homogeneous area that represents the chorion frondosum can be easily detected by ultrasonography. If CVS is performed before this period, the incidence of fetal loss and fetal anomaly increases. If it is performed afterwards, the gestational sac will ultimately occupy the entire uterine cavity, blocking the transcervical passage of instruments and increasing the possibility of amniotic membranes rupture. Although CVS is commonly performed in the first trimester (early CVS), Holzgreve and co-workers[9] proposed placental biopsy (late CVS) in the second and third trimesters in high-risk pregnancies.

Role of ultrasonography

Before performing CVS, a detailed ultrasonographic examination confirming the existence of fetal anomaly, missed abortion, multiple gestation and gestational weeks should be checked. During the procedure, the CVS catheter is guided to the chorionic frondosum where the umbilical cord inserts and appears as a hyperechoic homogeneous area ultrasonographically. After CVS, fetal viability as well as complications such as fetal death and subchorionic hematoma should be identified. The patient should be followed up for the detection of fetal anomaly and fetal growth restriction.

Transcervical chorionic villus sampling

The patient is placed in the lithotomy position. The vulva, vagina and cervix are aseptically prepared, and this is followed by speculum insertion. The CVS catheter is made of plastic with a central metal stylet. In the USA, a Portex catheter is commonly used, whereas in Europe, an Angiomed echogenic catheter is popularly used[10]. The CVS catheter should be bent according to the uterine curvature, and under ultrasonographic guidance the tip of the CVS catheter should be identified and directed to the chorion frondosum until resistance can be felt. After the chorionic frondosum is reached, the stylet is removed and a syringe filled with medium is attached. Negative pressure is applied through the syringe as the catheter and the attached syringe are slowly withdrawn (Figure 1). The obtained material should be put in a Petri dish for observation of the chorionic villi with their distinctive branched appearance. The mitotically active cytotrophoblastic buds are used for rapid direct karyotyping (short-term culture), whereas the mesenchymal core is used for tissue culture (long-term culture). Compared to the chorionic villus, the decidua that is derived from the maternal tissue appears to be more sheet-like and less vascular. Immediate separation of decidua from chorionic villi is recommended to avoid maternal cell contamination.

Transabdominal chorionic villus sampling

After 9 weeks' gestation, the uterine fundus is placed under the peritoneum so that the uterus can be approached without passing the bladder or intestine. Transabdominal CVS is carried out in two ways: the double needle technique[11] and the single needle technique[12] (Figure 1). Placental biopsy (late CVS) was performed by Holzgreve and associates[9] in the second or third trimester for the confirmation of abnormal results after early CVS or amniocentesis, suspicious ultrasound findings and unsuccessful amniotic fluid cell culture. Since the results of karyotyping can be obtained rapidly and its safety has been confirmed, with low complication and low spontaneous abortion rates after 12 gestational weeks, transabdominal CVS in the second trimester can also serve as a valuable alternative to early and mid-trimester amniocentesis[7].

Transcervical vs. transabdominal chorionic villus sampling

The overall sampling success rate in the study by Yang and colleagues[8] was 98.0%. According

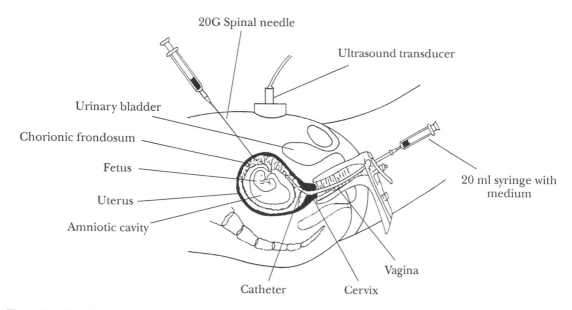

20G Spinal needle

Ultrasound transducer

Urinary bladder

Chorionic frondosum

Fetus

Uterus

Amniotic cavity

20 ml syringe with medium

Vagina

Catheter   Cervix

Figure 1   *Technique of ultrasonography-guided transcervical and transabdominal chorionic villus sampling*

to Brambati and associates[7], the sampling success rate for both transabominal and transcervical CVS by the second insertion was 99.8% and 99.2%, respectively. Some authors have observed a higher rate of bleeding, infection, fetal loss and maternal cell contamination in transcervical compared to transabdominal CVS[13,14]. Brambati and co-workers[7] chose transabdominal CVS because it succeeded in a higher number of cases at the first insertion (98% vs. 86.8%) and was associated with small samples (< 10 mg) in fewer cases (3.2% vs. 4.9%). The practitioner should be very familiar with both sampling techniques and apply the appropriate one according to the patient.

Transvaginal chorionic villus sampling

For the patient with a posterior placenta on a retroverted uterus with a cervical canal pointed anteriorly towards the mother's abdomen, transvaginal CVS is used; here, the biopsy needle is inserted through the cul-de-sac, as in culdocentesis.

Chorionic villus sampling in twin pregnancy

With the recent development of assisted reproduction techniques, the rate of twin pregnancy has increased, and as the advanced maternal age group has increased, the need for chromosomal analysis in twin pregnancy has also increased concomitantly. In the first trimester, the zygocity is easier to identify, selective reduction is possible and pregnancy termination is safer and more easily done. The accurate identification of the placental site is necessary for the recognition of twin status. If only one placenta exists, the biopsy should be performed in the nearest insertion site to the umbilical cord. A transcervical approach may cause sample contamination of the placental tissues, so a repeated transcervical approach should be avoided. A repeated transabdominal approach or a combination of transcervical and transabdominal approaches is recommended for CVS of twin pregnancy[15].

INDICATIONS

Cytogenetic analysis

Both short-term (direct preparation) and long-term culture methods are used for chromosomal analysis. The most common indication in CVS is maternal age over 35 years, previous birth with chromosomal anomaly, previous birth with congenital anomaly, perinatal death from unknown cause and a family history of anomalous birth[7,8,16,17].

DNA analysis

The obtained chorionic villi from CVS are used for DNA analysis by recombinant DNA technology for the detection of abnormalities at the gene level. Therefore, the chorionic villus is the sample to be studied in the prenatal diagnosis of Mendelian diseases such as thalassemia, Duchenne/Becker muscular dystrophy, hemophilia A/B and cystic fibrosis[7].

Enzyme analysis

Diseases due to abnormal enzyme activities, such as mucopolysaccharidosis, lipidosis, amino acid disorders, carbohydrate metabolism disorders and congenital adrenal hyperplasias, can also be detected by CVS[7].

CONTRAINDICATIONS

CVS is not performed in cases of missed abortion, before 9 gestational weeks, or in mothers with a previous history of neural tube defect, because this cannot be diagnosed using CVS. In the presence of uterine contractions, one should wait for the contractions to dissipate. The CVS catheter insertion is much more difficult in patients who have vaginismus, cervical stenosis or leiomyoma in the lower uterine segment, or who have previously undergone cryosurgery or cone biopsy, so the practitioner should be particularly careful in inserting the CVS catheter. Spontaneous abortion is possible when the patient has vaginal bleeding, so the procedure must be done at some other time or another method must be used. In the presence of vaginal infection, ascending infection is possible; therefore, a transcervical approach is not appropriate. The possibility of worsening rhesus isoimmunization in sensitized women is also a concern, since small transplacental hemorrhages caused by CVS may be sufficient to worsen the existing rhesus immunization, so CVS for these women is contraindicated[7,10,18].

SAFETY AND EFFICACY

The evaluation of safety in CVS has focused on the fetal loss rate, particularly on the spontaneous abortion rate after the adjustment of background loss. The safety of CVS as a first-trimester diagnostic procedure has been demonstrated in many studies, in which the mean spontaneous abortion rate was 4.1%[16,17,19], whereas Yang and colleagues[8] and Brambati and co-workers[7] reported the total fetal loss rate to be below 3%. The American collaborative report by Rhoads and colleagues[17] and the Canadian Collaborative Group[16] compared the results of amniocentesis with CVS, and no statistical differences were found in the rates of preterm birth, low birth weight or maternal complications. The factors compromising safety were the performing doctor's skill, maternal age, weeks of gestation, types of method and the frequency of catheter insertion.

The cytogenic analysis accuracy rate in previously published studies between 1988 and 1996 ranged from 97.5% to 99.7%[8,16,17,19], whereas in the latest report from Brambati and associates[7] (1998) it was 99.4%. As for the factors compromising efficacy, maternal cell contamination, placental mosaicism and the availability of a laboratory can be considered. The maternal cell contamination rate due to decidua was 1.9–3.8%[20,21], which was slightly higher with the transcervical approach.

The direct preparation of chorionic villi can avoid maternal cell contamination by decidua, while the culture of chorionic villi has a possibility of maternal cell contamination, but differentiation between the two is not difficult and false reports are rare. Another factor compromising the efficacy is placental mosaicism. Chromosomal mosaicism confined to the placenta in human conceptions was initially reported by Kalousek and Dill[22]. After that, placental mosaicism with a normal fetus was demonstrated; from a clinical standpoint, the interpretation of those cases was very confusing. In the Canadian

Collaborative Group[16] and the American collaborative report by Rhoads and associates[17], 0.6–0.8% of chorionic villus samples demonstrated mosaicism, but approximately three-quarters of follow-up analyses resulted in normal fetal karyotypes. Vejerslev and Mikkelsen[23] studied 11 000 specimens in which 1.3% of cases showed mosaicism, but about 70% of the mosaics were restricted to extraembryonic tissue. Brambati and colleagues[7] also reported mosaicism or rare trisomies in 1.3% of 10 000 specimens. The possible mechanism of placental mosaicism can be explained by the predominance of postzygotic non-disjunction limited to cytotrophoblast, because the majority of blastomeres in the early morula stage are destined for trophoblast formation, thereby affording more opportunities for postzygotic non-disjunction to occur[6]. In cases with placental mosaicism, mid-trimester amniocentesis should be offered, to confirm the fetal karyotype. In no case should a decision to terminate a pregnancy be based entirely on a CVS mosaic result.

COMPLICATIONS

Bleeding

After a transcervical CVS, vaginal bleeding or spotting occurs in 15–25% of patients, appearing a few hours after the procedure, but heavy bleeding is unusual. When severe vaginal bleeding occurs, it is mostly from damage to vessels in the decidua basalis underlying the chorion frondosum. Subchorionic hematoma can be observed after CVS, but most disappear spontaneously by 16 weeks of gestation, and are rarely associated with poor perinatal outcome[24].

Infection

When a transcervical approach is used, there is a possibility of ascending infection, and a 0.14% intrauterine infection rate has been reported[7]. No specific causative microorganism has been identified and prophylactic antibiotics have been of no use.

With a transabdominal approach, localized peritonitis is possible, but this usually heals without trouble. However, there is always a possibility of intestinal perforation and excessive bleeding during the CVS catheter insertion[25].

Fetomaternal transfusion

CVS is performed after fetomaternal circulation has occurred; therefore, when performing the test, fetal blood leakage is possible and the level of maternal serum α-fetoprotein may rise from 40% to 70%[10]. The frequency of catheter reinsertion and the amount of villi sampled may have a role in fetomaternal transfusion[10,18]. For the above reasons, rhesus-negative mothers who have not been sensitized should receive immunoglobulin. Mothers who have been sensitized should not undergo CVS because a boost in antibody reaction may result in fetal hemolysis.

Malformation

In 1991, Firth and colleagues[26] initially reported severe limb abnormalities in cases of CVS carried out before 9 weeks of gestation, and following this report, some reported a fetal malformation rate up to ten times higher than in the normal population[27]. In contrast, a collaborative USA study[17] and follow-up studies done by the WHO Registry[28] have reported no difference in digital deficiency between CVS and normal pregnancy groups. In a recent study by Brambati and colleagues[7], the fetal congenital malformation rate in CVS cases was 1.96%, and no statistical difference was found from the general Italian population included in the national hospital-based registry, with a rate of 1.9%. No increase in the frequency of transverse limb reduction defect was apparent in CVS carried out beyond 9 gestational weeks[7].

CONCLUSIONS

Early CVS performed at the proper time by experienced physicians and at the proper facility can be assumed to have no adverse effect on pregnancy. Late CVS (placental biopsies) carried out during the second or third trimester has also proven to be safe and efficient. Therefore, CVS can be considered as a valuable alternative to early and mid-trimester amniocentesis. In the future, with the progression of recently developed recombinant DNA technology, human gene mapping and other newly studied techniques, CVS may greatly contribute to prenatal genetic diagnosis.

References

1. Mohr J. Foetal genetic diagnosis: development of techniques for early sampling of foetal cells. *Acta Pathol Microbiol Scand* 1968;73:7377

2. Hahnemann N. Early prenatal diagnosis: a study of biopsy techniques and cell culturing from extraembryonic membranes. *Clin Genet* 1974;6: 294–306

3. Kazy Z, Rozovsky IS, Bakharev VA. Chorion biopsy in early pregnancy: a method of early prenatal diagnosis for inherited disorders. *Prenat Diagn* 1982;2:39–40

4. Ward RHT, Modell B, Petrou M, Karagozlu F, Ddouratos E. Method of sampling chorionic villi in first trimester of pregnancy under guidance of real time ultrasound. *Br Med J* 1983;286: 1542–4

5. Simoni G, Brambati B, Danesino C, *et al.* Efficient direct chromosome analysis and enzyme determinations from chorionic villi samples in the first trimester of pregnancy. *Hum Genet* 1983;63:349–57

6. Crane JP, Cheung SW. An embryogenic model to explain cytogenetic inconsistencies observed in chorionic villus versus fetal tissue. *Prenat Diagn* 1988;8:119–29

7. Brambati B, Tului L, Cislaghi C, Alberti E. First 10,000 chorionic villus samplings performed on singleton pregnancies by a single operator. *Prenat Diagn* 1998;18:255–66

8. Yang YH, Park YW, Kim SK, *et al.* Chorionic villus sampling: clinical experience of the initial 750 cases. *J Obstet Gynecol Res* 1996;22:143–9

9. Holzgreve W, Miny P, Gerlach B, Westendorp A, Ahlert D, Horst J. Benefits of placental biopsies for rapid karyotyping in the second and third trimesters (late chorionic villus sampling) in high-risk pregnancie. *Am J Obstet Gynecol* 1990; 162:1188–92

10. Holzgreve VW, Miny P. *Chorionzotten-diagnostik.* Weinheim, Germany: VCH, 1987:18–21,120–3

11. Smith-Jensen S, Hahnemann N. Transabdominal chorionic villi sampling for fetal genetic diagnosis: technical and obstetric evaluation of 100 cases. *Prenat Diagn* 1988;8:7

12. Brambati B, Oldrini A, Lanzani A. Transabdominal chorionic villus sampling: a free hand ultrasound-guided technique. *Am J Obstet Gynecol* 1987;157:134–7

13. Chueh JT, Goldberg JD, Wohlferd MM, Golbus MS. Comparison of transcervical and transabdominal chorionic villus sampling loss rates in 9000 cases from a single center. *Am J Obstet Gynecol* 1995;173:1277

14. Jackson LG, Zachary JM, Fowler SE, *et al.* Randomized comparison of transcervical and transabdominal chorionic villus sampling. *N Engl J Med* 1992;327:594–8

15. Catte LD, Liebaers I, Foulon W, Bonduelle M, Assche EV. First trimester chorionic villus sampling in twin gestations. *Am J Perinat* 1996;13: 413–17

16. Canadian Collaborative CVS–Amniocentesis Clinial Trial Group. Multicentre randomized clinical trial of chorionic villus sampling and amniocentesis. *Lancet* 1989;1:1–6

17. Rhoads GG, Jackson LG, Schlesselman SA, Desnick RJ, Golbus MS. The safety and efficacy of chorionic villus sampling for early prenatal diagnosis of cytogenetic abnormalities. *N Engl J Med* 1989;320:609–17

18. Yang YH, Lee MS, Park YW, *et al.* Studies on the prenatal chromosomal analysis and the changes of maternal serum alpha-fetoprotein following chorionic villi sampling. *Yonsei Med J* 1991;32:292–302

19. Ward RHT, Petrou M, Modell BM, Knott PD, Maxwell D, Hooker JG. Chorionic villus sampling in a high-risk population: 4 years experience. *Br J Obstet Gynaecol* 1988;95:1030–5

20. Ledbetter DH, Zachary JM, Simpson JL. Cytogenetic results from the U.S. collaborative study on CVS. *Prenat Diag* 1992;12:317–45

21. Lippman A, Tomkins DT, Shine J, Hamerton JL, and the Canadian Collaborative CVS–amniocentesis Clinical Trial Group. Canadian multicentre randomized clinical trial of chorion villus sampling and amniocentesis: final report. *Prenat Diagn* 1992;12:385–467

22. Kalousek D, Dill F. Chromosomal mosaicism confined to the placenta in human conceptions. *Science* 1983;221:665–7

23. Vejerslev LO, Mikkelsen M. The European collaborative study on mosaicism in chorionic villus sampling: data from 1986 to 1987. *Prenat Diagn* 1989;9:575–88

24. Brambati B, Oldrini A, Ferrazzi E, Ianzani A. Chorionic villus sampling: an analysis of the obstetrics experience of 1000 cases. *Prenat Diagn* 1987;7:157–69

25. Brambati B, Martarrelli M, Varotto F. Septic complications after chorionic villus sampling. *Lancet* 1987;1:1212–13

26. Firth HV, Boyd PA, Chamberain P. Analysis of limb reduction defects in babies exposed to chorion villi sampling. *Lancet* 1994;343:1069–71

27. Hsieh FJ, Shyu MK, Sher BC, Lin SP, Chen CP, Huang FY. Limb defects after chorionic villus sampling. *Obstet Gynecol* 1995;85:84–8

28. World Health Organization. *Chorionic Villus Sampling Safety.* Document EUR/ICP/MCH 123A. Copenhagen: WHO Regional Office for Europe, 1994

Prenatal diagnosis of hemoglobinopathies

19

S. T. Chasen

Hemoglobinopathies, the quantitative or qualitative alteration of the globin chains, are among the most common genetic disorders worldwide. They are typically inherited in an autosomal recessive fashion from parents who are healthy carriers, although transmission from affected parents does occur. Recently, it has been estimated that there are over 250 million carriers of hemoglobinopathy traits worldwide (4.5% of the world population), and over 300 000 affected newborns annually[1].

Sickle cell disorders and the thalassemias are the most common hemoglobinopathies. Although these hereditary anemias were initially confined to the tropics and subtropics, population migration has caused these hemoglobinopathies to appear worldwide[1]. Consequently, there are very few obstetricians who will not encounter patients who are at risk of transmitting these disorders. Hemoglobinopathies are well suited for prenatal screening, and a basic understanding of the pathophysiology and genetics of these disorders is important.

Hemoglobin, which is found in red blood cells, absorbs oxygen from the lungs, transfers it to tissues, and returns carbon dioxide to the lungs. The hemoglobin molecule is a tetramer of globin chains, each covalently bonded to a heme moiety. The heme moiety consists of an iron atom centrally placed in a protoporphyrin ring.

The globin component in the normal adult consists of two α-globin chains and two β-type globin chains. There are 141 amino acid residues in the α-chains, and 146 amino acid residues in the β-type chains. In normal adults, about 97% of hemoglobin is hemoglobin A_1 $(\alpha_2\beta_2)$. The remainder is hemoglobin A_2 $(\alpha_2\delta_2)$ and hemoglobin F $(\alpha_2\gamma_2)$, or fetal hemoglobin.

Hemoglobinopathies result from either reduced production of globin chains or production of abnormal globin chains. In the sickle cell disorders, mutations in the genes coding for β-globin chains lead to amino acid substitutions in the β-globin chains. This leads to hemoglobin molecules with abnormal configurations and reduced oxygen-carrying capacity. In the thalassemias, reduced globin chain production is the result of either gene deletions or mutations.

Table 1 *Compound heterozygous conditions associated with clinically significant hemoglobinopathies*

Hemoglobin SC
Hemoglobin SD
Hemoglobin SO^{ARAB}
Hemoglobin S-β-thalassemia
Hemoglobin E-β-thalassemia

SICKLING DISORDERS

Sickle cell disease is caused by the presence of mutations in both genes, located on the short arm of chromosome 11. Classical sickle cell disease is the homozygous presence of the substitution of valine for glutamic acid, resulting in hemoglobin SS. Other amino acid substitutions can lead to hemoglobin C, D, or O^{ARAB}, all of which can lead to a clinically significant compound-heterozygous state when inherited in conjunction with hemoglobin S (Table 1). When the hemoglobin S gene is inherited with a gene for β-thalassemia, sickle-thalassemia, a moderate-to-severe hemolytic anemia, is the result.

These amino acid substitutions cause the red blood cell to take an elongated form when lowered oxygen tension, dehydration, or acidosis is present. The altered configuration of the red blood cell causes a loss of flexibility, and clinical manifestations of sickle cell disease are due to vaso-occlusion and hemolytic anemia. The life expectancy is reduced, although there may be marked clinical heterogeneity among affected patients.

In general, compound heterozygotes (hemoglobin SC, SD, or SO[ARAB]) have milder forms of disease and may be asymptomatic. They may, however, have disease as severe as those homozygous for hemoglobin S. It should be noted that these mutations other than hemoglobin S are clinically significant only when inherited with hemoglobin S; those who are homozygous for these mutations are clinically asymptomatic.

Sickle cell disease is most common in Africa, with the carrier frequency for hemoglobin S as high as 25% in certain populations. In the USA the carrier frequency among those of African descent is approximately 8–10% for hemoglobin S and 2.5% for hemoglobin C[2]. Sickle cell disease is seen to a lesser extent in those of Mediterranean, Indian, Caribbean, Latin American and Middle Eastern descent.

Carriers of hemoglobin S may be detected by hemoglobin electrophoresis, peripheral smear, or solubility testing[3]. Hemoglobin electrophoresis involves the separation of different hemoglobins on cellulose acetate at an alkaline pH, with citrate agar at an acid pH used for confirmation. Carriers typically have 30–40% hemoglobin S on hemoglobin electrophoresis. On peripheral smear, sickled cells, target cells, basophilic stippling and nucleated red blood cells are seen. Solubility testing involves mixing a drop of peripheral blood with a reducing agent; under microscopy, sickle cells are seen. While any of these methods will detect carriers of hemoglobin S, only hemoglobin electrophoresis will diagnose carriers of other hemoglobin variants such as hemoglobin C, D, or O[ARAB] [4].

α-THALASSEMIA

α-Thalassemia is almost always caused by deletions in the gene on the short arm of chromosome 16 which codes for the α-globin gene. There are two genes on each chromosome, so a normal person has four genes coding for the α-globin chain. Those with gene deletions will make reduced amounts of α-globin, leading to decreased hemoglobin per red blood cell. The relative excess of β-chains will lead to the formation of β-tetramers, which transport oxygen poorly.

A person missing one gene will be a 'silent carrier', with normal hematological parameters. Those with two genes deleted will have a mild microcytic anemia. Those with three genes deleted will have an accumulation of β-tetramers, known as hemoglobin H. Hemoglobin H disease is a moderate-to-severe hemolytic anemia. When all four genes are deleted, severe intrauterine anemia will result, since no α-chains will be available to form fetal hemoglobin ($\alpha_2\gamma_2$). There is an accumulation of γ-tetramers, known as Bart's hemoglobin. This condition results in hydrops fetalis or early neonatal demise (Table 2).

The two-gene deletion associated with hemoglobin H disease or hydrops fetalis is almost exclusively seen among Southeast Asians. The single-gene deletion is seen in Southeast Asians, those of Mediterranean or African descent and Sephardic Jews.

Carrier screening for α-thalassemia is done with red blood cell indices. Carriers will generally have microcytosis, with a mean corpuscular volume (MCV) below 80 fl. Hemoglobin electrophoresis is usually normal in carriers of α-thalassemia. When a microcytic anemia is present in the absence of iron deficiency or other identifiable causes, α-thalassemia should be suspected. Confirmation is by DNA analysis[5-7].

β-THALASSEMIA

β-Thalassemia is usually caused by mutations in the genes on the short arm of chromosome 11 which code for β-globin chains. Mutations in these genes lead to errors in transcription

Table 2 *Characteristics of α- and β-thalassemia*

Condition	Hemoglobin electrophoresis	Population at risk	Clinical severity
Homozygotes			
α-Thalassemia (4 α-gene deletion)	hemoglobin Bart	Southeast Asian Mediterranean (rare)	hydrops fetalis
β$^+$-Thalassemia (β-globin chain ↓ 50–75%)	↑ hemoglobin A$_2$ (variable) ↑↑ fetal hemoglobin	Mediterranean, Middle Eastern, Indian, Southeast Asian, African	moderate-to-severe anemia
β^0-Thalassemia (β-globin chains absent)	no hemoglobin A$_1$ ↑ hemoglobin A$_2$ (variable) ↑↑↑ fetal hemoglobin	Mediterranean, Middle Eastern, Indian, Southeast Asian, African	severe anemia, transfusion, dependency, skeletal deformities, chronic organ damage
Heterozygotes			
α-Thalassemia trait (1 α-gene deletion)	normal	Southeast Asian, Mediterranean African, Sephardic Jews	silent carrier
α-Thalassemia trait (2 α-gene deletions)	normal	Southeast Asian, Mediterranean African, Sephardic Jews	mild anemia
Hemoglobin H disease (3 α-gene deletions)	hemoglobin H	Southeast Asian, Mediterranean (rare)	moderate anemia
β-Thalassemia trait (β-globin chain ↓ 25–50%)	hemoglobin A$_2$ > 3.5% ↑ fetal hemoglobin	Mediterranean, Middle Eastern, Indian, Southeast Asian, African	mild anemia

of RNA, which lead to decreased or absent production of β-globin. Deficiencies in β-globin chains cause compensatory increases in other β-type globin chains, such as δ-globin or γ-globin. Thus, while a deficiency in β-globin chains causes reduced production of hemoglobin A$_1$, an increase in hemoglobin A$_2$ ($α_2δ_2$) and fetal hemoglobin ($α_2γ_2$) can be seen. With decreased β-globin production, an accumulation of α-globin chains takes place. This is highly toxic to red blood cells, and leads to ineffective erythropoiesis and decreased survival of red blood cells.

As in α-thalassemia, reduced β-globin production causes reduced amounts of hemoglobin and a microcytic anemia. There are important differences, however. Unlike α-thalassemia, clinical manifestations of β-thalassemia are not apparent until several months after birth, as fetal hemoglobin is the predominant hemoglobin in the intrauterine and neonatal periods. Another important difference is that there will be increased amounts of hemoglobin A$_2$ and fetal hemoglobin F in those with β-thalassemia. Thus, even in Cooley's anemia, the severest form of β-thalassemia in which there is little or no hemoglobin A$_1$ production, compensatory increases in hemoglobin A$_2$ and fetal hemoglobin can modify the severity of the disease.

The severity of disease in β-thalassemia reflects the degree of β-globin chain deficiency. Those who are heterozygous for a mutation causing diminished but not absent β-globin production (β$^+$) are silent carriers, and may have only microcytosis and a mild anemia, as well as a slight increase in hemoglobin A_2 on hemoglobin electrophoresis. Those who are heterozygous for a mutation causing absent β-globin chain production ($β^0$) or homozygous for $β^+$ generally have more significant microcytosis and anemia, and increases in fetal hemoglobin as well as hemoglobin A_2 are seen on hemoglobin electrophoresis. Those who are homozygous for $β^0$ or inherit one $β^+$ and one $β^0$ will have more severe disease, and may be transfusion dependent. Other clinical manifestations of severe disease include skeletal abnormalities, hepatosplenomegaly and chronic organ damage from iron overload. These patients will have predominantly fetal hemoglobin on hemoglobin electrophoresis (Table 2).

β-Thalassemia is seen in those of Mediterranean, Middle Eastern, Indian, Pakistani, Southeast Asian, or Northern African descent. As in α-thalassemia, carrier screening is done with red blood cell indices. Carriers typically have a mild microcytic anemia. Unlike in α-thalassemia carriers, however, abnormalities such as elevated hemoglobin A_2 or fetal hemoglobin levels may be seen on hemoglobin electrophoresis[5,7].

It must be noted that all the clinical manifestations seen in β-thalassemia can be present in those who are compound heterozygotes for β-thalassemia and hemoglobin E. Hemoglobin E is caused by a mutation in the gene coding for β-globin chains, and results in an amino acid substitution of lysine for glutamic acid in the 26th position. It is the second most common hemoglobin variant worldwide, and it occurs frequently in the Southeast Asian population. Those who are heterozygous or homozygous for this mutation generally have no clinical manifestations, though they may have mild microcytosis[8].

PRENATAL DIAGNOSIS

In couples who are both carriers for a hemoglobinopathy trait that could result in an affected child, prenatal diagnosis is an option. Initially, fetal blood cells, obtained through either placental aspiration or cordocentesis, were necessary for the prenatal diagnosis of hemoglobinopathies. Fetal blood would be studied for the presence or absence of adult globin chains, which are present in small amounts in the second trimester[9-11].

Advances in molecular genetics have made the prenatal diagnosis of hemoglobinopathies easier. As the DNA mutations responsible for globin chain abnormalities were identified, prenatal diagnosis could be based on DNA analysis. The advent of the polymerase chain reaction has enabled DNA mutation analysis to be carried out expediently with relatively few fetal cells. Thus, chorionic villi and amniocytes, as well as fetal blood, can be used[12].

In the future, the prenatal diagnosis of hemoglobinopathies may be achieved with less invasive techniques than amniocentesis, chorionic villus sampling or cordocentesis, which carry a small but tangible risk of fetal loss. Trophoblast cells can be recovered from cervical mucus; in couples at risk for having a child with a hemoglobinopathy who underwent cervical mucus aspiration followed by chorionic villus sampling, concordant results were seen in a majority of cases in one small series[13]. There is also a small amount of fetal blood cells present in the maternal circulation. Techniques involving magnetic cell sorting and microdissection have enabled some investigators to isolate fetal erythroblasts, and identify point mutations in single gene disorders, including sickle cell disease and β-thalassemia[14].

HEMOGLOBINOPATHY SCREENING IN PREGNANCY

The majority of patients who transmit abnormal hemoglobin genes are asymptomatic carriers. Because prenatal diagnosis is available, it is important for the obstetrician to identify those who are at risk.

Different strategies for screening for hemoglobinopathy traits in pregnancy have been proposed. One strategy involves red blood cell indices on all patients and hemoglobin electrophoresis screening in those considered at risk[15]. Because solubility testing does not identify carriers of abnormal hemoglobins such as C, D, E, or O, which could result in a compound heterozygous state if inherited with a hemoglobin S gene (SC, SD, SO) or a β-thalassemia gene (β-thalassemia-E), this approach will identify more pregnancies at risk[16–18]. Although hemoglobin electrophoresis is more expensive than solubility testing, screening would not have to be repeated in subsequent pregnancies.

One recent study sought to determine which patients with abnormal hemoglobins would not have been identified if a screening protocol involving selective rather than universal hemoglobin electrophoresis had been used. In this population, 1% were carriers of hemoglobin C, D, or E, and two-thirds of these patients had normal red blood cell indices. These patients would not have been identified if they had been screened with red blood cell indices and solubility testing[19].

An alternative strategy relies on red blood cell indices in all patients and sickle solubility testing in those at risk for sickling disorders[20]. This strategy will identify those who carry genes for thalassemia as well as carriers of hemoglobin S. Proponents of this strategy cite the lower cost of solubility testing compared with electrophoresis, and the relatively low number of fetuses at risk for a hemoglobinopathy who would not be identified with this protocol. The relatively low risk of acceptance of prenatal diagnosis in those at risk and the institution of routine neonatal screening are other factors that may argue against using hemoglobin electrophoresis as the primary mode of screening in pregnancy[21,22].

Protocols that put on the obstetrician the burden of identifying couples who are 'at risk' are problematic. Because of large population migrations and mixing of different ethnic groups, this is becoming increasingly difficult[1,15]. Indeed, one large study in which hemoglobin electrophoresis was routinely performed on all pregnant women found that 7% of those with sickle cell trait were not black, and 22% of β-thalassemia carriers were not Mediterranean, Asian, or black[16]. Therefore, screening of all women, not just those considered 'at risk' because of a patient's stated ethnic group, may be indicated.

When a patient who is a carrier of an abnormal hemoglobin gene is identified, the partner must be tested. Importantly, the partner must not only be screened for the presence of the abnormal gene identified in the mother. The partner should have red blood cell indices as well as hemoglobin electrophoresis, to identify those fetuses at risk for compound heterozygous conditions. For instance, in a woman identified as a carrier of hemoglobin S, it would be inappropriate to perform only sickle solubility testing in her partner. He must undergo hemoglobin electrophoresis as well as red blood cell indices to exclude the possibility that he is a carrier of hemoglobin C, D, O^{ARAB} or β-thalassemia, as well as hemoglobin S.

Unfortunately, it is not uncommon for a partner to be unable or unwilling to be tested after the mother is identified as a carrier of a hemoglobinopathy trait. In these situations, the option of prenatal diagnosis should still be available to the patient. For example, if a woman is a carrier of hemoglobin S, and her partner is black, there is approximately a 10% chance that he is a carrier of hemoglobin S (or another β-chain variant). If this is the case, there is a 25% chance that the fetus has inherited an abnormal gene from each parent. Thus, there is an approximately 2.5% chance that the fetus is affected. Invasive testing is frequently performed to diagnose chromosomal abnormalities when a much lower a priori risk is present[17].

CONCLUSION

Hemoglobinopathies are ideally suited to prenatal screening. All pregnant women should be screened for these disorders, and those at risk should be offered prenatal diagnosis. If *in utero* stem cell therapy proves effective in the future, parents may have options other than pregnancy termination. The relative costs of different screening protocols in specific populations should be considered when instituting a protocol for hemoglobinopathy screening.

References

1. Angastiniotsis M, Modell B, Englezos P, Boulyjenkov V. Prevention and control of haemoglobinopathies. *Bull WHO* 1995;73:375–86
2. Motulsky AG. Frequency of sickling disorders in U.S. blacks. *N Engl J Med* 1973;288:31–3
3. Scott RB, Castro O. Screening for sickle cell hemoglobinopathies. *J Am Med Assoc* 1979;241:1145–7
4. Simmons A. *Hematology: a Combined Theoretical and Technical Approach*, 2nd edn. Boston: Butterworth-Heinemann, 1997: 84–6
5. The Thalassemia Working Party of the BCSH General Hematology Task Force. Guidelines for investigation of the alpha and beta thalassemia traits. *J Clin Pathol* 1994;47:289–95
6. Gehlbach DL, Morgenstern LL. Antenatal screening for thalassemia minor. *Obstet Gynecol* 1988;71:801–3
7. The General Hematology Task Force of the BCSH. The laboratory diagnosis of haemoglobinopathies. *Br J Haematol* 1998;101:783–92
8. Rees DC, Styles L, Vichinsky EP, Clegg JB, Weatherall DJ. The hemoglobin E syndromes. *Ann NY Acad Sci* 1998;850:334–43
9. Fischel-Ghodsian N. Prenatal diagnosis of hemoglobinopathies. *Clin Perinatol* 1990;17:811–28
10. Hollenberg MD, Kaback MM, Kazazian HH Jr. Adult hemoglobin synthesis by reticulocytes from the human fetus at midtrimester. *Science* 1971;174:698–702
11. Kan YW, Golbus MS, Klein P, Dozy AM. Successful application of prenatal diagnosis in a pregnancy at risk for homozygous beta-thalassemia. *N Engl J Med* 1975;292:1096–9
12. Embury SH. Advances in the prenatal and molecular diagnosis of the hemoglobinopathies and thalassemias. *Hemoglobin* 1995;19:237–61
13. Adinolfi M, el-Hashemite N, Sherlock J, Ward RH, Petrou MJ, Rodeck C. Prenatal detection of Hb mutations using transcervical cells. *Prenat Diagn* 1997;17:539–43
14. Cheung MC, Goldberg JD, Kan YW. Prenatal diagnosis of sickle cell anemia and thalassemia by analysis of fetal cells in maternal blood. *Nature Genet* 1996;14:264–8
15. American College of Obstetricians and Gynecologists. *Hemoglobinopathies in Pregnancy*. ACOG Technical Bulletin 220. Washington, DC: ACOG, 1996
16. Rowley PT, Loader S, Sutera CJ, Walden M, Kozyra A. Prenatal screening for hemoglobinopathies. *Am J Hum Genet* 1991;48:439–46
17. Bowman JE. Prenatal screening for hemoglobinopathies. *Am J Hum Genet* 1991;48:433–8
18. Fishleder AJ. Prenatal hemoglobinopathy screening. *J Am Med Assoc* 1992;268:266
19. Loeb-Zeitlin S, Chasen ST, Landsberger EJ. Prenatal screening for hemoglobinopathies. *Am J Obstet Gynecol* 1998;178:S64
20. American College of Obstetricians and Gynecologists. *Hemoglobinopathies in Pregnancy*. ACOG Technical Bulletin 185. Washington DC: ACOG, 1993
21. Schoen EJ, Marks SM, Clemons MM, Bachman RP. Comparing prenatal and neonatal diagnosis of hemoglobinopathies. *Pediatrics* 1993;92:354–7
22. National Institutes of Health Consensus Conference. Newborn screening for sickle cell disease and other hemoglobinopathies. *J Am Med Assoc* 1987;258:1205–9

Fetal cells in maternal blood: diagnostic aid or disease-causing culprit?

W. Holzgreve, C. Troeger, X. Y. Zhong, S. Schatt, C. van Kaisenberg and S. Hahn

INTRODUCTION

Hope has been put in the use of fetal cells enriched from the blood of pregnant women as a means of achieving a non-invasive alternative for prenatal diagnosis. Reports of the identification of fetal aneuploidies by use of such enriched cells and fluorescence *in situ* hybridization (FISH)[1-3], or single-gene defects by the single-cell polymerase chain reaction (PCR)[4,5], have helped to fuel clinical expectations. As current procedures are not sufficiently sensitive and specific, this transition into the clinic has not yet taken place. Here we report on our experiences in trying to optimize the system.

The research bestowed on trying to enrich fetal cells from maternal blood has opened up interesting new avenues regarding this trafficking of cells between mother and fetus. The longevity of fetal cells[6] in the maternal periphery after parturition has been implicated in the etiology of autoimmune disorders[7,8]. Furthermore, we have found that the number of fetal cells is significantly elevated in cases of pre-eclampsia[9], thereby providing further evidence for the possible involvement of fetal cells in disease.

OPTIMIZATION STRATEGIES

Most researchers in the field have focused their attention on fetal erythroblasts, since these are abundant in the early fetus, rare in normal adult blood and, because they are short-lived, there is no risk of obtaining cells derived from previous pregnancies. Further-more, they are readily identifiable by their distinct morphology, compact nucleus in a large cytoplasm the size of a normal erythro-cyte, and the presence of fetal hemoglobin.

Our pioneering enrichment protocol made use of a triple density gradient and subsequent magnetic separation with micromagnet, conjugated anti-CD71 antibodies and mini magnetic activated cell sorting (MACS) columns[10]. Although the purity of erythro-blasts obtained by this method was excellent, the yield was less than satisfactory. A further problem was that it required a large sample of maternal blood (40 ml), which was found to be a drawback. In order to simplify the protocol, thereby minimizing the number of steps during which cells could be lost, we opted for a less precise single density Ficoll gradient and a single round of miniMACS sorting.

The presence of male fetal cells was scored by X and Y chromosome-specific FISH. After our initial results indicated that no significant reduction in the sensitivity or specificity had occurred, barring that slightly more cells had to be analyzed per fetal cell scored, we adopted this procedure for future exami-nations. Furthermore, the maternal blood sample size was reduced to approximately 16 ml, thereby permitting us to recruit considerably more patients.

Our current experience with this protocol, by which we have processed more than 500 samples, has indicated that the enrichment procedure is not the only critical component, but rather that the examination by FISH requires considerable skill. In this way we were able to increase our level of detection efficiency from around 40%, which was comparable to that achieved with triple density gradient and two rounds of MACS sorting, to almost 80 %[11]. The high degree of insensitivity was largely due to the extent of contamination of the enriched preparation by maternal cells, whereby on average only 1–2 cells in 1000 were actually fetal. It is, hence, not surprising that problems which arise by background can easily lead to incorrect analyses.

This highlights one problem currently plagueing the use of automated dot counters to score for cells with anomalous numbers of FISH signals[12], as they will have great difficulty in discriminating between aberrant signals and those reflective of a true aneuploidy. This problem is probably best countered by using a specific fetal marker, such as immuno-histochemical staining for fetal hemoglobin and simultaneous FISH analyses. In this manner, the technician or automated scanner would first locate the fetal hemoglobin-positive cells and then examine the FISH signals in these cells only. Our experience with such an approach has indicated that most of those cells staining positive for fetal hemoglobin were also identified as being fetal on the basis of XY FISH[13].

In examining whether other modes exist of optimizing enrichment we recently observed that recovery is greatly influenced by the density of the Ficoll gradient used. This is probably a reflection of the rather amorphous nature of the differentiating erythroblasts which do not sediment at any given density. By using the heaviest gradient (1119) we observed the greatest yield, which was almost 5-fold that obtained with normal densities such as 1077 or 1110. Discontinuous Percoll gradients have recently been used successfully for the isolation of fetal erythroblasts[4]. Our preliminary results indicate that this is a viable alternative, but that the yields are considerably lower than those we achieve with MACS-based enrichment.

We examined whether we could further increase the yield by using antibodies that would be more specific for fetal erythroblasts than the transferring receptor (CD71). In order to maximize the yield, we would keep the first step, the Ficoll gradient, as unspecific as possible, but enhance the specificity of the second step, the antibody/magnet-mediated separation, to obtain the highest degree of purity. Our results showed that significantly more erythroblasts were obtained by the use of glycophorin A (GPA), than with any other antibodies tested, including CD36 (thrombo-spondin), HAE9 (anti-fetal liver) and the i blood group antigen. A complication that arises from the use of GPA is that this antibody promotes cell clumping (Figure1a) in contrast to CD71 (Figure1b), which we have found to be distracting in FISH analyses. Since the erythroblasts are frequently located in these clumps of erythrocytes, this method could actually be advantageous when using single microscopically manipulated cells for PCR.

PCR ON SINGLE CELLS AND SERUM DNA

Having shown that enriched fetal erythroblasts can be used for the detection of fetal aneuploidies[3], we next set about using such cells to look for the presence of single gene mutations, specifically β-thalassemias. Our approach was akin to that used by the laboratory of Kan[5], in that fetal erythroblasts were first immunohistochemically stained for zeta or gamma globin and then picked under the microscope using a micromanipulator.

Although fetus-specific genes, such as Y chromosome sequences (Figure 2), are easy to detect in picked single cells, the situation becomes somewhat more complicated when investigating the fetal genotype for single gene disorders, since here one has to be able to detect both the paternal and the maternal alleles.

In our experience, a major problem in using single or multiple cells for PCR is allele drop-out (ADO), a phenomenon whereby one allele of a pair is lost during the PCR process by being totally underamplified[15]. In our studies we have found ADO to be random and not to be affected by allele size. Indeed, we observed ADO to occur in alleles differing

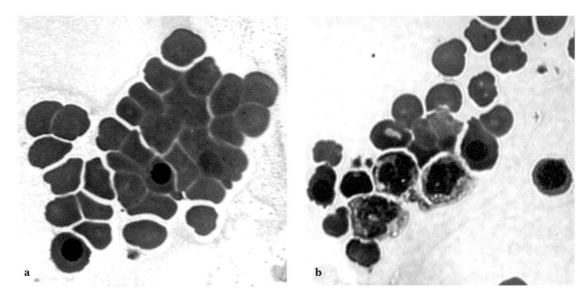

Figure 1 *(a) Enrichment with anti-glycophorin A leads to tight aggregates of erythrocytes, which frequently contain erythroblasts. This illustration also shows the high degree of purity attained by use of this antibody. (b) Loose aggregation of various cell types observed upon enrichment with anti-CD71, showing the low degree of specificity demonstrated by this antigen*

by a single nucleotide[16]. Furthermore, we were not able to overcome ADO by pooling cells, as we observed ADO to occur at levels of DNA comparable to ten genome equivalents. Procedures for random amplification of the genome, such as primer extension preamplification (PEP)[17] or degenerate oligonucleotide primer-PCR (DOP-PCR)[18], should also be used with some caution, as we have observed ADO to occur during this process[16]. Furthermore, by uneven amplification, these procedures can lead to the generation of artifacts, especially when using highly repetitive sequences, such as short tandem repeats (STRs). It is noteworthy that in the original publications these protocols were used either on single sperm, which by being haploid are not subject to ADO, or on amounts of DNA equal to several thousand genomes, and thereby not likely to be affected.

Another problem lies in the positive identification of the fetal erythroblast; none of the 'fetus-specific' antibodies are 100% specific, and since most of the erythroblasts are not of fetal but rather of maternal origin, one runs the risk of making a false diagnosis

by basing it on a wrongly identified cell. We hypothesized that this problem could be overcome by using the inherent and unique pattern of STRs located on each chromosome. In this manner, while the fetus would share one allele with the mother, it would be identifiable by the presence of a unique paternal allele.

To test whether this procedure would function despite the problem of ADO we used

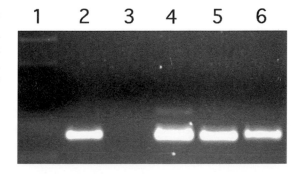

Figure 2 *Detection of Y chromosome-specific sequences by nested polymerase chain reaction from single microscopically manipulated cells. Lane 1, DNA molecular weight marker; lane 2, positive control; lane 3, negative control; lanes 4–6, single male cells*

a model system whereby cord blood erythroblasts were diluted into the corresponding maternal blood sample. Single erythroblasts were then microscopically picked and analyzed at those STR loci found to be informative for both mother and fetus[15]. Our results showed that such a procedure was indeed feasible if the identification was based on the presence of a unique paternal allele. Furthermore, by using multiplex PCR, a procedure whereby multiple PCR reactions are directly performed on the same sample, we could examine such positively identified cells at other loci. These studies showed that the problem of ADO is best overcome by examining multiple single cells and then basing the diagnosis on the pooled results. By such means, the results obtained from four cells will already yield a 98% degree of accuracy even with an ADO rate of over 60%[15].

The recent observation that fetal DNA can be obtained directly from maternal serum has raised the question of whether this can be used diagnostically. Since here no clear distinction would be possible between maternal and fetal DNA, one could only examine those genes which are absent from the maternal genome but which may be present in that of the fetus, e.g. with a rhesus D-negative mother and a rhesus D-positive father. We tested the efficacy of such DNA in predicting the gender of the fetus (S. Schatt and colleagues, submitted for publication). To optimize the efficiency, we first extracted the DNA from the maternal serum sample and then examined it by a sensitive nested PCR analysis that was specific for a Y chromosome sequence.

By using serum samples from those blood samples that were being enriched by MACS and analyzed by FISH, we were able to draw a direct comparison between the two methods. In our hands, we determined that PCR on serum DNA was less sensitive than on fetal cells enriched from maternal blood in determining fetal sex. Specificity, on the other hand, was higher, having a considerably lower false-positive rate. Interestingly, in several of the instances where we observed a 'false-positive' male signal, some of these women

had previous pregnancies with male offspring; in the others the pregnancy outcome was not noted. This raises the possibility that fetal DNA derived from previous pregnancies may be detected by this method. Nevertheless, we feel optimistic that, should one be able to increase the sensitivity of this method, it may be developed into a promising non-invasive alternative for the detection of the fetal rhesus status.

POSSIBLE INVOLVEMENT OF FETAL CELLS IN DISEASE

The report by Bianchi and colleagues that fetal progenitor cells could persist in the circulation of women for several decades postpartum[6] begged the question of what the effect of such cells was, and whether they could be involved in any disease processes, for instance in those autoimmune disorders, e.g. scleroderma, to which women after parturition are more prone. In following up their intriguing observation that a strong correlation existed between the susceptibility to scleroderma and the sharing of HLA antigens between mother and fetus[19], Artlett and co-workers recently demonstrated the presence of fetal cells in both lesion biopsies and peripheral blood samples obtained from patients affected by scleroderma[7]. In a seperate confirmatory report, Nelson and colleagues, by using the quantitative PCR procedure established by the laboratory of Bianchi, demonstrated the increased presence of male fetal cells in the peripheral blood of women suffering from scleroderma[8]. Since no similar increment was observed in their healthy sisters, these results strongly implicate the presence of elevated persisting fetal cells in the etiology of this disorder.

It is important to realize that the levels of fetal cells found in these patients are still at the microchimeric levels: Nelson and colleagues reported between zero and 61 fetal cell equivalents per 16 ml of blood, whereas Artlett and colleagues observed approximately two fetal cells in 3000 enriched lymphocytes, implying that there are only a few fetal cells in peripheral maternal blood.

This level of potential effector cells corresponds well with current thinking in the development of autoimmune disorders.

We have made a similar observation regarding the presence of fetal cells and a disease state, namely that of the gestational disorder pre-eclampsia, in which we noted significant increases in the numbers of erythroblasts when compared to normal controls. Since at that time we could not establish whether these cells were of fetal or maternal origin, we recently carried out a case controlled study in which we examined pregnancies carrying only male fetuses[9]. By use of X and Y chromosome FISH, we could compare both morphology-identified erythroblasts and the actual number of male fetal cells. Our study showed that both the number of erythroblasts and the number of fetal cells were significantly elevated in the blood of pre-eclamptic women when compared to the matched controls.

Since some aspects of pre-eclampsia, and especially the associated HELLP syndrome (hemolysis, elevated liver enzymes, low platelets), bear hallmarks of an overt or even autoimmune response, it is enticing to speculate that such aberrant cell trafficking might help elicit this immune dysfunction.

CONCLUSIONS

Although we will not be able to use fetal cells enriched from maternal blood for prenatal diagnosis in the next year, the constant stream of steady improvements means that the arrival of this methodology is no longer a matter of the distant future. The advantages of such a method are readily apparent: the ability to screen for fetal genetic abnormalities in a risk-free manner, thereby providing this type of testing for a broader population, including women of below 35 years of age. The inherent disadvantages should, however, also be borne in mind; these include the current inability to obtain full karyotypic information. We envisage that this test will be used complementarily to other practices, and that, as for ultrasound, anomalies will be confirmed by classical genetics on cells obtained by current invasive procedures. The advantage of this test is that it could help reduce the number of unnecessary invasive procedures which are performed because of the high false-positive rates of current non-invasive tests.

The ability to find and enrich fetal cells from the periphery of pregant women, and even mothers postpartum, has helped us to readdress the nature of the placental barrier and the possible physiological consequences such cells could elicit in their new host. It is likely that these points will gain in clinical importance.

ACKNOWLEDGEMENTS

This work was supported in part by Swiss National Science Foundation Grant Number: 3200-047112.96, NIH (USA) Contract Number: N01-HD-4-3202 and a grant from the Institute of Hormone and Fertility Research, Hamburg, Germany. C.T. is recipient of a stipend (Tr 452/1-1) from the German Research Foundation.

References

1. Elias S, Price J, Dockter M, *et al.* First trimester prenatal diagnosis of trisomy 21 in fetal cells from maternal blood. *Lancet* 1992;340:1033

2. Bianchi DW, Mahr A, Zickwolf GK, Houseal TW, Flint AF, Klinger KW. Detection of fetal cells with 47,XY,+21 karyotype in maternal peripheral blood. *Hum Genet* 1992;90:368–70

3. Gänshirt-Ahlert D, Börejesson-Stoll R, Burschyk M, *et al.* Detection of fetal trisomies 21 and 18 from maternal blood using triple gradient and magnetic cell sorting. *Am J Reprod Immunol* 1993; 30:194–201

4. Sekizawa A, Kimura T, Sasaki M, Nakamura S, Kobayashi R, Sato T. Prenatal diagnosis of Duchenne muscular dystrophy using a single fetal nucleated erythrocyte in maternal blood. *Neurology* 1996;46:1350–3

5. Cheung MC, Goldberg JD, Kan YW. Prenatal

diagnosis of sickle cell anaemia and thalassaemia by analysis of fetal cells in maternal blood. *Nature Genet* 1996;14:264–8

6. Bianchi DW, Zickwolf GK, Weil GJ, Sylvester S, Demaria MA. Male fetal progenitor cells persist in maternal blood for as long as 27 years postpartum. *Proc Natl Acad Sci USA* 1996;93: 705–8

7. Artlett CM, Smith JB, Jimenez SA. Identification of fetal DNA and cells in skin lesions from women with systemic sclerosis. *N Engl J Med* 1998;338: 1186–91

8. Nelson JL, Furst DE, Maloney S, *et al.* Microchimerism and HLA-compatible relationships of pregnancy in scleroderma. *Lancet* 1998;351:559–62

9. Holzgreve W, Ghezzi F, Di Naro E, Maymon E, Gänshirt D, Hahn S. Disturbed fetomaternal cell traffic in preeclampsia. *Obstet Gynecol* 1998;91: 669–72

10. Holzgreve W, Garritsen IIS, Ganshirt Ahlert D. Fetal cells in the maternal circulation. *J Reprod Med* 1992;37:410–18

11. Hahn S, Kiefer V, Brombacher V, Troeger C, Holzgreve W. Fetal cells in maternal blood: an update from Basel. *Eur J Obstet Gynecol Reprod Biol* 1998; in press

12. Netten H, Young IT, van Vliet LJ, Tanke HJ, Vroljik H, Sloos WCR. FISH and chips: automation of fluorescent dot counting in interphase cell nuclei. *Cytometry* 1997;28:1–10

13. Hahn S, Sant R, Holzgreve W. Fetal cells in maternal blood: current and future perspectives. *Mol Hum Reprod* 1998;4:515–21

14. Troeger C, Holzgreve W, Hahn S. A comparison of different density gradients and antibodies for the enrichment of fetal erythroblasts by MACS. *Prenat Diagn* 1999: in press

15. Garvin AM, Holzgreve W, Hahn S. Highly accurate analysis of heterozygous loci by single cell PCR. *Nucleic Acids Res* 1998; 26:3468–72

16. Hahn S, Garvin A, Di Naro E, Holzgreve W. Allele drop out can occur in alleles differing by a single nucleotide and is not alleviated by preamplification nor minor template increments. *Genet Test* 1998;2:351–5

17. Zhang L, Cui X, Schmitt K, Hubert R, Navidi W, Arnheim N. Whole genome amplification from a single cell: implications for genetic analysis. *Proc Natl Acad Sci USA* 1992;89:5847–51

18. Cheung VG, Nelson SF. Whole genome amplification using a degenerate oligonucleotide primer allows hundreds of genotypes to be performed on less than one nanogram of genomic DNA. *Proc Natl Acad Sci USA* 1996; 93:14676–9

19. Artlett CM, Welsh KI, Black CM, Jiminez SA. Fetal-maternal HLA compatibility confers susceptibility to systemic sclerosis. *Immunogenetics* 1997;47:17–22

Issues in multifetal pregnancy reduction   21

M. I. Evans, Y. Yaron, L. Littmann, C. Tapin and H. R. Belkin

INTRODUCTION

The past 20 years have seen an explosion of knowledge in the area of infertility. The days of infertile couples wanting children having either to remain childless or adopt a child are gone. Infertile couples now have options for treatment that were in the realm of science fiction not too many years ago. The treatment of infertile patients has become a common-place type of therapy, widely requested by patients and widely performed by physicians. Foremost in the treatment of these patients are fertility drugs such as human menopausal gonadotropin (Perganol®) or new agents (Metrodin®). These drugs help thousands of couples each year to conceive their own children. Advanced reproductive technologies including *in vitro* fertilization (IVF) and gamete intra-Fallopian transfer procedures (GIFT) have brought the promise of parenthood to many more childless couples. However, these drugs and advanced techniques have created one of the most bitter ironies in medicine. Women who were previously incapable of either becoming pregnant or carrying a fetus to term are suddenly faced with the prospect of bearing more fetuses than they can carry to viability, or that place them at significantly increased risk for perinatal mortality or morbidity[1,2].

In this chapter, we examine the technical, legal and ethical aspects of both multifetal pregnancy reduction and selective termination of pregnancy. After examining the history of these procedures and how they have developed over the past 20 years, we look at the specific techniques for performing these procedures and then examine the moral, legal and ethical underpinnings thereof, especially in light of classical United States Supreme Court rulings. It is interesting to note that many of these ethical issues were initially raised in an article written two decades ago, during a time when these techniques were just being developed[3]. Many of the issues raised by those authors are still important issues today.

Modern advanced prenatal care has greatly reduced the mortality associated with multiple pregnancies and to a lesser degree the associated morbidity[4-7]. However, the obstetric outcome for triplets or higher numbers of fetuses is much poorer than that of a singleton or even a twin pregnancy[1,4-7]. A woman's ability to carry four or five fetuses to term is greatly reduced and, despite the publicity attendant on very high-order pregnancies, those involving sextuplets or more are rarely successful. Although recent improvements in treatment and diagnosis have been associated with decreases in fetal mortality, particularly with triplets, long-term morbidity is still a significant issue[4,5].

Couples faced with multiple pregnancies have a dilemma that needs to be addressed. The dilemma is the fact that the couple, who have often desperately sought pregnancy, are now faced with a pregnancy of high order for which they may not be physically or emotionally prepared. Very often these pregnancies are a result of the use of the drugs and advanced obstetric techniques discussed above.

These couples have three options, none of which is entirely satisfactory. The first option is the termination of the entire pregnancy. In general, as these patients have spent a great deal of time, money and emotion in achieving the pregnancy, this is not an acceptable choice. The second option is continuation of the pregnancy with all of the fetuses. Although in cases of quadruplets or even quintuplets, survival of some or all is certainly realistic but problematic, the risk of complete loss of the pregnancy is much higher than in a singleton or twin pregnancy and, furthermore, there is a great risk of long-term morbidity. When the pregnancy is of sextuplets or higher, the chance of survival is extremely low. The past 10 years have given these couples another option: the use of multifetal pregnancy reduction (MFPR). Over the past decade, MFPR has become a staple in the management of infertility drug complications[8-14]. It is important to understand some of the terminology. A fetal reduction procedure performed for the purpose of reducing the number of fetuses, *per se*, is called MFPR. Procedures that reduce the number of fetuses present because of fetal abnormality are called selective termination.

It may also be instructive to recognize that the demographics of patients who present for MFPR may be quite different from those who present for selective termination. Most selective termination patients have twin pregnancies discordant for some type of anomaly. They have not necessarily had any type of fertility treatment. They come from a broad socioeconomic spectrum and are usually faced with making a decision about a problem of which they have only very recently become aware. In contrast, patients who present for MFPR are almost invariably patients who have undergone treatment for infertility and are usually of a fairly high economic level. Having been through what may be numerous rounds of treatment for their infertility, they are usually quite knowledgeable about treatment options and have often invested substantial amounts of time, money and emotion in their attempts to achieve pregnancy.

HISTORY OF FETAL REDUCTION

The first reported use of selective reduction was in 1978 as reported by Aberg and colleagues[15]. That was a case of a twin pregnancy discordant for Hurler's syndrome. This was a procedure performed at a time when ultrasound diagnostic technology was rather rudimentary. At that time, there was considerable concern surrounding the procedure. These worries included the possibility that the wrong fetus could be identified and terminated, that damage or death could occur to the normal fetus and that there remained a risk of disseminated intravascular coagulopathy (DIC) affecting the remaining fetus and/or the mother. There was also a good deal of concern that the procedure itself could act to induce preterm labor. Over the past two decades, the procedure has become widely performed with generally little media attention. However, a case reported in 1981 by Kerenyi and Chicaro involved selective birth in a twin pregnancy discordant for Down's syndrome[16]. The authors stated that they were 'blackmailed' by the mother into performing the procedure when she declared that, if they did not attempt the termination of the anomalous fetus, she would terminate the entire pregnancy. In 1981, Petres and Redwine reported that they had failed twice selectively to terminate a fetus diagnosed with Down's syndrome through the use of exsanguination[17]. There was appropriate concern that the trauma of the two failed procedures themselves would compromise the fetus even more than its original diagnosis. They made a third attempt at reduction through the use of intracardiac air embolization, which resulted in a successful termination. However, chorioamnionitis subsequently developed with the onset of preterm labor and delivery of the normal child at 28 weeks. This resulted in subsequent death of the normal neonate from prematurity. In 1982 and 1984, Rodeck and colleagues published six cases of selective terminations performed in the second trimester using intracardiac sterile air embolization under fetoscopic guidance[18,19]. Five of the six cases resulted in a normal liveborn twin. However, in the sixth case, preterm labor and delivery at 29 weeks occurred, and the fetus died at 1 month of age from necrotizing enterocolitis. In 1988, Golbus and co-workers reported selective termination procedures in 22 patients[20]. Of these, 19 were for a fetal abnormality found in a twin pregnancy. In 17 dichorionic pregnancies there was successful delivery of surviving singletons. However, for twins in five monochorionic pregnancies, there was only one successful delivery. Pregnancy loss occurred in the other four. It is interesting to note that six of 18 delivered pregnancies in their study were complicated by premature labor and delivery.

MULTIFETAL PREGNANCY REDUCTION: TECHNIQUES AND PROCEDURES

As awareness of the usefulness of MFPR has spread over the past 10 years, the number of cases performed has greatly increased. As more and more centers perform these procedures and as experience continues to accumulate, modifications to the procedures occur, results improve and the risks and benefits become better appreciated. Three different technical procedures have been reported[10-14]: transcervical, transvaginal and transabdominal.

Transcervical suction

The original 1986 report by Dumez and Oury discussed their technique of using transcervical, low-pressure suction to remove embryos at 8–11 weeks[10]. Ultrasound was used to guide mini-suction curettage. Technical success was achieved in the majority of cases; however, there was an approximately 50% loss of the entire pregnancy[1]. This technique eventually was largely abandoned; however, it has now re-emerged in a few centers.

Transvaginal aspiration

Transvaginal aspiration is a technique by which vaginal access is obtained. This procedure has been successfully performed on embryos as early as 6–7 weeks. Technically, the procedure is analogous in many respects to oocyte aspiration for IVF. It may be particularly useful in those cases in which it is desirable to perform the reduction very early in gestation.

The procedure is performed by inserting a speculum into the vagina. The vagina is then cleansed with Betadine®. Under ultrasound guidance, a long, sharp needle is passed through the vaginal wall into the uterine cavity. The needle is maneuvered into the chosen sac and placed up against the embryo. Suction is applied, and the embryo is aspirated or disrupted. The amniotic fluid is left in utero. If further embryos are to be reduced, the same needle is partially withdrawn and then repositioned as needed.

Transabdominal use of potassium chloride

This is considered by many to be the most feasible and practical technique utilized in fetal reduction. It involves the insertion of a spinal needle transabdominally under ultrasound guidance. This is generally a 22-gauge needle; however, in obese patients when the needle insertion has to go beyond about 3 inches (7.5 cm), we have found it best to use a 20-gauge 6-inch (15 cm) needle. The 6-inch 22-gauge needle is too flexible for easy control, and is not as easily visualized on ultrasound as is the 20-gauge needle.

The abdomen is prepared as it would be for amniocentesis. The approach varies depending upon the general style of the operator and whether or not the physician self-guides. Those who do self-guide will generally place the ultrasound transducer on the top of the abdomen and insert the needle from an angled position. As we have found that it is much less uncomfortable to the patient when the needle is inserted directly downward and scanning is done from the side, we use a transverse rather than a longitudinal scan approach.

The insertion site must be chosen with a great deal of care. One needs to attempt a direct, vertical, downward approach to the fetus. Using careful technique, the operator confirms the position of the needle over the fetal heart (Figure 1) and thrusts it into the thorax. It is important to use a reasonable amount of force in this technique because, if it is done too gently, the embryo will simply bounce away from the needle, necessitating

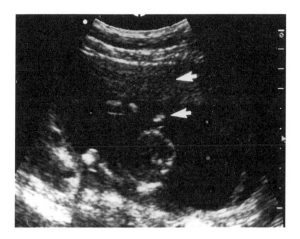

Figure 1 *Needle coming in from 1 o'clock, hovering over cardiac chamber*

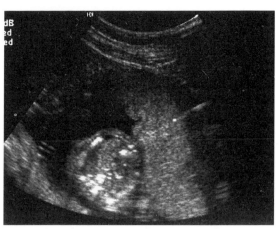

Figure 2 *10-Week fetus with tip of needle in heart*

repositioning. When repositioning is needed, it is rarely necessary to remove the needle completely. Although one does aim for the heart, inserting the needle anywhere within the fetal thorax is acceptable during the first trimester. Care must be taken to make sure that the needle is not accidentally placed intra-abdominally. Placement of the needle below the diaphragm will often lead to failure.

Once the operator feels that the needle is properly positioned, the inner stylet must be removed, and a 3-ml syringe attached, with the plunger gently pulled back. This allows the operator to confirm the location of the needle. A properly positioned needle will result in negative pressure or the return of a small amount of blood from the heart into the syringe. The return of amniotic fluid indicates improper positioning and requires repositioning.

After the position of the needle has been confirmed, a small dose of potassium chloride (about 0.5–1.5 ml) is injected. With ideal positioning, cardiac standstill occurs within a minute of the injection and can be clearly seen on ultrasound. Generally, one can also detect the formation of a pleural or cardiac effusion (Figure 2). The needle is left in the thorax until cardiac asystole is confirmed for 2 or 3 min. This is to guard against the possibility of resumption of cardiac activity, which has occasionally been known to occur if the needle is withdrawn too soon, particularly if there is not a persistent pleural effusion. The gestational sac will eventually be resorbed.

EMBRYO SELECTION AND TIMING

Embryo selection

When performing a MFPR procedure, the initial question always involves which embryos should be selected for reduction. This is not always an easy question to answer and may require many factors to be taken into account. One must first look at the fetuses and try to make whatever appropriate judgements one can about them from their ultrasound appearance. The choice of fetuses is made easier if an abnormality is discovered on ultrasound. Certain abnormalities, including acrania or ventral wall defects, may be detectable as early as 9–10 weeks. Nuchal membranes can often be seen early through the use of ultrasound. Nuchal membranes or significant size discrepancies are markers for increased risks of aneuploidy. Another consideration may be whether the pregnancy involves any monoamniotic twins. Mono-amniotic twins are subject to great risks and should generally be reduced. With mono-zygotic/diamniotic twins, they need to be either both kept or both reduced. However, in many cases no abnormalities will be seen.

In these cases the choice of which embryo to reduce is based upon the practical consideration of ease of approach. Our experience suggests that, in general, it is better not to choose the embryo closest to the cervix, as persistent vaginal bleeding is likely.

Timing

Generally, transabdominal cases are performed between 9 and 12 weeks of pregnancy. It appears likely that trans-abdominal attempts prior to 8 weeks would generally be more technically difficult to perform. The use of a transvaginal approach will probably give better results at very early gestational ages. However, it must be kept in mind that, at earlier gestational ages, there is still a chance of a 'natural' spontaneous loss of remaining embryos. This therefore adds to the risk of losing some or all of the remaining embryo(s)[21,23]. After approximately 13 weeks' gestational age, the chance of spontaneously losing the pregnancy becomes greatly reduced. There are at least theoretical risks of infectious necrosis arising from the remaining tissue mass or the development of DIC. However, these risks may remain merely theoretical, as there have been no known cases to date.

Number

It has been our experience that patients and physicians almost always wish to reduce the pregnancy to twins. We believe that by leaving twins there will still be some 'margin for error' that would be absent in a singleton pregnancy. There are other advantages to leaving twins. Although the obstetric outcome for twins is not quite as good as that for singleton pregnancies, it is considerably better than for triplets or more. Furthermore, virtually all obstetricians are familiar and comfortable with the delivery of twins. There have been many cases in which, after reduction, triplets have been left[8,9], with an extremely satisfactory outcome. However, the risks attendant on a triplet pregnancy, including prematurity and morbidity, are certainly much greater than those with twins. It is essential that the couple understands these risks and accepts them in making their decision to retain three fetuses. If the couple does understand these risks and accepts the fact that during the pregnancy there will probably be a significant lifestyle change, along with the increased risk of an unsatisfactory outcome, then the risks are justified. The importance of a well-informed patient cannot be overemphasized.

Although pooled collaborative data suggest that singleton pregnancies are associated with longer gestational periods and a slightly lower morbidity rate than are non-singleton pregnancies, it is our opinion that leaving only one fetus is generally not the best medical decision. This is based mainly on the fact that, in the event of there being a problem with the one remaining fetus, then the entire pregnancy will be lost. One must be conscious of the fact that, especially for couples who have undergone a great deal of treatment for infertility, the loss of the entire pregnancy could be truly devastating. Generally speaking, these couples want the safety of having that second fetus. They would in general greatly prefer taking home twins to losing an entire pregnancy. However, there are certainly medical exceptions to the above. These would include a woman with diethylstilbestrol-induced uterine malformations, cervical incompetence, or very significant medical disease such as cardiac failure. In these conditions and others, the added burden of a multiple gestation might prevent a viable pregnancy from being carried to term altogether, and therefore these conditions must be given overriding importance in the decision of how many fetuses to carry. When we began treating these patients, for the first few years of our experience, we would not reduce a pregnancy to fewer than two fetuses. However, as with most things in life, as we performed more and more of these procedures and talked to our patients, not only did our experience in performing the procedures safely increase, but we also realized the importance of patient autonomy in the decision-making process.

The truly small decrease in the risk of morbidity for a singleton makes our policy of not reducing past twins less justifiable. By the mid 1990s, there was an increasing percentage of patients over 40 years of age, and many of them were using donor eggs. Particularly for these patients, reducing to a singleton is very common, and understandable.

We have recently published a report that examined 143 patients seen over a 10-year period in order to determine whether or not MFPR improves pregnancy outcome in reductions of three to two[24]. We found there to be a significant reduction in the miscarriage rate with three to two reductions, resulting in a 6.2% rate, versus 25% in the expectantly managed unreduced triplets. This rate is similar to rates previously reported. Very premature infants were seen in only 4.9% of the three to two reduction group, but in 25% of the expectantly managed unreduced triplets. The MFPR group had an average gestational age of 35.6 ± 3.1 weeks at birth, while the non-reduced triplets were born at 32.9 ± 4.7 weeks. The mean birth weight of the three to two twins was 2381 ± 602 g, as compared to the triplets of 1636 ± 645 g. This study demonstrated that when MFPR is utilized to perform a three to two reduction, there is a significant difference in the outcome variables described above. This study also allows the clinician to give specific information about a procedure to a patient.

RECENT ADVANCES IN MULTIFETAL PREGNANCY REDUCTION

As mentioned above, the past decade has seen an explosion in the use of MFPR. It is now performed in many centers and has truly become integrated into the practice of fertility medicine. It has emerged as a staple of infertility therapy. Over the past 15 years the number of procedures performed on a yearly basis have increased geometrically. Whereas these procedures were at one time limited to use by certain academic medical centers, their use has now expanded to that limited number of centers known internationally for considerable experience, and also to other

physicians with less experience[8–10,12–14,23,25–27]. Published collaborative reports have documented this increased utilization of MFPR[23,26]. It is our belief that the improved outcomes that have been observed to occur since the early 1990s are a direct result of both the learning curve and the use of more sophisticated ultrasound equipment. These factors, along with increased patient and physician awareness of the availability of the procedure, has led to the improvements in MFPR.

In 1993, the first collaborative report covering the years 1988 to early 1991 was published[23]. This report included cases that were all performed by the transabdominal insertion of a needle with potassium chloride injection into the fetal thorax. The data showed an overall 16.4% pregnancy loss rate up to 24 weeks' gestation. Our collaborative paper[26] focused on cases that were performed between mid-1991 and 1993. This report demonstrated that there was a significant drop in the overall pregnancy loss rate. Of cases performed transabdominally, the rate decreased by 50%, from 16% in the first series, to 8% in the second series. Transcervical and transvaginal cases were also included in the second series. These cases demonstrated a loss rate of approximately 13%. The percentages of patients having very early premature deliveries, i.e. at 25–28 weeks, were approximately 5.5% for both approaches. Approximately 10% of these patients delivered between 29 and 32 weeks . Nearly 50% of all patients reached 37 weeks of gestation.

In our second report, we examined in detail the differences between the transabdominal and transvaginal/transcervical approaches. We found that, in general, transvaginal/transcervical procedures tended to be carried out at an earlier stage and also tended to have fewer fetuses to start and finish[28]. The earlier gestational age increased our losses and the lower numbers decreased the losses. These factors tended to cancel each other out.

Next, we embarked on reporting about the third series of patients. The third series doubled the total number of cases added to the registry, including those cases with the procedure performed in 1993 and 1994, and also added two new centers to the consortium. The purpose of our study was to examine a procedure that had in the time since the initial series become mature, in order to determine whether further progress is still being made and to provide outcome data to aid in patient counselling. The fact that we had so many cases available allowed us, for the first time, to develop relatively smooth risk curves. It furthermore has given us enough cases in each category to document incremental risks with fetal number.

As we now have almost a decade of experience, we can see improvements in the outcomes. Overall pregnancy loss rates have decreased to 11.7% with early premature deliveries at 4.5%. These numbers are both substantially better than untreated cases of multifetal pregnancies[12-14,23,25-28]. There continues to be a strong correlation among the starting number, finishing number and the likelihood of poor outcomes for both losses and prematurity (Tables 1 and 2). Pregnancy loss rates exceeded 20% for patients starting with sextuplets or more. These fell to a minimum of 7.6% for triplets reduced primarily to twins ($\chi^2 = 32.1$, $p < 0.0001$) (Table 1). Similarly, there was a corresponding relationship for those cases of early premature deliveries, i.e. for sextuplets: 11.5% delivered between 25 and 28 weeks. The rate fell to 3.3% for triplets ($\chi^2 = 19.4$, $p < 0.0001$).

The finishing number data were interesting. They showed the lowest pregnancy loss rates for those cases reduced to twins, with increasing losses for singletons, followed by triplets. The rate of early premature delivery was, as one might suspect, highest with triplets followed by twins and then singletons. Also, as would be expected, the mean gestational age at delivery was lower for higher-order cases (Table 2).

Our comparison of transabdominal with transvaginal/transcervical cases paralleled our findings from our earlier study, that is there were no consistent differences. We found no pattern among gestational age at

procedure, average starting or finishing number as a function of method, when cases were lost or their gestational age at delivery.

Our data suggest that, over the past decade, MFPR has become a well established and integral part of infertility therapy. MFPR also attempts to deal with the sequelae of aggressive infertility management. A decade ago, one could have had no idea about all the risks and benefits of the procedure[8,9]. Because of the collaborative nature of our investigations, we now have very clear and precise data on the risks and benefits of these procedures. We furthermore understand that the risks attendant on these procedures increase substantially as the starting and finishing number of fetuses in multifetal pregnancies increase. These new data suggest that a plateauing of risks and benefits of the procedure occurs. This suggests that the learning curve is very substantial, but that it eventually flattens out. We now have numbers that can be discussed with patients in order to give them and the practitioners a guide to the risks. The collaborative loss rate numbers, i.e. 7.6% for triplets, 13.8% for quadruplets, 17.1% for quintuplets and 22.9% for septuplets or more, are reasonable to present to patients for the procedure when performed by an experienced operator (Table 1). The results obtained by less experienced practitioners, as our own experiences and anecdotal reports from other groups have suggested, are, as one might expect, that less experienced operators have worse outcomes.

Although it may be the most dramatic, pregnancy loss is not the only poor outcome possible. The risk of very early premature delivery and the problems involved with this is the other main issue with which one must be concerned. Again, in our cases, there was an increasing rate of poor outcomes that correlated with the starting number. The finishing numbers are also critical. As discussed above, twins had the best outcomes. Triplets and singletons did not do as well (Table 2).

There is another group of patients who have been examined. This is the subset of patients whose fetuses were reduced from two

Table 1 *Collaborative data. Pregnancy losses and deliveries as a function of starting number*

Starting number	Total (n)	Losses at < 24 weeks		Deliveries								Mean gestational age (weeks)
				25–28 weeks		29–32 weeks		33–36 weeks		37+ weeks		
		n	%	n	%	n	%	n	%	n	%	
Total	1789	209	11.7	81	4.5	161	9.0	584	32.6	754	42.1	35.6
6+	96	22	22.9	11	11.5	11	11.5	33	34.4	19	19.8	33.6
5	170	29	17.1	9	5.3	21	12.4	55	32.4	56	32.9	34.5
4	653	90	13.0	32	4.9	68	10.4	221	33.8	242	37.1	35.0
3	759	58	7.6	25	3.3	57	7.5	263	34.7	356	46.9	35.5
2	111	10	9.0	4	3.6	4	3.6	12	10.8	81	73.0	35.6

Table 2 *Pregnancy losses and deliveries as a function of finishing number*

Finishing number	Total (n)	Losses at < 24 weeks		Deliveries								Mean gestational age (weeks)
				25–28 weeks		29–32 weeks		33–36 weeks		37+ weeks		
		n	%	n	%	n	%	n	%	n	%	
3	68	12	17.6	5	7.4	21	30.9	23	33.8	7	10.3	32.9
2	1437	156	10.9	66	4.6	127	8.8	528	36.7	560	39.0	35.3
1	284	39	13.7	8	2.8	11	3.9	33	11.6	193	68.0	37.6

to one for reasons other than fetal anomalies. This group comprised 111 patients, of whom ten lost their pregnancies before 24 weeks and four delivered between 25 and 28 weeks. While the numbers, in absolute terms, are not large as compared to the other categories, they suggest a somewhat higher loss rate than that seen for reduction from three to two. The reasons for the two to one reduction were quite varied. In about half of these cases, there was a medical indication for the procedure – e.g. maternal cardiac disease, prior twin pregnancy with severe prematurity or uterine abnormality. In the other half, the patient expressed a significant fear of multiple pregnancy. In many cases, these patients stated that they would terminate the entire pregnancy if they could not reduce to a singleton. The data thus reflect the fact that in many cases the compelling medical reasons above did influence pregnancy outcome. As one might imagine, performance of a two to one reduction might be controversial. Among

nine centers in our collaborative study, there were differing attitudes towards performing procedures of two to one reduction. These varied from complete refusal to perform the procedure to what might be called a conditional willingness, depending upon varying conditions of medical and social need. This issue is one that will probably be debated for many years to come.

OUTCOME OF MULTIFETAL PREGNANCY REDUCTION

It is possible to achieve a 100% technical success rate in the performance of MFPR. Composite data from the most experienced centers suggest that the success rate, defined as the live birth of an infant, is approximately 85–90%. This must be viewed against the background risks of multifetal pregnancy which are about 10% for twins in the first trimester. Complications are primarily a function of the initial starting number of

Table 3 *Incidence of chromosomal abnormalities in at least one fetus in a multifetal gestation, according to approximate maternal age*

Maternal age (years)	Singleton risk	Risk equivalent age (years)	Twin risk	Risk equivalent age (years)	Triplet risk
20	1/526	≈ 34	1/263	≈ 36	1/175
25	1/476	≈ 34	1/238	≈ 36	1/150
30	1/385	≈ 35	1/192	≈ 37	1/128
35	1/192	≈ 38	1/96	≈ 40	1/64
40	1/66	≈ 43	1/33	≈ 45	1/22

fetuses[23] (Table 1). It is thus not surprising that a three to two reduction would be less risky than a six to two reduction.

GENETIC TESTING AND MULTIFETAL PREGNANCY REDUCTION

As patients and physicians become more aware of the availability of fertility treatment, more women of increasing maternal age seek such treatment. Many women requesting infertility service are over 30 years of age. It is especially important for these patients to understand the risk of genetic anomalies. It must first be realized that most multiple pregnancies are not monozygotic; the risk that one twin is genetically abnormal is essentially twice the singleton risk at the same age (Table 3). There has been some controversy about the role and risks of genetic testing with MFPR. This has often centered on the need for or appropriateness of pre-MFPR chorionic villus sampling (CVS) for karyotype examination. Some programs advocate CVS prior to the performance of MFPR in order to guarantee that euploid fetuses are left. We believe that, in those cases in which a singleton is to be left, this may be the best approach, but studies have demonstrated that both the error rate and the loss rates may be higher this way[29]. In our experience we have found it preferable first to reduce to twins and then perform CVS or early amniocentesis 1–2 weeks later. Only twice in more than 10 years have we had to go back to reduce an abnormal twin left behind. While one report suggested a higher risk of amniocentesis loss, our data have confirmed the safety of the procedure.

MANAGEMENT OF PREGNANCIES AFTER MULTIFETAL PREGNANCY REDUCTION

Management of patients after MFPR is basically the same as the management of naturally occurring twin pregnancies. However, it must be kept in mind that there is a correlation between the starting number of fetuses and the increasing risks of pregnancy losses (up to 24 weeks) and increasing risks of prematurity[23,30,31]. There have not yet been any documented risks of coagulopathies.

TREATMENT OF INFERTILITY AND MULTIPLE PREGNANCY

High-order pregnancies can be very problematic. Nearly all pregnancies of an order of quadruplets or higher are iatrogenic. Many of these result from the overuse of medical treatment, from poorly controlled medical treatment, or from IVF and embryo transfer of large numbers of embryos. With the development of cryopreservation, the incidence of IVF multiple gestations has been decreasing[32].

A decrease in these cases may come in response to malpractice litigation initiated by patients who have had poorly controlled Pergonal cycles. However, it is clear that, with about 20 000 patients in the USA receiving Pergonal or equivalents annually, multifetal pregnancies can and will occur occasionally. It is important to note that these cases are not necessarily limited to those physicians who intentionally or unintentionally fail to retain adequate control of treatment. They may occur even with excellent physicians using the best of equipment, skill and intent. There are some patients for whom there exists a very narrow margin of medication use between no response and hyperstimulation. Although MFPR is by no means intended as a routine 'correction' for overtreatment, its availability allows the physician to take 'calculated' risks for patients who otherwise would probably not become pregnant.

In our opinion it is extremely important for both physicians and patients to be aware of the potential for overuse of treatment for infertility by relying upon MFPR to correct the overuse. Furthermore, this is not a concern that is of recent vintage. In an examination of the early discussions of the issues regarding the potential abuses that were considered in the developing years of these procedures, the only one later deemed an 'epidemic'[33] was the potentially aggressive use of fertility treatment resulting in multiple pregnancies[28].

PRENATAL DIAGNOSTIC TECHNIQUES

The early 1970s witnessed the development of amniocentesis, the first truly advanced prenatal diagnostic technique. This was followed by the development of fetoscopy, by sophisticated ultrasound and, ultimately in the 1980s, by CVS and fetal blood sampling[34]. These techniques have truly revolutionized obstetric practice. They allow the physician to provide couples with an assessment of fetal health during pregnancy. They give patients the option of considering termination of pregnancy when fetal abnormalities are detected. This option would not be available but for changes that occurred in the law over the past 25 years. The history of the availability of pregnancy termination is both interesting and instructive. Laws in place in most of the USA since the early years of the 20th century were extremely restrictive of a woman's ability to obtain a pregnancy termination. In 1973, in response to challenges of these laws, in two separate United States Supreme Court decisions (Roe vs. Wade and, later, Doe vs.

Bolton), the Supreme Court decided that the due process clause of the Constitution had what was described as a 'penumbra' of rights. This included a right to privacy under which a woman had the absolute right to decide upon continuation or termination of pregnancy in the first trimester. Prior to fetal viability, the state's only interest in this matter was to insure that such procedures were done under safe and acceptable conditions. Termination at a time after fetal viability could be performed only for the health and welfare of the mother. Laws in many other countries underwent similar changes in the 1970s, although in a few countries such as Germany, laws have tended to become more restrictive in the 1980s and 90s.

Before the development of fetal reduction techniques, in the case of a multifetal pregnancy, advanced prenatal diagnostic techniques created a new dilemma. A patient might have discovered after testing that one of the fetuses she was carrying had an abnormality and the other was most likely to be normal. This resulted in an impossible situation. The couple was faced with the choice of either continuing with both or terminating both fetuses. Faced with such quandaries, couples were forced to choose between two very difficult options. The development of fetal reduction procedures have greatly alleviated these problems.

RISKS OF ANOMALIES

It has been recognized for many years that the incidence of certain structural abnormalities such as neural tube defects, cardiac defects and chromosomal defects are more commonly seen in twin gestations than in singletons[1,35,36] (Table 4). Monozygotic twins in particular are prone to develop defects of laterality such as situs inversus. The incidence of abnormalities in monoamniotic twins is even higher than that in monochorionic/diamniotic fetuses.

The incidence of chromosome abnormalities in monozygotic twins parallels age-related risks for singleton gestations. Furthermore, there should be essentially

Table 4 *Incidence (%) of major and minor malformations in monozygotic and dizygotic twins and in singletons*

Race	Twins						Singletons	
	Monozygotic		Dizygotic					
	Major	Minor	Major	Minor			Major	Minor
White	10.49	9.09	6.06	3.41				
Black	11.54	12.50	8.56	7.65				
Total	10.72	10.99	7.78	5.51			7.10	7.26

100% concordance between the twins who formed from the fertilization of one egg with one sperm and divided into twins after fertilization. Most twins, however, are dizygotic. Dizygotic twins are created when two eggs are fertilized by two sperm. Thus, the risk of either twin being aneuploid is independent of the risk of the other twin being aneuploid. An example would be in the case of a patient of age 35. The risk of this woman having a baby with a chromosome abnormality is approximately one in 190[35,37]. If there are two fetuses, the risk is essentially doubled, i.e. two in 190 or one in 95. A one in 95 risk corresponds to the risk of a singleton for a 38-year-old woman. We have thus aged our 35-year-old patient by 3 years. Similarly, the risk for a 30-year-old woman with a singleton is one in 380. With twins the risk is approximately two in 380, i.e. the risk of a 35-year-old woman, an aging of 5 years. It is important to note that traditionally one in three twins are said to be monozygotic. However, that proportion has steadily fallen secondary to the use of fertility drugs, as described below (Table 3).

Reproductive medicine has been extremely successful. As these technologies become more advanced and successful, the number of multiple gestations has grown. From 1973 to 1990 twin births increased at twice the rate of singletons and triplets, and triplet and higher births rose seven-fold faster than singletons[38]. The rate of twins in the USA increased from one in 55 births to one in 43, and the rate of triplets and higher births from one in 3323 to one in 1343[38]. This is a significant increase. Along with the increasing number of multiple gestations there is an increasing incidence of congenital anomalies diagnosed in these gestations. In dizygotic twins the likelihood of finding an anomaly in at least one twin is slightly more than twice the risk of finding an anomaly in a singleton pregnancy. However, in monozygotic gestations for whom the rate of Mendelian and chromosomal abnormalities is equivalent to that of a singleton pregnancy, there is a significantly increased risk for structural malformations. This is primarily the result of defects of laterality[25]. Discordancy for structural and genetic anomalies is common in both monozygotic and dizygotic twins. For example, in a dizygotic pregnancy at risk for an autosomal recessive disorder such as cystic fibrosis or Tay–Sachs disease, the chance that at least one of the twins will be affected is not 25% but 44%. This raises several issues regarding pregnancy management including termination of the pregnancy, expectant management and, more recently, selective termination of the anomalous fetus.

ETHICS

The development of the procedures that reduce the number of a pregnancy has been wrought with controversy. Many people steadfastly feel that any deliberate termination of a fetus is *prima facie* ethically unpermissible. Examining these issues requires one to look both at the similarities between selective termination of an anomalous fetus and at the reduction of the number of fetuses in a multifetal pregnancy. There are many parallels when comparing selective termination to MFPR in terms of the ethics of the procedure[39]. There are, however, distinct differences between these procedures and the performance of an elective or voluntary termination of pregnancy. A woman undergoes a voluntary termination of pregnancy because she does not want to have a child at this time. It is a procedure specifically intended to terminate a pregnancy in its entirety. Selective termination and MFPR are performed for quite different reasons. Patients who have these procedures performed fully intend to carry a pregnancy to term. These patients desire to have one or more healthy children and want their pregnancy to proceed in such a way as to give that child or those children the best possible chance of a good outcome. A woman undergoes MFPR because of the large number of fetuses, greatly reducing her chances of a happy outcome. A selective termination is performed in order to prevent a tragedy, the birth of an abnormal child. Before the development of these procedures, in the case of one anomalous twin, there was only the option of either terminating the entire pregnancy or keeping both fetuses and committing oneself to care of a potentially severely handicapped infant. The development of selective termination has allowed couples faced with this extremely difficult situation to attempt to have a presumably healthy infant while being spared the emotional and financial trauma incurred with the birth of a severely handicapped infant. The Ethics Committee of the American College of Obstetricians and Gynecologists has endorsed the ethical probity of offering selective termination under such circumstances[40]. In a society that legally permits abortion, there is no ethical justification and probably no legal basis for attempting to impose legal sanctions against selective termination as have been proposed in a number of jurisdictions in the USA.

Chervenak and colleagues discuss the underlying ethical justifications for selective termination[41]. The first occurs when one seeks the delivery of one or more healthy liveborn infants. The second seeks the delivery of one or more infants whose anomalies, although present, could not have been detected prenatally. The third ethical justification is that of a pregnancy that results in a singleton live birth, through the use of multifetal reduction. These three outcomes are supported primarily by two ethical principles: the first is the importance that we give to the autonomy of the pregnant woman; and the second is the autonomy and beneficence of the pregnant woman herself. With each of these two principles, it is the mother who confers independent status on the pre-viable fetus. These principles are in direct opposition to an ethical belief that the fetus has an independent status from the point of conception forward. This latter belief is inconsistent with the laws of the USA, at least until the point of viability. It was initially our opinion that, because of the complexity of the procedure and the risk to the remaining fetus(es), these procedures should not be performed 'frivolously', but only for well-defined medical indications[8]. However, we eventually realized the importance of autonomy and free choice in the patient's desire to have these procedures performed. Our feeling now is that, within the confines of the law and ethics, the choice of treatment must ultimately reside in the hands of the patient. This brings up the question of the physician who does not ethically wish either to provide these services to patients or to offer these patients a referral to a physician who will do so. A basic legal and ethical principle is that, with the exception of medical emergencies, a patient's individual right to treatment does not supercede a physician's right of conscience to refrain from acting in a manner that he or she finds unacceptable[42]. There is no legal or ethical obligation for a doctor to perform a fetal reduction, as it is not an emergency procedure. However, it is the obligation of each physician to educate their patients regarding treatment options.

Fetal reduction procedures have been performed for only approximately 20 years, a relatively short time. As with all procedures, as physicians gain experience in their performance and the safety of the procedure becomes more recognized, the appropriate indications for the procedure will be likely to become more clearly delineated. Neither selective termination nor MFPR should be performed for frivolous reasons, merely for convenience or without serious individual examination of the appropriateness of the procedures. The issue of reduction to singleton still remains controversial. Preliminary data from the International Registry of Multifetal Pregnancy Reductions suggest that there is a slightly better outcome for multifetal pregnancies reduced to a singleton as opposed to those reduced to twins[43]. An important issue is that twins on average are delivered about 4 weeks prematurely and have a 5% incidence of long-term problems. This is as opposed to a 2–3% incidence in a singleton pregnancy. It could be argued that this difference alone might be sufficient to make fetal reduction to singleton ethically appropriate in selected circumstances. We believe that, in a pluralistic society such as the one in which we live, intelligent and well-meaning people can look at the same facts and reach completely opposite conclusions. It is therefore our belief that, in the appropriate cases, selective termination of a multifetal pregnancy to a singleton can be justified on ethical and scientific grounds. There appears to be a more favorable fetal outcome. This is particularly true if there are mediating circumstances that would make even a twin pregnancy difficult for the mother to carry. A great deal of thought and consideration must go into the decision to reduce to a singleton pregnancy. As long as the decision for reduction to a singleton is not based on convenience or sex selection, we believe that it can be considered ethical under appropriate circumstances. It is our feeling, however, that in the majority of instances, reduction of multifetal pregnancies to twins is probably the more appropriate course. We would thus strongly argue against routine reduction of twins to a singleton. The difference in outcome between twin and singleton pregnancies in the USA does not justify the utilization of this invasive procedure in an effort to improve the favorable outcome by reduction of uncomplicated twin pregnancies to singletons.

CONCLUSION

The science and practice of obstetrics has been changed radically over the past 20 years by the development of advanced reproductive technologies. These medical advances have, however, created a bitter irony. Women who previously could not achieve a successful pregnancy now are suddenly faced with the prospect of bearing more fetuses than they are likely to carry successfully. It has been known for many years that the obstetric outcome for triplets or higher-order pregnancies is significantly worse than that of the singleton. These patients now have three options available to them. They may choose to end the pregnancy. However, with the time, emotion and finances spent on becoming pregnant, this option is quite unsatisfactory. They may continue with the entire pregnancy, knowing that the likelihood of complete success is low. The last option is that they may reduce the number of fetuses. Multifetal pregnancy reduction (MFPR) is now a realistic option. It is performed in the late first trimester. The most common technique used involves the intrathoracic injection of potassium chloride with a technical success rate approaching 100% in experienced hands. The procedure-related pregnancy loss rates depend upon the number of fetuses terminated and range from 6 to 12%. We continue to hope that MFPR will become obsolete as better control of ovulation agents and assisted reproductive technologies make multifetal pregnancies uncommon.

Selective termination is the procedure that has been developed in order to manage a twin gestation discordant for fetal anomalies. As most anomalies are diagnosed and confirmed by 14 weeks' gestational age, this procedure is most often performed in the second trimester. As with MFPR, intrathoracic potassium chloride is used. Selective terminations should, when possible, be performed before 20 weeks' estimated gestational age. This acts to reduce the rate of preterm delivery noted when the procedure was performed at more than 20 weeks' gestational age. As in all medical procedures, patients need to be counselled individually regarding their procedural risks.

The development of these procedures has caused a great deal of discussion to occur in the area of medical ethics. In the case of obstetric ethics, the principles of autonomy and beneficence give the pregnant mother the right to bestow independent status on her pre-viable fetus. As with any aspect of medical practice, the physician has no obligation to perform a procedure that violates his or her own personal ethics, except in the case of a life-threatening emergency. However, all physicians have the obligation to inform patients of legally available procedures that could be potentially beneficial.

References

1. Bronsteen RA, Evans MI. Multiple gestation. In Evans MI, Fletcher JC, Dixler AO, Schulman JD, eds. *Fetal Diagnosis and Therapy: Science, Ethics and the Law.* Philadelphia: JB Lippincott, 1989: 242–65

2. Lunefeld B, Lunenfeld E. Ovulation induction: HMG. In Seibel MM, ed. *Infertility: A Comprehensive Text.* Norwalk, CT: Appleton & Lange, 1992:311–23

3. Evans MI, Dixler AO. Human *in vitro* fertilization: some legal issues. *J Am Med Assoc* 1981;245:22, 2324–7

4. MacLennan AH. Multiple gestations. In Creasy RK, Resnik R, eds. *Maternal Fetal Medicine: Principles and Practice,* 3rd edn. Philadelphia: WB Saunders, 1994:589–601

5. Newmann RB, Hamer C, Miller C. Outpatient triplet management: a contemporary review. *Am J Obstet Gynecol* 1989;161:547–55

6. Collins MS, Bleyl JA. Seventy one quadruplet pregnancies: management and outcome. *Am J Obstet Gynecol* 1990;162:1384–92

7. Petrokovsky B, Vintzileos A. Management and outcome of multiple pregnancies of higher fetal order: literature review. *Obstet Gynecol Surv* 1989;44:578

8. Evans MI, Fletcher JC, Zador IE, Newton BW, Quigg MG, Struyk CD. Selective first trimester termination in octuplet and quadruplet pregnancies: clinical and ethical issues. *Obstet Gynecol* 1988;71:289–96

9. Berkowitz RL, Lynch L, Chitkara U, *et al.* Selective reduction of multifetal pregnancies in the first trimester. *N Engl J Med* 1988;318:1043

10. Dumez Y, Oury JF. Method for first trimester selective abortion in multiple pregnancy. *Contrib Gynecol Obstet* 1986;15:50

11. Kanhai HH, VanRijssel EJC, Meerman RJ, *et al.* Selective termination in quintuplet pregnancy during first trimester. *Lancet* 1986;2:1447

12. Lynch L, Berkowitz RL, Chitkara U, *et al.* First trimester transabdominal multiple pregnancy reduction: a report of 85 cases. *Obstet Gynecol* 1990;75:735

13. Tabsh KM. Transabdominal multifetal pregnancy reduction: report of 40 cases. *Obstet Gynecol* 1990; 75:739

14. Evans MI, May M, Drugan A, *et al.* Selective termination: clinical experience and residual risks. *Am J Obstet Gynecol* 1990;162:1568–75

15. Aberg A, Miterian F, Cantz M, Geliler J. Cardiac puncture of fetus with Hurler's disease avoiding abortion of unaffected co-twin. *Lancet* 1978;2: 990–1

16. Kerenyi T, Chitkara U. Selective birth in twin pregnancy with discordancy for Down's syndrome. *N Engl J Med* 1981;304:1525–7

17. Petres R, Redwine F. Selective birth in twin pregnancy. *N Engl J Med* 1981;305:1218–19

18. Rodeck C, Mibashan R, Abramowitz J, Campbell S. Selective feticide of the affected twin by fetoscopic air embolization. *Prenat Diagn* 1982;2:189–94

19. Rodeck C. Fetoscopy in the management of twin pregnancies discordant for a severe abnormality. *Acta Genet Med Gemellol* 1984;33:57–60

20. Golbus MS, Cunningham N, Goldberg JD, Anderson R, Filly R, Callen P. Selective termination of multiple gestations. *Am J Med Genet* 1988;31:339–48

21. Varma TR. Ultrasound evidence of early pregnancy failure in patients with multiple conceptions. *Br J Obstet Gynaecol* 1979;86:290

22. Gindoft PR, Yeh MN, Jewelewicz R. The vanishing sac syndrome. *J Reprod Med* 1986;31:322

23. Evans MI, Dommergues M, Wapner RJ, *et al.* Efficacy of transabdominal multifetal pregnancy reduction: collaborative experience of the world's largest centers. *Obstet Gynecol* 1993;82: 61–6

24. Yaron Y, Bryant-Greenwood PK, Dave N, *et al.* Multifetal pregnancy reductions (MFPR) of triplets to twins: comparison with non-reduced triplets and twins. *Am J Obstet Gynecol* 1999;in press

25. Wapner RJ, Davis GH, Johnson A. Selective reduction of multifetal pregnancies. *Lancet* 1990;335:90–3

26. Evans MI, Dommergues M, Timor-Tritsch I, *et al.* Transabdominal versus transcervical and transvaginal multifetal pregnancy reduction: international collaborative experience of more than one thousand cases. *Am J Obstet Gynecol* 1994; 170:902–9

27. Timor-Tritsch IE, Peisner DB, Monteagudo A, Lercner JP, Sharma S. Multifetal pregnancy reduction by transvaginal puncture: evaluation of the technique used in 134 cases. *Am J Obstet Gynecol* 1993;168:799–804

28. Evans MI, Littman L, St Louis L, *et al.* Evolving patterns of iatrogenic multifetal pregnancy generation: implications for aggressiveness of infertility treatments. *Am J Obstet Gynecol* 1995; 172:1750–3

29. Brambati B, Tului L, Baldi M, Guercilena S. Genetic analysis prior to selective fetal reduction in multiple pregnancy: technical aspects and clinical outcome. *Hum Reprod* 1995;10:818–25

30. Evans MI, Goldberg JD, Dommergues M, *et al.* Efficacy of second trimester selective termination for fetal abnormalities: international collaborative experience among the world's largest centers. *Am J Obstet Gynecol* 1994;171:90–4

31. Evans MI, Dommergues M, Wapner RJ, *et al.* International collaborative experience of 1789 patients having multifetal pregnancy reduction: a plateauing of risks and outcomes. *J Soc Gynecol Invest* 1996;3:23–6

32. Cohen J, DeVane GW, Elsner CW, *et al.* Cryopreservation of zygotes and early cleaved human embryos. *Fertil Steril* 1988;49:283–9

33. Hecht BR, Magoon MW. Can the epidemic of iatrogenic multiples be conquered? *Clin Obstet Gynecol* 1998;41:127–37

34. Evans MI, Quigg MH, Koppitch FC III, Schulman JD. First trimester prenatal diagnosis. In Evans MI, Fletcher JC, Dixler AO, Schulman JD, eds. *Fetal Diagnosis and Therapy: Science, Ethics and the Law.* Philadelphia: JB Lippincott, 1989:17–35

35. Luke B. Monozygotic twinning as a congenital defect and congenital defects in monozygotic twins. *Fetal Diagn Ther* 1990;5:61–9

36. Evans MI, Johnson MP, Isada NB, Holzgreve W. Selective termination. In Brock DJH, Rodeck CH, Ferguson-Smith MA, eds. *Prenatal Diagnosis and Screening.* New York: Churchill Livingstone, 1992: 689–95

37. Verp MS. Antenatal diagnosis of chromosomal abnormalities. In Sciarra JJ, ed. *Gynecology and Obstetrics*, vol 5. Philadelphia, JB Lippincott, 1988:1–8

38. Luke B. The changing pattern of multiple births in the United Sates: maternal and infant characteristics, 1973 and 1990. *Obstet Gynecol* 1994;84:101–6

39. Evans MI, Fletcher JC, Rodeck C. Ethical problems in multiple gestations: selective termination. In Evans MI, Fletcher JC, Dixler AO, Schulman JD, eds. *Fetal Diagnosis and Therapy: Science, Ethics and the Law.* Philadelphia: JB Lippincott, 1989:266–76

40. Committee on Ethics, American College of Obstetricians and Gynecologists. *Ethics Statement: Multifetal Pregnancy Reduction and Selective Fetal Termination.* Washington: ACOG, 1990

41. Chervenak FA, McCullough LB, Wapner R. Three ethically justified indications for selective termination in multifetal pregnancy: a practical and comprehensive management strategy. *J Assist Reprod Med* 1995;12:531–6

42. McCullough LB, Chervenak FA. *Ethics in Obstetrics and Gynecology.* New York: Oxford University Press, 1994

43. Dumez Y, Evans MI, Wapner RJ, *et al.* Efficacy of multifetal pregnancy reduction (MFPR): collaborative experience of the world's largest centers. *Society of Perinatal Obstetricians, 11th Annual Meeting*, San Francisco, January 28–February 2, 1991

Antepartum testing of fetal well-being 22

K. B. Lescale and M. Y. Divon

INTRODUCTION

The concept of antepartum fetal surveillance was first introduced three decades ago. Following the inception of the electronic fetal monitor in the 1960s, the contraction stress test (CST) was the first technique introduced to assess fetal well-being[1,2]. Subsequently, various other techniques have been developed, including maternal assessment of fetal activity, the non-stress test (NST), the fetal biophysical profile and Doppler velocimetry. Although initially intended to evaluate the fetus' potential for labor, the primary goal of antepartum fetal surveillance is to detect fetal hypoxia and acidosis (common causes of fetal death) and, if possible, to avoid fetal death by initiating timely interventions[3]. Indications for antepartum fetal surveillance include maternal and fetal conditions associated with increased rates of intrauterine fetal death, such as suspected intrauterine growth restriction (IUGR), hypertension, diabetes mellitus, prolonged pregnancy, decreased fetal movement and history of previous stillbirth. Despite their recent popularity and widespread use, few randomized controlled trials have been performed to assess any of these techniques in an adequate fashion. In fact, the majority of data have shown improved pregnancy outcome by way of descriptive clinical studies[4]. This chapter reviews each of the above techniques, with emphasis on the evidence available to validate their efficacy in clinical practice.

THE CONTRACTION STRESS TEST

As the use of intrapartum electronic fetal monitoring became more widespread, it was noted that late fetal heart rate (FHR) decelerations were associated with 'utero-placental insufficiency' and subsequent fetal hypoxia[5]. A late FHR deceleration was recently defined as an apparent gradual decrease and return to baseline FHR associated with a uterine contraction. The decrease is calculated from the most recently determined portion of the baseline. The deceleration is delayed in timing, with the nadir of the deceleration occurring after the peak of the contraction. In most cases, the onset, nadir and recovery of the deceleration occur after the beginning, peak and ending of the contraction, respectively[5]. From these observations the CST was developed[6]. The CST is performed with the patient in the semi-Fowler's position with left lateral uterine displacement. With the use of a standard Doppler ultrasound transducer and tocodynamometer, a baseline tracing is obtained for 10–20 min. Uterine contractions are induced if adequate spontaneous contractions (at least three contractions of 40-s duration or more in a 10-min period) are not observed. Contractions are induced either by nipple stimulation or by a low-dose infusion of oxytocin. The CST is considered positive when late decelerations are seen following 50% or more of uterine contractions. When no decelerations are observed, the test is interpreted as negative. With intermittent late or significant variable decelerations (defined as an abrupt decrease in the FHR below the baseline which may begin before, during or after the onset of the contraction), the CST is labeled equivocal[7]. When the equivocal test is repeated within 24 h, the second test is rarely positive[8].

Although numerous observational and retrospective studies have been performed evaluating the CST[9-13], only one prospective and blinded study has been published. In 1972, Ray and colleagues[14] described their experience with the oxytocin challenge test and noted three fetal deaths in 15 patients with a positive CST. They also noted a 53% incidence of low Apgar scores in the group with a positive CST. However, the overall false-positive rate of the CST was greater than 50% in combined studies. The false-negative rate was very low, with an incidence of stillbirth occurring within 1 week of a negative test at 0.4 per 1000 high-risk patients[15]. The CST is contraindicated in those patients at high risk for preterm labor, premature rupture of membranes, placenta previa and previous classical Cesarean section.

In summary, despite a high false-positive rate, the negative CST is highly predictive of a non-asphyxiated fetus. It is, however, not widely used currently, primarily because of its drawbacks, which include the possible needs for oxytocin infusion and relative proximity to a labor and delivery unit as well as the relative contraindications mentioned above.

THE NON-STRESS TEST

The NST, which was first described by Hammacher[16] in 1968, is the most widely used primary antepartum fetal surveillance technique. It is based on the premise that the presence of FHR accelerations associated with fetal body movements is indicative of a fetus that is not acidotic or neurologically depressed[16]. Patient positioning and electronic fetal monitoring are similar to those in the CST; however, the NST is less invasive, simple to perform and interpret and often less time consuming. The NST is considered reactive if two or more FHR accelerations (defined as 15 beats/min above the baseline lasting for 15 s) are observed within a 20-min period. A non-reactive tracing is one without sufficient FHR accelerations over a 40-min period[17].

There have been four controlled trials that have evaluated the efficacy of the NST[18-21]. Because of their small sample size, none was able to show a benefit from the use of the NST in preventing perinatal mortality. It has been stated that, in order to detect a reduction in perinatal death from 15/1000 pregnancies to 10/1000 pregnancies, one would have to study more than 19 000 fetuses[22].

A large collaborative trial by Freeman and co-workers[23] compared the efficacy of the NST to that of the CST in 1542 high-risk patients. Although the perinatal mortality was significantly higher for the NST than for the CST (3.2/1000 vs. 1.4/1 000), they were both considered extremely low and acceptable for a high-risk population.

Similarly to the CST, the NST has a false-positive rate of greater than 50%. However, the false-negative rate is higher, at 5/1000 for weekly testing and approximately 2/1000 for semi-weekly testing[24]. Still, it is less time consuming than the CST and has relatively no contraindications. As both tests have a high false-positive rate, they should be used as a screening test only in indicated high-risk pregnancies at increased risk for perinatal morbidity and mortality.

MATERNAL ASSESSMENT OF FETAL ACTIVITY

Regarded as an inexpensive and simple technique, maternal assessment of fetal activity has been studied since the early 1970s as an effective form of antepartum fetal surveillance[25,26]. Numerous protocols have been outlined in prospective studies, all with different time intervals for movements counted and number of movements counted per interval.

In one prospective controlled study by Neldam[27], 1562 pregnant patients at 32 weeks' gestation were asked to count fetal movements three times weekly for 2 h after meals. Further evaluation by ultrasound or the NST was performed in patients who noted fewer than three fetal movements per hour. A total of 1549 pregnant patients served as controls and were not asked to monitor fetal activity. Ten stillbirths were noted in the control group as compared to one in the monitored group.

Using the 'count to ten' approach, Moore and Piacquadio[28] illustrated, in a prospective trial in 1989, a 50% decrease in fetal deaths in monitored vs. non-monitored pregnancies. In this protocol, pregnant women were asked to monitor fetal activity daily for up to 2 h or until ten movements were observed. Further evaluation was performed in women who did not perceive ten movements in 2 h. During an expanded period, in a study of nearly 6000 pregnant women, the fetal death rate dropped from 8.7/1000 to 3.6/1000. Only one of 290 patients who presented with a complaint of decreased fetal movement had already suffered a fetal death.

In summary, maternal assessment of fetal activity is a simple, inexpensive and non-invasive form of antepartum surveillance. As with the NST and the CST there is a high false-positive rate combined with a relatively low (i.e. approximately 10%) false-negative rate[4]. One advantage over other antepartum tests is the convenience of performing fetal movement counts at home.

THE FETAL BIOPHYSICAL PROFILE

The biophysical profile was first introduced in the early 1980s by Manning and co-workers[29]. It was the outgrowth of prior studies which were able to predict perinatal outcome based on the presence or absence of fetal breathing movements[30]. Five components make up the original test and consist of ultrasound monitoring of fetal body movements, fetal tone, fetal breathing, assessment of amniotic fluid volume and FHR reactivity by electronic fetal monitoring. The biophysical profile is based on the association between changes in these five parameters with respect to chronic fetal compromise. Each parameter is given a score of 2 when normal or a score of 0 when abnormal for a total of 10 possible points[29]. A score of ≥ 8 out of 10 is normal while a score of ≤ 4 is abnormal. A score of 6 is considered equivocal and should be repeated within 12–24 h[17]. The presence of oligohydramnios in patients with intact membranes is considered ominous regardless of the overall score. In addition, gestational age should be taken into account when intervention is entertained on the basis of a biophysical profile score.

In the original prospective blinded study of 216 high-risk patients, Manning and colleagues observed no perinatal deaths when all five variables were normal[29]. A perinatal mortality rate of 60% was observed in fetuses with a score of zero. Unfortunately, since its introduction more than 18 years ago, fewer than 3000 pregnancies have been studied in randomized trials[31–34]. When compared with conventional fetal monitoring (NST or CST), the use of the biophysical profile resulted in no obvious improvement on pregnancy outcome relative to the NST or the CST. In other words, the biophysical profile may be used interchangeably with the NST or CST to achieve a similar perinatal outcome. The false-positive rate for the biophysical profile has not been easily ascertainable from the available data. However, available data on fetal breathing movements have demonstrated a false-positive rate of 75% and a false-negative rate of 4%, which are comparable to those of the NST[35]. Some authors have suggested a 'modified biophysical profile' based on the combination of the NST and sonographic assessment of amniotic fluid volume[33]. This has been shown to be as reliable as the CST when performed twice weekly.

Unlike the NST or CST, which result in a retrievable document, the biophysical profile cannot be reviewed unless videotaped. There are no known contraindications to performing a biophysical profile; however, its cost is commonly higher than that of the NST and possibly similar to that of the CST.

UMBILICAL ARTERY DOPPLER VELOCIMETRY

Doppler techniques have been studied in obstetrics since the initial report of successful recording of blood flow signals from the umbilical artery by Fitzgerald and Drumm[36] in 1977. This is based on the premise that an insufficient uterine, placental or fetal circulation results in adverse pregnancy outcome and that these abnormalities can be defined with the use of Doppler velocimetry.

Under normal physiological conditions the placenta presents as an area of low vascular impedance, thus the umbilical artery demonstrates a peak in systole (S) with a large amount of end-diastolic (D) flow. Throughout the third trimester of a normal pregnancy there is a progressive increase in diastolic flow, leading to a gradual decrease in the S/D ratio. Beyond 30 weeks' gestation the umbilical artery S/D ratio is generally between 2.0 and 3.0. Elevated placental impedance is associated with low, absent or even reversed end-diastolic blood flow.

Despite the fact that Doppler velocimetry is the newest modality to assess fetal well-being, it has been the subject of more randomized trials than any other biophysical test of fetal growth or well-being[4]. Management and perinatal intervention based on abnormal umbilical artery Doppler velocimetry remain unclear. It is reasonable to consider extremely abnormal umbilical arterial flow patterns (i.e. absent or reversed umbilical flow) in the context of other abnormal test results in formulating a management plan[4].

Recently, Giles and Bisits[37] evaluated the clinical utility of umbilical artery velocimetry in the management of high-risk pregnancies by performing a meta-analysis of published, peer-reviewed and randomized controlled trials. Six studies were reviewed with 2102 patients in the Doppler group and 2133 patients in the control (non-Doppler) group. The analysis was based on 'intention to treat' and perinatal death was defined as the primary outcome variable. The meta-analysis revealed a significant reduction in perinatal mortality in the Doppler group without an increase in the rate of inappropriate obstetric interventions. Specifically, the analysis demonstrated a reduction in the incidence of intrauterine death in normally formed fetuses, with a typical odds ratio of 0.54 and a 95% confidence interval of 0.32–0.89. A similar conclusion was reached by Alfirevic

and Neilson[38] who reviewed 12 published and unpublished randomized controlled trials of Doppler ultrasonography of the umbilical artery in high-risk patients.

A cumulative meta-analysis of eight published and peer-reviewed randomized controlled trials of 6838 patients revealed that the availability of umbilical artery Doppler studies significantly decreased perinatal mortality with an odds ratio of 0.66 and a 95% confidence interval of 0.46–0.94 ($p = 0.013$)[39]. Repeating the analysis after exclusion of the malformed fetus did not drastically change these results. Thus, the author concluded that no further randomized trials were needed.

Despite the absence of unified management protocols based on Doppler velocimetry[40], there are ample data which indicate that the availability of umbilical artery Doppler velocimetry in high-risk patients (especially those complicated by hypertension or suspected fetal growth restriction) is associated with a significant decrease in perinatal mortality without a concomitant increase in maternal or neonatal morbidity. At a minimum, an abnormal result of an umbilical artery Doppler study should be added to the current list of indications for intensive fetal surveillance[39].

CONCLUSION

The concept of antepartum fetal surveillance was introduced over three decades ago. With the support of numerous descriptive clinical trials and very few randomized controlled trials it has become a major component in the effort to maximize pregnancy outcome and minimize perinatal morbidity and mortality in high-risk pregnancies. As all of the currently available techniques are associated with a high false-positive rate, they should be applied only in pregnancies believed to benefit from their use.

References

1. Caldeyro-Barcia R, Mendez-Bauer C, Posiero JJ, *et al.* Fetal monitoring in labor. In Wallace HM, Gold EM, Lis EF, Thomas CG, eds. *Maternal Child Health Practices: Problems, Resources, and Methods of Delivery.* Springfield, IL: Third Party Publishing, 1994:332–94

2. Hon EH. Fetal heart rate monitoring for evaluation of fetal well-being. *Postgrad Med* 1977; 61:139

3. Vintzileos AM. Antepartum fetal surveillance. In Pitkin RM, Scott JR, eds. *Antepartum Fetal Surveillance. Clinical Obstetrics and Gynecology.* Philadelphia: JB Lippincott, 1995:1–3

4. Thacker SB, Berkelman RL. Assessing the diagnostic accuracy and efficacy of selected antepartum fetal surveillance techniques. *Obstet Gynecol Surv* 1986;41:121–41

5. Parer JT, Quilligan EJ. Electronic fetal heart rate monitoring: research guidelines for interpretation. *J Obstet Gynecol Neonatal Nursing* 1997;26:635–40

6. Pose SV, Castillo JB, Mora-Rojas EO, *et al.* Test of fetal tolerance to induce uterine contractions for the diagnosis of chronic distress: perinatal factors affecting human development. *Pan Am Health Organ Sci Publ* 1969;185:96–104

7. Lagrew DC Jr. The contractions stress test. In Pitkin PM, Scott JR, eds. *Antepartum Fetal Surveillance. Clinical Obstetrics and Gynecology.* Philadelphia: JB Lippincott, 1995:11–25

8. Bruce SL, Petrie RH, Yeh SY. The suspicious contractions stress test. *Obstet Gynecol* 1978;51:415

9. Nageotte MP, Towers CV, Asrat T, *et al.* The value of a negative antepartum test: contraction stress test and modified biophysical profile. *Obstet Gynecol* 1994;84:231

10. Freeman R, Garite T, Modanlou H, *et al.* Postdate pregnancy: utilization of contraction stress testing for primary fetal surveillance. *Am J Obstet Gynecol* 1981;140:128

11. Druzin ML, Karver ML, Wagner W, *et al.* Prospective evaluation of the contraction stress test and non stress tests in the management of post-term pregnancy. *Surg Gynecol Obstet* 1992;174: 507

12. Gabbe SG, Mestman JH, Freeman RK, *et al.* Management and outcome of diabetes mellitus, classes B-R. *Am J Obstet* 1977;129:723

13. Legrew DC, Pircon RA, Towers CV, *et al.* Antepartum fetal surveillance in patients with diabetes: when to start. *Am J Obstet Gynecol* 1993; 168:1820

14. Ray M, Freeman R, Pine S, *et al.* Clinical experience with the oxytocin challenge test. *Am J Obstet Gynecol* 1972;114:1

15. Everston L, Gauthier R, Collea J. Fetal demise following negative contraction stress tests. *Obstet Gynecol* 1978;51:671

16. Hammacher K. The clinical significance of cardiotocography. In Huntingford J, Hunter ES, Saling E, eds. *Perinatal Medicine.* New York: Academic Press, 1968:80–93

17. American College of Obstetricians and Gynecologists. *Antepartum Fetal Surveillance.* ACOG Technical Bulletin 138. Washington: ACOG, 1994

18. Brown VA, Sawers RS, Parsons RJ, *et al.* The value of antenatal cardiotocography in the management of high-risk pregnancy: a randomized controlled trial. *Br J Obstet Gynaecol* 1982;89:716

19. Flynn AM, Kelly J, Mansfield H, *et al.* A randomized controlled trial of non-stress antepartum cardiotocography. *Br J Obstet Gynaecol* 1982;89:427

20. Granat M, Lavie P, Adar D, Sharf M. Short-term cycles in human fetal activity. I. Normal pregnancies. *Am J Obstet Gynecol* 1979;134:696

21. Lumley LA, Anderson I, Renou P, Wood C. A randomized trial of weekly cardiotocography in high-risk obstetric patients. *Br J Obstet Gynaecol* 1983;90:1018

22. National Center for Health Statistics/National Center for Health Services Research. *Health United States, 1981.* Publication no. (PHS) 82-1332. Hyattsville, MD: DHHS, 1981:112

23. Freeman R, Anderson G, Dorchester W. A prospective multi-institutional study of antepartum fetal heart rate monitoring. II. Contraction stress test versus nonstress test for primary surveillance. *Am J Obstet Gynecol* 1982; 143:778

24. Boehm FH, Salyer S, Shah DM, *et al.* Improved outcome of twice weekly nonstress testing. *Obstet Gynecol* 1986;67:566

25. Rosen MG, Hertz RH, Dieker LJ Jr, *et al.* Monitoring fetal movement. *Clin Obstet Gynecol* 1979;6:325

26. Sadovsky E, Yaffe H. Daily fetal movement recording and fetal prognosis. *Obstet Gynecol* 1973; 41:845

27. Neldam S. Fetal movements as an indicator of fetal well being. *Lancet* 1980;1:1222

28. Moore TR, Piacquadio K. A prospective evaluation of fetal movement screening to reduce the incidence of antepartum fetal death. *Am J Obstet Gynecol* 1989;160:1075

29. Manning F, Platt L, Sipos L. Antepartum fetal evaluation: development of a fetal biophysical profile. *Am J Obstet Gynecol* 1980;136:787

30. Platt L, Manning F, Lemay M, Sipos L. Human fetal breathing: relationship to fetal condition. *Am J Obstet Gynecol* 1978;132:514

31. Alfirevic Z, Walkinshaw SA. A randomized controlled trial of simple compared with complex antenatal fetal monitoring after 42 weeks of gestation. *Br J Obstet Gynaecol* 1995;102:638–43

32. Manning FA, Lange IR, Morrison I, Harman CR. Fetal biophysical profile score and the nonstress test: a comparative trial. *Obstet Gynecol* 1984;64:326–31

33. Nageotte MP, Towers CV, Asrat T, Freeman RK. Perinatal outcome with the modified biophysical profile. *Am J Obstet Gynecol* 1994;170:1672–6

34. Platt LD, Walla CA, Paul RH, *et al.* A prospective trial of the fetal biophysical profile vs the nonstress test in the management of high-risk pregnancies. *Am J Obstet Gynecol* 1985;153:624–33

35. Manning FA, Platt LD, Sipos L, *et al.* Fetal breathing movements and the nonstress test in high-risk pregnancies. *Am J Obstet Gynecol* 1979;135:511

36. Fitzgerald DE, Drumm JE. Non-invasive measurement of human fetal circulation using ultrasound, a new method. *Br Med J* 1977;2:1450–1

37. Giles WB, Bisits A. Clinical use of Doppler in pregnancy: information from six randomized trials. *Fetal Diagn Ther* 1993;8:247–55

38. Alfirevic A, Neilson JP. Doppler ultrasonography in high-risk pregnancies: systemic review with meta-analysis. *Am J Obstet Gynecol* 1995;172:1379–87

39. Divon MY. Randomized controlled trials of umbilical artery Doppler velocimetry: how many are too many? [Editorial]. *Ultrasound Obstet Gynecol* 1995;6:377–9

40. Divon MY, Girz BA, Lieblich R, Langer O. Clinical management of the fetus with markedly diminished artery end diastolic flow. *Am J Obstet Gynecol* 1989;161:1523–7

Doppler flow studies and fetal heart rate variability

23

G. P. Mandruzzato, L. Fischer-Tamaro, Y. J. Meir and G. Conoscenti

The acronym ARED indicates a Doppler velocity waveform characterized by the absence of detectable flow at the end of diastole or by the presence of reversed flow during diastole. This particular pattern is observable in about 10% of fetuses affected by intrauterine growth restriction (IUGR) and in some cases of fetal abnormalities[1,2]. The observation of ARED flow always indicates a critical condition, as these fetuses are hypoxemic and/or acidemic[3]. This condition is the consequence of a severe reduction of maternal–fetal exchange due to the alterations of the vascular bed of the placenta[4,5]. The clinical outcome is very poor, as this hemodynamic condition is frequently observed at an early gestational age and is associated with increased frequency of fetal abnormalities.

Perinatal mortality and morbidity, immediate and late, are excessively high, but differ according to the characteristics of the Doppler velocity waveform. The clinical aspects and outcome are largely different in the two conditions, absent or reversed flow, being significantly better in the former condition. The outcome is markedly influenced by many other factors, such as gestational age, birth weight, fetal lung maturity and the level and duration of fetal hypoxemia and acidemia. Taking into account all these variables, the timing of the delivery and the choice of the management, active or not, is always difficult and should be based on the evaluation, besides other factors, of the level of hypoxemia. Cordocentesis has been proposed for accurate assessment of the level of fetal oxygenation and acidemia, but the procedure is invasive and carries an increased risk of fetal demise. The availability of a non-invasive technique is preferable for assessing, with sufficient accuracy, the presence and the level of fetal hypoxemia. Fetal heart function is also influenced by hypoxemia and/or acidemia, and its evaluation is the oldest and still the most widely used method for assessing fetal conditions. Cardiotocography (CTG) has been introduced into clinical practice, both intrapartum and antepartum, but, owing to large interobserver and intraobserver variability, its clinical usefulness, particularly when evaluating the compromized fetus, has been disappointing. By traditional eyeball evaluation, alterations of the record are often noticeable too late to be useful in clinical application[6].

In order to overcome these limitations a computerized system for evaluating CTG has been proposed[7]. Among many other parameters offered by this system, fetal heart rate variability is observable on-line. Both long-term and short-term variability are expressed in milliseconds by using different algorithms. The relationship between the two values is very high, exceeding 0.9. Moreover, it has been shown that fetal heart rate variability is significantly reduced in hypoxemic/acidemic fetuses[8].

The aim of our study was to assess the characteristics of fetal heart rate variability in the presence of ARED flow.

MATERIALS AND METHODS

A total of 64 fetuses presenting ARED flow in the umbilical artery and/or the thoracic descending aorta underwent repeated

Table 1 *Clinical characteristics and outcome of 64 fetuses presenting with absent or reversed flow on the Doppler velocity waveform at end-diastole*

	Absent or reversed flow ($n = 64$)	Absent flow ($n = 34$)	Reversed flow ($n = 30$)	Significance
Gestational age at delivery (weeks)	31.73 (23–40)	32.85 (26–40)	30.46 (23–37)	$p < 0.05$
Birth weight (g)	1211 (455–3150)	1341 (550–3150)	1065 (455–2780)	$p < 0.01$
Birth weight (centile)				
< 5th	54 (84.3%)	27 (79.41%)	27 (90%)	NS
5–10th	4 (6.25%)	3 (8.82%)	1 (3.33%)	NS
11–25th	1 (1.56%)	—	1 (3.33%)	
26–50th	1 (1.56%)	1 (2.94%)	—	
> 90th	4 (6.25%)	3 (8.82%)	1 (3.33%)	NS
Fetal abnormalities	8 (12.5%)	3 (8.82%)	5 (16.66%)	NS
Perinatal deaths	28 (43.75%)	5 (14.70%)	23 (76.66%)	$p < 0.01$
fetal	25 (39.06%)	4 (11.76%)	21 (70%)	$p < 0.01$
neonatal	3 (4.68%)	1 (2.94%)	2 (6.66%)	NS
Handicaps (among survivors)	4 (11.11%)	3 (10.34%)	1 (14.28%)	NS
Intact survival	32 (50%)	26 (89.65%)	6 (85.71%)	NS
Days in intensive care	44.37	38.1	70	

computerized CTG. The clinical characteristics and the outcome are presented in Table 1.

Doppler velocity waveforms were obtained in the fetal thoracic descending aorta and the umbilical arteries in a floating part of the cord. At least 10 cycles were studied during periods of fetal apnea and in the absence of fetal movements. The equipment used was an Acuson 128 PX machine (Mountain View, CA) with a probe frequency of 5 MHz, and the high-pass filter set at the minimum possible level in order to avoid false-positive results. The Doppler investigation was repeated daily until delivery or intrauterine fetal demise.

Computerized analysis of the CTG was obtained by using the Oxford System 8000 and the software has been developed by Dawes and co-workers[7]. The long-term fetal heart rate variability was considered as abnormal if values below 20 ms were recorded in more than one trace. The examination was repeated daily or twice a day until delivery or intrauterine fetal demise occurred. Rapid karyotyping by cordocentesis was carried out in 13 cases. In case of fetal or neonatal death, necroscopy was performed in order to confirm the characteristics of the fetal/neonatal anatomy.

At birth, an accurate neonatological examination was undertaken and follow-up of the survivors was performed for not less than 12 months.

RESULTS

In Table 2 the characteristics of the Doppler velocity waveforms are presented with regard to whether they were observed in the aorta only or also at the level of the umbilical arteries. The number of fetal/neonatal deaths in each subgroup and the rates of perinatal mortality are also indicated. The perinatal mortality rate was lower when ARED flow was present only in the aorta, and higher when the umbilical arteries were also involved; the difference was statistically significant ($p < 0.01$), particularly when reversed flow was observed (also reaching the level of significance; $p < 0.01$). The perinatal mortality

Table 2 *Absent or reversed flow in the fetal descending aorta or also in the umbilical arteries, shown by the Doppler velocity waveforms at end-diastole*

	Absent or reversed flow	Perinatal death	Absent flow	Perinatal death	Reversed flow	Perinatal death	Significance
Aorta	23 (35.93%)	2 (8.69%) ↕ $p < 0.01$	18 (52.94%)	2 (11.1%) ↕ NS	5 (16.66%)	0 ↕ $p < 0.01$	NS
Umbilical arteries	41 (64.06%)	26 (63.41%)	16 (47%)	3 (18.75%)	25 (83.33%)	23 (92%)	$p < 0.01$
Total	64	28 (43.75%)	34	5 (14.7%)	30	23 (76.66%)	$p < 0.01$

Table 3 *Absent or reversed flow on Doppler velocity waveform at end-diastole according to normal or abnormal fetal heart rate variability*

Fetal heart rate variability	Absent or reversed flow ($n = 64$)	Perinatal death	Absent flow ($n = 34$)	Perinatal death	Reversed flow ($n - 30$)	Perinatal death	Significance
Normal (≥ 20 ms)	39 (60.93%)	11 (28.2%) ↕ $p < 0.05$	28 (82.35%)	4 (14.29%) ↕ NS	10 (33.3%)	7 (70%) ↕ NS	$p < 0.01$
Abnormal (< 20 ms)	25 (39.06%)	17 (68%)	6 (17.64%)	1 (16.66%)	20 (66.6%)	16 (80%)	$p < 0.01$

rate in the subgroup presenting absent end-diastolic flow did not differ significantly between cases in which only the aorta was involved and those in which the umbilical arteries were also involved.

In the subgroup presenting absent end-diastolic flow only in the aorta, two cases of perinatal death occurred. The first was a case of neonatal death at 20 days due to a congenital heart abnormality and situs viscerum inversus. The second was a case of intrauterine death at 26 weeks; after counselling with the family, a non-active management had been chosen, owing to the estimated low fetal weight. At birth, the weight was 550 g. Among the 16 survivors, late sequelae are present in two cases: one of lobar emphysema and one of retinopathy.

In the group of five cases presenting reversed flow only in the aorta, no deaths were recorded, but one of the survivors presents a handicap (cerebral palsy).

Perinatal mortality was significantly higher when reversed flow was observed, particularly in the umbilical arteries, as compared to cases presenting absence of end-diastolic flow ($p < 0.01$). In the subgroup with absence of end-diastolic flow in the umbilical arteries, three deaths were recorded among 16 cases (18.75%). These were all cases in which non-active management had been chosen: because of malformation in two cases (hydrops) and because of early gestational age and low estimated fetal weight in one case. The difference in perinatal mortality rate with the group of absent flow observed only in the aorta was not significant.

In the subgroup of 25 cases presenting reversed flow in the umbilical arteries also, 23 cases of perinatal death were recorded (92%), and the difference compared to those observed in cases of absent flow in the umbilical arteries was significant. It was also significant when compared with the subgroup with reversed flow present only in the aorta. In two cases, neonatal death occurred (at 8 days and at 9 months, respectively). In the other 21 cases intrauterine death was recorded, owing to the choice of non-active management related to the presence of fetal malformations (five cases) or early gestational age and/or a low estimated fetal weight.

In Table 3 the characteristics of the fetal heart rate variability are presented in relation

Table 4 *Sequelae in four survivors with absent or reversed end-diastolic flow in the fetal aorta or umbilical arteries*

Case	Gestational age (weeks)	Birth weight (g)	Centile	Aorta	Umbilical arteries	Fetal heart rate variability (ms)	ICU stay (days)	Handicap
1	31	1370	11–25	absent 3 days; reversed 1 day	absent 4 days	21.9	42	cerebral palsy
2	36	1630	< 5	absent 2 days	PI > 2 SD 2 days	46.7	39	retinopathy
3	33	1260	< 5	PI > 2 SD 12 days; absent 2 days	PI > 2 SD 14 days	16.8	38	lobar emphysema
4	28	755	< 5	PI < 2 SD	absent 10 days	31	156	tetraparesis and deafness

ICU, intensive care unit; PI, pulsatility index

to the hemodynamic patterns (absent or reversed flow) divided into normal (mean values ≥ 20 ms) or abnormal in more than one record (mean values < 20 ms). The cases of death and the perinatal mortality rate are also presented for each subgroup. Fetal heart rate variability was within the range of normality in 60.93% of the study group.

When considering the groups presenting absent or reversed flow separately, a significant difference was observed in the distribution of normal or abnormal fetal heart rate variability values. In the first group, the values were normal in 82.35% of cases, while it was reduced to 33.3% in the second group presenting more severe hemodynamic patterns. The perinatal mortality rate was also significantly different in the whole study group according to the characteristics of fetal heart rate variability, being 28.2% when values were normal and 68% when abnormal ($p < 0.05$). No significant difference in perinatal mortality rate was found between cases presenting normal or abnormal fetal heart rate variability when absent and reversed flow cases were considered separately. The four cases of death observed in cases with absent flow presenting normal fetal heart rate variability were related in three cases to fetal abnormalities (two intrauterine deaths with non-immunological hydrops, one neonatal death presenting heart malformation and situs viscerum inversus) and in one case to

the decision of the family to avoid active management.

In the subgroup of reversed flow with fetal heart rate variability in the range of normality, seven cases of death were observed. They were all intrauterine demise, in one case associated with fetal abnormality (non-immunological hydrops and trisomy 21) and in the other cases due to the choice of non-active management. Of the 16 perinatal deaths observed in the subgroup presenting abnormal fetal heart rate variability values, two were cases of neonatal death at the ages of 8 days and 9 months, respectively. In the 14 cases of intrauterine death, fetal malformations were associated in four cases. In all the cases of malformations, necroscopy confirmed the prenatal diagnosis.

Looking now at the problem of late sequelae in survivors, as already shown, four such cases were observed in this study group: three in the group of with absent end-diastolic flow (10.34%) and one in the group with reversed flow (14.28%). The difference is not statistically significant. The characteristics of each case are presented in Table 4. Case 1 presented absent end-diastolic flow for 3 days preceding the appearance of reversed flow in the aorta. At the level of the umbilical arteries, absence of flow was observed for 4 days. The fetal heart rate variability was 21.9 ms and therefore not in the range of frank abnormality, but questionable. The fetus was delivered by Cesarean section immediately after the appearance of reversed flow. He is now suffering cerebral palsy.

Case number 2 showed absence of end-diastolic flow in the aorta for 2 days and, during the same period in the umbilical arteries, the values of the pulsatility index (PI) were over 2 SD but with diastolic flow present. The fetal heart rate variability was within the range of normality, but the baby is now suffering from retinopathy.

Case number 3 showed PI values over 2 SD in the aorta for 12 days that preceded the absence of flow in diastole that lasted 2 days. During the same period, PI values in the umbilical arteries were over 2 SD but with diastolic flow. Fetal heart rate variability values were in the last record in the range of abnormality. The baby is now suffering from lobar emphysema.

In case number 4, absent end-diastolic flow was observed only at the level of the umbilical arteries for 10 days and during the same period, surprisingly, the aorta constantly showed PI values in the range of normality (< 2 SD). The fetal heart rate variability also showed normal values, but now the baby is suffering from tetraparesis and deafness.

Owing to the small number of cases it is impossible to draw any conclusion regarding the possible prognostic validity of fetal heart rate variability in terms of neonatal sequelae. Moreover, it is not easy to identify precisely the origin and cause of handicaps: whether they were due to adverse intrauterine life or to difficult neonatal adaptation.

DISCUSSION

From Table 1 it is clear that, in the group of fetuses presenting ARED flow, large differences exist between cases presenting absence of end-diastolic flow and those with reversed flow. In particular, there was a statistically significant difference in the mean birth weight and the gestational age at delivery. As a consequence, the clinical outcome was also significantly different, considering the rates of perinatal death ($p < 0.01$), of late sequelae and of the duration

of stay in the neonatal intensive care unit. Therefore, in the difficult clinical approach to these fetuses, it is necessary to consider the choice of management, whether active or not, according to the flow patterns in diastole (absent or reversed). Moreover, in order to draw prognostic conclusions, it is wise to assess which vascular district is involved. From Table 2 it is clear that a large difference in perinatal mortality rate exists between cases presenting ARED flow only in the fetal aorta and those showing this pattern also at the level of the umbilical arteries. This difference is also evident when cases with absent flow and these with reversed flow are considered separately.

In the group showing absent flow only in the aorta, two cases of perinatal death occurred. In one case after counselling with the family, taking into consideration the low gestational age (26 weeks) and the low estimated fetal weight (550 g at birth), non-active management was undertaken and intrauterine death occurred after 3 days. In the other case, the newborn, delivered by Cesarean section at 35 weeks with a birth weight of 3150 g, died after 20 days, being affected by heart malformation and situs viscerum inversus. Therefore, the corrected neonatal mortality was 0. In cases presenting ARED in the aorta only, the neonatal mortality was also 0. On the other hand, when ARED was present at the level of the umbilical arteries also, perinatal mortality was significantly higher, being much higher in the presence of reversed end-diastolic flow.

These differences have a logical background. The characteristics of the Doppler velocity waveform are mainly influenced in diastole by the peripheral resistance downstream of the investigated segment of the vessel. Evidence has been given that the alterations of the sonogram are proportional to the obliteration of the placental vascular bed[9] and that not less than 60% must be obliterated before the alterations in the sonogram become evident[10]. Characteristic morphological alterations have been shown in the placenta of fetuses presenting ARED flow. Particularly, maldevelopment of the tertiary villi has been described[4], as has infarction and massive perivillous fibrin deposition[5]. Both conditions can explain the increase of impedance to blood flow in the umbilical arteries. As a consequence, it is possible to say that Doppler flow velocity waveforms in the umbilical arteries reflect, when altered in diastole, the reduction of maternal–fetal exchange, leading to fetal hypoxemia and/or acidemia.

As reversed flow is caused by a very high increase of the resistance at the level of the placenta, as compared to that with absent flow, it seems logical to expect a higher rate of fetal/neonatal complications with reversed flow. In contrast, Doppler flow velocity waveforms at the level of the fetal thoracic aorta reflect the increase of peripheral resistance mainly in somatic vessels, as caused by the redistribution of the circulation – the mechanism of adaptation of the fetus when faced with hypoxemia. How long the hypoxemic fetus can sustain this severe hemodynamic condition, without harm, is the major problem. In this study group, the five survivors presenting reversed flow in the aorta were delivered by Cesarean section at the first observation of this hemodynamic pattern, but one is affected by cerebral palsy. In the 16 survivors in the group presenting absent end-diastolic flow only in the aorta, this pattern was recorded from a minimum of 1 day to a maximum of 9 days. Two of these infants are suffering handicaps, both related to neonatal life (one retinopathy and one lobar emphysema).

In Table 3 the values of the fetal heart rate variability in the groups are presented. These were considered as abnormal if they presented long-term variability of < 20 ms. Evidence has been given regarding fetal heart rate variability values and the metabolic status of the fetus[8]. When abnormal values are recorded, the likelihood of the fetus being hypoxemic and/or acidemic is significantly higher than that for fetuses presenting values over this threshold. It is clear that the distribution of normal and abnormal fetal heart rate variability is different according to the severity of the hemodynamic patterns. In fact, 60 (93%) of

the cases of ARED showed fetal heart rate variability within the range of normality, but with a significant difference if the pattern was that of absent or of reversed flow. In the first group, normal values were present in 82.35% of the cases, while in the second group they were normal in only 33.3 %. No significant difference has been found in perinatal mortality rate within the two subgroups, but a significant difference was observed in that regard in the whole group of ARED in relationship to the characteristics of the fetal heart rate variability. The four cases of death observed in the group of absent flow and normal fetal heart variability values were in particular related to intrauterine demise in three and neonatal death in one. Of the intrauterine deaths, two were associated with fetal abnormality (non-immune hydrops) and one was the consequence of the choice of the family to avoid active management (the fetus died after 11 days). In the case of neonatal death a cardiac abnormality and a situs viscerum inversus was associated. After excluding these four cases, the neonatal corrected mortality rate in this subgroup became 0. In the group presenting fetal heart rate variability values within the range of normality and associated with reversed flow, seven cases of death occurred. In six cases, non-active management was chosen in accordance with the family's wishes and in one case fetal abnormality was present (hydrops and trisomy 21). Of the three survivors, two are normal at follow-up while one is suffering cerebral palsy. After excluding these 11 cases, the corrected neonatal mortality rate becomes 0.

It is interesting that the neonatal corrected mortality rate is the same in ARED cases if only the fetal thoracic aorta is involved or if normal values of fetal heart rate variability are recorded. This is not surprising, because the hemodynamic patterns in fetal vessels reflect the phenomenon of adaptation to hypoxemia for fetal heart function. From a practical point of view, it is possible to consider that fetal heart rate variability, assessed by the System 8000, offers the same information of diagnostic and prognostic value as is given by Doppler flow velocity waveform investigation of the fetal thoracic descending aorta.

CONCLUSIONS

The recognition of ARED flow always indicates a critical fetal condition. These fetuses are hypoxemic and/or acidemic and, moreover, the situation is usually complicated by prematurity and severe IUGR. Not only is the perinatal mortality rate excessively high, but also the rate of late sequelae is increased. As a consequence, after careful evaluation of all the clinical characteristics of any single case, the crucial point in the clinical management is the choice between the non-active approach or the active, and the timing. Possible adjunctive information, of practical clinical utility, is offered by the assessment of fetal heart function and particularly of the fetal heart rate variability, as is possible by using computerized evaluation of the CTG. This parameter and its alterations reflect some aspects of fetal adaptation to hypoxemia, as Doppler investigation of fetal vessels offers information about the redistribution of the circulation. On the other hand, Doppler study of the umbilical arteries informs about possible alterations of maternal–fetal exchanges that are the cause of the fetal hypoxemia. In order to assess the prognostic value of any clinical element in ARED cases, it seems unwise to refer to the perinatal mortality rate, as too many factors influence this. In particular the high rate of mal-formations and the frequent choice to avoid active management are responsible for an excessive rate of intrauterine deaths. It seems more logical, therefore, to refer to neonatal outcome. According to our experience, the following elements should be taken into account in order to optimize the timing of the delivery and to obtain a better neonatal outcome after exclusion of contraindications to active management.

(1) Is absent or reversed end-diastolic flow present? The outcome is more favorable if no reversed flow is detected, and therefore active management is a reasonable option.

(2) Is absent or reversed end-diastolic flow observed in the fetal vessel or in the umbilical arteries also? In the case of ARED only in the aorta, the outcome is better in both absent and reversed flow, and therefore active management can be considered. In the case of reversed flow, the delivery should occur at the first appearance of the pattern, while in the case of absent flow, immediate action is not always advisable. When reversed flow is present in the umbilical arteries also, the outcome is very poor and active management cannot be recommended.

(3) When fetal heart rate variability is within the range of normality in the presence of ARED flow, the neonatal outcome is more favorable. Looking at this parameter and particularly at its trend, it is possible to optimize the timing of the delivery.

References

1. Mandruzzato GP, Bogatti P, Fischer Tamaro L, Gigli C. The clinical significance of absent or reverse end-diastolic flow in the fetal aorta and umbilical artery. *Ultrasound Obstet Gynecol* 1991; 1:192–6

2. Mandruzzato GP, Fischer Tamaro L, Meir YJ. Doppler velocimetry in intrauterine growth restriction. In Kurjak A, ed. *Textbook of Perinatal Medicine*. Carnforth, UK: Parthenon Publishing, 1998:447–51

3. Nicolaides KH, Bilardo CM, Soothill PW, Campbell S. Absence of end diastolic frequencies in umbilical artery: a sign of fetal hypoxia and acidosis. *Br Med J* 1988;297:1026–7

4. Krebs C, Macara LM, Leiser R, Bowman A, Greer IA, Kingdom JCP. Intrauterine growth resctriction with absent end-diastolic flow velocity in the umbilical artery is associated with maldevelopment of the placental terminal villous tree. *Am J Obstet Gynecol* 1996;175:1534–42

5. Montenegro N, Laurini R, Brandao O, *et al.* Placental findings in fetuses with absent or reversed end-diastolic flow in the umbilical artery (ARED flow): a reappraisal. *J Matern Fetal Invest* 1997;7:175–9

6. Trimbos JB, Keirse MJNC. Observer variability in the assessment of antenatal cardiotocograms. *Br J Obstet Gynaecol* 1978;85:900

7. Dawes GS, Redman CWG, Smith J. Improvements in the registration and analysis of fetal heart rate records at the bedside. *Br J Obstet Gynaecol* 1985; 92:317

8. Smith JH, Anand KJS, Cotes PM, *et al.* Antenatal fetal heart rate variation in relation to the respiratory and metabolic status of the compromised human fetus. *Br J Obstet Gynaecol* 1988;95:980–9

9. Giles W, Trudinger B, Baird P. Fetal umbilical artery flow velocity waveforms and placental resistance: pathological correlations. *Br J Obstet Gynaecol* 1985;92:31

10. Trudinger B, Cook CM. Doppler umbilical and uterine flow waveforms in severe pregnancy hypertension. *Br J Obstet Gynaecol* 1997;97:142

Fetal behavior: integrity of brain stem apparatus

24

T. Koyanagi, T. Takashima and H. Nakano

INTRODUCTION

Over the past two decades, an ever increasing number of studies on cardiotocographic and real-time ultrasound observation has given rise to the organization of *in utero* behavior in the human fetus, in order to elucidate the ontogeny of somatic activities in connection with the functional development of the fetal central nervous system[1,2].

In this chapter, we consider several fetal motor activities and integrate the correlation of their age-specific patterns with developing brain stem function.

PATTERNS OF FETAL MOVEMENT

Fetal heart rate variation patterns

Analysis of fetal heart rate (FHR) variation described using the probability distribution matrix[3] (see Appendix) results in good agreement[4-6] with the generally accepted characterization of the age-related profile when assessed by visual recognition, conventionally using the cardiotocographic chart:

(1) The mean FHR, with almost the same value of standard deviation, decreases from 11 to about 30 weeks' gestation;

(2) From 26–28 weeks' gestation onwards, a large rise in the number of accelerations is apparent with episodes of high FHR baseline variability and associated fetal movement;

(3) A rest–activity cycle occurs, starting at around 34 weeks' gestation.

Fetal stomach movement patterns

The fetal stomach emerges, demonstrating rhythmic movement, at the latest by 27 weeks' gestation and clearly manifests such movement from 29 weeks' gestation onwards. Superimposing these movements, the fetal stomach adds a different movement, indicating the onset of a rest–activity cycle from 31 weeks' gestation onwards[7-9] (Figure 1).

Fetal eye movement/no eye movement patterns

The duration of the fetal eye movement period (d_{EM}) is constant by 29–30 weeks' gestation, and then increases to 37–38 weeks' gestation, whereas the duration of the no eye movement period (d_{NEM}) is constant by 31–32 weeks' gestation, and then increases to 37–38 weeks' gestation. The alternation of d_{EM} and d_{NEM} becomes stable after the same gestational age of 37–38 weeks[10] (Figure 2).

DISCUSSION

Somatic activities in the human fetus illustrated here appear to run on an innately decided course, albeit slightly different in onset, from temporal changes with duration of several seconds (acceleration in FHR variation at 26–28 weeks' gestation and rhythmic contraction in the stomach at 27 weeks' gestation) first manifested and later followed by the rest–activity cycle (FHR variation at 34 weeks, gastric movement at 31 weeks and d_{EM}/d_{NEM} alternation at 37 weeks).

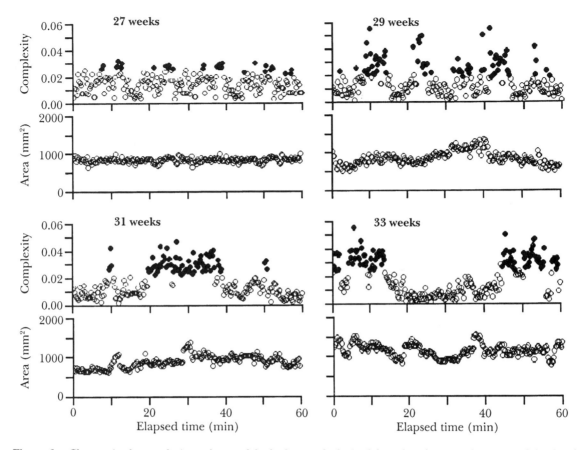

Figure 1 *Changes in the complexity and area of the fetal stomach obtained from three fetuses with congenital duodenal obstruction at 27–33 weeks' gestation (described in detail elsewhere). Closed and open circles among the stomach complexity measurements indicate the outlying points and non-outlying points, respectively, when assessed using the least median of square of regression analysis. No significant time series correlation was found between the complexity and the area. Modified from reference 9, with permission*

Just as the caudal brain stem follows the development of the spinal cord, the function of the central nervous system begins, anatomically, in the caudal segments and then is seen in the rostral segments[11].

Study of movement in anencephalic fetuses demonstrates that a lack of normal movement patterns in fetuses with major defects in the neural tube provides convincing evidence of the necessity of normally ordered neurons, even though they may be sparse or have a limited number of connections[12]. With regard to which brain segment would control FHR variation in anencephalic fetuses, a critical age is evident between 27–28 and 29–30 weeks' gestation. In the early period, the medulla function, *per se*, relates to FHR regulation,

whereas in the latter period, the brain cephalad to the medulla also appears to participate[13] (Figure 3). The nucleus tractus solitarii and ventrolateral medulla are two brain stem sites involved in the regulation of function[14]. Thus, the fact that fetal motor activities become manifest with their temporal changes in the early third trimester of gestation implies neural control of the autonomic nervous system.

Rapid eye movement (REM) sleep and non-rapid eye movement (NREM) sleep in the human fetus begin to manifest at 33 and 35 weeks' gestation[15,16], respectively, indicating that the pontine and thalamocortical connection area neurons start functioning at this time[17,18]. In the human fetus, therefore,

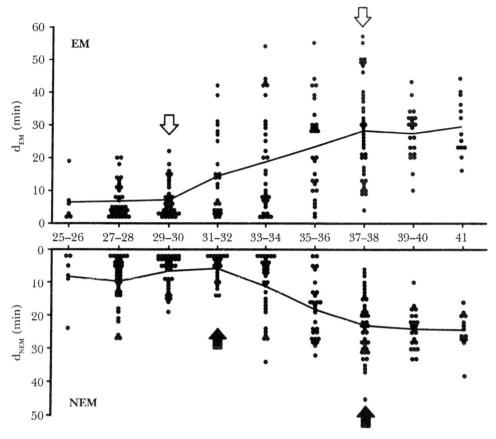

Figure 2 *Changes in duration of the eye movement period (d_{EM}) and duration of the no-eye movement period (d_{NEM}) obtained from 240 fetuses from 25 to 41 weeks' gestation. The age group (weeks) is indicated along the horizontal axis. The vertical axis indicates the duration in 1-min epochs. The solid line indicates the mean value for each age group. Open and solid arrows indicate the statistically critical points in d_{EM} and d_{NEM}, respectively, when assessed using piecewise linear regression analysis. Modified from reference 10, with permission*

this period around 35 weeks' gestation or more marks the time that various somatic activities reach maturation.

Based on observations of human infants, Kleitman[19] first proposed the hypothesis that the alternation of REM and NREM sleep is the manifestation of a fundamental ultradian rhythm of the central nervous system and is not affected by time of day. He referred to this as the basic rest–activity cycle (BRAC). The posterior hypothalamus is the likelier candidate of the brain site in charge of ultradian rhythm; however, there still remain ambiguities[20]. The medulla also has the capacity for generating ultradian rhythmicities which may contribute to the control of BRAC and REM/NREM sleep cycles[21]. In this way,

the ultradian rhythm-specific generator may not be single but multiple, and localized from the medulla to the hypothalamus. Furthermore, it may not be in the form of a signal-pulsing pacemaker but in the form of a circuit functioning as a clock by rotating the signal around the neurons concerned. Nevertheless, the functional integrity of the broad area from the medulla to the hypothalamus or higher level of the brain is seemingly required to manifest ultradian rhythm.

The mechanism determining the duration of REM sleep periods is dissociable from the switching mechanism of REM sleep to NREM sleep and vice versa[22]. Likening this to the case seen in this text, d_{EM} and d_{NEM} increase with

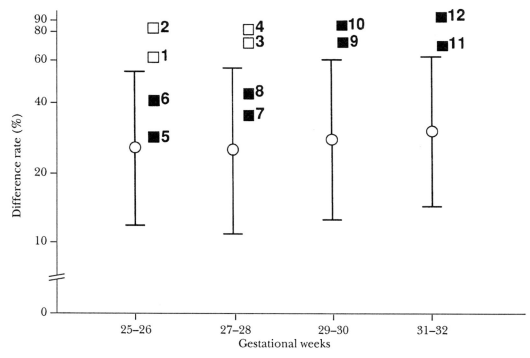

Figure 3 *The 95% confidence ranges (circles, mean values) of the difference rates (see Appendix) of 165 uncomplicated fetuses (control group) and the difference rates of five individual anencephalic fetuses in corresponding age groups (described in detail elsewhere; see Appendix) from 25–26 to 31–32 weeks' gestation: Open squares, cases with only the spinal cord present; closed squares, cases with both the spinal cord and the medulla present. When assessed using the Smirnoff test, until 27–28 weeks' gestation, there were significantly higher values in the difference rates of anencephalic fetuses with only the spinal cord preserved, whereas the difference rates of those fetuses with both spinal cord and medulla preserved demonstrated no significant differences. From 29–30 weeks' gestation thereafter, the difference rates of anencephalic fetuses, with both the spinal cord and the medulla preserved, had significantly higher values than uncomplicated fetuses. Modified from reference 13, with permission*

gestational age from the early third trimester until 37 weeks' gestation. The gestational age at which increases in d_{EM} and d_{NEM} begin, however, from relatively constant levels at the end of the second trimester, is not the same. The d_{EM} increases from the critical point at 29–30 weeks' gestation, whereas the d_{NEM} increases after 31–32 weeks' gestation. This discrepancy between the gestational ages at the critical points where increases in d_{EM} and d_{NEM} begin could imply the start of the development of two separate mechanisms, one for maintaining the d_{EM} and another for the d_{NEM}. Both switching and maintaining mechanisms responsible for ultradian rhythm of the d_{EM} and d_{NEM} have matured by 37 weeks' gestation[10]. When attempting to make a study from the viewpoint of chronobiology, one must keep these underlying mechanisms in mind.

We hypothesize that the somatic activities in the human fetus are programmed in such a way that early temporal changes under control of the autonomic nervous system come under the control of BRAC rhythm at critical periods and this principle can be generalized for other physical activities including respiratory movement, the esophageal phase of swallowing, blood pressure variation and the plasma level of substances (e.g. melatonin, somatomedin)[23], as observed in adults and infants.

APPENDIX

Probability distribution matrix

The probability distribution matrix we devised is a matrix with FHR in rows, DFHR (the

Probability distribution matrix I   Probability distribution matrix II

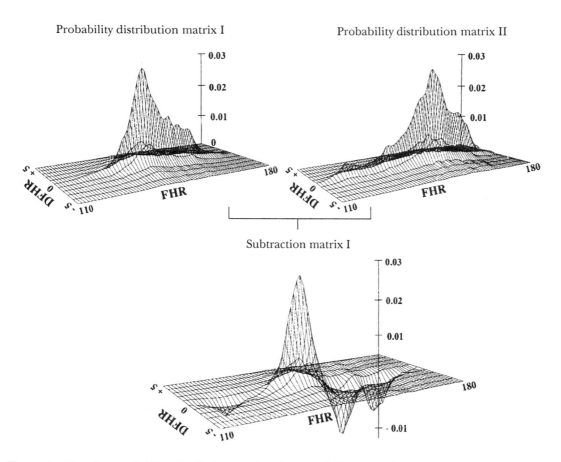

Figure 4 *Two given probability distribution matrices, I (x_{ik}) and II (y_{ik}) (top)[3]. The subtraction matrix (bottom) is obtained by subtracting probability distribution matrix I from probability distribution matrix II, where both residue distribution II (derived from the probability distribution II and plus (+) in value) and residue distribution I (from probability distribution matrix I and minus (−) in value) are equal to each other in distribution pattern. FHR in rows, fetal heart rate; DFHR in columns, difference between two successive heart rates; and probability value in elements*

difference between the two consecutive rates) in columns and probability representing a quantifying scale from any given FHR to the next FHR in corresponding elements (Figure 4). Thus, the resulting two-dimensional pattern of FHR vs. DFHR indicates the distribution of probability, thereby enabling quantitatively equivalent intergroup or intersubject comparison.

In the text, probability distribution matrices for each consecutive 2-week interval between 23 and 40 weeks' gestation previously obtained from a total of 10 934 604 recordings of FHR in 743 uncomplicated singleton fetuses are considered as a standard reference used for the subsequent analysis[3].

Difference rate

The difference between any two probability distribution matrices, I (x_{ik}) and II (y_{ik}) can be quantified as follows[3]:

$$\text{Difference rate} = \frac{\sum\sum|(y_{ik}) - (x_{ik})|}{2} \times 100$$

ACKNOWLEDGEMENTS

We thank L. Saza for help with manuscript preparation. This study is supported by a Grant-in-Aid for Scientific Research (No. 09470361) from the Ministry of Education, Science, Sports and Culture, Japan.

References

1. Nijhuis JG, Martin CB, Prechtl HFR. Behavioural states of the human fetus. In Prechtl HFR, ed. *Continuity of Neural Functions from Prenatal to Postnatal Life*. London: Spastics International Medical Publications, 1984:65–78

2. Koyanagi T, Nakano H. Functional development of the fetal central nervous system. In Levene MI, Lilford RL, eds. *Fetal and Neonatal Neurology and Neurosurgery*, 2nd edn. London: Churchill Livingstone, 1995:31–44

3. Koyanagi T, Yoshizato T, Horimoto N, *et al*. Fetal heart rate variation described using a probability distribution matrix. *Int J Biol Med Comput* 1994;35:25–37

4. Wheeler T, Murrills A. Patterns of fetal heart rate during normal pregnancy. *Br J Obstet Gynaecol* 1978;85:18–27

5. Dawes GS, Houghton CRS, Redman CWG, Visser GHA. Pattern of the normal human fetal heart rate. *Br J Obstet Gynaecol* 1982;89:276–84

6. Timor-Tritsch IE, Dierker LJ, Hertz RH, Deagan NC, Rosen MG. Studies of antepartum behavioral state in the fetus at term. *Am J Obstet Gynecol* 1978;132:524–8

7. Nagata S, Koyanagi T, Fukushima S, Akazawa K, Nakano H. Change in the three-dimensional shape of the stomach in the developing human fetus. *Early Hum Dev* 1994;37:27–38

8. Devane SP, Soothill PW, Candy DCA. Temporal changes in gastric volume in human fetus in late pregnancy. *Early Hum Dev* 1993;33:109–16

9. Hussein SM, Yoshizato T, Fukushima S, Koyanagi T, Akazawa K, Nakano H. Rhythmic changes in the stomach movement of the human fetuses with congenital duodenal obstruction during the third trimester of pregnancy. *Early Hum Dev* 1999; 54:1–13

10. Koyanagi T, Horimoto N, Takashima T, Satoh S, Maeda H, Nakano H. Ontogenesis of ultradian rhythm in the human fetus, observed through the alternation of eye movement and no eye movement periods. *J Reprod Infant Psychol* 1993;11:129–34

11. Humphrey T. Function of the nervous system during prenatal life. In Stave U, ed. *Perinatal Physiology*. New York: Plenum Press, 1978: 651–83

12. Visser GHA, Laurini RN, de Vries JIP, Bekedam DJ, Prechtl HFR. Abnormal motor behaviour in anencephalic fetuses. *Early Hum Dev* 1985;12: 173–82

13. Yoshizato T, Koyanagi T, Takashima T, Satoh S, Akazawa K, Nakano H. The relationship between age-related heart rate changes and developing brain function: a model of anencephalic human fetuses *in utero*. *Early Hum Dev* 1994;36:101–12

14. Rao H, Jean A, Kessler JP. Postnatal ontogeny of glutamate receptors in the rat nucleus tractus solitarii and ventrolateral medulla. *J Auton Nerv Syst* 1997;65:25–32

15. Horimoto N, Koyanagi T, Satoh S, Yoshizato T, Nakano H. Fetal eye movement assessed with real-time ultrasonography: are there rapid and slow eye movements? *Am J Obstet Gynecol* 1990;163: 1480–4

16. Horimoto N, Koyanagi T, Nagata S, Nakahara H, Nakano H. Concurrence of mouthing movement and rapid eye movement/non-rapid eye movement phases with advance in gestation of the human fetus. *Am J Obstet Gynecol* 1989;161: 344–51

17. Sakai K. Anatomical and physiological basis of paradoxical sleep. In McGunity DJ, Drucker-Colin R, Morrison A, eds. *Brain Mechanisms of Sleep*. New York: Raven Press, 1985:111–37

18. Watanabe K, Iwase K. Spindle-like fast rhythms in the EEGs of low-birth weight infants. *Dev Med Child Neurol* 1972;14:373–81

19. Kleitman N. Basic rest-activity cycle – 22 years later. *Sleep* 1982;5:311–17

20. Grass K, Prast H, Phillipu A. Influence of mediobasal hypothalamic lesion and catechol-amine receptor antagonists on ultradian rhythm of EEG in the posterior hypothalamus of the rat. *Neurosci Lett* 1996;207:93–6

21. Siegel JM, Tomaszewski KS, Nienhuis R. Behavioral states in the chronic medullary and midpontine cat. *Electroencephalogr Clin Neurophysiol* 1986;63:274–88

22. Sitaram N, Moore AM, Gllin CJ. Experimental acceleration and slowing of REM sleep ultradian rhythm by cholinergic agonist and antagonist. *Nature (London)* 1978;274:490–2

23. Brandenberger G, Charloux A, Gronfier C, Otzenberger H. Ultradian rhythms in hydro-mineral hormones. *Horm Res* 1998;49:131–5

The development of the senses   25

B. Arabin, R. van Lingen, W. Baerts and J. van Eyck

INTRODUCTION

The development of the senses is a multidimensional process incorporating sensory, emotional, affective, cognitive and evaluative abilities. For a long time it was rather a philosophical than a scientific question how early such abilities are acquired. Aristotle already anticipated the phenomenon that sensory development is a quiet process of the prenate gradually responding to the extrauterine world. However, negative thinking about prenatal sensory capabilities was more common: Rousseau referred to the fetus as a 'witless tadpole' isolated from the agitation of the world. Even first scientific approaches by Preyer in 1885 led to doubtful conclusions about fetal sensory capacities[1]. The advent of technical advances allowed access to the unborn in the womb and the study of mainly behavioral responses. Prechtl[2] can be regarded as the pioneer of integrating observations of endogenously evoked behavior into neonatal and prenatal surveillance. He stressed the clinical importance and provided us with a tool appropriate for the investigation of developmental responses towards internal and external stimuli. Reactive behavioral patterns towards touch, sound (including maternal noise), vibration, light, taste and odor have been observed and may be integrated into a cohesive whole, to describe developmental sensitivity. Besides behavioral reactions, responses may be mediated by physiological, hormonal or metabolic processes. Although the fetal brain can organize and elaborate stimulus information and encode in memory the activation of reflex responses, it is still difficult to define how far the 'memories' are or become conscious, reflect the present or contribute to future sensory development.

This chapter tries to summarize some essential aspects and eventual clinical implications.

SENSITIVITY AND THE EXPERIENCE OF PAIN

Anatomy, sensory physiology and responsiveness

Cutaneous sensory receptors appear in the perioral area of the human fetus in the 7th week, spread to the face, hands and feet at around 11 weeks, to the trunk, arms and legs at around 15 weeks and to all cutaneous and mucous surfaces at around 20 weeks. The spread of cutaneous receptors is accompanied by the development of synapses between sensory fibers in the dorsal horn of the spinal cord, which first appear at around 6 weeks. Sensory nerves first grow into the spinal cord at 14 weeks' gestation. Development of the fetal neocortex begins at 8 weeks. Most sensory pathways to the neocortex have synapses in the thalamus. Between 20 and 24 weeks thalamocortical fibers establish synaptic connections with dendritic processes of neocortical neurons. After that time it is more likely that the fetus might not only react towards but also 'experience' touch and pain. *In vivo* measurements of glucose utilization have shown that maximal metabolic activity is located in sensory areas of the neonatal brain, suggesting the functional maturity. The existence of neurotransmitters, endogenous opioids released pre- and perinatally in response to fetal stress and of stereospecific opiate receptors at spinal and supraspinal levels as well as behavioral reactions have further increased our knowledge of sensory

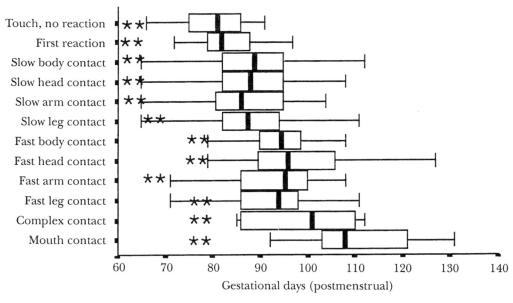

Figure 1 *Onset of prenatal contacts in 20 dichorionic and five monochorionic diamniotic twin pairs (box and whisker plots) compared to two cases of monoamniotic twins (*). Ultrasound observations at 1-week intervals*

or painful sensation and offered implications for treatment (summary by Anand and Hickey[3]).

As supposed for motor activities[4], sensitivity to touch may develop before the response to relevant biological or psychological sensory input. Hooker was the first to describe reactions towards the cutaneous stimulation of embryos after therapeutic terminations of pregnancy by hysterotomy, maintaining them in an isotonic fluid bath[5]. With the introduction of real-time ultrasound, it became possible to observe early prenatal movements and behavior[6]. To study reactions of single fetuses towards touch *in utero* would be combined with ethical and practical restraints. However, twins are naturally exposed to cutaneous stimulations of the co-twin, enabling us to study the onset of reactions towards touch *in vivo*.

Multiple pregnancies for study of reactions to cutaneous stimulation *in vivo*

The onset of reactions towards touch can ideally be investigated in monoamniotic multiplets, since the first reactions towards touch are observed earlier than in mono-chorionic diamniotic multiplets and again earlier than in dichorionic multiplets (Figure 1). As described *in vitro*[5] we found *in vivo* that monoamniotic multiplets responded to tactile stimulation between 8 and 9 weeks[7]. Early contacts in monoamniotic and mono-chorionic twin pregnancies are also more numerous than in dichorionic pregnancies because the membranes may prevent early reaching and touching *in utero*[7]. The development of reactions towards cutaneous stimulations of a co-twin *in utero* reveals different qualities. Up to 16 weeks, we have meanwhile analyzed several contact patterns according to the speed of initiatives and reactions or the part of the body involved[7]. In advanced pregnancy, it is more difficult to differentiate fetal reactions to touch by conventional ultrasound methods. Three-dimensional real-time ultrasound may facilitate observations in the future. From early fetal heart rate (FHR)/fetal movement analysis of singletons compared to twins, one can conclude that inter-twin reactions contribute to an increased number of simultaneous FHR accelerations.

Gender differences have been reported for cognition, aggression and sociability in humans. Explanations have focused on neuroanatomical differences and exposure to steroid hormones. We have analyzed twin pairs with different gender combinations between 8 and 16 weeks. In the group of only male twins, fast initiatives combined with fast reactions and the number of complex contacts were significantly increased compared to only female or mixed twin pairs[7]. It is suggested that differences of testosterone levels might have an impact on early development *in utero*. Limitations in the interpretation of our twin studies include difficulties in differentiating reactions to touch from a parallel onset of endogenously evoked movements, and passive from active reactions.

It was speculated that the tactile stimuli of multiplets might improve their development during early follow-up examinations up to the age of 6 years, when multiplets scored better than singletons[7], and that it is not only activity that promotes growth and dendritic branching of individual neurons, but similarly, that sensation from receptor cells might promote the development of the neural system[8].

FETAL PAIN

Pain includes feeling, suffering and learning (memory). The increasing number of prenatal techniques and of operations in premature neonates has given rise to controversial discussions about how early and how far fetuses and neonates feel pain. This has implications for professionals who provide abortions. Fetal responses to invasive techniques were observed as blood flow redistribution from 18 weeks[9] and as an increase of cortisol and β-endorphin from at least 23 weeks of gestation[10]. Nevertheless, the most rational approach is to make an informed guess based on knowledge of the development of the nervous system or measurements and observations in preterm infants. Some authors argue for placing the onset of pain sensation at somewhere between 6 and 12 weeks after conception[11]. Others define recorded responses before 26 weeks

as reflexes without conscious appreciation, suggesting that, only then, is it likely that the fetus not only reacts towards a stimulus but also experiences pain[12]. It seems to be accepted that the thalamus may assume some functions to contribute to fetal awareness of pain, but it is still not known when the brain is mature enough to register pain.

To avoid suffering and long-term effects, it is considered advisable to provide the fetus with analgesia. Suffering during termination of pregnancy is also a question of concern. The Royal College of Obstetricians and Gynaecologists recommends that practitioners who undertake diagnostic or therapeutic surgical procedures upon the fetus at or after 24 weeks consider the requirements of fetal analgesia and sedation, either by agents given to the mother or directly[13]. Before performing late terminations of pregnancy it is suggested that feticide be considered. Maternal analgesia which transfers across the placenta is supposed to be sufficient in cases with early terminations of pregnancy. Research is needed to determine how the detection and treatment of pain can be extended to the fetal patient in a direct way.

The preterm infant of 23 weeks' gestation shows reflex responses to noxious stimuli. A variety of physiological, hormonal, metabolic and behavioral changes have been observed after painful procedures; these include cardiovascular variables, palmar sweating, increase of renin, epinephrine (adrenaline), norepinephrine (noradrenaline), catecholamines and glucocorticoids, which are related to the intensity of the stimulus[6]. Stimulation of the cutaneous flexor reflex showed that reflex thresholds were proportionally related to increasing gestational age[14]. Therefore, infants under 32 weeks might need even more analgesia to avoid stress responses and pain experience. In our group we score neonates from 24 weeks onwards according to the neonatal infant pain score (NIPS) looking at cry patterns, breathing, body language and facial expressions[15]. If we suspect that infants experience pain from ventilation or invasive procedures we start treatment with morphine or acetaminophen (APAP). We take advantage of the increased half-life due to decreased clearance of the drug in preterm infants to reach higher concentrations according to the supposed lower pain threshold[16] (Figure 2). Little attention is given to the experience of pain during vacuum or forceps delivery. Newborns born by either of these procedures in our unit receive pain treatment directly after birth.

HEARING

The onset and development of fetal hearing are dated by extrapolation from animal studies or from measurements in premature babies and by studying prenatal reactions to acoustic stimuli. References to the extensive detailed literature on fetal hearing development can be obtained in a previous publication[17].

Anatomy and acoustic physiology

From 10 weeks onwards the external ear and later even the tympanic membrane are visualized by ultrasound. The outer ear collects sound energy and shapes it towards the tympanic membrane. The ossicles of the middle ear develop between 4 and 6 gestational weeks and reach full size by 18 weeks. Only then do they become ossified; they are of adult size by 8 months of gestation. At 7 weeks, the Eustachian tube and the tympanic cavity are formed. In the middle ear, acoustic energy is transduced into mechanical energy. The inner ear consists of a membranous labyrinth inside a bony labyrinth. Ossification does not occur until each portion has attained adult size. Hair cell differentiation, synaptogenesis and ciliogenesis of the membranous labyrinth are completed at around 24 weeks. The basis of the frequency-related regional displacement of the entire cochlear partition was revealed by the classic Nobel laureate von Bekesy. With the entry of the acoustic nerve into the brainstem, auditory neurons multiply and project the information to the auditory cortex. Many

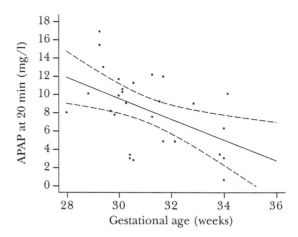

Figure 2 *Linear regression analysis with confidence limits of gestational age on acetaminophen (APAP) concentrations at 20 min after administration. From reference 16*

auditory abilities are attributable to subcortical processing. Therefore, decorticated animals are capable of detecting the intensity and frequency of sounds, and anencephalic fetuses demonstrate behavioral reactions to external stimuli.

Sound is created by a vibratory source, causing molecules to be displaced. The amplitude is measured in pascals (Pa). Sound pressure level and frequency is given in decibels (dB) and hertz (Hz), respectively. The range of 20–20 000 Hz is the bandwidth of human hearing. Information about intrauterine hearing conditions are obtained from sheep experiments or from pregnancies with ruptured membranes: a bone conduction route is assumed, whereby sound energy is diminished by 10–20 dB for frequencies of < 250 Hz and by 40–50 dB for > 500 Hz.

A second reason for fetal 'sound isolation' is the sound pressure attenuation. Thereby, transmission losses range from 39 dB at 500 Hz to 85 dB at 5000 Hz. It has been shown that sound attenuation decreases during late gestation. In humans, sound of at least 65–70 dB is transmitted with attenuation of 30 dB in sound pressure level for tones of up to 12 kHz. Frequencies of 200 Hz are even enhanced. The sound environment *in utero* is dominated by frequencies of < 500 Hz and mean sound pressure levels of 90 dB caused by vessel pulsations, intervillous injections and maternal digestion or breathing. It might have an 'imprinting' and a masking effect for the fetus. 'Intelligibility' reflects the ability to distinguish complex sounds: music and voices are distinguishable from the basal noise by 8–12 dB. The male voice with a mean frequency of 125 Hz is better transmitted, but emerges in the range with high internal noise. Female voices with an average of 220 Hz receive greater attenuation, but emerge in a range with low internal noise.

Prenatal and postnatal auditory responsiveness

Studies of fetal response to sound have used a variety of stimuli, not always with rationale. Studies with airborne and vibroacoustic stimuli (VAS) providing vibration and airborne sound should be differentiated. The electronic artificial larynx used for VAS has a spectrum between 0.5 and 1 kHz and a sound pressure level averaging 135 dB. The first responsiveness to pure tones was detected at 23 weeks at 500 Hz, by 27 weeks up to 500 Hz and only at 31 weeks were responses observed to 1000–3000 Hz. The sound pressure level required is 20–30 dB less at 35 than at 23 weeks. With the use of a habituation–dishabituation technique, a fetus aged 35 weeks was found to discriminate between frequencies of 250 and 500 Hz and different speech sounds; fetuses of 27 weeks were unable to make this differentiation.

Non-invasive recordings of auditory responses are based on compound potentials representing the activity of many cells; these recordings use the electroencephalographic (EEG) or magnetoencephalographic (MEG) methods. Human EEG responses to acoustic signals have been obtained after ruptured membranes. In MEG recordings neuromagnetic auditory brainstem responses are measured with intact membranes. Short stimuli are produced in a room guaranteeing electrical radio frequency shielding. Thus, we succeeded in recording stimulus-related auditory evoked neuromagnetic fields through the mothers' abdomen at 34 weeks

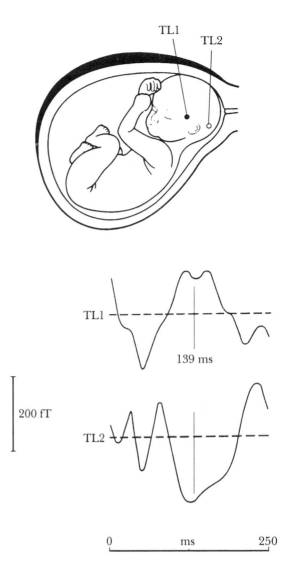

Figure 3 *Waveforms obtained from brainstem recordings after click stimulation at 34 weeks, using one-channel magnetoencephalography. TL, temporal lateral; fT, fentotesla. From reference 17*

(Figure 3). Latency shifts of brainstem components are proposed to reflect early brain maturation. Use of multi-channel magnetoencephalography specifically designed for the prenate might be expected to extend the window of observation.

Fetal auditory abilities can be examined by behavioral reactions. Problems arise when the fetus does *not* react, since we cannot say that the stimulus is not sensed. In general, reactions towards acoustic stimuli do not occur before 24 weeks. Fetal movement and FHR responses may be classified into immediate short (blinking, reflex movements) and long-term changes of activity and FHR patterns. With increasing gestational age, an increasing number of long reactions are observed after VAS. FHR baseline changes more dramatically than FHR variability. Fetal responses to speech were studied at 26–34 weeks' gestation, during periods of low FHR variability. A decrease in FHR was found, as the only demonstration of prenatal responses to speech stimuli. Female fetuses responded earlier than males. Twins are ideal models to differentiate the simultaneous influence of gestational age, state before stimulation, individual disposition (zygosity), position and sex of the prenates by analyzing inter-twin differences of FHR/fetal movement patterns towards vibroacustic stimulation (VAS).

The detection of cortical potentials and auditory evoked potentials as early as 25 weeks before birth indicates functional maturity of the auditory pathway. Electrophysiological responses from the cochlea, the eighth nerve and the auditory brainstem are similar to those of the adult by 32–36 gestational weeks. In neonates, broadband sounds (speech) are likely to elicit responses depending on states of hunger and sleep–wakefulness. Newborns differentiate band-width, duration, inter-stimulus interval, frequency and sound pressure levels: signals of < 4 kHz evoke responses more often than signals in the higher range. Lower frequencies generally evoke gross motor activity; high frequencies evoke freezing reactions.

Effects of prenatal hearing on postnatal development

While habituation reflects short-term memory, there is also proof of long-term memory from pre- to postnatal life, as observed by studies of behavioral modifications of neonates presented with stimuli with which they have been confronted prenatally. Newborns showed a preference for the voice of their mother and, with a baby's pacifier (dummy) connected to a tape

recorder, they were able to distinguish between their mother speaking in her native or an unfamiliar language, and they preferred a lullaby that had been read twice a day by the mother during the last weeks of pregnancy to a new story. All this suggests the possibility of prenatal acquisitions and antenatal discrimination, however elementary it might be.

Settings of talking, music and meditation were performed during pregnancy. Postnatally, for talking only 58% of behavioral variables were identified as positive, 16% as ambiguous and 26% as negative (e.g. crying for obscure reasons, needing constant supervision). Music and meditation, however, correlated in 90–100% with positive attitudes. It is speculated that variations of timbre and hormonal changes associated with the content of speech may evoke associations in the infant. Hearing has a close relation to the kinetic system: the 'auditory–vocal–kinetic channel'. Vocal expression can be heard in immature newborns and follows unpleasant maneuvers. Newborn 'cryprints' are as unique as fingerprints. The fetus seems to store maternal speech features: even newborns born at 28 weeks had similar voice performance features to those of their mothers.

Prenatal acoustical responsiveness as a test for fetal well-being

The ability of VAS to elicit FHR accelerations has been well established. In this context, VAS was proposed to assess fetal well-being and to discriminate between 'non-reactive' non-stress tests (NST) due to hypoxia and a quiet state. FHR reactions are reduced after VAS in fetuses with intrauterine growth restriction (IUGR). The conclusion, that nutritional deprivation is associated with delayed sensory maturation, is not necessarily true, since even when there is no reaction, the stimulus might well be received.

We compared the clinical value of the NST, the ratio of cerebral versus umbilical blood flow, VAS and the contraction stress test (CST) to predict poor outcome for IUGR and post-term pregnancies: Doppler velocimetry and the NST were superior to VAS and the CST. In the only controlled trial, in which VAS was compared to the NST, false-positive tests were slightly lowered and performance reduced from a mean of 27 to 23 min. The question remains of whether 4 min justifies frightening – or only wakening – an innocently sleeping fetus. For the time being, we recommend VAS only under controlled conditions, but not for routine use, as proposed by others.

Possible damage from environmental hazards during pregnancy

Fetal noise-induced hearing loss has been a matter of concern regarding the working or living conditions of pregnant women supposing that noise can adversely change fetal hearing. From sheep experiments it was found that noise sources with low-frequency components and high intensity impulses had temporary effects, whereas long-term effects are still unknown. In summary, the Committee on Hearing, Bioacoustics and Biomechanics attempting to protect fetal hearing suggested that pregnant women should avoid noise exposures greater than 90 dB.

OLFACTION AND TASTE

Anatomy and physiology of nasal and oral flavor reception

About 1–2% of the human genome is allocated to receptors for the olfactory epithelium[18]. Olfactory receptors mediate the sense of flavor arising from volatile substances pumped into the nasal cavity during inhalation, swallowing or chewing. They also mediate neuroendocrine responses[18,19].

The primary neuronal cells of the main olfactory system are embedded in the upper part of the nasal cavity. Their dendrites merge into the mucus and bear receptor-binding compounds. The receptor binding elicits in the neuron an electrical signal, which is transmitted along the axon penetrating the lamina cribrosa to meet in one of the paired olfactory bulbs, and via a neuronal network to the paleocortex including the hippocampus[18]. Impulses reaching the thalamic nuclei project to the frontal cortex where the conscious perception of smell takes place; pathways to the limbic system mediate affective and neuroendocrine responses. The vomeronasal organ with sensory cells on the nasal septum mediates endocrine responses activated by pheromones. More studies are required to determine the specific function in humans. By the third trimester all chemosensory receptors seem ready to be functional. The nostrils have become patent and amniotic fluid is swallowed and inhaled. Taste buds are found as early as 12 weeks and displayed over the oral cavity, concentrating at birth on the tongue and on the anterior palate[20].

Prenatal and postnatal olfactory responsiveness

Olfactory responses have been demonstrated in premature babies of 6 months. In the sheep, intranasal injections of odorant components induced FHR changes[19]. Intra-amniotic injection of a saccharine solution led to increased swallowing; injection of bitter or acid solutions reduced fetal swallowing, signifying awareness of different tastes during pregnancy even influencing fetal behavior[20].

The newborn may retain an olfactory memory trace: during the initial attempt to locate the mother's nipple, newborns preferred a breast with the areola moistened with amniotic fluid over an untreated breast[18]. The scent of amniotic fluid even has a calming effect shortly after birth, as measured by infants' rate of crying[21]. There is also evidence that babies recognize their mother by her scent, because 6-day-old infants turned preferentially in the direction of their own mother's odor pad rather than towards an alien breast odor. Neonates respond to scents by changes in respiration, facial expression and orientation. Even at less than 2 days old, they developed preferences (based on formation of new synapses) and oriented towards an odor that had been present in their nursery for the preceding 24 h. This phenomenon was still evident 2 weeks after the exposure was discontinued[18].

Knowledge about olfaction and taste may have not only diagnostic but also therapeutic implications, such as the initiation and stabilization of breast feeding, newborn adaptation, attachment and social interaction as well as the reduction of apneic episodes[21]. We therefore try to provide the newborns admitted to our intensive care unit with some accessories of their mothers.

VISION

Anatomy and physiology of visional function

Different parts of the eye develop from different origins: the retina, iris and optic nerve are of neuroectodermal origin; the lens and cornea are of ectodermal origin; and the choroid, sclera, ciliary body and ocular blood vessels are of mesodermal origin. Neuroblastic cells differentiate into photoreceptor cells, which later secrete interstitial retinol-binding protein, which plays a role in the defense against free radicals by binding vitamin E[22]. After 18 weeks, synapses appear on the eye rods. From 20 to 24 weeks, fetal eyelids may open. Macula and photoreceptors start development, which is not completed before birth and lasts for several postnatal months[20]. The retinal surface area doubles between 6 months and term[23]. Birnholz was the first to describe prenatal ocular structures as seen by ultrasound[24]. He described periods of active growth between 12 and 20 and between 28 and 32 weeks. At term, the eye is well developed, growing only three times compared to 20 times for the rest of the body to reach adult size. Myelination of the optic nerve starts between 6 and 8 months; myelination of the posterior visual pathway and superior colliculus starts just before term[23].

Prenatal and postnatal visual responsiveness

More than sound, light is attenuated by the maternal abdomen. Transmission of external light was detected to be around 2% at 550 nm

and to reach 10% at around 650 nm[20]. In addition, the fetal position might prevent even a limited amount of light from reaching the fetal retina. The restricted and irregular visual input impairs profound studies about behavioral responses to light *in utero*. Nevertheless, prenatal responses have been reported from 25 weeks onwards[24]. We have observed movements of the bulbs ('twinkling') by ultrasound as well as reactions of FHR and fetal movements towards stimulation with a flashlight from 28 weeks onwards, comparable to behavioral patterns towards VAS[8]. However, probably owing to the described problems, reactions of FHR/fetal movement patterns were recorded in only around 10%. Stimulations with light that was introduced during amnioscopy directly into the uterine cavity were more successful[20].

After delivery, the newborn is suddenly exposed to light, and we do not know how this sudden impression is experienced. Recordings of visual responses based on compound potentials can be applied in preterm newborns such as the electro-retinogram (ERG) or the visual evoked potential (VEP). The latter can be elicited even at 23 weeks; with increasing age the latency of the response signal decreases and its morphology gets more complex, signifying visual pathway maturation[23]. Behavioral tests have been introduced, such as the blink response and the registration of awareness and fixation. Dubowitz and Dubowitz used the ability of the preterm infant to focus, to follow and to track in order to draw conclusions about the developing visual system[25]. They also observed that newborns frequently do not open their eyes in the presence of strong lighting[25].

Further studies have used 'preferential looking'-based tests of visual acuity measurement. Although the visual development of preterm infants at different gestational ages lags behind that of the term infant, when this is corrected for the degree of prematurity, both groups behave similarly. Preterm infants sometimes exhibit more rapid development than term infants[23]. All in all, around 50% of infants with very low birth weight show visual impairments across a range of functions[26]. The highest incidence was found at around 6 months; beyond this age fewer deficits were observed, suggesting delayed rather than permanently impaired visual development. Visual abnormality is frequently related to neurological impairment, suggesting that it is of cerebral rather than of ophthalmological origin (Figure 4). Still, in time these infants may show progress, thanks to neural plasticity.

Possible damage during and after pregnancy

The very small premature infant spends his/her first weeks in a constantly illuminated environment. Light is transmitted even through the eyelid at a rate of 1–10%, predominantly at the red end of the spectrum[23]. Exposure to light has been demonstrated to cause retinal damage in animals even at intensities encountered in neonatal intensive care units. It is an intriguing question how far this can be extrapolated to humans, and might require that light be reduced or adapted to the sleep–wakefulness rhythms of the neonates. Retinal photodamage mainly occurs by a raise of oxygen tension, occurring unnaturally for the very premature infant. At present, retinopathy is the most common ocular disease, being characterized by abnormal proliferation of the immature retina, which can progress to retinal scarring and visual handicap up to blindness (for review, see reference 24).

CONCLUSIONS

An increasing amount of data demonstrate that learning abilities of the newborn organism reflect continuity from prenatal life. The long history of denial and the short history of limited research relating to prenatal perception and the implications for further life highlight our ignorance of the effects of early sensory development. The use of modern technology in order to understand pathophysiological processes and to create stimulative interventions, but even more important our own respect and awareness

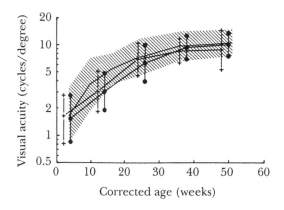

Figure 4 *Development of binocular acuity in infants of very low birth weight with neurologically normal (circles) and abnormal (crosses) development at the time of testing, compared to mean low-risk preterm acuity. Vertical lines indicate 2 SD. From reference 26 with permission*

towards the unborn and newborn infant are prerequisite to discover that this topic represents a wealth for ongoing and future research. Early capabilities reflect complex neurological development and thus one of the most important objectives of perinatal care. It is our responsibility to avoid unnecessary stress of the fetus and newborn from overstimulation by unnatural exposure to light or sound and to treat pain as effectively as we do in adult patients. However, health is understood as the physical, mental and social well-being that goes much further than just the absence of suffering or illness. As important as it is to teach children abilities at certain times, it might favor the development or prevent sensory retardation to create integrated stimulations for the unborn or newborn. This should be a matter of concern for public health projects. Encouragement and avoidance of stimuli have to be considered and balanced in observational or interventional projects according to critical developmental phases. Whether we go so far as to found prenatal universities is of secondary importance, as long as we strive to understand the physiology and pathophysiology of early sensory development and to create designs suitable to induce a comprehensive expression of all our genetic potential.

References

1. Preyer W. *Spezielle Physiologie des Embryo.* Leipzig: Grieben, 1885
2. Prechtl HFR. The behavioural states of the newborn infant. *Brain Res* 1974,76:185–212
3. Anand KJS, Hickey PR. Pain and its effects in the human neonate and fetus. *N Engl Med J* 1987; 387:1321–9
4. Prechtl HFR. Continuity and change in early neural development. In Prechtl HFR, ed. *Continuity of Neural Functions from Prenatal to Postnatal Life. Clinics in Developmental Medicine,* vol 94. Oxford: Blackwell Scientific, 1984:1–15
5. Hooker D. *The Prenatal Origin of Behavior.* Kansas: University of Kansas Press, 1952
6. Hepper PG. Fetal psychology: an embryonic science. In Nijhuis JG, ed. *Fetal Behaviour. Developmental and Perinatal Aspects.* Oxford, New York, Tokyo: Oxford University Press, 1992: 130–56
7. Arabin B, Bos R, Rijlarsdam R, van Eyck J. The onset of inter-human contacts. Longitudinal ultrasound observations in twin pregnancies. *Ultrasound Obstet Gynecol* 1996;8:166–73
8. Arabin B, Mohnhaupt A, van Eyck J. Intrauterine behaviour of multiplets. In Kurjak A, ed. *Textbook of Perinatal Medicine.* Carnforth, UK: Parthenon Publishing, 1998:1506–31
9. Giannakoulopoulos X, Sepulveda W, Kourtis W, Glover V, Fisk NM. Fetal plasma cortisol and β-endorphin response to intrauterine needling. *Lancet* 1994;334:77–81
10. Teixeira J, Fogliani R, Giannakoulopoulos X, Glover V, Fisk NM. Fetal haemodynamic stress response to invasive procedures. *Lancet* 1996; 347:624
11. McCullagh P. Do fetuses feel pain? *Br Med J* 1997; 314:302–3
12. Lloyd Thomas AR, Fitzgerald M. Reflex responses do not necessarily reflect pain. *Br Med J* 1997; 313:797–8
13. The Royal College of Obstetricians and Gynaecologists. Fetal awareness – report of a working party. London: RCOG Press, 1997
14. Fitzgerald M, Shaw A, MacIntosh N. The postnatal development of the cutaneous flexor reflex: a comparative study in premature infants and newborn rat pups. *Dev Med Child Neurol* 1988;30:520–6
15. Lawrence J, Alcock D, McGrath P, Kay J, MacMurry SB, Dulberg C. The development of a tool to assess neonatal pain. *Neonatal Network* 1993;12:59–66
16. Van Lingen RA, Deinum JT, Quak JME, Kuizenga AJ, van Dam JG, Anand KJS, Tibboel D, Okken A. Pharmacokinetics and metabolism of rectally administered paracetamol in preterm neonates. *Arch Dis Child Fetal Neonatal Ed* 1999;80:F59–63
17. Arabin B, van Straaten I, van Eyck J. Fetal hearing. In Kurjak A, ed. *Textbook of Perinatal Medicine.* Carnforth, UK: Parthenon Publishing, 1988: 756–75
18. Winberg J, Porter RH. Olfaction and human neonatal behaviour: clinical implications. *Acta Paediatr* 1998;87:6–10
19. Beauchamp GK, Mennella JAS. Sensitive periods in the development of human flavor perception and preference. *Ann Nestle* 1998;56:19–31
20. Lecanuet JP, Schaal B. Fetal sensory competencies. *Eur J Obstet Gynecol Reprod Biol* 1996;68: 1–12
21. Garcia AP, White-Traut R. Preterm infants' responses to taste/smell and tactile stimulation during an apneic episode. *J Pediatr Nurs* 1993;8: 24–52
22. Baerts W, Fetter WP. Retinopathy of prematurity. In Kurjak A, ed. *Textbook of Perinatal Medicine.* Carnforth, UK: Parthenon Publishing, 1998: 129–40
23. Fielder AR, Moseley MJ, Ng YK. The immature visual system and premature birth. In Whitelaw A, Cooke RWI, eds. *The Very Immature Infant Less than 28 weeks Gestation.* London, New York: Churchill Livingstone, 1998:1094–118
24. Birnholz JC. Ultrasonic fetal ophthalmology. *Early Hum Dev* 1985;12:198–209
25. Dubowitz L, Dubowitz V. *The Newborn Assessment of the Preterm and Full-term Newborn Infant. Clinics in Developmental Medicine,* no 79. Suffolk: Lavenham Press, 1981:48–50
26. Groenendaal F, van Hof-van Duin J, Baerts W, Fetter WPF. Effects of perinatal hyopxia on visual development during the first year of (corrected) age. *Early Hum Dev* 1989;20:267–79

Fetal hemodynamics and behavioral states

26

G. Clerici, A. Cutuli and G. C. Di Renzo

Behavior is the interaction of an organism with its environment. The behavioral states in the newborn were described in the 1960s. After 20 years, Nijhuis and colleagues[1,2] demonstrated the existence of fetal behavioral states. These were defined as physiological and behavioral variables that characterize an organism at a given moment and they classified the behavioral states into four conditions (from 1F to 4F) based on the characteristics of three main parameters – fetal body movements, fetal eye movements and fetal heart rate (FHR) pattern – as follows:

(1) State 1F is a quiescent state with the FHR pattern showing oscillatory bandwidth.

(2) State 2F is characterized by frequent gross body movements, continuous eye movements and the FHR pattern showing a wider oscillatory bandwidth and accelerations.

(3) State 3F is one of co-ordination; body movements are absent, but eye movements are present continuously. The FHR pattern shows a more regular wide oscillatory frequency than in state 2F, with no accelerations.

(4) State 4F is one vigorous body movement with continuous eye movements; the FHR exhibits long-lasting accelerations and even sustained tachycardia.

Subsequently the response of a normal fetus to a single stimulus, more commonly an acoustic stimulus, was studied. After the stimulus a mean increase in the FHR is noted from 26 weeks of gestation. After 30 weeks there is also a significant increase in the basal FHR which is not observed previously to this

gestation. Habituation is recognized as a simple and common learning pattern. The standard behavior of a normal term fetus is to habituate to a stimulus, that is to cease to respond on repeated exposure to the stimulus. The rate of habituation becomes significantly faster as gestational age increases. This decrement in the rate of fetal habituation is thought to reflect the maturation of the neural circuitry responsible for this form of learning[3].

Because the fetal behavioral states are represented fundamentally by 1F 'quiet sleep' (60–65% of the time) and 2F 'active sleep' (20–25% of the time), it was possible to study, with sonography, the characteristics of these two fetal situations and, with Doppler technology, the related fetal hemodynamic changes to these conditions (Table 1).

However, several studies have shown that quite a few vascular fetal districts are affected in their velocimetric patterns during 'physiological' conditions such as the fetal behavior states. During state 2F there is a significant increase of left ventricular output (LVO) associated with a concomitant decrease of right ventricular output (RVO), which is primarily the result of modifications in stroke volume. This evidence suggests a redistribution of cardiac output in favor of the left side of the heart during state 2F. Possible explanations for these findings include modifications of the venous return to the heart (preload) or selective changes in the vascular resistance against which ventricles eject (afterload). The former hypothesis seems unlikely, on the basis of the unchanged combined ventricular output (CVO) and of the absence of evident modifications of the

Table 1 *Definition of the fetal behavioral states (FBS) 1F and 2F. Coincidental states present for at least 3 min. From reference 2*

FBS 1F ('quiet sleep)
No eye movements

Quiescence, which can be interrupted by brief gross body movements, mostly startles

Fetal heart rate pattern A: stable heart rate pattern with a small oscillation bandwidth of less than 10 beats/min; isolated accelerations do occur, but are strictly related to fetal movements

FBS 2F ('active sleep')
Eye movements are continuously present

Frequent and periodic gross body movements, mainly stretches and retroflexions and movements of the extremities

Fetal heart rate pattern B: oscillation bandwidth of mone than 10 beats/min; frequent accelerations during movements

E/A ratio (early ventricular filling/atrial contraction), an index believed to be influenced by the preload of the heart. The latter explanation is consistent with results of animal studies which showed a significant increase of cerebral blood flow during active sleep. This hypothesis could be sustained by studies in the human fetus that showed a decrease of vascular resistance at the cerebral level and a reduction of peak flow velocity in the ductus arteriosus during state 2F. In fact, it was demonstrated that systolic peak flow velocity waveforms in the fetal ductus arteriosus were markedly reduced during behavioral state 2F as compared with state 1F, suggesting a redistribution in the left and right ventricular output in favor of the left side of the heart[4]. Moreover, van Eyck and colleagues[5] showed an increase in the average flow velocity at the foramen ovale level during active sleep, resulting in an increased right-to-left shunt. The increased foramen ovale blood flow during ventricular contraction may be explained by the fact that a closed tricuspid valve prevents superior vena cava blood flow from entering the right ventricle, leading to a raised right-to-left atrial pressure gradient. The upward movement of the tricuspid leaflets during ventricular contraction further contributes to this increased pressure gradient.

The ductus venosus also acts as an important shunt for well-oxygenated blood to be directed through the foramen ovale into the left heart. During state 1F there is a decrease of approximately 30% of peak systolic and peak diastolic flow velocities, these fndings suggesting decreased volume flow through the ductus venosus during this behavioral state. More volume flow through the ductus venosus during behavioral state 2F as compared with state 1F would be consistent with earlier reports of a behavioral state-related rise in volume flow at the foramen ovale and mitral valve levels, thus comfirming an increased volume through the left heart to ensure raised cerebral blood flow during fetal behavior state 2F[6].

All these findings show an increased fetal cardiac output in relation to state 2F, suggesting a redistributed cardiac output in favor of well-oxygenated blood from the left heart during this sleep state in the human fetus[7]. All the described hemodynamic mechanisms produced an improved venous return and an increased preload in the left ventricle.

Whereas in normal pregnancies the pulsatility index (PI) in the lower thoracic part of the fetal descending aorta and fetal internal carotid artery depicts significant changes with respect to the fetal behavioral state, this is not seen in the umbilical artery. Van Eyck and co-workers[8] established a decrease in the PI in the umbilical artery and fetal descending aorta with increased fetal heart rate. Hu and colleagues[9] observed that the pulse wave velocity in the fetal aorta was lower in state 2F than in 1F and that it seemed to suggest a reduction of the systemic blood pressure in this 'quiet sleep' state, perhaps by peripheral vasodilatation.

The behavioral state has been shown to influence cerebral blood flow in animals, adult humans, neonates and fetuses. Some authors have demonstrated a decrease in PI and an increase in the systolic peak, mean and end-diastolic velocities in the internal carotid artery during behavioral state 2F[10,11]. All these findings suggest a reduction in vascular resistance in the fetal brain. The increased systolic peak and mean velocity could be explained by an increased contraction force of the heart and/or a redistribution of blood flow during 2F in favor of the left heart, as is demonstrated with increasing volume flow at the foramen ovale and mitral valve levels. Increased volume flow through the left heart would be necessary to ensure raised cerebral blood flow during fetal behavioral state 2F which has been demonstrated in animal studies. For example, in the fetal lamb there was a significant increase in cerebral oxidative metabolism during the low-voltage electrocortical state (active sleep) which was sustained by a rise in cerebral blood flow; this was most pronounced in the subcortex and brainstem areas[10].

In fetal behavioral state 2F the systolic peak, averaged and end-diastolic velocities of the anterior cerebral artery are significantly increased. This observation coupled with the presence of rapid eye movements suggests raised electrocortical activity in the frontal lobes. An increase in the systolic peak and averaged velocities but not in tlle end-diastolic velocity in the posterior cerebral artery takes place during behavioral state 2F.

Noordam and colleagues[10] found no significant hemodynamic changes in the middle cerebral artery related to different fetal behavioral states. This could be attributed to the fact that the middle cerebral artery supplies the neocerebrum, where myelinization is still incomplete and the number of synapses is still increasing in term fetuses. However, we obtained different findings in our recent study[12] in which we evaluated the PI in the middle cerebral artery and its different portions supplying different areas of the fetal brain that are supposed to be activated in different behavioral states. The rationale of our study was based on the following considerations:

(1) The activation of metabolism in some areas of the brain may produce biochemical modifications such as the production of metabolites and some vasoactive substances that can induce vasodilatation of the cerebral vessels.

(2) The cerebral centers that regulate the vital and essential functions are located in the sub-cortical areas of the brain.

(3) The cerebral centers that regulate the functions of life are located in the cortical areas of the brain.

(4) The middle cerebral artery is the main vessel that supplies, with its proximal portion, some sub-cortical areas and, with its distal portion, 80% of the whole cerebral cortex.

(5) During different fetal behavioral states, the activation of metabolism in some cerebral areas may produce hemodynamic changes in the cerebral vessels, particularly in the main vessel, the middle cerebral artery and in its different portions, which supply different cerebral districts.

We found a positive correlation between the middle cerebral artery-M1 and FHR during the quiet phase ($r = 0.288$) and during the active phase ($r = 0.234$). There was a positive correlation between the middle cerebral artery-M2 and FHR during the quiet phase ($r = 0.341$) and a negative correlation during the active phase ($r = -0.075$) (Figure 1).

Figure 2 shows that the mean PI of the middle cerebral artery was lower during 2F than 1F both in the M1 segment and in the M2 segment; nevertheless, in the latter, the decrease of the PI value was significantly greater.

The variations (mean ± SD) registered in percentage of PI values going through the quiet phase to the active phase were -8.71 ± 11.28 for the M1 segment versus -24.72 ± 11.98 for the M2 segment ($p < 0.01$). These observations show a direct correlation between fetal behavioral states and cerebral hemodynamics, demonstrating a significant decrease in the impedance values to the flow during fetal behavioral state 2F in the main cerebral vessel, the middle cerebral artery and

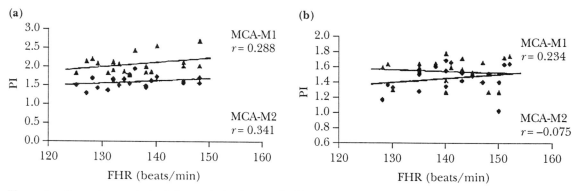

Figure 1 *Regression analysis of the correlation between fetal heart rate (FHR) and pulsatility index (PI) in the middle cerebral artery (MCA)-M1 and MCA-M2 in fetal behavioral states 1F (a) and 2F (b)*

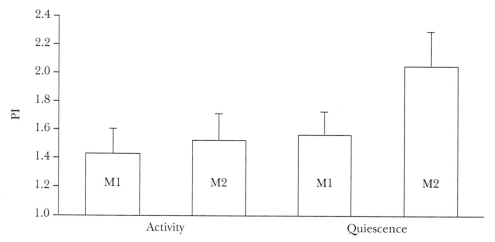

Figure 2 *Pulsatility index (PI) values in the M1 and M2 segments of the middle cerebral artery (MCA) during behavioral states 2F (activity) and 1F (quiescence). Mean ± SD of the PI of the MCA-M1: 1F, 1.5865 ± 0.150; 2F, 1.441 ± 0.172 ($p < 0.05$). MCA-M2: 1F, 2.0615 ± 0.256; 2F, 1.53 ± 0.176 ($p < 0.01$)*

particularly in its sub-cortical segment (M2). This is probably due to the metabolic activation of the cortical areas during state 2F ('active sleep') of the fetal brain which induces vasodilatation probably by local mechanisms (endothelium-derived relaxing factor/nitric oxide system, prostaglandins, pH, etc.).

The study of fetal hemodynamics is used for the evaluation of fetal conditions during pathology: understanding of the mechanisms which are involved in the regulation of the physiological hemodynamic adaptations to different fetal behavioral states may help in the differentiation between physiology and

pathology. Moreover, to disregard these aspects may produce misunderstandings in the evaluation of fetal well-being with potential severe fetomaternal complications mainly due to inappropriate obstetric management.

Finally, the study of fetal behavior must be considered, with other tools such as Doppler technology, in the evaluation of fetal well-being and, prospectively, in the assessment of fetal neurological status *in utero*, which may be compromised in several fetomaternal pathological conditions such as growth restriction, congenital abnormalities or diabetes.

References

1. Nijhuis JG. Fetal behavior and biophysics as observed by ultrasound. *J Perinat Med* 1991; 19(Suppl 1):145–50
2. Nijhuis JG, Prechtl HFR, Martin CB Jr, Bots RSGM. Are there behavioral states in the human fetus? *Early Hum Dev* 1982;6:177–95
3. Vindla S, James D. Fetal behavior as a test of fetal wellbeing. *Br J Obstet Gynaecol* 1995;102:597–600
4. Rizzo G, Arduini D, Valensise H, Romanini C. Effects of behavioral state on cardiac output in the healthy human fetus at 36–38 weeks of gestation. *Early Hum Dev* 1990;23:109–15
5. Van Eyck J, Stewart PA, Wladimiroff JW. Human fetal foramen ovale flow velocity waveforms relative to behavioral sates in normal term pregnancy. *Am J Obstet Gynecol* 1990;163:1239–42
6. Huisman TWA, Brezinca C, Stewart PA, Stijnen T, Wladimiroff JW. Ductus venosus flow velocity waveforms in relation to fetal behavioral states. *Br J Obstet Gynaecol* 1994;101:220–4
7. Richardson BS. The effect of behavioral state on fetal metabolism and blood flow circulation. *Semin Perinatol* 1992;16:227–33

8. Van Eyck J, Wladimiroff JW, Van Den Wijngaard JAGW, Noordam MJ, Prechtl HFR. The blood flow velocity waveform in the fetal internal carotid and umbilical artery; its relation to fetal behavioral states in normal pregnancy at 37–weeks. *Br J Obstet Gynaecol* 1987;94:736–41
9. Hu J, Nijhuis IJM, Hof JT, Gennser G. Dependence of aortic pulse wave assessment on behavioral state in normal term fetus. *Early Hum Dev* 1997;48:59–70
10. Noordam MJ, Hoekstra FME, Hop WCJ, Wladimiroff JW. Doppler color flow imaging of fetal intracerebral arteries relative to fetal behavioral states in normal pregnancy. *Early Hum Dev* 1994;39:49–56
11. Shono M, Shono H, Ito Y, Muro M, Uchiyama A, Sugimori H. The effect of behavioral states on fetal heart rate and middle cerebral artery flow-velocity waveforms in normal and full-term fetuses. *Int J Gynecol Obstet* 1997;58:275–80
12. Clerici G, Cutuli A, Di Renzo GC. Fetal cerebral hemodynamics and behavioral states. *Am J Obstet Gynecol* 1999;180:S155

In utero treatment: state of the art 27

M. I. Evans, A. W. Flake, M. P. Johnson, H. R. Belkin, A. Johnson
and M. Harrison

INTRODUCTION

The past two decades have demonstrated some extremely remarkable advances in the science that underlies maternal–fetal therapy. Numerous diagnostic techniques have been developed that allow physicians to detect fetal anomalies that heretofore were undetectable prenatally. The advances in therapy for these abnormalities are equally astounding. Fetuses now are treated both medically and surgically in ways that could not even have been imagined 25 years ago. Anomalies can now be detected whether they originate structurally, biochemically or functionally. These early diagnoses allow couples to choose the option of either pregnancy termination when legally permissible or, where possible, fetal therapy to correct early-diagnosed abnormalities. In general, structural abnormalities are treated surgically, whereas metabolic and biochemical abnormalities receive pharmacological or genetic treatment. The past several years have shown numerous advances in both surgical and medical treatment.

Since its inception in the early 1980s, open fetal surgery has been performed basically in one medical center and has spread as graduates of that program have assumed leadership positions at other centers. The main limitation in the use of open fetal surgery is the concern for maternal risk and, in some instances, poor results. As a rule, quite rigorous selection criteria have been used, also limiting the number of patients who are appropriate candidates for treatment. As experience with the procedures expands, results naturally have improved significantly. There has been a great deal of innovation in this area. This was necessitated by practical, clinical need. Investigators wanted to improve both the usefulness and the safety of open fetal surgery

for both mothers and fetuses. At the present time, many techniques have become standardized, including methods used to open and close the uterus, and to monitor the fetus during the procedure while maintaining oxygenation, hemostasis and homeostasis. Many of the operative techniques are also relatively standardized. These factors will in the future lead to a greater and more widespread usage of fetal surgical procedures.

OPEN SURGICAL APPROACHES

The fetal operation

Introduction

The initial consideration in the treatment of a fetus through a surgical procedure is the question of when the surgical procedure should be performed. Deciding upon the exact timing of a fetal operation is complex. It is dependent upon several factors, including the specific anomaly being treated, the pathophysiology of the abnormal fetus, the estimated gestational age and various maternal factors. Small size is a significant factor in the fetus that is less than approximately 18 weeks' gestational age. At the other end of the spectrum, the fetus which has reached approximately 30 weeks' gestational age is generally delivered and treated *ex utero*. In addition, with a later gestational age of the fetus, there is naturally less time for the intervention to achieve the desired effect. For example, a late operation performed in order to allow lung growth in the fetus will have less time to permit that lung growth if the fetus is at 29 rather than 19 weeks. There is also the unproven, but anecdotally recognized impression that, as the term of a pregnancy increases, the uterine reactivity increases, and the higher the risk of preterm labor. Because of this, open fetal procedures are generally limited to being performed on fetuses who are between 18 and 30 weeks' gestation. One must also consider the fact that some procedures are quite significant and bring with them a great deal of fetal stress. Minor procedures that can be performed rapidly through a small hysterotomy incision are much less likely to cause any derangement to the fetus or uteroplacental complex than are prolonged, major fetal operations with their increased likelihood of causing secondary preterm labor or fetal demise.

Monitoring and fetal homeostasis

One key to the successful completion of these procedures is accurate monitoring of the mother and fetus during the surgical procedure. This intraoperative monitoring has presented a rather difficult problem to solve. There are numerous issues that need to be addressed in the consideration of the techniques of intraoperative monitoring. The first consideration is that there is not much room in which one can work. This is compounded by the small physical size of the developing fetus. These difficulties, combined with the poor tissue integrity of the fetus, make sutured electrodes generally a poor choice. Although not a perfect procedure, pulse oximetry has been successfully utilized. However, pulse oximetry has the twin problems of reliability and accuracy. There is also the fact that, because this is being used in a fetus, the inherent limitations of pulse oximetry are amplified. A fetus is small, there is a minimal pulse pressure and the environment is wet and dark. All of these factors reduce the reliability of pulse oximetry and thus its usefulness. This is especially true unfortunately at times when it is most essential, that is when one is working with an unstable, hypotensive fetus. Physical exposure of the extremity can, even in the best of cases, be difficult. If one uses this technique, a great deal of care must be taken

in its application. The entire fetal hand must be dried and kept dry with an appropriate dressing. A foil wrap must be used to shield the area from light. As one can readily imagine, keeping such a small area perfectly dry during a surgical procedure is quite challenging. Several solutions have been attempted, chiefly the development of radiotelemetry units. These systems allow various fetal parameters such as heart rate, temperature, intra-amniotic pressure and potentially parameters such as pH and tissue oxygenation to be monitored. The surgeon attaches a small radiotelemetry unit to the fetal skin with suture material. The unit sends a continuous signal to an outside antenna. Another advantage of this unit is the fact that it can be left in place postoperatively for monitoring. Importantly, as a device that remains intrauterine, it is more sensitive for detection of uterine contraction than is standard tocodynamometry. However, no matter how accurate this type of unit appears to be, experience has demonstrated that intraoperative ultrasound is still the most reliable method of assessing fetal status. Intraoperative ultrasound can provide a wide variety of information, including fetal heart rate, volume status and contractility.

Maintaining fetal homeostasis through the protection of uteroplacental blood flow remains key to the successful treatment of the fetus. This is done by the maintenance of uterine relaxation. One must also carefully monitor and control maternal volume status and blood pressure. A common cause of decreased uteroplacental blood flow is umbilical cord compression. This may occur at the margins of the hysterotomy or in those cases where there is an inadequate amount of amniotic fluid. It is essential to maintain intra-amniotic volume by exteriorizing only the parts of the fetus actually necessary for the procedure, and by using a continuous high-volume perfusion of the amniotic space with warm Ringer's lactate solution. Loss of amniotic fluid can lead to loss of uterine volume. Loss of uterine volume can in many cases stimulate uterine contraction, with devastating effects to the fetus.

Congenital diaphragmatic hernia

The first reported case of an attempted repair of congenital diaphragmatic hernia (CDH) was in 1986 and the first success in 1989. In the 10 years since that procedure was performed, it has evolved significantly. Definitive repair of CDH has generally proved disastrous. Definitive repair is a complex procedure and includes the reduction of viscera from the chest, diaphragmatic patch placement and abdominal silo construction. The goal is to return the viscera to a more physiological location, while reducing intra-abdominal pressure. This has proven to be extremely difficult, and is associated with an extremely high mortality rate. This is particularly true in those cases wherein the liver has herniated into the chest. Our group has abandoned definitive repair as an option for CDH. Quite recently, a novel technique has been developed. This is the procedure that uses *in utero* tracheal occlusion. Access is obtained and clips are placed on the fetal trachea in order to occlude the egress of fluids formed in the lungs. This forces the build-up of fluid to occur within the lung itself. Tracheal occlusion induces lung growth. This, in turn, physically reduces the herniated viscera from the chest, thus alleviating lung hypoplasia. The procedure involved in placing the tracheal occlusion is relatively simple. The surgeon exposes the fetal neck, dissecting the trachea circumferentially (avoiding causing injury to the recurrent laryngeal nerves) and places occlusive hemoclips. The surgeon then replaces the fetus in the uterus and closes the incision. Further experience will be necessary before it can be determined whether or not tracheal occlusion will improve on the results of conventional treatment of CDH.

Congenital cystic adenomatoid malformation

Congenital cystic adenomatoid malformation (CCAM) is a congenital cystic lung lesion. As with any large space occupying lesion of the lung, if it grows large enough, it can cause lung compression, mediastinal shift and reduction of venous return to the heart, resulting in fetal hydrops. The development of hydrops is an extremely serious consequence. Fetuses with CCAM who develop hydrops have a mortality approaching 100%. Fetal surgery in such a case can be life-saving to the fetus. Surgical resection of CCAM in the fetus causes a reversal of the hydrops condition. Fetal survival is dramatically improved. A hysterotomy is performed and the arm and chest wall on the side of the lesion are exposed. The procedure performed on the fetus includes the creation of a large thoracotomy through the mid-thorax of the fetus. The surgeon then exteriorizes the lobe containing the CCAM. Blunt dissection is used to detach the lobe from adjacent normal tissue. The lobar hilum is divided by application of a stapler or a bulk ligature and the thoracotomy is quickly closed. This procedure is significantly simpler to perform than is a CDH repair, and operative time is short compared to that of CDH repair. Fetal blood loss and stress are relatively minimal. Fetal and maternal outcomes have been quite good to date.

Sacrococcygeal teratoma

Fetal sacrococcygeal teratoma (SCT) arises from the presacral space. It may grow to such an enormous size that in some fetuses high-output cardiac failure will occur from vascular steal by the tumor. There will generally be an associated placentomegaly and fetal hydrops. This combination of SCT and high-output cardiac failure is uniformly fatal. This is a condition ideally situated for fetal surgical treatment. As the basic pathophysiological problem is the vascular steal, it is logical to think that, if this steal is ligated, the high-output cardiovascular situation will terminate, resulting in a correction of the aberrant physiology. In this procedure, the fetal buttocks are exteriorized and the tumor is exposed. It is important to make every attempt to keep the head, torso and lower extremities of the fetus in the uterus. A problem may arise because of the size of the tumor. Often these tumors can be much larger than the fetus itself. When the tumor is removed, there can be a significant loss of uterine volume and the occurrence of uterine contraction. One must be aware of and prepared for this possibility. The surgeon must identify the anus and incise the fetal skin posterior to the anorectal sphincter complex. This is essential in order to avoid damaging this area, leading to fecal incontinence. A tourniquet is then applied to the base of the tumor and brought down gradually as the tumor is finger fractured down to its vascular pedicle. The tumor pedicle is then ligated using either sutures or staples. This entire procedure can be performed on the fetus in less than a quarter of an hour. The amount of blood loss should be minimal. Hemodynamics may be significantly affected by the loss of the tumor. It is important to be aware of the fact that fetal hemodynamics will change after the procedure. The tumor is a very low-resistance area and its removal from the circulation may significantly increase the afterload. It is therefore necessary to monitor the fetal cardiovascular status closely, both during and immediately following the ligation, by ultrasound. Any needed interventions must be performed rapidly.

The ex utero intrapartum treatment

As many of the fetal procedures result in a situation that would lead to a compromise of fetal oxygenation if a normal delivery were attempted, other techniques of delivery have been developed. One of these is the *ex utero* intrapartum treatment (EXIT) procedure. This is a modification of delivery and may be applied to deliver a fetus after certain surgical procedures have been performed on the fetus. These would include procedures that reduce the ability to oxygenate in neonatal life, such as tracheal ligation. The EXIT procedure can also be used on fetuses with problems that compromise the airway, including massive cervical teratomas or cystic hygromas. As the EXIT procedure is performed in fetuses with compromised airways, fetal blood oxygenation must be maintained through the placental attachment to the mother until the fetal airway is patent.

It is essential that, during the performance of the EXIT procedure, uteroplacental perfusion be maintained until the fetal airway is secured and ventilation is established. To this end, it is also essential to maintain the maternal uterus in a relaxed condition in order to provide the fetus with as much perfusion as possible. This is exactly opposite to the situation in vaginal delivery and surgical delivery, in which uterine contraction for hemostasis is desired. During the EXIT procedure, tocolytics are used to ensure uterine relaxation. Thus, while the fetal procedure is being performed, maternal circulation is still supporting the fetus, as it was when the fetus was *in utero*. Clips can be removed, bronchoscopy performed and an airway established in what otherwise would be almost impossible circumstances. Once the airway is stabilized, the delivery can be completed.

Closing the uterus

About the only similarity between fetal surgery and a Cesarean section is that both involve surgery on a pregnant woman. There are numerous significant differences. The most obvious difference is that the fetus is returning to the uterus and will remain there for the duration of the pregnancy in order for the procedure to succeed. Therefore, there must be an adequate closure of the uterus allowing for the containment of both the fetus and the amniotic fluid without leaks. The closure must be strong enough both to contain the fetus and amniotic fluid and not to burst or leak under the pressure of contractions. The proper closing procedure has been described in detail in the literature. This technique has been used many times and has resulted in tight closures with minimal risk of leakage of amniotic fluid.

Initially, one places an appropriate number of large interrupted full-thickness mono-filament retention sutures over the entire length of the wound. This elevates the wound edges and minimizes bleeding. In order to freshen the wound edges, one then cuts away the staple lines, allowing apposition of muscle tissue. Membranes are closed using a fine running monofilament. It is important to leave in the amniotic space a small catheter that can be used in order to reconstitute amniotic fluid. This catheter can also be used as a port through which one can instil antibiotics before completing the closure. The myometrium is then closed with a second running layer of larger monofilament absorbable suture. Retention sutures are placed in order both to relieve tension on the wound and to provide more strength. Last, the skin is closed in an appropriate manner. The final action of the surgeon is to reconstitute the amniotic fluid volume with warm lactated Ringer's solution under ultrasound guidance and instil the appropriate antibiotics just before placing the final suture and removing the catheter.

Summary

Open fetal surgery has come a long way since its inception. The techniques used in the various procedures have been refined over the past decade. Fetal surgery is now performed in several centers within the USA. In general, results have been quite good for most procedures; however, the application of fetal surgery remains controversial in certain instances. This is particularly true in the case of CDH where results, as yet, have not unequivocally supported the use of fetal surgery. As in many areas of surgery, in fetal surgery, there is a trend towards less invasive approaches to the treatment of fetal disease, including an increased use of endoscopy and ultrasound. It is anticipated that the continued expansion of their use will further reduce the use of the open approach. An example of this is seen in the use of endoscopic or bronchoscopic tracheal occlusion. This may one day eliminate the need for open fetal surgery in the treatment of CDH. However, open fetal surgery, for the time being, remains a valuable part of the armamentarium. In selected cases, it is the best or sometimes the only option available. Fetal surgery is now being performed much more safely, rapidly and accurately than ever before and with a greater likelihood of success.

ENDOSCOPIC APPROACHES

Lower obstructive uropathy

The development of an endoscopic approach to the treatment of certain fetal anomalies has added a new dimension to fetal therapy. Procedures that at one time required an open approach or could not be performed at all can currently be performed with a minimally invasive endoscopic approach. Endoscopy combined with sonography provide visualization equal to, if not superior to, that of conventional open procedures. A prime example of the application of these procedures is in the treatment of fetal lower urinary tract obstruction (LUTO). LUTO affects 1 : 5000–8000 males and, if left untreated, may lead to renal dysplasia, hydronephrosis and perinatal death. Prenatally diagnosed cases of posterior urethral valves have a 30–50% mortality with death generally being attributable to pulmonary hypoplasia and/or renal dysplasia.

The initial indication that LUTO may be present is generally obtained during a routine ultrasonic examination of the pregnant patient. Certain sonographic features typify LUTO. These include the presence of a dilated and thickened bladder, hydroureters, hydronephrosis and oligohydramnios. Depending upon the gestational age at which the diagnosis is made, the oligohydramnios may be quite severe. The gender of the fetus also has a relationship to the positive predictive value of these signs. These findings, in a male fetus, are suggestive of the presence of posterior urethral valves. There are, however, other anomalies that can present with identical findings. These are such findings as urethral stricture, urethral atresia, urethral agenesis, ureteral reflux, persistent cloaca and megalourethra. Although prenatally, one can limit the differential diagnosis to these several abnormalities, the precise diagnosis can be made only after delivery and birth of the infant.

Once the ultrasound findings have been made, the issue of management arises. In most of these cases, the discovery of LUTO indicates that there will be a need for complex management of the patient. Perhaps the most important action is to perform a thorough, careful sonographic examination in order to rule out any associated congenital anomalies. One must also look for any sonographic evidence of renal cystic dysplasia or oligohydramnios. One need be concerned not only with anatomical but also with functional abnormalities. The best way to assess function is through the use of serial vesicocenteses. It should be noted that a single vesicocentesis may not adequately reflect the renal reserve, as two consecutive samples may be on different sides of the normal cut-off level.

Once the diagnosis has been made, issues of management must then be addressed. Obviously in the case of patients with LUTO, some relief of the obstruction and bladder fluid build-up must be achieved. This is generally done through the use of a shunting procedure. Vesicoamniotic shunts placed with ultrasound guidance have been suggested since 1982 for the treatment of fetuses with LUTO. This serves two purposes. It relieves the pressure within the bladder, which is causing urine back-up, and potential organ dysfunction and also acts to increase the volume of amniotic fluid, potentially relieving the associated oligohydramnios. This additionally provides for normal fetal lung development. Animal studies have demonstrated that, when the ureters or the urethra and urachus of fetal lambs were ligated during mid-gestation, renal dysplasia and pulmonary hypoplasia resulted. When the ligation was removed, the urinary obstruction resolved and the animals demonstrated improved pulmonary status at birth. Clinical experience has shown some success also. The use of percutaneous vesicoamniotic shunting in humans, from data collected at the International Fetal Surgery Registry, shows a 5% procedure-related loss, and a 48% survival rate (40 of 83 treated fetuses). Of the treated fetuses, 74% with posterior urethral valves survived, in contrast to a 45% fetal loss rate reported in untreated fetuses with posterior urethral valves. Survivors with total urethral

obstruction, as with urethral atresia or agenesis, are extremely rare. This is a significant increase in survival, but it is hoped that, with further experience in the field, the survival rate can be increased to an even greater degree.

There are several limitations to the treatment of fetuses afflicted with LUTO. First, these procedures are not definitive. Rather they are temporary, palliative measures designed to defer final treatment until the infant is born. Second, as with any type of shunt, vesicoamniotic shunts may become obstructed or displaced. This obviously would require an additional procedure in order to replace the shunt. These complications occur in up to 25% of all cases. Some investigators have proposed the use of fetal vesicostomy or ureterostomy performed through the use of open fetal surgery in order to overcome these problems. There has not been a great deal of support for these approaches.

We wished to build upon the advantages of performing procedures without open fetal surgery and thus have introduced the concept of performing percutaneous fetal cystoscopy in order to evaluate fetuses with LUTO. Percutaneous fetal cystoscopy uses the same techniques and requires the same skills as does fetal vesicocentesis. A needle or trocar is placed in the appropriate manner and a thin endoscope is passed through the lumen. Thus, one is able to observe the fetal bladder at the time of the vesicocentesis. The anatomy of the trigone is identified, and the operator can thus determine the presence or absence of posterior urethral valves. After the endoscope is removed, the bladder is drained. Fetal cystoscopy may also be used in a therapeutic manner. Our group has performed ablation of posterior urethral valves in a fetus at 24 weeks of gestation. This was accomplished with the use of an operating endoscope positioned towards the posterior urethra. We next advanced an electrode through the operating channel of the endoscope. The valves were identified and cauterized through the use of direct endoscopic visualization. We then immediately confirmed urethral patency by the use of a transurethral instillation of physiological solution into the amniotic cavity. We have also used YAG laser energy to ablate the valves, again with documentation of urethral patency. These are exciting new procedural techniques with a good deal of potential for future use. We believe that, although these techniques are still in the early learning phase, as we gain experience in their use it will be possible to compare these new techniques against more established shunt procedures.

From our work to date, it appears that the use of percutaneous fetal cystoscopy may allow one to make a more precise prenatal diagnosis and prognosis in fetuses with LUTO. A great advantage to this procedure is the fact that it can be performed at the time of diagnostic vesicocentesis. Therefore, it should not pose additional risks to the standard assessment of fetal renal function. Most importantly, it is a procedure whereby the obstruction is completely eliminated *in utero*. It seems probably that such early *in utero* relief of obstruction may help these fetuses to fare better in the long run. This type of procedure avoids the complications of both vesicoamniotic shunts and open fetal surgery.

Other endoscopic approaches

We feel that endoscopic fetal surgery will prove to be useful in many varied areas of maternal–fetal therapy. Endoscopic fetal surgery is being developed in our center and others for many purposes, in cases previously only correctable by open surgery, if at all. These include cases that involve the treatment of umbilical cord ligation in acardiac twins, and laser ablation in twin to twin transfusion. Future developments include its use for early fetal blood sampling and as an adjunct to *in utero* fetal muscle biopsy.

The advances that it is hoped will take place over the next several years may prove to be very exciting. Procedures will be developed and modified, bringing a new level of safety and reliability to current techniques. With simplification of existing techniques, learning curves should flatten, bringing the use of these procedures to many more medical centers throughout the world. It is likely that many applications of open fetal surgery will in fact be modified to be done endoscopically, reducing the need for and therefore the potential complications of open fetal surgery.

MEDICAL THERAPY

Overview

Fetal therapy has been part of medical practice for over three decades. The initial experiments in fetal therapy were performed by Wiley in the 1960s, when he first attempted intraperitoneal transfusion. A decade and a half later, fetoscopic blood sampling began to be used for the diagnoses of genetic disorders, and for fetal transfusions. In the late 1970s, techniques had advanced to such a degree that attempts to correct obstructive hydrocephalus and obstructive uropathies with shunt therapy were begun. At that time, animal experiments were establishing the model for open fetal surgery. In the 1980s, open fetal surgery was first performed on human fetuses. Open fetal surgery at this time ultimately succeeded in the repair of diaphragmatic hernia and congenital cystic adenomatous malformations. The 1980s and 1990s have also demonstrated advances in the use of metabolic fetal therapies. These have been used for the treatment of congenital adrenal hyperplasia, methylmalonic aciduria, cardiac arrhythmias and neural tube defects. One of the greatest advances of the current decade in maternal–fetal therapy has been the dramatic increase in the use of endoscopy. Endoscopy has emerged as a procedure that can be used to reduce the incision size in open surgery. Furthermore, in the past 10 years, hematopoietic stem cell transplants have become possible. These appear to be potentially successful in appropriately chosen cases.

The history of medical treatment of pregnant women has been fraught with dramatic successes and failures. Drugs and other agents have been administered to pregnant women for many years in order to attempt to treat various fetal disorders. Well-known examples include Rhogam injections to prevent Rh disease, exchange transfusionons to treat Rh disease, the administration of corticosteroids for the prevention of respiratory distress syndrome in premature infants and the administration of phenobarbital prior to birth in the hope of inducing liver enzymes for postnatal reduction of serum bilirubin concentration. These are medical treatments that are delivered to the patient prenatally. We now wish not merely to treat these conditions medically, but to treat the genetic causes prenatally. There are, however, currently only a very few examples of attempted prenatal treatments for genetically determined metabolic defects.

Congenital adrenal hyperplasia

The most frequently diagnosed adrenal anomaly that affects the fetus is congenital adrenal hyperplasia (CAH). CAH is a group of disorders, all of which devolve in an autosomal recessive manner. They are characterized by an absolute or relative deficiency in one or more of the enzymes required for adrenal cortisol biosynthesis. The most common abnormality, responsible for > 90% of cases of CAH, is caused by a deficiency of the enzyme 21-hydroxylase (21-OH), also known as p450c21. Diminished 21-OH activity results in accumulation of 17-hydroxyprogesterone (17-OHP) due to a decrease in its conversion to 11-deoxycorticosterone. The excess 17-OHP is then converted via androstenedione to androgens, the levels of which increase by as much as several hundred-fold. The excess androgens have many untoward effects upon the developing fetus, especially on developing female fetuses. These excess hormones will frequently cause masculinization of the undifferentiated female external genitalia, resulting in a wide range of conditions. The degree of masculinization may vary from slight clitoral hypertrophy to complete

formation of a phallus and scrotum. Depending on the specific enzyme missing in CAH, in addition to ambiguous genitalia, the absence of certain adrenal enzymes may cause the infant to have either a moderate degree of hypertension or a salt-wasting condition. This is therefore an extremely important condition to diagnose and treat prenatally.

Since discovery and mapping of the allelic variants in the 1980s, direct DNA analysis has become the routine approach to diagnosis. This condition may be diagnosed inadvertently through the use of routine ultrasonic examination. The sonographic detection of an abnormally enlarged phallus should alert the physician to investigate for CAH.

The objective in the treatment of CAH is to reduce the amount of androgens that are being produced. The basic physiology behind the disease is the absence of a cortisol end product, preventing feedback inhibition to the pituitary's production of adrenocorticotropic hormone (ACTH). With no feedback inhibition, pituitary formation of ACTH continues to stimulate adrenal cortical production of androgens. By replacing the missing cortisol, the physician can cause the pituitary's production of ACTH to become suppressed. This stops the cycle and should reduce the aberrant hormonal levels back to normal. The fetal adrenal gland can be pharmacologically suppressed by maternal replacement doses of dexamethasone. In an attempt to prevent female genital birth defects, Evans and colleagues first administered dexamethasone at a dose of 0.25 mg four times a day to a mother known to be at risk for CAH, beginning at 10 weeks of gestation.

The difficulty arises in the fact that fetal external genitalia differentiation begins at about 7 weeks of gestation, much earlier than diagnosis by amniocentesis or even chorionic villus sampling (CVS) can be made. Thus, diagnosis generally comes too late to prevent at least some degree of masculinization. Therefore, for patients at risk of having an affected fetus, pharmacological therapy must be initiated prior to diagnosis. The issue is to decide which patients are at risk of having a fetus with CAH. This implies that therapy needs to be administered to all patients at risk despite the fact that the chance of an affected female fetus for carrier parents is only 1 in 8 (i.e. 1 in 4 affected × 1 in 2 female). This will result in some fetuses receiving treatment that does not turn out to be necessary. However, there should be no untoward effects on the developing fetus with therapy provided for a short period of time. Direct DNA diagnosis or linkage studies may then be performed by CVS in the first trimester. Therefore, in the cases of seven out of eight patients, CAH will be ruled out and therapy can be discontinued. In the one out of eight patients in whom the fetus is found to be an affected female, therapy is continued throughout the pregnancy. It is important to remember that the stress of labor will require the addition of stress-doses of corticosteroids given to the mother. These steroids will then be slowly tapered postpartum.

There have been, to date, several dozen infants who otherwise would have been born masculinized, born with normal genitalia because they were treated by this protocol. In a few cases some degree of masculinization has still been observed following this regimen when it was begun at 9 weeks. Therefore, we currently begin the protocol at 7 weeks. The efficacy of this change is still being evaluated. These events represent the first prenatal attempt to prevent a birth defect and we believe that they serve as a model for other attempts at pharmacological fetal therapy.

Hypothyroidism

Fetal hypothyroidism is an extremely serious disease, the consequences of which may indeed be fatal. Goiter can result in fetal esophageal obstruction, polyhydramnios and preterm delivery. Fetal goiter can also cause extension of the fetal neck, leading to dystocia during delivery, requiring intervention by the physician, with increased potential for trauma to the child during delivery. If fetal hypothyroidism is not treated, postnatal growth delay and severe mental retardation can ensue.

Ultrasound generally gives the first indication of goiter. Generally, the indication for the ulrasonographic scan is a fundal height discrepancy. The uterus is found to be greater than expected from gestational age. This is caused by polyhydramnios that has resulted from the esophageal obstruction, impaired swallowing and the attendant failure of the fetus to reduce the volume of amniotic fluid present. Again, as in other types of fetal functional disorders, early treatment after diagnosis is the key to a successful outcome. *In utero* treatment was initially suggested by Van Herle and colleagues, using intra-muscular injection of levothyroxine sodium. Subsequent studies, however, have indicated that intra-amniotic administration of thyroxine is superior. The doses commonly used for treatment range from 200 to 500 mg intra-amniotically every week. More recently, it has been recommended that more accurate dosage can be determined by adjusting for fetal weight. The dose of 10 mg/kg, similar to the recommended dose for neonates, has been used with success. With this regimen, fetal goiters have been shown to regress, and fetal and newborn thyroid stimulating hormone levels have normalized.

Hyperthyroidism

Neonatal hyperthyroidism is much less common than is neonatal hypothyroidism. The reported incidence of this disorder ranges from approximately 1 : 4000 to 1 : 40 000 live births. In the majority of these cases, fetal thyrotoxic goiter is secondary to maternal autoimmune disease, generally Graves' disease or Hashimoto's thyroiditis. It is hypothesized that maternal antithyroid antibodies traverse the uteroplacental barrier, and cause an immunological reaction in the fetus. For this reason, adequate counselling is extremely important for any pregnant patients who present with histories of these diseases as to the potential fetal consequences.

Once the diagnosis of fetal hyperthyroidism is confirmed, treatment should be begun.

Several different protocols have been reported in the literature. Many investigators have reported treating fetal hyperthyroidism by delivering anti-thyroid drugs to the mother. Porreco used maternally delivered propyl-thiouracil (PTU) to treat fetal thyrotoxicosis, with a reported good outcome. He initially dosed the mother at 100 mg orally three times a day. This was later decreased to 50 mg orally three times a day. Wenstrom and co-workers described using methimazole delivered to the mother with a favorable outcome. This was performed in a patient who could not tolerate PTU. Hatjis also treated fetal goiterous hyperthyroidism with a maternal dose of 300 mg PTU. This patient, however, required supplemental synthroid to remain euthyroid, but a good outcome was reported. At the present time, there appear to be several treatments with potentially good outcomes. Clinical judgement will determine which is most appropriate for a specific patient.

Methylmalonic acidemia

Methylmalonic acidemia is a metabolic disease that is related to a functional vitamin B_{12} deficiency. Coenzymatically active vitamin B_{12} is required for the conversion of methylmalonyl-coenzyme A (Co-A) to succinyl-Co-A. Without an adequate amount of coenzymatically active vitamin B_{12}, methylmalonyl-Co-A is not transformed properly to succinyl-Co-A. Excessive amounts of methylmalonyl-Co-A are excreted in the urine, where it is detected. The presence of this disease in the fetus can have significant consequences.

Prenatal treatment with maternally injected vitamin B_{12} can improve both the fetal and the maternal biochemistry. It is difficult to assess whether or not there is any significant clinical benefit to the fetus by *in utero* treatment. It does, though, seem likely that reducing the fetal burden of methylmalonic acid should have some beneficial effect on fetal development and could reduce the risks in the neonatal period. However, further investigation would be necessary in order to determine whether this is accurate.

Multiple carboxylase deficiency

Biotin-responsive multiple carboxylase deficiency is another biochemical disorder with potentially serious consequences to the newborn. This disorder is an inborn error of metabolism in which several mitochondrial enzymes have decreased levels of activity. These include the mitochondrial biotin-dependent enzymes, pyruvate carboxylase, propionyl-Co-A carboxylase and β-methylcrotonyl-CoA carboxylase. These patients present in the newborn or early childhood period with dermatitis, severe metabolic acidosis and a characteristic pattern of organic acid excretion. Biotin supplementation can restore metabolism in patients or in their cultured cells. There have been at least two reports of prenatal administration of biotin to fetuses affected with this disorder.

Galactosemia

Galactosemia is an autosomally recessive inborn error of metabolism that is a result of the diminished activity of the enzyme galactose-1-phosphate uridyltransferase, resulting in the accumulation of metabolic intermediates in many bodily tissues. The disease results in cataracts, growth deficiency and ovarian failure. It can be diagnosed prenatally by study of cultured amniocytes and chorionic villi. The disease clinically presents in the neonatal period, most commonly with growth deficiency. The effects of this disease can be largely ameliorated if galactose is eliminated from the diet. Unfortunately, in the female infants, galactosemia irreversibly damages oocytes long before birth. Cellular damage in galactosemia is thought to be mediated by accumulation of galactose-1-phosphate intracellularly and of galactitol in the lens.

Galactosemia may be a disease in which prenatal treatment is extremely important. It has been suggested that even the early postnatal use of a low galactose diet may not be sufficient to ensure normal development. Some have speculated that prenatal damage to galactosemic fetuses could contribute to subsequent neurological devdopment and to lens cataract formation. For these reasons, the prenatal treatment of galactosemia appears to be extremely important.

Neural tube defects

The studies surrounding the relationship between folic acid and neural tube defects are an example of what seems to be an extremely successful public education initiative. In 1991, a randomized double-blind trial designed by the Medical Research Council Vitamin Study Research Group demonstrated that folate given preconceptionally reduced the risk of recurrence of fetal neural tube defects in high-risk patients. It has been subsequently shown that preparations containing folate and other vitamins also reduce the occurrence of first-time neural tube defects. In response to these findings, public health guidelines were issued calling for consumption of 4.0 mg/day of folic acid by women with a prior child affected with a neural tube defect, for at least 1 month prior to conception through the first 3 months of pregnancy. In addition, it is now recommended that all women planning to become pregnant begin to take 0.4 mg/day folic acid daily.

PRENATAL HEMATOPOIETIC STEM CELL TRANSPLANTATION

The potential for treatment of diseases involving the hematological system using transplanted hematopoietic stem cells (HSCs) is significant. The engraftment and clonal proliferation of a relatively small number of normal HSCs can sustain lifelong hematopoiesis. This observation forms the scientific basis behind bone marrow transplantation (BMT). It is now supported by thousands of long-term survivors of BMT who otherwise would have succumbed to lethal hematological disease. We have not to date come anywhere near to the realization of the full potential of BMT. As a threshold problem, there remains a critical shortage of immunologically compatible donor cells.

Furthermore, we are unable to control the recipient or donor immune response. Coupling these problems with the requirement for recipient myeloablation to achieve engraftment, one can readily see the difficulties faced. Human leukocyte antigen (HLA) matching is essential. The greater the degree of mismatch, the greater the risk of failure. Failure includes the development of graft failure, graft-versus-host disease (GVHD) and delayed immunological reconstitution. This is further complicated by the fact that current methods of myeloablation have unacceptably high levels of morbidity and mortality. These combined problems severely limit the number of patients who could successfully receive BMT. Early research seems to indicate that it is at least theoretically possible to use the *in utero* transplantation of HSCs in order to overcome many of the limitations of BMT. This approach is potentially applicable to any congenital hematopoietic disease that can be diagnosed prenatally and can be cured or improved by engraftment of normal HSCs.

Rationale for *in utero* transplantation

In utero transplantation takes advantage of an opportunity created by normal ontogeny. There is a period of time during fetal developing that exists prior to the time that bone marrow has become populated and self-antigens have been processed by the thymus, when the fetus theoretically should be receptive to engraftment of foreign HSCs. Theoretically, as the immune response has not yet been developed by the fetus, this should be accomplished without rejection and without the need for myeloablation. In effect, the fetus will recognize the foreign HSCs as self and not reject the transplant. In the human fetus, the ideal window of opportunity would appear to be prior to 14 weeks' gestation. This is a time before release of differentiated T lymphocytes into the circulation and while the bone marrow is just beginning to develop hematopoietic sites. It certainly may extend beyond that in immunodeficiency states, particularly when

T-cell development is abnormal. As this is the stage of thymic processing that involves negative selection, the presentation of foreign antigen by thymic dendritic cells theoretically should result in clonal deletion of reactive T cells. This type of treatment is a perfect example of the importance of mutual advances in both the early diagnosis and the treatment of genetic disease. Many congenital diseases can now be diagnosed as early as the first trimester of pregnancy. Advances in fetal intervention make transplantation possible by 10 to 12 weeks' gestation. The ontological window of opportunity falls well within these diagnostic and technical constraints, making application of this approach a realistic possibility. Thus, the possibilities of treating many diseases that heretofore were untreatable is now a realistic goal.

The advantages of prenatal HSC transplantation are immediately obvious. Most importantly, there would be no requirement for HLA matching. This would result in an enhanced number of donors. It would also result in the transplanted cells not being rejected, space being available in the bone marrow. This would thus eliminate the need for toxic immunosuppressive and myeloablative drugs. As the fetus remains in the uterus, it is engulfed in an excellent ultimate sterile isolation chamber. This eliminates the need for and expense of the 2 to 4 months of isolation required after postnatal BMT and prior to immunological reconstitution. Perhaps, most importantly, with prenatal transplantation, the disease would not become clinically manifest. The problems of multiple and recurrent infections, growth retardation, the need for multiple transfusions and the suffering attendant thereto would not arise.

Source of donor cells

With the theoretical possibilities of the use of HSCs, the issue becomes that of obtaining an adequate number of donor cells. Although cross-matching is no longer a problem, an adequate supply of these cells is essential. The source of donor cells may be critical to the success of engraftment. Fetal cells have distinct advantages. The most obvious advantage of the use of fetal cells is the decreased risk for the occurrence of GVHD due to the minimal number of mature T cells in fetal liver-derived populations prior to 14 weeks' gestation. This also avoids the necessity of T-cell depletion, something which detrimentally influences engraftment.

While it is true that there may be important technical advantages to the use of fetal cells, there are practical and ethical advantages to the use of cord blood or postnatal HSC sources. There are legitimate ethical concerns regarding the use of fetal tissue for transplantation that must be addressed. Would we as a society agree to the use of fetuses conceived specifically for that purpose? What about anencephalics? Can the parent of a fetal donor specify to whom the harvested cells will be donated? These and other ethical questions will probably continue to be asked for many years to come. In addition to the ethical questions, practical issues abound. Furthermore, the methods generally utilized to obtain fetal tissue risk a high degree of microbial contamination, potentially rendering the tissue unusable. If a bacterial, viral or fungal disease were transplanted, there could be disastrous results for both the fetus and the mother. The small size of the fetal liver also limits total cell yield, and currently the specific donor cells are not renewable. The use of adult-derived cells bypasses most of these ethical and technical issues. Adult-derived cells would allow a renewable, relatively infection-free, much more ethically acceptable source of donor cells. One potential strategy would be tolerance induction by the *in utero* transplantation of highly purified adult bone marrow HSCs from a living related donor, followed by a single or multiple postnatal 'booster' injections.

Diseases amenable to prenatal treatment

As stated above, the potential uses for this type of treatment are almost staggering. A target disease would have to be able to be diagnosed early enough in pregnancy for treatment to make a difference, capable of being improved by BMT and not satisfactorily treated postnatally. This would include some of the most devastating diseases that affect mankind. There are three different categories of diseases that would fit this description. They would include the hemoglobinopathies, immunodeficiency disorders and inborn errors of metabolism. It is particularly important to note that, in many of the target diseases, engrafted normal cells should have a significant survival advantage over diseased cells. This would clinically result in the amplification of the level of engraftment in the peripheral circulation. In addition, other immunological factors would be advantageous. Even in cases that involved merely minimal levels of engraftment, specific tolerance for donor antigen would probably be induced. This would result in the recipient's immune system allowing additional cells from the same donor to be given to the tolerant recipient after birth with no rejecting immune response.

Hemoglobinopathies

Sickle cell anemia and the thalassemias make up the largest group of diseases potentially treatable by prenatal stem cell transplantation. Both groups can be diagnosed within the first trimester and can be potentially cured by postnatal BMT. However, BMT is not recommended routinely, because of both its prohibitive morbidity and mortality, and the relative success of modern medical management. If used, the success of BMT is indirectly related to the the age of the patient at the time of BMT and the morbidity of the disease. In other words, the younger the patient, the fewer transfusions he or she has received, with therefore less organ compromise from iron overload and thus better results from BMT. The threshold questions relevant to both of these diseases are the same. First, what levels of normal peripheral cell expression are necessary to alleviate clinical disease? Second, can adequate levels of donor cell engraftment be

achieved by *in utero* HSC transplantation? At present only indirect evidence exists to answer these questions. Further investigation is necessary.

In sickle cell disease (SCD) the pathophysiology is directly related to the defect in the β-hemoglobin chain. This causes an increase in the concentration of hemoglobin S (HbS) within red cells, causing the typical sickling noted on light microscopy and marked rheological abnormality, including hyperviscosity, cellular adherence and sickling, with resulting vaso-occlusion and tissue ischemia. These cause the typical crises so common in patients with sickle cell anemia. These vaso-occlusive crises also cause splenic infarction, resulting in functional asplenia and consequent increased susceptibility to certain bacterial infections. In examining the *in vitro* relationships between hematocrit and viscosity using mixtures of sickle and normal red blood cells (RBCs), Schmalzer observed that the primary determinant of viscosity was the sickle hematocrit (fraction of RBCs that contain HbS). Adverse effects of the hematocrit on viscosity were seen at a sickle hematocrit level in the low 20s. Oxygen delivery, as gauged by the maximum point on the hematocrit versus viscosity curve, was markedly improved by exchanging normal for sickle RBCs (even when the total hematocrit was held constant). The clinical correlative of this *in vitro* information is chronic exchange transfusion therapy, which is indicated after cerebrovascular accidents in SCD. Maintenance of the HbS below 30% reduces the risk of recurrent stroke from 60–90% to less than 10%. The maximum HbS that effectively prevents stroke is unknown, but a transfusion regimen maintaining a HbS of 50% was found to be effective in preventing recurrent stroke in a small study group of SCD.

There are several varieties of thalassemia. Clinical manifestations range from none to fetal death. The clinical manifestations most frequently observed are those that arise secondary to hypoxia related to severe anemia and ineffective erythropoiesis. It is now standard therapy to transfuse patients with thalassemia major chronically from an early age. This suppresses endogenous erythropoiesis and maintains oxygen delivery. When instituted at an early age this effectively prevents the bone marrow expansion and secondary bony changes that otherwise often occur with this disease. It also prevents the hemodynamic and cardiac manifestations of the disease, including moderate to severe anemia and potentially high-volume cardiac failure. The necessary normal hemoglobin level required is controversial, but good results have been achieved with maintenance of 9 g/dl.

These diseases are prime examples of disorders that could benefit greatly from HSC transplantation. Although the levels of normal hemoglobin are higher than have been achieved experimentally (30% donor hemoglobin is maximal), there would be a significant survival advantage of normal cells in both diseases. In SCD, erythrocytes have a circulating half-life of 10 to 20 days (normal half-life 120 days) prior to destruction. The presence of a significant number of normal red blood cells would significantly increase the average circulating half-life of the cells. It would also increase the oxygen-carrying potential of the blood. In thalassemia, most cells (80%) never leave the bone marrow and also have shortened survival in the periphery. Therefore, engraftment of even a few normal stem cells could result in significantly amplified levels of peripheral donor cell expression.

Immunodeficiency diseases

This group of diseases demonstrates the potential benefit of HSC transplantation in diseases that involve the immune system and white blood cells. These represent an extremely heterogeneous group of diseases, which differ in their likelihood of cure by achievement of hematopoietic chimerism. The diseases that are most amenable to treatment from donor cell transplantation are those in which a survival benefit exists for normal cells. The best example of this situation is the diseases collectively known as severe combined immunodeficiency syndrome (SCID). Several different molecular causes of SCID have been identified, with approximately two-thirds of cases being of X-linked recessive inheritance (X-SCID). The genetic basis of X-SCID has been defined recently as a mutation of the gene encoding the common γ chain (γc), which is a common component of several members of the cytokine receptor superfamily, including those for interleukin-2 (IL-2), IL-4, IL-7, IL-9, IL-15 and possibly IL-13. Children affected with X-SCID therefore have simultaneous inactivation of multiple cytokine systems, resulting in a block in thymic T-cell development and diminished T-cell response. B cells, although present in normal or even increased numbers, are dysfunctional, either secondary to the lack of helper T-cell function or owing to an intrinsic defect in B-cell maturation. The end result of affliction with SCID is decreased ability to fight off infections that require the use of either cell-mediated or antibody-mediated immunity.

Another form of SCID is secondary to adenosine deaminase (ADA) deficiency. There has been some successful treatment of these patients. Clinical experience with HLA-matched sibling bone marrow or fetal liver or thymus transplantation generally has been successful without myeloablative therapy. This suggests that the lymphoid progeny of relatively few engrafted normal HSCs have a selective growth advantage *in vivo* over genetically defective cells. The competitive advantage of non-affected cells in X-SCID is best supported by the discovery of skewed X-inactivation in female carriers. Only T cells containing the normal X chromosome are present in the circulation. Evidence that ADA production confers a survival advantage derives from the early experience with gene therapy for ADA-deficient SCID. ADA-gene-corrected autologous T cells have persisted for prolonged periods despite discontinuation of T-cell infusions. Transfer of ADA-gene-corrected cells versus uncorrected cells from the same SCID patient into an immuno-deficient BNX mouse results in survival of the corrected cells and death of the uncorrected cells, confirming a survival advantage for ADA-producing cells even when there is normal ADA production in the surrounding environment. Unfortunately, this type of competitive advantage would not be present in all diseases. A disease such as chronic granulomatous disease would not be expected to provide any competitive advantage for donor cells. However, the mere introduction of a number of properly functioning cells, reconstructing the defective component, should ameliorate at least partially the clinical manifestations of the disease and should result in donor-specific tolerance. If higher levels of engraftment are needed, further HSC transplants from the same donor could be performed after birth without fear of rejection, potentially leading to a significant decrease in untoward disease outcome.

In our department, we have successfully treated a fetus with X-linked SCID in a family where a previously afflicted child died at 7 months of age. Diagnosis by CVS during the second pregnancy showed another affected male. For this couple termination was not an option. After lengthy discussions with the couple, their informed consent was obtained and paternal bone marrow was harvested. The paternal T cells were depleted, and bone marrow was injected intraperitoneally into the fetus beginning at about 16 weeks of gestation. Subsequent injections were performed at 17 and 18 weeks. The fetus was delivered and, subsequent to birth, at present shows a split chimerism. All of his T cells have devolved from his father and most of his B cells are his. He has achieved normal milestones and immune progress through 3 years of age. An Italian group replicated this success for shorter X-linked SCID cases. Other disorders have recently been tried using higher T-cell concentrations, but have ended in fetal demise. Many details still remain to be worked out, but there is a good deal of promise in this therapy.

Inborn errors of metabolism

Inborn errors of metabolism are a widely heterogeneous group of diseases caused by the deficiency of one or more specific lysosomal hydrolases. This absence results in the accumulation of substrates such as mucopolysaccharide, glycogen or sphingo-lipid. Depending on the specific enzyme abnormality and the compounds that accumulate, specific identifiable patterns of tissue damage and organ failure occur. These are generally quite serious and include central nervous system (CNS) deterioration, growth failure, dysostosis multiplex and joint disability, hepatosplenomegaly, myocardial or cardiac disease, upper airway obstruction, pulmonary infiltration, corneal clouding and hearing loss. The end result of these inborn errors of metabolism is often disastrous. The potential efficacy of prenatal HSC transplantation for the treatment of these diseases must be considered on an individual disease basis. BMT has been used to treat many of these diseases. The purpose of BMT in the treatment of these diseases is to provide HSC-derived mononuclear cells that can repopulate various organs in the body. These include the liver (Kupffer cells), skin (Langerhans cells), lung (alveolar macro-phages), spleen (macrophages), lymph nodes, tonsils and the brain (microglia). Patients who have been corrected by postnatal BMT, such as those with Gaucher's disease or Maroteaux–Lamy syndrome (minimal CNS involvement), are certainly reasonable candidates for prenatal treatment. In many cases postnatal BMT has corrected the peripheral manifestations of the disease and has arrested the neurological deterioration, but has not reversed the neurological injury that is present in disorders such as metachromatic leukodystrophy and Hurler's disease. In these cases the neurological injury may begin well before birth. This factor is one that makes the *in utero* use of HSCs especially attractive. Postnatal maturation of blood–brain barrier restricts access to the CNS by transplanted cells or the deficient enzyme, but this is not a factor prenatally. These considerations suggest that these diseases may possibly be cured through the use of prenatal therapy. The primary question is whether donor HSC-derived microglial elements would populate the CNS, providing the necessary metabolic correction within the blood–brain barrier. In the authors' opinion, these represent the least likely group of diseases to benefit from *in utero* HSC transplantation.

SUMMARY

The advances made in fetal therapy over the past three decades have been dramatic. Diseases that once could not even be detected until after birth can now not only be diagnosed, but treated as well. Treatment ranges from open fetal surgery to surgery performed through an endoscope or cystoscope, using minimally invasive surgical techniques. Metabolic diseases are now also being treated prenatally. Many of these diseases are treated with medical techniques, correcting biochemical anomalies that otherwise would greatly reduce the life span or quality of life of the newborn. Perhaps the most exciting development in prenatal treatment is the use of hematopoietic stem cell transplantation. The potential uses of this technique could cause diseases such as sickle cell anemia, thalassemia and the numerous inborn errors of metabolism to become relegated to medical history books. These developments and future advances may result in the elimination of suffering for millions.

Bibliography

Abuhamad AZ, Fisher DA, Warsof SL, *et al.* Antenatal diagnosis and treatment of fetal goitrous hypothyroidism: case report and review of the literature. *Ultrasound Obstet Gynecol* 1995;6:368–71

Adzick N, Harrison M, Flake A, Glick P, Bottles K. Automatic uterine stapling devices in fetal surgery: experience in a primate model. *Surg Forum* 1985;XXXVI:479–81

Adzick NS, Harrison MR, Flake AW, Howell LJ, Golbus MS, Filly RA. Fetal surgery for cystic adenomatoid malformation of the lung. *J Pediatr Surg* 1993;28:806–12

Albanese CT, Harrison MR. Surgical treatment for fetal disease. The state of the art. *Ann NY Acad Sci* 1998,847:74–85

Almeida-Porada GD, Hoffman R, Manalo P, Gianni AM, Zanjani ED. Detection of human cells in human/sheep chimeric lambs with *in vitro* human stroma-forming potential. *Exp Hematol* 1996;24:482–7

Archer DR, Turner CW, Yeager AM, Fleming WH. Sustained multilineage engraftment of allogeneic hematopoietic stem cells in NOD/SCID mice after *in utero* transplantation. *Blood* 1997;90:3222–9

Benachi A, Dommergues M, Delezoide AL, Bourbon J, Dumez Y, Brunnelle F. Tracheal obstruction in experimental diaphragmatic hernia: an endoscopic approach in the fetal lamb. *Prenat Diagn* 1997;17:629–34

Bernstein J, Boyle DW, Srour EF, *et al.* Variation in long-term engraftment of a large consecutive series of lambs transplanted *in utero* with human hematopoietic cells. *Biol Blood Marrow Transplant* 1997;3:247–54

Bruner JP, Dellinger EH. Antenatal diagnosis and treatment of fetal hypothyroidism. A report of two cases. *Fetal Diagn Ther* 1997;12:200–4

Bruner JP, Tulipan NE, Richards WO. Endoscopic coverage of fetal open myelomeningocele *in utero* [Letter; comment]. *Am J Obstet Gynecol* 1997;176:256–7

Bui TH, Jones DR. Stem cell transplantation into the fetal recipient: challenges and prospects. *Curr Opin Obstet Gynecol* 1998;10:105–8

Calvano CJ, Moran ME, Mehlhaff BA, Sachs BL, Mandell J. Amnioscopic endofetal illumination with infrared-guided fiber. *J Endourol* 1997;11:259–61

Calvano CJ, Moran ME, Mehlhaff BA, Sachs BL, Mandell J. Assessment of access strategies for fetoscopic urologic surgery: preliminary results. *J Endourol* 1997;11:49–53

Calvano CJ, Reddy PP, Moran ME, *et al.* Initial studies of holmium : YAG laser creation of spinal defects in fetal rabbits: model for urologic effects of myelomeningocele. *J Endourol* 1998;12:199–203

Carrier E, Lee TH, Busch MP, Cowan MJ. Recruitment of engrafted donor cells postnatally into the blood with cytokines after *in utero* transplantation in mice. *Transplantation* 1997;64:627–33

Coplen DE. Prenatal intervention for hydronephrosis. *J Urol* 1997;157:2270–7

Cowan MJ, Golbus M. *In utero* hematopoietic stem

cell transplants for inherited diseases. *Am J Pediatr Hematol Oncol* 1994;16:35–42

Crombleholme TM, Bianchi DW. *In utero* hematopoietic stem cell transplantation and gene therapy. *Semin Perinatol* 1994;18:376–84

Crombleholme TM, Dirkes K, Whitney TM, Alman B, Garmel S, Connelly RJ. Amniotic band syndrome in fetal lambs. 1. Fetoscopic release and morphometric outcome. *J Pediatr Surg* 1995;30:974–8

Deprest JA, Lerut TE, Vandenberghe K, *et al.* Operative fetoscopy: new perspective in fetal therapy? *Plast Reconstr Surg* 1998;101:287–96

Deprest JA, Lerut TE, Vandenberghe K. Operative fetoscopy: new perspective in fetal therapy? *Prenat Diagn* 1997;17:1247–60

Deprest JA, Van Schoubroeck D, Van Ballaer PP, Flageole H, Van Assche FA, Vandenberghe K. Alternative technique for Nd : YAG laser coagulation in twin-to-twin transfusion syndrome with anterior placenta. *Ultrasound Obstet Gynecol* 1998;11:347–52

Dracker RA. Cord blood stem cells: how to get them and what to do with them. *J Hematother* 1996;5: 145–8

Dumic M, Brkljacic L, Plavsic V, *et al.* Prenatal diagnosis of congenital adrenal hyperplasia (21-hydroxylase deficiency) in Croatia. *Am J Med Genet* 1997;72:302–6

Evans MI, ed. *Reproductive Risks and Prenatal Diagnosis.* Norwalk, Connecticut: Appleton & Lange, 1992

Evans MI, Adzick NS, Johnson MP, Flake AW, Quintero R, Harrison MR. Fetal therapy – 1994. *Curr Opin Obstet Gynecol* 1994;6:58–64

Evans MI, Duquette DA, Rinaldo P, *et al.* Modulation of B12 dosage and response in fetal treatment of methylmalonic aciduria (MMA); titration of treatment dose to serum and urine MMA. *Fetal Diagn Ther* 1997;12:21–3

Evans MI, Sacks AL, Johnson MP, Robichaux AG III, May M, Moghissi KS. Sequential invasive assessment of fetal renal function, and the *in utero* treatment of fetal obstructive uropathies. *Obstet Gynecol* 1991;77: 545–50

Evrard VA, Verbeke K, Peers KH, *et al.* Amnioinfusion with Hartmann's solution: a safe distention medium for endoscopic fetal surgery in the ovine model. *Fetal Diagn Ther* 1997;12:188–92

Feitz WF, Steegers EA, Aarnink RG, Arts T, De Vries JD, Van de Wildt B. Endoscopic intrauterine fetal therapy: a monkey model. *Urology* 1996;47:118–19

Fisher DA. Fetal thyroid function: diagnosis and management of fetal thyroid disorders. *Clin Obstet Gynecol* 1997;40:16–31

Flake AW, Puck JM, Almieda-Porada G, *et al.* Successful *in utero* correction of X-linked recessive severe combined immuno-deficiency (X-SCID): fetal intraperitoneal transplantation of CD34 enriched paternal bone marrow cells (EPPBMC). *N Engl J Med* 1996;335:1806–10

Flake AW, Roncarolo MG, Puck JM, *et al.* Treatment of X-linked severe combined immunodeficiency by *in utero* transplantation of paternal bone marrow [see comments]. *N Engl J Med* 1996;335:1806–10

Flake AW, Zanjani ED. *In utero* hematopoietic stem cell transplantation. A status report. *J Am Med Assoc* 1997;278:932–7

Flake AW, Zanjani ED. *In utero* transplantation for thalassemia. *Ann NY Acad Sci* 1998;850:300–11

Flake AW. Fetal sacrococcygeal teratoma. *Eur J Med* 1993;2:113–20

Ford WD. Fetal intervention for congenital diaphragmatic hernia. *Fetal Diagn Ther* 1994;9:398–408

Freedman AL, Bukowski TP, Smith CA, Evans MI, Johnson MP, Gonzalez R. Fetal therapy for obstructive uropathy: specific outcomes diagnosis. *J Urol* 1996;156:720–4

Gibbs DL, Piecuch RE, Graf JL, *et al.* Neuro-developmental outcome after open fetal surgery. *J Pediatr Surg* 1998;33:1254–6

Hajdu K, Tanigawara S, McLean LK, Golbus MS. *In utero* allogeneic hematopoietic stem cell trans-plantation to induce tolerance. *Fetal Diagn Ther* 1996;11:241–8

Hanley FL. Fetal cardiac surgery. *Adv Card Surg* 1994;5:47–74

Harrison M, ed. *The Unborn Patient.* Philadelphia: WB Saunders, 1991

Harrison MR, Adzick NS, Bullard KM, *et al.* Correction of congenital diaphragmatic hernia *in utero*: VII. A prospective trial. *J Pediatr Surg* 1997;32:1637–42

Harrison MR, Adzick NS, Flake AW, *et al.* Correction of congenital diaphragmatic hernia *in utero*: VI. Hard-learned lessons. *J Pediatr Surg* 1993;28:1411–17; discussion 1417–18

Harrison MR, Adzick NS. Fetal surgical techniques. *Semin Pediatr Surg* 1993;2:136–42

Harrison MR, Longaker MT, Adzick NS, *et al.* Successful repair *in utero* of a fetal diaphragmatic hernia after removal of herniated viscera from the left thorax. *N Engl J Med* 1990;322:1582–4

Harrison MR, Mychaliska GB, Albanese CT, *et al.* Correction of congenital diaphragmatic hernia *in utero*: IX. Fetuses with poor prognosis (liver herniation and low lung-to-head ratio) can be saved by fetoscopic temporary tracheal occlusion. *J Pediatr Surg* 1998;33: 918–20

Hecher K, Hackeloer BJ, Ville Y. Umbilical cord coagulation by operative microendoscopy at 16 weeks' gestation in an acardiac twin. *Ultrasound Obstet Gynecol* 1997;10:130–2

Hecher K, Hackeloer BJ. Intrauterine endoscopic laser surgery for fetal sacrococcygeal teratoma [Letter]. *Lancet* 1996;347:470

Hedrick MH, Estes JM, Sullivan KM, *et al.* Plug the lung until it grows (PLUG): a new method to treat congenital diaphragmatic hernia *in utero*. *J Pediatr Surg* 1994;29:612–17

Jennings RW, Adzick NS, Harrison MR. Fetal surgery. In *Reproductive Risks and Prenatal Diagnosis*. Norwalk, Connecticut: Appleton & Lange, 1992:311–20

Jennings RW, Adzick NS, Longaker MT, Lorenz HP, Estes JM, Harrison MR. New techniques in fetal surgery. *J Pediatr Surg* 1992;27:1329–33

Jennings RW, Adzick NS, Longaker MT, Lorenz HP, Harrison MR. Radiotelemetric fetal monitoring during and after open fetal operation. *Surg Gynecol Obstet* 1993;176:59–64

Johnson MP, Bukowski TP, Reitlerman C, Isada NB, Pryde PG, Evans MI. *In utero* surgical treatment of fetal obstructive uropathy: a new comprehensive approach to identify appropriate candidates for vesicoamniotic shunt therapy. *Am J Obstet Gynecol* 1994; 170:1770–9

Johnson MP, Flake AW, Quintero RA, Evans MI. Shunt procedures. In Evans MI, Johnson MP, Moghissi KS, eds. *Invasive Outpatient Procedures in Reproductive Medicine*. New York: Raven Press, 1997

Jones DR, Bui TH, Anderson EM, *et al. In utero* haematopoietic stem cell transplantation: current perspectives and future potential. *Bone Marrow Transplant* 1996;18:831–7

Jones DR, Bui TH. Fetal therapy: prospects for transplantation early in pregnancy. *In Utero Stem Cell Transplantation and Gene Therapy: Second International Meeting*, Nottingham, UK, September 1997. *Mol Med Today* 1998;4:10–11

Kimber C, Spitz L, Cuschieri A. Current state of antenatal *in utero* surgical interventions. *Arch Dis Child Fetal Neonatal Ed* 1997;76:F134–9

Kohl T, Szabo Z, Suda K, *et al.* Percutaneous fetal access and uterine closure for fetoscopic surgery. Lessons learned from 16 consecutive procedures in pregnant sheep. *Surg Endosc* 1997;11:819–24

Luks FI, Deprest JA, Gilchrist BF, *et al.* Access techniques in endoscopic fetal surgery. *Eur J Pediatr Surg* 1997;7:131–4

Luks FI, Gilchrist BF, Jackson BT, Piasecki GJ. Endoscopic tracheal obstruction with an expanding device in a fetal lamb model: preliminary considerations. *Fetal Diagn Ther* 1996;11:67–71

Luks FI, Johnson BD, Papadakis K, Traore M, Piasecki GJ. Predictive value of monitoring parameters in fetal surgery [In Process Citation]. *J Pediatr Surg* 1998;33:1297–301

Luks FI, Peers KH, Deprest JA, Lerut TE, Vandenberghe K. The effect of open and endoscopic fetal surgery on uteroplacental oxygen delivery in the sheep. *J Pediatr Surg* 1996;31:310–14

Monni G, Ibba RM, Zoppi MA, Floris M. *In utero* stem cell transplantation. *Croat Med J* 1998;39:220–3

Mychaliska GB, Rice HE, Tarantal AF, *et al. In utero* hematopoietic stem cell transplants prolong survival of postnatal kidney transplantation in monkeys. *J Pediatr Surg* 1997;32:976–81

New MI. Diagnosis and management of congenital adrenal hyperplasia. *Annu Rev Med* 1998;49:311–28

Oberg KC, Robles AE, Ducsay C, *et al.* Endoscopic excision and repair of simulated bilateral cleft lips in fetal lambs. *Plast Reconstr Surg* 1998;102:1–9

Papadakis K, Luks FI, Deprest JA, *et al.* Single-port tracheoscopic surgery in the fetal lamb. *J Pediatr Surg* 1998;33:918–20

Porreco RP, Chang JH, Quissell BJ, Morgan MA. Palliative fetal surgery for diaphragmatic hernia [see comments]. *Am J Obstet Gynecol* 1994;170:833–4

Quintero RA, Hume RF, Smith C, *et al.* Percutaneous fetal cystoscopy and endoscopic fulguration of posterior urethral valves. *Am J Obstet Gynecol* 1995;172: 206–9

Quintero RA, Johnson MP, Romero R, *et al. In utero* percutaneous cystoscopy in the management of fetal lower obstructive uropathy. *Lancet* 1995;346:537–40

Quintero RA, Reich H, Romero R, Johnson MP, Goncalves L, Evans MI. *In utero* endoscopic devascularization of a large chorioangioma. *Ultrasound Obstet Gynecol* 1996;8:48–52

Quintero RA, Romero R, Reich H, *et al. In utero* percutaneous umbilical cord ligation in the management of complicated monochorionic multiple gestations. *Ultrasound Obstet Gynecol* 1996;8:16–22

Sack J, Weller A, Rigler O, Rozin A. A simple model for studying the correction of *in utero* hypothyroidism in the rat. *Pediatr Res* 1995;37:497–501

Simpson TJ, Golbus MS. *In utero* fetal hematopoietic stem cell transplantation. *Semin Perinatol* 1985;9: 68–74

Sistino JJ. Foetal bypass: concepts and controversies. *Perfusion* 1998;13:111–17

Skarsgard ED, Bealer JF, Meuli M, Adzick NS, Harrison MR. Fetal endoscopic ('Fetendo') surgery:

the relationship between insufflating pressure and the fetoplacental circulation. *J Pediatr Surg* 1995;30:1165–8

Takeyama Y, Uehara S, Okamura K, Yajima A. *In-utero* transplantation of fetal hematopoietic cells in the mouse: the effect of donor and recipient gestation maturity. *Tohoku J Exp Med* 1997;183:113–22

Touraine JL, Raudrant D, Laplace S, Roncarolo MG. Immunological tolerance following stem cell transplantation in human fetuses *in utero*. *Transplant Proc* 1997;29:2477

Touraine JL. *In utero* transplantation of fetal liver stem cells into human fetuses. *J Hematother* 1996;5:195–9

Touraine JL. *In utero* transplantation of stem cells in humans. *Nouv Rev Fr Hematol* 1990;32:441–4

Touraine JL. Treatment of human fetuses and induction of immunological tolerance in humans by *in utero* transplantation of stem cells into fetal recipients. *Acta Haematol* 1996;96:115–19

Van Loon AJ, Derksen JT, Bos AF, Rouwe CW. *In utero* diagnosis and treatment of fetal goitrous hypothyroidism, caused by maternal use of propylthiouracil. *Prenat Diagn* 1995;15:599–604

VanderWall KJ, Bruch SW, Meuli M, *et al.* Fetal endoscopic ('Fetendo') tracheal clip. *J Pediatr Surg* 1996;31:1101–3; discussion 1103–4

VanderWall KJ, Meuli M, Szabo Z, *et al.* Percutaneous access to the uterus for fetal surgery. *J Laparoendosc Surg* 1996;6(Suppl 1):S65–7

VanderWall KJ, Skarsgard ED, Filly RA, Eckert J, Harrison MR. Fetendo-clip: a fetal endoscopic tracheal clip procedure in a human fetus. *J Pediatr Surg* 1997;32:970–2

Vicens-Calvet E, Potau N, Carreras E, Bellart J, Albisu MA, Carrascosa A. Diagnosis and treatment *in utero* of goiter with hypothyroidism caused by iodide overload. *J Pediatr* 1998;133:147–8

Ville Y, Hecher K, Gagnon A, Sebire N, Hyett J, Nicolaides K. Endoscopic laser coagulation in the management of severe twin-to-twin transfusion syndrome. *Br J Obstet Gynaecol* 1998;105:446–53

Weinzweig N. Constriction band-induced vascular compromise of the foot: classification and management of the intermediate stage of constriction-ring syndrome. *Plast Reconstr Surg* 1995;96:972–7

Wengler GS, Lanfranchi A, Frusca T, *et al. In-utero* transplantation of parental CD34 haematopoietic progenitor cells in a patient with X-linked severe combined immunodeficiency (SCIDXI). *Lancet* 1996;348:1484–7

Westgren M, Ringden O, Eik-Nes S, *et al.* Lack of evidence of permanent engraftment after *in utero* fetal stem cell transplantation in congenital hemoglobino-pathies. *Transplantation* 1996;61:1176–9

Wu SY, Fisher DA, Huang WS, *et al.* Urinary compound W in pregnant women is a potential marker for fetal thyroid function. *Am J Obstet Gynecol* 1998;178:886–91

Yang EY, Adzick NS. Fetoscopy. *Semin Laparosc Surg* 1998;5:31–9

Yuh DD, Gandy KL, Hoyt G, Reitz BA, Robbins RC. Tolerance to cardiac allografts induced *in utero* with fetal liver cells. *Circulation* 1996;94:II304–7

Zanjani ED, Almeida-Porada G, Ascensao JL, MacKintosh FR, Flake AW. Transplantation of hematopoietic stem cells *in utero*. *Stem Cells* 1997;15(Suppl 1):79–92; discussion 93

Zhang YY, Bailey RR. Treatment of vesicoureteric reflux in a sheep model using subureteric injection of cultured fetal-bladder tissue. *Pediatr Surg Int* 1998; 13:32–6

Current perspectives on twin-to-twin transfusion syndrome

28

D. W. Skupski

Twin-to-twin transfusion syndrome (TTTS) is a syndrome that occurs in multifetal pregnancies, usually in twin gestations. This syndrome has many names (Table 1). The end result, without treatment, is almost always delivery from premature labor at gestational ages prior to viability[1,2]. Even with treatment, the fetal/neonatal death rate averages 40–60%[3–5]. Despite much enthusiasm for the various treatments for this syndrome, little is known about the etiology, and salvage for these fetuses is less than optimal. This chapter reviews the pathophysiology, clinical course and the treatments for TTTS, focusing on the limitations of our knowledge of this severe disease.

PATHOPHYSIOLOGY

Vascular anastomoses are present in virtually 100% of monochorionic twin pregnancies, but are rare in dichorionic twin gestations[6–8]. TTTS is present only in monochorionic twins (with rare exceptions)[6–10] and occurs in 5–10% of monochorionic pregnancies[11]. It is believed that vascular connections (in the placenta) between twins are necessary for TTTS to develop[12,13]. The progressive nature of TTTS *in utero* is thought to be due to chronic fetofetal transfusion; one twin (the donor) slowly pumps blood to the other (the recipient) through the placental vascular anastomoses. The placenta, including its maternal and fetal vasculature, is in dynamic change throughout pregnancy. The establishment of new vessels, and thus vascular connections between twins, even in a dichorionic gestation with a single placental mass, should not be surprising. The reason

Table 1 *Alternative terminology for the twin-to-twin transfusion syndrome*

1. Twin–twin transfusion syndrome
2. Stuck twin syndrome
3. Twin oligohydramnios–polyhydramnios sequence
4. Fetofetal transfusion
5. Chorioangiopagus twins

for the occurrence of TTTS in only a small proportion of monochorionic twin pregnancies with vascular anastomoses is unknown; the etiology of TTTS is unknown.

A recent study has elucidated details about the anastomoses in the placentas of TTTS twins that may provide a clue to the etiology[14]. In a study of ten monochorionic pregnancies diagnosed with TTTS and ten monochorionic pregnancies without TTTS, placental vascular anastomoses were characterized by immediate post-delivery placental injection studies. This study suggested that the development of vascular anastomoses of the arteriovenous type running from the donor to the recipient deep within the placenta that are uncompensated by arteriovenous anastomoses running in the reverse direction could be implicated in the etiology of TTTS. However, the numbers in this study were small. What causes the development of these uncompensated anastomoses in only a small proportion of monochorionic twin pregnancies is unknown.

TTTS is a slowly progressive disease. The gestational age of initial presentation of TTTS has been reported to be 13–29 weeks, but with availability of more routine obstetric ultrasound, the gestational age range in which the syndrome will begin to manifest itself is

Table 2 *The use of ultrasound in the diagnosis of twin-to-twin transfusion syndrome (TTTS)*

Second- or third-trimester diagnostic criteria for TTTS
Monochorionic gestation
    same gender
    single placental mass
    thin dividing membrane
    lack of lambda or twin peak sign
Abnormal amniotic fluid volume*
    one sac with oligohydramnios, deepest vertical pocket ≤ 2.0 cm
    one sac with polyhydramnios, deepest vertical pocket ≥ 8.0 cm
Persistent urinary bladder findings*
    small or no bladder visualized in twin with oligohydramnios
    large bladder visualized in twin with polyhydramnios

Other ultrasound findings helpful in the diagnosis
Estimated fetal weight discordance (≥ 20% of larger twin's estimated weight)
Appearance of a 'stuck twin'*
Hydrops fetalis (presence of one or more of the following in either twin)
    skin edema (≥ 5 mm thickness)
    pericardial effusion
    pleural effusion
    ascites
Membrane folding at 14–17 weeks of gestation

First-trimester findings suspicious for the later development of TTTS
Monochorionic gestation
Nuchal translucency measurement > 3 mm at 10–14 weeks of gestation
Poor crown–rump length growth of one fetus
Membrane folding at 10–13 weeks of gestation

*Serial scanning may be necessary

known to be 17–26 weeks. The clinical course is varied; preterm delivery may occur quickly after the diagnosis or several months later. Progressive oligohydramnios in one sac and polyhydramnios in the other sac is the rule.

DIAGNOSIS

The classic neonatal findings of birth weight difference, hematocrit difference, and plethora in the recipient and pallor in the donor do not apply to the prenatal diagnosis of TTTS[15]. TTTS is a diagnosis made by prenatal ultrasound examination. Great strides have been made in the ultrasound identification of TTTS. The hallmarks of the diagnosis are:

(1) Monochorionic gestation;

(2) Same-sex twins identified by ultrasound;

(3) The combination of polyhydramnios in

one sac and oligohydramnios in the other sac (Table 2).

A monochorionic gestation is identified by the combination of a single placental mass, same-sex fetuses and the lack of the twin peak or lambda sign at the point where the intertwin membrane meets the placental chorionic plate (Figure 1). Growth discrepancy or differences in estimated fetal weight are not universally present in TTTS[16]. The persistent finding of a small or non-visualized bladder in the donor and a large bladder in the recipient has also been used in the diagnostic criteria for some recent studies[5,17]. The recent publication of normal values for the measurement of amniotic fluid in twin gestations has allowed the use of the upper and lower limits of normal in making a diagnosis of oligohydramnios and polyhydramnios rather than the subjective impression of the sonographer (Table 2)[18].

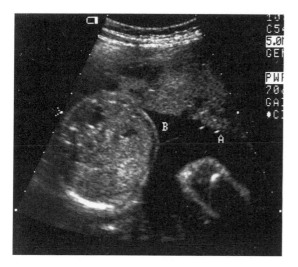

Figure 1 *Ultrasound image of a twin gestation showing the characteristic 'T-junction' or lack of the lambda sign at the junction of the intertwin membrane and the placental chorionic plate*

Serial ultrasound scanning is necessary for any cases in which the diagnosis is entertained but the criteria are not met; TTTS may subsequently appear. A careful search for fetal anomalies should also be undertaken.

Perhaps the severest form of TTTS is where there is no amniotic fluid visualized by ultrasound in the donor's sac. This has been termed the 'stuck twin syndrome'. It may be difficult to distinguish the stuck twin syndrome from a monoamniotic twin gestation, because the intertwin membrane is closely wrapped against the donor twin and cannot be visualized by ultrasound. If one fetus remains pressed in one place against the uterine wall over the course of one or more examinations, and the character of the movements is somewhat constricted, this is likely to be a stuck twin.

In addition to the above second-trimester diagnostic criteria, there can be ultrasound findings in the first trimester that are associated with the subsequent development of TTTS (Table 2)[19].

TREATMENT

TTTS has a wide range of severity and outcomes. This is evidenced by the survival

Table 3 *Published experience*

First author	Year	Treatment	Survival (%)
Bebbington[11]	1989	none	47
Bebbington[11]	1989	amnioreduction*	0
Mahoney[25]	1990	none	20
Mahoney[25]	1990	amnioreduction	69
Urig[2]	1990	none	0
Urig[2]	1990	amnioreduction	39
Gonsoulin[40]	1990	amnioreduction	21
Elliott[27]	1991	amnioreduction	79
Saunders[3]	1992	amnioreduction	37
Pinette[41]	1993	none	75
Pinette[41]	1993	amnioreduction	83
Fries[42]	1993	amnioreduction	50
Reisner[26]	1993	none	40
Reisner[26]	1993	amnioreduction	74
Ville[5]	1995	FLOC	52
De Lia[4]	1995	FLOC	53
Ville[43]	1996	amnioreduction	50
Dennis[20]	1997	none	50
Dennis[20]	1997	amnioreduction	82
Mari[24]	1998	amnioreduction	66
Saade[17]	1998	septostomy	83

FLOC, fetoscopic laser occlusion of chorioangiopagus placental vessels; *amnioreduction used only for maternal respiratory compromise

Table 4 *The treatment options of twin-to-twin transfusion syndrome*

1. Careful antenatal assessment by ultrasound, Doppler blood flow analysis, fetal echocardiography and fetal cardiotocography or non-stress testing, with tocolysis for preterm labor
2. Serial amniotic fluid volume reduction (amnioreduction)
3. Fetoscopic laser occlusion of chorioangiopagus placental vessels
4. Septostomy

rates during the past decade of 0–83% in various published series (Table 3). There are currently four options for treatment available (Table 4).

The option of careful antenatal assessment and tocolysis for preterm labor is generally used in all cases as an adjunct to other invasive treatments. Despite the normalization of amniotic fluid volumes after other treatments, in some cases of severe TTTS there will be progression of hypertension and hypervolemia in the recipient and hypotension and hypovolemia in the donor, leading to death *in utero* (of either twin). Careful, intensive and frequent antenatal assessment may allow an iatrogenic decision for delivery, and prevent death *in utero*.

Amnioreduction (serial amniotic fluid volume reduction) was the earliest therapy available[21] and is currently the most widespread treatment. An 18- or 20-gauge needle is placed into the polyhydramniotic sac and fluid is drained to restore a normal level of fluid in this sac. The amount of fluid drained at a single procedure has been reported to be 1–7 l[22]. Multiple procedures may be necessary. Complications of the procedure occur in about 8% of cases and include chorioamnionitis, preterm labor and delivery, preterm premature rupture of the amniotic membranes and abruptio placentae[22]. Despite extensive experience, there is not a clear indication in the literature that amnioreduction is beneficial to fetal or neonatal survival[23]. A large registry of TTTS patients undergoing amnioreduction has shown that an earlier presentation of the disease and a greater number of procedures are associated with poorer outcome[24].

Fetoscopic laser occlusion of chorioangiopagus placental vessels (FLOC) is a therapy designed to interrupt the vascular anastomoses within the placenta, and is attractive to many patients and physicians because it appears at least to try to get to the root of the problem. FLOC requires general anesthesia, a laparotomy and a larger-bore puncture of the uterus, and, thus, is a more invasive procedure than other treatments. Survival rates for fetuses in large series of TTTS pregnancies undergoing FLOC therapy show no difference from those of amnioreduction (Table 3). This may attest to the severity of the disease of TTTS, the differences in diagnostic criteria between studies, the lack of diagnostic criteria in some studies, the technical difficulties encountered in the use of FLOC, the lack of complete ablation of anastomosing vessels in many cases where FLOC is used, which may allow continued fetofetal transfusion, or other unknown factors.

Septostomy is the puncture of the intertwin membrane or septum, designed to allow amniotic fluid to circulate between the two amniotic cavities[17]. The development of septostomy was based on the observation that a single amnioreduction in some cases of TTTS led to normal amniotic fluid volumes around both twins, sometimes for many weeks or longer[28]. It has been postulated that the intertwin membrane or septum was pressed against the uterine wall by the polyhydramnios in the recipient's sac, and thus could not be visualized by ultrasound. This intertwin membrane was then punctured during amnioreduction therapy, leading to the normalization of amniotic fluid volumes between the two sacs. Septostomy can lead to a large hole in the intertwin membrane that continues to enlarge as gestation advances (pseudomonoamniotic twins) and a risk of umbilical cord entanglement[29]. A smaller-gauge needle (22 gauge) can be used without the complication of a pseudomonoamniotic gestation[17]. The most recent report showed a fetal/neonatal survival rate of 83% in 13 pregnancies undergoing septostomy[17].

NEUROLOGICAL OUTCOME

Neurological injury is common in survivors of TTTS[30]. Antenatal neurological injury in survivors of TTTS occurs at an increased rate compared to that of other monochorionic pregnancies[31]. There are several theories that have been developed to explain this finding. The first is that, following one fetal death, the acute hemorrhage of the surviving fetus into the dilated vascular system of the dead fetus results in hypotension and cerebral ischemia in the surviving fetus[32]. However, antenatally acquired neurological injury occurs in cases where both twins have survived[30]. Therefore, alternative hypotheses are necessary. These include vascular sludging due to an extremely high hemoglobin concentration in the recipient[30] and anemia and hypoxemia in the donor (which are common findings in the donor fetus *in utero*[33]). The high incidence of antenatally acquired central nervous system injury in survivors of TTTS argues for cranial imaging studies in the immediate neonatal period (< 48 h after birth) and careful neurodevelopmental follow-up[30]. In addition, when the initial diagnosis of TTTS is made, this high incidence of neurological injury needs to be included when counselling patients.

CRITICAL ANALYSIS

None of the treatments for TTTS has been subjected to a randomized controlled trial. Indeed, there have been only three controlled trials of any treatment for TTTS, and all three of these studies have compared historical controls to those undergoing amnio-reduction[2,3,25]. Several studies have shown an exaggeration of the treatment effect in studies using historical controls[34–37]. In studies using historical controls, there appears to be a selection bias favoring a better outcome for patients in later time periods (the treated patients). This exaggeration of the treatment effect can be up to 30–40%[38]. This effect is also seen in the recent obstetric literature[36,37]. In the three controlled trials of amnioreduction for TTTS, although the p values range from 0.04 to 0.000 000 1, the treatment effect is 30–40% (risk ratio for fetal or neonatal death 0.60–0.66)[23]. Thus, the effectiveness of serial amnioreduction has not been adequately demonstrated.

Each of the therapies for TTTS has shown increasing survival rates with successive publications (Table 3), suggesting a different cause for the apparent success – namely, advances in neonatal care. An analysis of the deaths in the three controlled trials above shows that two-thirds were neonatal and only one-third fetal, allowing for this possibility. However, the only study addressing this issue suggested a possible benefit of amnioreduction over and above the increased survival due to advances in neonatal care for those TTTS twins delivered at ≤ 27 weeks of gestation[39].

We are in need of randomized controlled trials to demonstrate the effectiveness of these treatments for TTTS. At the current time, the counselling of patients is based upon a subjective determination of the most promising treatment. These women, and their fetuses as patients, deserve better.

References

1. Wittmann BK, Baldwin VJ, Nichol B. Antenatal diagnosis of twin transfusion syndrome by ultrasound. *Obstet Gynecol* 1981;58:123–7

2. Urig MA, Clewell WH, Elliott JP. Twin–twin transfusion syndrome. *Am J Obstet Gynecol* 1990; 163:1522–6

3. Saunders NJ, Snijders RJM, Nicolaides KH. Therapeutic amniocentesis in twin–twin transfusion syndrome appearing in the second trimester of pregnancy. *Am J Obstet Gynecol* 1992; 166:820–4

4. De Lia J, Kuhlmann RS, Harstad TW, Cruikshank DP. Fetoscopic laser ablation of placental vessels in severe previable twin–twin transfusion syndrome. *Am J Obstet Gynecol* 1995;172:1202–11

5. Ville Y, Hyett J, Hecher K, Nicolaides K. Preliminary experience with endoscopic laser surgery for severe twin–twin transfusion syndrome. *N Engl J Med* 1995;332:224–7

6. Robertson EG, Neer KJ. Placental injection studies in twin gestation. *Am J Obstet Gynecol* 1983;147:170–4

7. Strong SJ, Corney G. *The Placenta in Twin Pregnancy.* Oxford: Pergamon Press, 1966

8. Blickstein I. The twin–twin transfusion syndrome. *Obstet Gynecol* 1990;76:714–21

9. King AD, Soothill PW, Montemagno R, Young MP, Sams V, Rodeck CH. Twin-to-twin blood transfusion in a dichorionic pregnancy without the oligohydramnios–polyhydramnios sequence. *Br J Obstet Gynaecol* 1995;102:334–5

10. Rodriguez JG, Porter H, Stirrat GM, Soothill PW. Twin-to-twin blood transfusion in a dichorionic pregnancy without the oligohydramnios polyhydramnios sequence. *Br J Obstet Gynaecol* 1995;102:334–5

11. Bebbington MW, Wittman BK. Fetal transfusion syndrome: antenatal factors predicting outcome. *Am J Obstet Gynecol* 1989;160:913–15

12. Rausen AR, Seki M, Strauss L. Twin transfusion syndrome. *J Pediatr* 1965;66:613–28

13. Tan KL, Tan R, Tan SH, Tan AM. The twin transfusion syndrome: clinical observations on 35 affected pairs. *Clin Pediatr Phil* 1979;18:111–14

14. Bajoria R, Wigglesworth J, Fisk NM. Angioarchitecture of monochorionic placentas in relation to the twin–twin transfusion syndrome. *Am J Obstet Gynecol* 1995;172:856–63

15. Wenstrom KD, Tessen JA, Zlatnik FJ, *et al.* Frequency, distribution and theoretical mechanisms of hematologic and weight discordance in monochorionic twins. *Obstet Gynecol* 1992;80:257–61

16. Brennan JN, Diwan RV, Rosen MG, *et al.* Fetofetal transfusion syndrome: prenatal ultrasonographic diagnosis. *Radiology* 1982;143:535–6

17. Saade GR, Belfort MA, Berry DL, *et al.* Amniotic septostomy for the treatment of twin oligohydramnios–polyhydramnios sequence. *Fetal Diagn Ther* 1998;13:86–93

18. Chau AC, Kjos SL, Kovacs BW. Ultrasonographic measurement of amniotic fluid volume in normal diamniotic twin pregnancies. *Am J Obstet Gynecol* 1996;174:1003–7

19. Sebire NJ, D'Ercole C, Hughes K, Carvalho M, Nicolaides KH. Increased nuchal translucency thickness at 10–14 weeks of gestation as a predictor of severe twin-to-twin transfusion syndrome. *Ultrasound Obstet Gynecol* 1997;10:86–9

20. Dennis LG, Winkler CL. Twin-to-twin transfusion syndrome: aggressive therapeutic amniocentesis. *Am J Obstet Gynecol* 1997;177:342–9

21. Danziger RW. Twin pregnancy with acute hydramnios treated by paracentesis uteri. *Br Med J* 1948;2:205–6

22. Moise KJ. Polyhydramnios: problems and treatment. *Semin Perinatol* 1993;17:197–209

23. Skupski, D. Amnioreduction for twin to twin transfusion syndrome. *Israel J Obstet Gynecol* 1997; 8:39–41

24. Mari G. Amnioreduction in twin–twin transfusion syndrome – a multicenter registry evaluation of 579 procedures. *Am J Obstet Gynecol* 1998;178:S28

25. Mahoney BS, Petty CN, Nyberg DA, Luthy DA, Hickok DLE, Hirsch JH. The 'stuck twin' phenomenon: ultrasonographic findings, pregnancy outcome, and management with serial amniocenteses. *Am J Obstet Gynecol* 1990;163: 1513–22

26. Reisner DP, Mahoney BS, Petty CN, *et al.* Stuck twin syndrome: outcome in thirty-seven consecutive cases. *Am J Obstet Gynecol* 1993;169: 991–5

27. Elliott JP, Urig MA, Clewell WH. Aggressive therapeutic amniocentesis for treatment of twin–twin syndrome. *Obstet Gynecol* 1991;77:537–40

28. Wax JR, Blakemore KJ, Blohm P, *et al.* Stuck twin with cotwin nonimmune hydrops: successful treatment by amniocentesis. *Fetal Diagn Ther* 1991;6:126–31

29. Megory E, Weiner E, Shalev E, Ohel G. Pseudo-monoamniotic twins with cord entanglement following genetic funipuncture. *Obstet Gynecol* 1991;78:915–17

30. Denbow ML, Batten MR, Cowan F, Azzopardi D, Edwards AD, Fisk NM. Neonatal cranial ultrasonographic findings in preterm twins complicated by severe fetofetal transfusion syndrome. *Am J Obstet Gynecol* 1998;178:479–83

31. Bejar R, Vigliocco G, Gramajo H, *et al.* Antenatal origin of neurologic damage in newborn infants. II. Multiple gestations. *Am J Obstet Gynecol* 1990; 162:1230–6

32. Benirschke K. The biology of the twinning process: how placentation influences outcome. *Semin Perinatol* 1995;19:342–50

33. Berry SM, Puder KS, Bottoms SF, Uckele JE, Romero R, Cotton DB. Comparison of intra-uterine hematologic and biochemical values between twin pairs with and without stuck twin syndrome. *Am J Obstet Gynecol* 1995;172:1403–10

34. Sacks HS, Chalmers TC, Smith H. Sensitivity and specificity of clinical trials: randomized v historical controls. *Arch Intern Med* 1983;143: 753–5

35. Chalmers TC, Celano P, Sacks HS, Smith H. Bias in treatment assignment in controlled clinical trials. *N Engl J Med* 1983;309:1358–61

36. Riduan JM, Hillier SL, Utomo B, Wiknjosastro G, Linnan M, Kandun N. Bacterial vaginosis and prematurity in Indonesia: association in early and late pregnancy. *Am J Obstet Gynecol* 1993;169: 175–8

37. Joesef MR, Hillier SL, Wiknjosastro G, *et al.* Intravaginal clindamycin treatment for bacterial vaginosis: effects on preterm delivery and low birth weight. *Am J Obstet Gynecol* 1995;173:1527–31

38. Schulz K. Chalmers I, Hayes RJ, Altman DG. Empirical evidence of bias. Dimensions of methodological quality associated with estimates of treatment effects in controlled trials. *J Am Med Assoc* 1995;273:408–12

39. Skupski DW. Changes in survival of preterm singletons versus twins delivered after twin–twin transfusion syndrome over the calendar years 1970–1994. *Fetal Diagn Ther* 1999; in press

40. Gonsoulin W, Moise KJ Jr, Kirshon B, Cotton DB, Wheeler JM, Carpenter RJ. Outcome of twin–twin transfusion diagnosed before 28 weeks of gestation. *Obstet Gynecol* 1990;75:214–16

41. Pinette MG, Yuqun P, Pinette SG, Stubblefield PG. Treatment of twin–twin transfusion syndrome. *Obstet Gynecol* 1993;82:841–6

42. Fries MH, Goldstien RB, Kilpatrick SJ, Golbus MS, Callen PW, Filly RA. The role of velamentous cord insertion in the etiology of twin–twin transfusion syndrome. *Obstet Gynecol* 1993;81: 569–74

43. Ville Y, Sideris I, Nicolaides KH. Amniotic fluid pressure in twin-to-twin transfusion syndrome: an objective prognostic factor. *Fetal Diagn Ther* 1996;11:176–80

Fetomaternal transfusion: state of the art

29

I. Szabó and Z. Papp

INTRODUCTION

Spontaneous transplacental passage of fetal erythrocytes into the maternal circulation has been described, but the amount of bleeding is less than 0.1 ml in 75–98% of cases[1,2]. It has been estimated that a fetomaternal transfusion of over 30 ml of fetal blood occurs in normal pregnancies with a frequency of about 1 in 300[3]. Massive fetomaternal transfusion has been defined as bleeding in which more than 150 ml of fetal blood is found in the maternal circulation[4]. However, the frequency of fetomaternal transfusion remains largely unknown. In a small series, fetomaternal transfusion was the unexpected cause of death in 13.8% of otherwise unexplained fetal deaths[5].

It is difficult to define the clinically important massive fetomaternal transfusion, because there are no large, prospective multicenter studies or comprehensive registries available. Some articles have considered more than 30 ml as indicative of massive fetomaternal transfusion, because Rh-negative women who had experienced transplacental hemorrhages of 30 ml of Rh-positive fetal blood needed a larger than standard (300 µg) dose of rhesus immune globulin for rhesus prophylaxis[6]. Almeida and Bowman[7] considered massive fetomaternal transfusion to be 80 ml of blood or more, because at this level neonatal anemia appeared in the examined population. Giacoia[8] reviewed all cases of fetomaternal transfusion that were published up to 1997. This review focused exclusively on cases with a transfusion of 50 ml or more, because 50 ml of fetal blood was likely to affect the outcome of the pregnancy.

Table 1 *Etiology of fetomaternal transfusion*

Placental and cord abnormalities
Abruptio placenta
Vasa previa/membranous insertion
Chorioangioma/choriocarcinoma
Thrombus of the umbilical vein

Maternal trauma
Direct trauma to the abdomen
Motor vehicle accident
Other trauma

Procedures or operations
Amniocentesis
External cephalic version

Unknown

Table 1 summarizes the possible causes of fetomaternal transfusion. Since this disease was hypothesized by Wiener[9] in 1948 and proven by Chown[10] in 1954, many case reports and several series with approximately 134 cases have been reported[8]. In 82% of the cases, no cause could be found. Furthermore, most fetomaternal transfusions occurred late in gestation. Only 35 of the 134 reviewed cases (26.1%) were infants born preterm. There were 33 (24.6%) stillbirths, and 11 (8.2%) died in the neonatal period.

SUSPICION AND RECOGNITION

Table 2 shows the most frequent signs and symptoms which can lead to the diagnosis of fetomaternal transfusion. Maternal reports of decreased or absent fetal body movements have been described as a premonitory non-specific sign in 24–25% of cases of fetomaternal transfusion[8,11,12]. The absence of fetal body movements was reported in 11–12%

Table 2 *Signs and symptoms leading to the diagnosis of fetomaternal transfusion*

Decreased or absent fetal body movements
Sinusoidal fetal heart rate pattern
Non-reactive fetal heart rate tracing with or without late deceleration
Intrauterine atrial fibrillation
Hydrops fetalis
Intrauterine growth restriction
Increased α-fetoprotein

Unexpected stillbirths
Anemia at birth

of cases for a period ranging from 24 h to 7 days[8].

Attempts have been made to use the fetal heart rate (FHR) tracing as a diagnostic aid in cases of massive fetomaternal transfusion. A pathological sinusoidal heart rate pattern associated with fetomaternal transfusion was described first by Modanlou and co-workers[11]. Sinusoidal heart rate patterns associated with massive fetomaternal transfusion have now been associated with several cases of severe neonatal anemia, and sinusoidal heart rate has been described as another non-specific sign in 15–16% of cases of fetomaternal transfusion[8]. Sinusoidal heart rate patterns together with decreased fetal body movements have been reported in 9–10% of cases[8]. A non-reactive FHR tracing with or without late decelerations has also been described in several newborns with profound anemia caused by fetomaternal transfusion[8,12] and one case of intrauterine atrial fibrillation has been associated with fetomaternal transfusion[8].

The literature suggests that decreased fetal body movements and sinusoidal heart rate patterns are two non-specific signs that can help in diagnosing fetomaternal transfusion. Decreased fetal body movements associated with decreased or absent variability may also be an indicator of fetomaternal transfusion.

In 8–9% of cases, sonographic demonstration of hydrops fetalis has been reported as the indicator of chronic fetal anemia associated with massive fetomaternal transfusion[8]. Excessive (acute) and persistent

or recurrent (chronic) fetal erythrocyte loss can both lead to fatal outcome, although the fetal adaptation to acute anemia differs from that seen in chronic anemia. In acute anemia there is a redistribution of blood flow to the brain and heart while blood flow and oxygen delivery to the kidneys, intestines, muscles and skin decreases[13]. In contrast, prolonged fetal anemia is associated with decreased vascular resistance to all tissues (except the placenta)[13]. Also, chronically anemic fetal lambs exhibit an increase in venous return, explaining observations of increased cardiac output with normal atrial pressure and increased coronary, aortic and cerebral blood flow. Unless low viscosity is an explanation for the hyperdynamic circulation, increased cardiac contractility could play a role as a compensatory mechanism. In severe anemia, however, despite successful cardiac adaptation, an increase in hydrostatic pressure leads to edema and hydrops fetalis[14].

Ultrasound indices such as placental thickness, umbilical vein diameter, abdominal circumference, or intraperitoneal volume fail to predict the severity of chronic anemia. A reliable prediction of chronic anemia by ultrasound is only possible if fetal hydrops is present, i.e. the fetal hematocrit is less than 15%[15], and the duration of persistent blood loss has allowed for cardiovascular adaptation by the fetus. In the cases of massive fetomaternal transfusion in which intrauterine transfusion was performed, hydrops fetalis was only present approximately 50% of the time[8]. Fetal hemoglobin concentration was between 2.1 and 5.4 g/dl in those fetuses with hydrops. In fetuses without signs of hydrops fetalis the fetal hemoglobin level ranged from 2.2 g/dl to 5.7g/dl[8].

Recently, Doppler ultrasound techniques have been applied to the characterization of hemodynamic changes in the anemic fetus[16–18]. The pathophysiological concept for identifying anemic fetuses by Doppler evaluation is based on a decrease in blood viscosity and a decrease in the fetal red blood cell count. Decreased viscosity should result in an increase of peak blood velocity measurable by Doppler. In addition, the fetal compensatory mechanism for anemia includes an increased cardiac output[14]. Furthermore, it is likely that this effect would be pronounced in the central part of the cardiovascular system, the cardiac inflow and outflow tracts. In previous studies a clear relationship has been reported between fetal aortic and middle cerebral artery peak systolic velocities as well as ductus venosus flow velocities and hematocrit[16–18]. Non-invasive Doppler studies can help to identify the early stages of chronic fetal anemia caused by persistent fetomaternal transfusion and may have the potential to be used in further management.

The acid elution test (Figure 1) described by Kleihauer and colleagues[19] in 1957 is generally accepted for recognition of fetomaternal transfusion and estimation of fetal blood loss volume. The test uses acid elution of maternal cells and the subsequent staining of fetal cells. Maternal erythrocytes are ruptured and appear as ghost cells, whereas the fetal red blood cells stain strongly because of the stability of the fetal hemoglobin in an acid medium. The value of the Kleihauer–Betke test for demonstrating fetal red blood cells in the maternal circulation is indisputable, but the precise estimation of the volume of fetomaternal transfusion is difficult and this test has a number of limitations[20].

The following factors can influence the accuracy of the Kleihauer–Betke test[8]:

(1) The differential hemoglobin elution is sensitive to temperature, pH and time;

(2) The quantitation of the amount of fetal blood depends on subjective interpretation;

(3) The number of cells counted, the thickness of smears and the intermediate staining of cells greatly influence the results (the increase in hemoglobin F occurring during pregnancy produces the so-called maternal F cells or intermediate staining cells);

(4) The acid elution test is uninterpretable in cases of hereditary persistence of fetal hemoglobin;

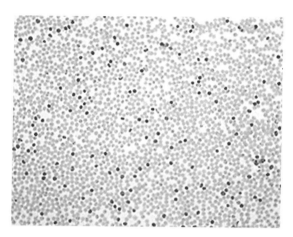

Figure 1 *Positive Kleihauer–Betke test. Peripheral maternal blood smear. Adult cells show as faint ghosts whilst fetal cells remain darkly stained. (Acid elution technique, 30×)*

(5) Various reagents have a short half-life;

(6) The estimation of the volume of fetomaternal transfusion is significantly influenced by the formula used to determine the amount of fetal blood.

Because of the multiplicity of factors influencing the results, the acid elution test may underestimate or overestimate the magnitude of the fetomaternal transfusion as well as show a large inter-observer and inter-hospital variation in interpretation[8,20]. Furthermore, the Kleihauer–Betke test cannot be used in patients who have received intrauterine transfusion, because donor red cells are not identifiable as fetal cells in the maternal circulation[8].

Increased maternal serum α-fetoprotein has also been interpreted as a non-specific sign in 9–10% of cases of fetomaternal transfusion[8]. Together with a positive Kleihauer–Betke test it has diagnostic value in the recognition of fetomaternal transfusion[21]. Furthermore, measurement of the maternal serum concentration of α-fetoprotein is another method used to estimate fetomaternal transfusion[21], by the formula: $AB/C\,(1-P)$ where A = increase in maternal α-fetoprotein concentration; B = estimated maternal plasma volume; C = fetal α-fetoprotein concentration; and

P = estimated fetal packed red blood cell volume.

The advantages of the α-fetoprotein measurements over the Kleihauer technique are the stability of α-fetoprotein under different storage conditions and the fact that α-fetoprotein is not influenced by the agglutination of fetal red blood cells. On the other hand, maternal serum concentrations of α-fetoprotein vary greatly during pregnancy and within a given pregnancy. Consequently, maternal blood samples before and after a potential fetomaternal transfusion would be needed to estimate the volume of fetal blood[8,21].

Several other methods applicable to all pregnancies have been developed to estimate fetomaternal transfusion as an alternative to the Kleihauer method[22,23]. The progress in monoclonal antibody technology may make it possible to develop an enzyme-linked antiglobulin test or a flow cytometry test that is capable of analyzing a large number of cells with objectivity and reproducibility[22]. Recently it has been suggested that a well-performed Kleihauer–Betke test would still appear to be useful as a screening technique for the detection of fetomaternal transfusion. However, accurate quantitation of the size of the fetomaternal transfusion is more reliably determined by flow cytometry[23].

Previous studies[7,8] have reported various infant health conditions at birth. Anemia was the most frequent symptom and was found in 47%[8] to 87%[7] of cases. No significant difference was found in the survival of patients whose pretransfusion hemoglobin level was either more or less than 6 g/dl[8]. When survival was related to the estimated fetomaternal transfusion, no statistically significant difference was found between those cases whose estimated volume was ≥ 200 ml and those whose volume was < 200 ml. For the whole reviewed population, a modest negative correlation was found between pretransfusion hemoglobin and estimated fetomaternal transfusion[8].

The major complications resulted from asphyxia and shock. Central nervous system dysfunction was reported in 14–15% of cases[8].

Within this group the following conditions were present: hypoxic ischemia, intraventricular bleeding, periventricular cysts and seizures due to cerebral infarction. Intrauterine insult to the fetal brain has been found in a handful of cases reviewed retrospectively by Giacoia[8]. The prevalence of this complication is unknown, for lack of systematic imaging studies of the brain at birth and long-term follow-up of patients.

DISCUSSION

Massive fetomaternal transfusion, although uncommon, is not rare. The frequency of such an event has been reported to be as high as one in 1000 deliveries[7]. The diagnosis of severe fetomaternal transfusion, however, remains elusive in most cases because of its silent nature. Unexpected anemia at birth or unexplained stillbirths are often the presenting manifestations.

When the condition has been diagnosed *in utero*, maternal reports of decreased or absent fetal body movements, detection of a sinusoidal heart rate pattern or non-reactive FHR tracing with or without late deceleration and sonographic demonstration of hydrops fetalis were the most frequent symptoms. This syndromic triad is usually a late manifestation in a fetus that has been bleeding into the maternal circulation for a considerable period of time, as judged by estimated volume of hemorrhage or fetal anemia. During the past few years, large fetomaternal transfusions have been diagnosed more frequently and the recognition of these three signs has been prevalent[8].

Fetal responses and survival after severe fetomaternal transfusion are insufficiently known. Previous studies[7,8] have reported some discrepancy between the fetal outcome and the estimated volume of fetal blood loss. Outcomes ranged from one asymptomatic newborn who bled 435 ml, representing more than his total fetoplacental blood volume, to a severely ill newborn with a poor outcome who bled 80 ml, representing 20% of his blood volume[7]. There appear to be two important factors in the clinical outcome: the amount and the rate of bleeding. In experimental data using fetal sheep as models, Brace[24] showed that removal of 30% of the total blood volume over a 2-h period was tolerated by the fetuses, with the fetal blood volume returning to normal within 3 h. When the same volume was removed in 10 min[25], the fetuses took an average of 6 h to restore their blood volumes, and three of ten died. Acute blood loss greater than 40% of the total blood volume resulted in fetal death.

The large fetomaternal transfusion in many of the cases reported by Almeida and Bowman[7] and reviewed retrospectively by Giacoia[8] occurred over a period of time, allowing for cardiovascular adaptation. High erythroblast and reticulocyte blood counts suggest an interval of time sufficient to stimulate the bone marrow. It is not known, however, how long after the fetomaternal transfusion those indices increase. Non-lethal, massive fetomaternal transfusion may occur over prolonged periods of time. It is possible that intermittent bleeding episodes may be superimposed over a chronic leakage of fetal blood into the maternal circulation[8].

Fetomaternal transfusion is a poorly understood condition. Although specific causes have been identified, the etiopathogenesis of most of the cases remains unknown. Pregnancies complicated by fetomaternal transfusion develop normally until signs of fetal decompensation begin to appear. Because massive fetomaternal transfusion can occur without prior risk factors, this diagnosis should be considered in any patient with decreased fetal body movements and a sinusoidal or non-reactive FHR pattern. A positive Kleihauer–Betke test as evidence of fetomaternal transfusion should warrant consideration of prompt delivery if the gestational age is consistent with neonatal viability. The neonatal team should be alerted to the possibility of intensive neonatal care and immediate transfusion. If the fetus is previable, confirmation of fetal anemia by cordocentesis is necessary to determine the need for intrauterine transfusion. Both procedures require experience not available in many centers. Early recognition of large fetomaternal transfusion should permit the referral of patients to a center experienced in these procedures.

An acute fetomaternal transfusion constitutes an unexpected medical emergency. Future efforts should concentrate on the early recognition of subacute and chronic fetomaternal transfusion which may improve the chances for a successful outcome. Cost-effective methods of detecting a large volume of fetal cells in the maternal circulation and extensive use of Doppler velocimetry during pregnancy to detect decreases in blood viscosity may lead to early detection.

References

1. Jorgensen J. Feto-maternal bleeding. *Acta Obstet Gynecol* 1977;56:487–90
2. Bowman JM, Pollock JM, Penston LE. Fetomaternal transplacental hemorrhage during pregnancy and after delivery. *Vox Sang* 1985;51: 117–21
3. Sebring ES, Polesky HF. Fetomaternal hemorrhage: incidence, risk factors, time occurrence, and clinical effects. *Transfusion* 1990; 30:344–57
4. Willis C, Foreman CS. Chronic massive fetomaternal hemorrhage: a case report. *Obstet Gynecol* 1988;71: 459–61
5. Laube DW, Schauberger CW. Fetomaternal bleeding as a cause for 'unexplained' fetal death. *Obstet Gynecol* 1982;60:649–51
6. Pollack W, Ascari WQ, Kochesky RJ, O'Connor RR, Ho-Ty, Tripodi D. Studies on Rh prophylaxis. I. Relationship between doses of anti-Rh and size of antigenic stimulus. *Transfusion* 1971;11:333–9
7. Almeida V, Bowman JM. Massive fetomaternal hemorrhage: Manitoba experience. *Obstet Gynecol* 1994;83:323–8
8. Giacoia GP. Severe fetomaternal hemorrhage: a review. *Obstet Gynecol Surv* 1997;52:372–80
9. Wiener AS. Diagnosis and treatment of anemia

of the newborn caused by occult placental hemorrhage. *Am J Obstet Gynecol* 1948;56:717–22

10. Chown B. Anemia from bleeding of the fetus into the mother's circulation. *Lancet* 1954;1:1213

11. Modanlou HD, Freeman RK, Ortiz O, Hinkes P, Pillsbury G. Sinusoidal fetal heart rate pattern and severe fetal anemia. *Obstet Gynecol* 1977; 49:537–41

12. Kosasa TS, Ebesugava I, Nakayama RT, Hale RW. Massive fetomaternal hemorrhage preceded by decreased fetal movement and a nonreactive fetal heart rate pattern. *Obstet Gynecol* 1993;82: 711–14

13. Davis LE, Hohimer R. Hemodynamics and organ blood flow in fetal sheep subjected to chronic anemia. *Am J Physiol* 1991;30:R1542–8

14. Davis LE, Hohimer AR, Giraud GD, Reller MD, Morton MJ. Right ventricular function in chronically anemic fetal lamb. *Am J Obstet Gynecol* 1996;174:1289–94

15. Grannum PA, Copel JA, Moya FR, *et al.* The reversal of hydrops fetalis by intravascular intrauterine transfusion in severe isoimmune fetal anemia. *Am J Obstet Gynecol* 1988;158:914–19

16. Steiner H, Chaffer H, Spitzer D, Batka M, Graf AH, Staudach A. The relationship between peak velocity in the fetal descending aorta and hematocrit in rhesus immunization. *Obstet Gynecol* 1995;85:659–62

17. Mari G, Adrignolo A, Abuhamad AZ, *et al.* Diagnosis of fetal anemia with Doppler ultrasound in the pregnancy complicated by maternal group immunization. *Ultrasound Obstet Gynecol* 1995;5:400–5

18. Oepkes D, Vandenbussche FP, Bel FV, Kanhai HH. Fetal ductus venosus blood flow velocities before and after transfusion in red-cell alloimmunized pregnancies. *Obstet Gynecol* 1993;82:237–41

19. Kleihauer E, Brauch H, Betke K. Demonstration of fetal hemoglobin in erythrocytes of a blood smear. *Klin Wochenschr* 1957;35:637–43

20 Duckett JRA, Constantine G. The Kleihauer Technique: an accurate method of quantifying fetomaternal haemorrhage? *Br J Obstet Gynaecol* 1997;104:845–6

21. Van Selm S, Kanhai HH, Van Loo AJ. Detection of fetomaternal hemorrhage associated with cordocentesis using serum alpha-fetoprotein and the Kleihauer technique. *Prenat Diagn* 1995; 15:313–16

22. Bayliss KM, Kueck BD, Johnson ST. Detecting fetomaternal hemorrhage: a comparison of five methods. *Transfusion* 1991;31:303–7

23. Bromilow IM, Duguid JK. Measurement of fetomaternal hemorrhage: a comparative study of three Kleihauer techniques and two flow cytometry methods. *Clin Lab Haematol* 1997;19: 137–42

24. Brace RA. Mechanism of fetal blood volume restoration after slow fetal hemorrhage. *Am J Physiol* 1989;256:R1040–3

25. Brace RA, Cheung CY. Fetal blood volume restoration following a rapid fetal hemorrhage. *Am J Physiol* 1990;259:H567–73

Perinatal cytomegalovirus infection

30

G. Nigro, M. Mazzocco and E. V. Cosmi

VIROLOGY

Cytomegalovirus (CMV) is a large (approximately 200 nm), enveloped, double-stranded DNA virus, belonging to the herpesvirus family, which shares several important properties, including persistence in human cells with alternation of latency and reactivation. The viral genes are expressed in a regulated temporal sequence designated as immediate early, early and late CMV genes. There are no distinct serotypes of CMV but numerous different strains, which are genetically homologous though not identical, and reinfection of a CMV-seropositive individual is possible in spite of pre-existing and cross-reacting antibodies. Although CMV infects primarily epithelial tissues *in vivo*, culture is possible in only human fibroblasts[1,2].

EPIDEMIOLOGY

The infection is very common worldwide, although the prevalence is influenced by many factors, including age, geographical distribution, socioeconomic status and childbearing practices. In developed countries, the seroprevalence is 40–60% in adult populations of mid to upper income and more than 80% in lower status groups[3]. In developing countries, 80% of children acquire CMV by the age of 3 years[4]. However, the epidemiology of CMV is complex, and many aspects are still poorly understood. Viral transmission is due to human reservoirs, since CMV-infected subjects are capable of excreting CMV in urine, saliva, semen, cervical secretions and breast milk, particularly in the young and middle aged. The main routes are: direct human-to-human or indirect contact (via contaminated items); vertical transmission from mother to infant;

and transfusion or transplantation-associated transmission from seropositive donors[2].

During pregnancy, CMV DNAemia is detected in 3–6% of women, viruria is present in 3–12% and cervical viral shedding increases as gestation advances: 0–5% in the first trimester, 6–10% in the second trimester and 11–28% in the third trimester[3]. The low viral shedding in the first trimester, during which organogenesis occurs, is correlated with a low rate of fetal abnormalities. In fact, viral shedding is better correlated with intrapartum than prenatal transmission. Primary CMV infection occurs in 0.7–4.1% of pregnancies with an annual seroconversion rate in women of childbearing age of about 2% in higher socioeconomic groups and about 6% in lower groups. The annual rate of primary infection in pregnancy appeared to be correlated with socioeconomic status, being higher in women of low income than in those of mid to upper income (6.8% vs. 2.5%), in spite of a higher seropositivity rate (64.5% vs. 23.4%)[5]. Significant risk factors for primary infection during pregnancy are the presence of young children attending daycare centers, young maternal age and mid to upper income[3]. Once one family member has seroconverted, almost half of the other susceptible household members acquire CMV infection within 6 months. Infectious viral particles persist for hours on plastic surfaces, such as toys. Overall, a quarter of the serious congenital infections occurring each year are attributable to the daycare setting. The role of sexual transmission in primary CMV infection is unclear and varies with the populations: young age, lower socioeconomic status, number of sexual partners and other sexually transmitted diseases are risk factors for sexual

CMV transmission. Saliva also is a significant source of viral transmission in this setting[5].

Approximately 0.5–2.5% of infants show cytomegaloviruria in the neonatal period. Intrapartum and immediately postnatal (through the breast milk or other sources) transmission accounts for an additional 10–15% of infants acquiring CMV infection in the first 4–8 weeks of life. Approximately half of the infants born to mothers with cervical CMV shedding who are uninfected at birth and not breastfed and 70% of infants of mothers excreting CMV in the milk will be infected perinatally[4]. In low-birth-weight infants, blood transfusions are an important source of infection[2].

PATHOGENESIS

Infection with CMV is differentiated as primary or recurrent, including reactivation of a pre-existing viral strain or reinfection by an exogenous strain. During active infection, CMV can be isolated directly from peripheral blood; monocytes are probably cellular sites at which the virus persists in normal subjects. Following primary maternal infection, CMV may be transmitted to the fetus by viremia and spread of infected leukocytes across the placenta; or by placentitis with spread to amniotic cells, which are swallowed by the fetus. Twin fetuses can respond differently, probably because the placentas play a role in transmitting the infection. After CMV replication in the fetal oropharynx, there is hematogenous spread to target tissues such as tubular epithelium, which appears to be a major site of replication. Maternal–fetal CMV transmission as well as neonatal disease expression may be enhanced by transient cellular and humoral immunodepression occurring in the second and third trimesters. Although gestational age appears to have little influence on the frequency of fetal infection, it probably influences the severity of disease: early CMV transmission seems to be correlated with poor outcome.

The prevalence of infections following recurrent CMV infections in pregnancy is considered to be 1–2%, but it is probably higher than is commonly believed. Pre-existing humoral immunity, although useful, does not completely protect seropositive women against reinfection or reactivation, which is probably common in pregnancy, like herpes simplex recurrence.

Although the pathogenic mechanisms of tissue damage are not completely clear, they seem to be:

(1) Direct tissue injury by persistent CMV replication in the infected cells, probably associated with a high viral concentration, resulting in clinically evident tissue injury;

(2) Ischemic tissue damage (vasculitis), related to the viral presence in the endothelial cells of vessels in several organs, including the placenta and the brain;

(3) Immune-mediated tissue injury by immune complex deposition.

Neuropathological processes, which are the most severe and characteristic features of congenital CMV infection, include meningo-encephalitis, periventricular calcifications, microcephaly, polymicrogyria and other migrational alterations. Viral predilection for the periventricular area may relate to the proximity to the cerebrospinal fluid (CSF) pathway, through which CMV probably spreads, and to the actively proliferating subependymal germinal matrix cells, which are particularly vulnerable to CMV. Microcephaly relates to encephaloclastic viral effects and possible neuroproliferative troubles due to CMV interference. Migrational alterations show that teratogenic effects of CMV may also occur in the second trimester of pregnancy, when neuronal migration takes place. In fact, CMV is the only congenitally transmitted pathogen causing altered gyral development, the pathogenesis of which includes both teratogenic and encephaloclastic mechanisms[6].

CMV INFECTION IN PREGNANCY

Approximately 10% of pregnant women with primary infection may have a mononucleosis-like syndrome with persistent fever as the prominent clinical feature, pharyngitis, cervical or generalized lymphadenopathy, fatigue, headache, myalgias, nausea and diarrhea. Rarely, hepatosplenomegaly or rash can occur. Laboratory findings include lymphopenia or lymphocytosis with atypical lymphocytes, thrombocytopenia and slightly increased aminotransferase levels. CMV culture or CMV DNA detection from blood, urine, saliva or cervicovaginal secretions may be positive but is sometimes negative, probably because the virus is confined to organs in the reticuloendothelial system. Primary CMV infection may be followed by early abortion, and recurrent infection has been associated with habitual abortion[7]. Intrauterine growth restriction is frequent in primary infection; about one-third of infected infants have a gestational age lower than 38 weeks[1-4].

CONGENITAL CMV INFECTION

CMV is the most common and serious congenital infection, and is associated with important neurological sequelae, although the majority of infants are asymptomatic at birth. Congenital CMV infection may occur in approximately 40% (range 24–75%) of infants born to mothers with primary infection; of these, 10–12% are symptomatic at birth and have a remote likelihood of developing normal intelligence and hearing. Congenital infection consequent on recurrent maternal disease is asymptomatic in the majority of cases, and less than 10% of infected infants have long-term sequelae. Apart from monolateral hearing loss, the only neurological sequela shown by infants born to mothers with recurrent infection was microcephaly. However, the presence of maternal antibodies could blunt the presentation and severity of fetal infection[3-5].

In symptomatic congenital infection, reticuloendothelial involvement, including jaundice, hepatosplenomegaly and thrombocytopenia, is predominant. Liver abnormalities generally disappear completely, although fatal cirrhosis can occur. Pneumonia

and a purpuric rash may also be present. Ocular manifestations include chorioretinitis, which is prevalent in premature infants, microphthalmia and cataract. Among numerous other manifestations occurring in infants with symptomatic congenital CMV infection, inguinal hernia is the most frequent (approximately 25%). Neurological syndromes, including seizures, hyper- or hypotonia, microcephaly and periventricular calcifications, are the most serious consequence of congenital CMV infection and occur in 30–50% of symptomatic infants[6]. Approximately 20% of these also develop sensorineural hearing loss, which is probably the most common handicap caused by congenital CMV infection, and is now considered one of the major causes of deafness in childhood. In some reports, hearing loss is considered to occur in approximately half of the infants with symptomatic and about 15% of the infants with asymptomatic congenital CMV infection[4]. The majority of patients have cerebrospinal (CSF) signs of encephalitis (e.g. pleocytosis, elevated protein concentration); diabetes insipidus may also occur. Children who are asymptomatic at birth may also have mental retardation or character troubles (about 10% of cases), which usually present during the first 2 years of life, but may escape detection until school age.

DIAGNOSIS

Primary CMV infection in pregnancy is shown by seroconversion of CMV-specific IgG antibodies from negative to positive. When both IgM and IgG antibodies are positive, they could represent primary infection (CMV IgM antibody generally persists for about 3 months, with range between 2 weeks and 6 months) but CMV recurrence or false-positive results (by cross-reaction with other herpesviruses or rheumatoid factor and/or by polyclonal B-cell activation) are more likely.

Prenatal diagnosis of fetal CMV infection, which may be obtained by viral isolation or CMV detection with the polymerase chain reaction (PCR) of DNA in the amniotic fluid, does not predict an adverse fetal outcome. Fetal CMV infection should be closely monitored by ultrasound examination for evidence of intrauterine growth restriction, oligohydramnios or polyhydramnios, ascites or hydrops, cerebral ventriculomegaly or hydrocephalus, microcephaly, pseudo-meconium ileus, pleural or pericardial effusion, hepatosplenomegaly, or necrotic, cystic or calcified periventricular lesions in the brain, liver or placenta[3,5]. Some of these manifestations, such as ascites or effusions, may resolve *in utero*[8]. Cordocentesis may be a useful adjunct to amniocentesis, since fetal blood can be tested for the viral genome or culture and IgM together with hematological, immunological and enzymatic examinations. However, umbilical cord sampling implies an increased procedural morbidity and the need to delay sampling until at least 20 weeks' gestation, when the vein is large enough to puncture and the immune system to produce IgM antibodies. If CMV initially infects the placenta, chorionic villus sampling offers the potential for first-trimester diagnosis[5]. The reliability of prenatal diagnosis of CMV infection may be affected by important variables, mainly including the time interval between maternal infection and amniocentesis or fetal sampling, and factors (e.g. cell-mediated immunity, other infections) influencing viral transmission.

Congenital CMV infection is diagnosed by viral isolation or CMV DNA detection from urine or blood within 2 weeks from birth. Electron microscopic demonstration of viral particles and detection of CMV antigens by immunofluorescence may also be useful, providing diagnostic information in 1–3 days. CMV must be detected within 2 weeks after birth to differentiate congenital from perinatal infection. Neurological involvement can be demonstrated by viral presence in the CSF. CMV infection can also be diagnosed by detecting specific IgM antibodies in cord or neonatal blood specimens, but false-positive or particularly false-negative results may occur. Detection of CMV IgA antibodies may be a complementary diagnostic tool[3–5].

Ultrasonography can show abnormalities consisting of periventricular cysts, ventriculo-megaly, periventricular echolucencies due to leukomalacia and thalamic echodensities representing arteries, but more precise definition of calcifications and cerebral damage can be obtained by computerized tomography (CT). Magnetic resonance imaging is very useful in revealing altered neuronal migration, parenchymal loss, delayed myelinization or cerebellar hypoplasia[6]. In symptomatic as well as asymptomatic infants, testing of brain stem auditory evoked potentials could reveal abnormalities. Possible ocular involvement should be investigated by ophthalmoscopic examination and visual evoked potentials.

PROGNOSIS

The combination of abnormal ultrasound findings and positive amniotic fluid culture appears to predict a worse neonatal outcome, although fetal signs do not always predict severe involvement at birth and do not necessarily predict an adverse long-term outcome[5]. In children with symptomatic congenital CMV infection, the outcome is closely related to the severity of the neurological syndrome. In fact, approximately 95% of the infants with microcephaly, periventricular calcifications or chorioretinitis may have major neurological sequelae such as severe mental retardation, seizures, deafness or spasticity[3–6]. A CT scan of the brain is particularly important to document the extent of neurological involvement. Children with microcephaly without calcifications may not have mental retardation. The clinical course is generally slow, but progressive encephaloclastic disease or hearing loss may occur[6]. Viruria persists in about 50% of patients at 5 years of age[3].

Among children with asymptomatic congenital infections, approximately 10–15% have been reported to develop mental retardation or hearing loss, which may not be diagnosed until serious language impairment occurs. However, hearing loss may not be detectable before the first year of life, being related to a direct and progressive lesion of the cochlear cells and of the neurons of the eighth cranial nerve. Late onset and reactivation of chorioretinitis in children with congenital CMV infection may also occur. Therefore, clinical and laboratory follow-up is essential[3].

PREVENTION

Since CMV is a major cause of childhood deafness and neurological handicap, routine antepartum screening should be very useful, but it appears to be impracticable. To avoid difficulties in differentiating recurrent from primary infections and problematic counselling when positive IgM antibodies are detected, serial examinations of CMV-specific IgG and IgM antibodies may be suggested, at least in the first two trimesters, particularly in women at high risk, such as daycare workers. It would then be feasible to reveal, as soon as possible, both primary infections (by seroconversion and high IgM levels) and recurrent infections (by significant IgG increase concomitantly or not with positive IgM antibodies). To prevent possible viral transmission to the fetus, primary maternal infection could be treated with CMV hyperimmune immunoglobulins, but data from the literature are lacking, probably because of the difficulty in detecting these infections. Termination of pregnancy should be considered if fetal CMV disease (not only infection) is confirmed.

Appropriate hygienic measures (e.g. handwashing, avoidance of contact with oral secretions) can prevent CMV transmission. The most efficient preventive approach requires the counselling of parents with seropositive children in daycare centers: seronegative parents should be instructed in frequent handwashing after handling diapers and material contaminated with secretions and cautioned about the potential risk of intimate contact, especially mouth-to-mouth. Seronegative women with multiple sexual partners and a history of sexually transmitted diseases should be counselled about the use of condoms.

Vaccines, using both live attenuated virus (Towne 125) and subunit or recombinant proteins, have been evaluated. However, a suitable CMV vaccine, particularly for women in the childbearing age, has not yet been developed. For prevention of transfusion-acquired CMV infections, fewer units, red blood cells or CMV-seronegative blood or deglycerolized and frozen cells should be used[9].

THERAPY

Antiviral therapy for infants with severe CMV disease can be attempted with ganciclovir or foscarnet, which are capable of inhibiting CMV replication by inactivation of viral DNA polymerase with different mechanisms. Clinical benefit (e.g. loss of hepatospleno-megaly, improvement in tone) has been associated with a ganciclovir regimen based on an initial course with a high dosage and a long maintenance course, to inhibit CMV replication for as long as possible[10]. Since the detection of CMV DNA in CSF has been associated with developmental delay, this evaluation could be used in the future to identify infants who are at risk for neurodevelopmental problems and who may therefore benefit from antiviral therapy[5]. The efficacy of hyperimmune immunoglobulins in the treatment of neonates with congenital CMV disease has not been evaluated. Because of their high content in neutralizing anti-CMV IgG antibodies, commercial anti-CMV immunoglobulins could be useful for the treatment of fetal infection following primary infection.

ACKNOWLEDGEMENTS

This work was supported in part by the Italian Research Council (CNR), and by the Ministry of University, Research & Technology (MURST).

References

1. Naraqi S. Cytomegaloviruses. In Belshe RB, ed. *Textbook of Human Virology*, 2nd edn. St Louis: Mosby Year Book, 1991:889–924
2. Ho M. *Cytomegalovirus: Biology and Infection.* New York: Plenum Press, 1991
3. Stagno S. Cytomegalovirus. In Remington JS, Klein JO, eds. *Infectious Diseases of the Fetus and Newborn Infant*, 4th edn. Philadelphia: WB Saunders, 1995:312–53
4. Demmler GJ. Congenital cytomegalovirus infection and disease. *Adv Pediatr Infect Dis* 1996; 12:135–62
5. Raynor BD. Cytomegalovirus infection in pregnancy. *Semin Perinatol* 1993;17:394–402
6. Volpe JJ. Viral, protozoan, and related intracranial infections. In *Neurology of the Newborn*, 3rd edn. Philadelphia: WB Saunders, 1995:675–729
7. Van Lunschoten G, Stals F, Evers JLH, *et al.* The presence of cytomegalovirus antigens on karyotyped abortions. *Am J Reprod Immunol* 1994; 32:211–20
8. Nelson CT, Demmler GJ. Cytomegalovirus infection in the pregnant mother, fetus, and newborn infant. *Clin Perinatol* 1997;24: 151–60
9. Adler SP. Cytomegalovirus and pregnancy. *Curr Opin Obstet Gynecol* 1992;4:670–5
10. Nigro G, Scholz H, Bartmann U. Ganciclovir therapy for symptomatic congenital cytomegalovirus infection in infants: a two-regimen experience. *J Pediatr* 1994;124:318–21

Laboratory and clinical diagnosis of intrauterine infection of the fetus

31

I. Sziller and Z. Papp

DEFINITIONS AND PREVALENCE

Intra-amniotic infection occurs when bacteria gain access to the fetal membranes, decidua and amniotic fluid[1]. In a later stage of primarily maternal infection, the fetus might also be involved. Micro-organisms in the amniotic fluid may induce the biosynthesis of proinflammatory cytokines, which may lead to the development of a fetal systemic inflammatory response[2]. This condition is similar to that observed in adults with multiple organ failure associated with generalized sepsis[3].

Bacterial invasion of the intrauterine cavity and fetus will in many but not all cases result in histological, laboratory and clinical evidence of infection. Accordingly, intra-amniotic infection can be described using histopathological, bacteriological or clinical definitions. The histopathological definition of intra-amniotic infection is based upon an acute, diffuse inflammatory process in the extraplacental membranes, chorionic plate of the placenta and umbilical cord[4]. If bacteria are recovered from the amniotic fluid, the condition is defined as amniotic fluid infection[5]. Both chorioamnionitis and amniotic fluid infection may be present with or without clinical signs of infection in the mother and the fetus. Clinical intra-amniotic infection (or chorioamnionitis) is reserved for the cases when febrile pregnant women present with labor or rupture of membranes, and supporting clinical evidence is not explained by other sources of infection. Silent (unrecognized or subclinical) intra-amniotic infection is reserved for the cases in which bacterial invasion of the amniotic fluid or histological chorioamnionitis are not associated with clinical markers of infection[6].

Until the late 1970s intact fetal membranes were considered to be a barrier to infection of the amniotic fluid, thus providing a sterile environment for the growing fetus *in utero*[7]. Bacterial colonization of the amniotic fluid was supposed to develop only after initiation of labor or rupture of the membranes at or close to term[8]. The condition was found to occur in 10% of term pregnancies with intact membranes, and in about 30% of term pregnancies with ruptured membranes.

Clinical intra-amniotic infection is an uncommon condition if related to all pregnancies, with an overall incidence of 0.5–1%. Among patients with microbial invasion of the amniotic fluid, only 15–55% of women have overt clinical signs of infection. Thus, the mere presence of bacteria in the amniotic cavity is not sufficient to cause intra-amniotic infection or preterm labor[9].

Histological chorioamnionitis is far more frequent than the clinically evident intra-uterine infection. At term, its prevalence is about 20%, but significantly higher rates (up to 50%) are documented in preterm pregnancies[4].

The prevalence of silent intra-amniotic infection is between these two extremes. It is generally accepted that intra-amniotic infection is the most common cause of preterm labor wherever it has been studied around the world and appears to be responsible for about one-third of all preterm deliveries[4]. Between 0% and 25% of women in preterm labor with intact membranes have positive amniotic fluid culture. In contrast, micro-organisms are rarely recovered from women not in labor[1]. Bacterial invasion of the amniotic fluid might occur as early as the beginning of the second trimester of pregnancy. The rate of positive amnitoic fluid cultures among afebrile, asymptomatic pregnant women undergoing diagnostic transabdominal amniocentesis was reported to vary between 5% and 13%, and adverse pregnancy outcomes were reported for those with amniotic fluid infection[10,11].

MATERNAL AND FETAL MORBIDITY

Infection of the amniotic cavity and its contents is a serious complication in pregnancy affecting both the mother and her fetus. Possible additional obstetric complications include dystocia, oxytocin supplementation to achieve adequate uterine activity, slow progress of cervical dilatation, higher frequency of Cesarean delivery and postpartum uterine atony[12].

Maternal consequences of intra-amniotic infection include an increased risk for febrile morbidity during labor, postpartum endometritis and sepsis. In cases of abdominal delivery, maternal infectious morbidity is further increased by a higher risk for post-Cesarean endometritis, pelvic inflammatory disease and wound infection[12].

Microbial contamination of the amniotic cavity is a significant contributor to perinatal morbidity and mortality[13]. It has long been known that the morbidity of neonates prematurely born to mothers with intra-amniotic infection includes congenital pneumonia, omphalitis, meningitis, respiratory distress syndrome, low Apgar scores, recurrent apnea and fetal or neonatal sepsis, with bronchopulmonary dysplasia and necrotizing enterocolitis as possible late consequences. Fetal morbidity in these cases is a combined effect of prematurity of the organs, prenatal hypoxic damage to the lungs and sometimes the destruction of surfactant by aspirated bacteria[14,15]. Moreover, recent reports have suggested that long-term consequences of fetal infection might manifest in severe neurological abnormalities including cerebral palsy, periventricular leukomalacia and intraventricular hemorrhage[2,16]. Severe neonatal central nervous system damage is supposed to be caused by maternal mediators of infection: pro-inflammatory cytokines (interleukin (IL)-1, IL-6, IL-8, tumor necrosis factor-α(TNF-α)) and bacterial endotoxin[17]. The effects of fetal infection on the central nervous system have been reported in both term and preterm births[16].

PATHOGENESIS

There are three possible routes of intra-amniotic infection: ascension of bacteria from the lower genital tract, hematogenous spread of bacteria from maternal sources and iatrogenic bacterial invasion of the amniotic fluid at the time of invasive diagnostic procedures[1].

Most cases of intra-amniotic infection are ascending in origin. Endogenous flora of the lower genital tract might gain access to the amniotic cavity most commonly after prolonged rupture of the membranes and labor. However, passage of cervicovaginal bacteria may also occur in patients with intact fetal membranes[1].

The source of blood-borne intra-amniotic infection is maternal bacteremia. *Listeria monocytogenes*, group A streptococci and *Campylobacter* have been reported to cause hematogenous intra-amniotic infection[12].

Iatrogenic bacterial invasion of the amniotic cavity is associated either with invasive prenatal diagnostic procedures including amniocentesis, intrauterine transfusion and percutaneous umbilical blood sampling or with internal fetal monitoring after rupture of the fetal membranes[12].

Microbial invasion of the amniotic cavity might induce a host inflammatory response that causes release of cytokines from placental tissue, decidua, chorion and amnion[2]. Proinflammatory cytokines (IL-1, IL-6, IL-8, TNF-α) may stimulate the production of prostaglandins, which increase myometrial contractility, resulting in preterm labor[18].

Most fetuses that are exposed to microbial invasion of the amniotic fluid aspirate some of the infected fluid, leading to the biosynthesis of cytokines also by the fetus. These mediators of infection are thought to play a significant role in altered biophysical activity and the development of a systemic inflammatory response in the fetus[2].

MICROBIOLOGY

The micro-organisms involved in intra-amniotic infection are similar to those in other obstetric infections. In general, two groups of micro-organisms were noted in the amniotic fluid of patients with intra-amniotic infection. The first group of micro-organisms include members of the bacterial vaginosis-associated bacteria (*Gardnerella vaginalis*, genital mycoplasmas and anaerobes) while the second group consists of the gut-associated aerobic bacteria (*Escherichia coli*, Gram-negative rods and Gram-positive cocci)[19,20]. The overall prevalence of gut-associated bacteria in the amniotic fluid from patients with intra-amniotic infection seems to be lower than that of vaginosis-associated bacteria; however, two-thirds of maternal and/or fetal morbidity is associated with the former group of organisms[19,20]. The association of gut-associated bacteria with neonatal death due to sepsis is even more striking. These data might suggest that intra-amniotic infection with anaerobic bacteria is more likely to result in preterm labor or premature rupture of the membranes, whereas aerobic infection is more likely to cause serious maternal, fetal or neonatal morbidity.

DIAGNOSIS

The diagnosis of intra-amniotic infection is extremely difficult except for the clinically evident cases when a pregnant woman presents with preterm premature rupture of membranes with prolonged duration, fever and maternal and fetal tachycardia. However, a substantial proportion of cases are subclinical, with preterm labor being the only sign of intrauterine infection. In addition, the diagnosis is difficult because the signs and symptoms of infection lack specificity. To date, no satisfactory test for diagnosing intra-amniotic infection has been found.

Therefore, diagnosis of intra-amniotic infection rests on a high level of suspicion from the clinician in all cases when pregnant women with preterm labor who have at least one possible sign of infection present for evaluation. Since intra-amniotic infection affects the mother, her fetus and the whole intrauterine environment, diagnostic activities of the physician are aimed at collecting as much information as possible from the mother, the amniotic fluid, the fetus and – after delivery – the neonate, placenta and chorioamnion.

Clinical criteria

The classical signs and symptoms of clinical intra-amniotic infection have been fever before delivery (37.8 °C or more) without other known sites of infection, together with maternal and/or fetal tachycardia, uterine tenderness, leukocytosis in maternal peripheral blood and foul odor either of the amniotic fluid or of the vaginal discharge or the neonate. The clinical diagnosis is appropriate if the patient is febrile and two or more of these signs are present[12].

Reported prevalence of maternal fever in documented cases of intra-amniotic infection is higher than 90%. The diagnostic evaluation of a febrile pregnant woman should include a search for extragenital sources of infection with the highest probability of urinary tract infection. The specificity of maternal fever during labor might be altered by maternal dehydration.

Maternal and fetal tachycardia is an early sign of intra-amniotic infection; however, its sensitivity (30–80%) is less than that of maternal fever[21]. Besides infection, prematurity, fetal hypoxia, heart block and medication during labor can cause tachycardia in the fetus, whereas medication, dehydration and anxiety may be responsible for the condition in the mother.

Uterine tenderness is probably the least sensitive clinical sign of intra-amniotic infection, and is found in about 25% or less of patients with the disease. However, if tenderness of the myometrium also includes preterm uterine activity, this sign is more valuable in making the diagnosis.

In most cases, foul-smelling amniotic fluid and neonate is a strong clinical sign of established intrauterine infection. Involvement of anaerobic bacteria should always be considered.

Clinical criteria

The clinical approach to assessing the fetal condition in patients with suspected or established intra-amniotic infection before delivery involves two major methods: cardiotocography and ultrasound.

Cardiotocography is used to evaluate the fetal heart rate pattern at admission and for monitoring it during intrauterine life. Slight fetal tachycardia defined as above 160 beats/min represents an early sign of fetal infection. In addition, a non-reactive non-stress test (NST) is also pathognomonic [21,22].

Clinical data have shown that combined evaluation of fetal biophysical activities – fetal movements, fetal breathing movements and fetal tone – and the NST by cardiotocography are useful to demonstrate the systemic inflammatory response syndrome of the fetus in patients after preterm premature rupture of the membranes[2,22,23]. Unfortunately, very limited information is available in patients with intra-amniotic infection and intact membranes. Fetal breathing movements lasting for at least 30 s seem to be the best indication of absence of intra-amniotic infection. If fetal breathing movements last for less than 30 s, the degree of loss in fetal movements predicts fetal compromise. If both parameters are absent, intra-amniotic infection is present in 100% of cases. Thus, in clinical practice, biophysical assessment of the fetus by ultrasound is particularly valuable among patients with preterm premature rupture of the membranes to confirm or rule out fetal infection[22,23].

The etiology of depressed fetal biophysical activity is associated with the direct effects of maternal cytokines on the fetal central nervous system[2].

Laboratory criteria

Evaluation of laboratory tests is aimed at confirming or excluding maternal, amniotic fluid or fetal infection.

Laboratory evaluation of the mother

The most widely used tests include leukocyte count and differential white cell counts. Normal pregnancy is associated with a significant rise in white blood cells. Therefore, sensitivity and specificity are dependent on the cut-off value set to define normal ranges. Patients with clinical intra-amniotic infection often have a moderate leukocytosis (between 12 000 and 15 000/mm^3). Moreover, a shift towards immature leukocytes is also seen in the differential peripheral blood.

Erythrocyte sedimentation rate is not feasible for the diagnosis or monitoring of intra-amniotic infection because the changing concentration of plasma globulins during pregnancy will falsely increase the rate.

C-reactive protein is an acute phase protein which is produced by the liver in response to infection or tissue necrosis. Several studies have demonstrated that the use of this infection marker is valuable in the early diagnosis of intra-amniotic infection, and probably in screening for silent chorioamnionitis[7].

A wide range of bacteria present in the female lower genital tract have been linked with prematurity, preterm labor and premature rupture of membranes. Consequently, bacteriological examination of the cervix and vagina is always recommended in pregnant women with suspected intra-amniotic infection.

Laboratory evaluation of the amniotic fluid

The greatest specificity in the diagnosis of intra-amniotic infection is offered by laboratory examination of the amniotic fluid. Transabdominal amniocentesis under direct ultrasonic guidance will allow appropriate samples to be obtained for bacteriological culture, Gram staining, microscopy and biochemical tests.

Gram staining is performed from an uncentrifuged specimen of amniotic fluid to demonstrate the presence of bacteria. Despite contradictory results with regard to the association between a positive Gram stain and diagnosis of infection in unselected populations, a positive result is a valuable measure in the diagnosis of intra-amniotic infection[5,6,8]. A positive test is a sensitive method to detect a high inoculum size (10^5 CFU/ml) of microbes in the amniotic fluid.

The identification of polymorphonuclear leukocytes in the amniotic fluid has also been advocated for the diagnosis of intra-amniotic infection[5,6,8]. A correlation between leukocytic infiltration of amniotic fluid and clinical intra-amniotic infection and postpartum infectious morbidity has been reported by many authors. Other investigators, however, were unable to demonstrate this association. Recent studies have demonstrated that at least a proportion of polymorphonuclear leukocytes found in the amniotic fluid were fetal in origin[24].

Amniotic fluid culture for aerobic and anaerobic bacteria and genital mycoplasmas may offer the strongest evidence for the bacterial invasion of the amniotic cavity and a high risk for fetal infection. In clinical practice, however, waiting for the identification of the organisms involved might delay adequate therapeutic decisions. Therefore, bacteriological culture serves rather as further confirmation of data obtained through Gram staining and microscopy of amniotic fluid. Recently, the polymerase chain reaction to detect bacteria in amniotic fluid samples of patients with preterm labor has been reported to be a more sensitive method than culture[25].

Biochemical analysis of amniotic fluid in patients with suspected intra-amniotic infection is aimed to demonstrate either infectious markers produced by the maternal host and the fetus or the metabolites produced by the invading organisms. Maternal markers of infection include proinflammatory cytokines (IL-1α, IL-1β, IL-6, IL-8, TNF) and prostaglandin (PG)E$_2$.

Elevated levels of amniotic fluid cytokines and PGE$_2$ predict preterm delivery within 1 week of evaluation, amniotic fluid infection and histological chorioamnionitis[18]. Of these cytokines, IL-6 is the strongest predictor of adverse maternal and fetal outcome even in the absence or low level of microbial invasion or histological chorioamnionitis.

Biochemical analysis of amniotic fluid for the presence of bacterial metabolites includes the leukocyte-esterase test and detection of endotoxin. Both methods have been found to be simple and sensitive markers of infection. In addition, low levels of amniotic fluid glucose and the presence of organic metabolites of pathogenic bacteria of the lower genital tract diagnosed through gas liquid chromatography have also been reported as markers of intra-amniotic infection[12].

Laboratory evaluation of the fetus

An inflammatory response of the fetus to intra-amniotic infection may be detected by evaluation of infection markers in fetal blood collected by cordocentesis. Analysis of fetal blood gases, pH, complete white blood cell count, platelet count and differential cell count may be useful in assessing fetal involvement. Recent data suggest that elevated fetal plasma IL-6 is the best independent predictor of a systemic inflammatory response and neonatal morbidity[2].

CONCLUSIONS

In summary, intra-amniotic infection is a serious complication in pregnancy with potential maternal and fetal morbidity. Early diagnosis is essential to minimize late sequelae to both mother and fetus. A careful evaluation of all pregnant women presenting with either labor or membrane rupture, most notably before 37 completed weeks of gestation, and identification of possible risk factors for genital, genitourinary and intra-amniotic infection might result in suspicion of intra-amniotic infection. Once a presumptive diagnosis is established, diagnostic procedures should involve all available clinical and laboratory tests to assess maternal and fetal condition.

If intra-amniotic infection is clearly established, delivery is attempted with intrapartum antibiotic prophylaxis or treatment. At present, this seems to be the safest way to obtain access, to allow aggressive treatment of the neonate and the drainage of the infected uterine cavity.

References

1. Romero R, Sirtori M, Oyarzun E, *et al.* Prevalence, microbiology, and clinical significance of intraamniotic infection in women with preterm labor and intact membranes. *Am J Obstet Gynecol* 1988;161:817–24

2. Gomez R, Romero R, Ghezzi F, *et al.* The fetal inflammatory response syndrome. *Am J Obstet Gynecol* 1998;179:194–202

3. Rangel-Frausto M, Pittet D, Costigan M, *et al.* The natural history of the systemic inflammatory response syndrome (SIRS): a prospective study. *J Am Med Assoc* 1995;273:117–23

4. Naeye RL, Ross SM. Amniotic fluid infection syndrome. *Clin Obstet Gynecol* 1982;9:593–607

5. Bobitt JR, Hayslip CC, Damato JD. Amniotic fluid infection as determined by transabdominal amniocentesis in patients with intact membranes in premature labor. *Am J Obstet Gynecol* 1981; 140:947–52

6. Bobitt JR, Ledger WJ. Unrecognized amnionitis and prematurity: a preliminary report. *J Reprod Med* 1977;19:8–12

7. Hameed C, Tejani N, Verma U, *et al.* Silent chorioamnionitis as a cause of preterm labor refractory to tocolytic therapy. *Am J Obstet Gynecol* 1984;149:726–31

8. Listwa HM, Dobek AS, Carpenter J, *et al.* The predictability of intrauterine infection by analysis of amniotic fluid. *Obstet Gynecol* 1976;48:31–4

9. Greci LS, Gilson GJ, Nevils B, *et al.* Is amniotic fluid analysis the key to preterm labor? A model using interleukin-6 for predicting rapid delivery. *Am J Obstet Gynecol* 1998;179:172–8

10. Goldstein I, Zimmer EZ, Merzbach D, *et al.* Intraamniotic infection in the very early phase of the second trimester. *Am J Obstet Gynecol* 1990; 163:1261–3

11. Cassell GH, Davis RO, Waites KB, *et al.* Isolation of *Mycoplasma hominis* and *Ureaplasma urealyticum* from amniotic fluid at 16–20 weeks of gestation: potential effect on outcome of pregnancy. *Sex Transm Dis* 1983;10:294–302

12. Gibbs RS, Duff P. Progress in pathogenesis and management of clinical chorioamnionitis. *Am J Obstet Gynecol* 1991;164:1317–26

13. Morales WJ. The effect of chorioamnionitis on the developmental outcome of preterm infants at one year. *Obstet Gynecol* 1987;70:183–6

14. Naeye RL, Maisels MJ, Lorenz RP, Botti JJ. The clinical significance of placental villous edema. *Pediatrics* 1983;71:588–94

15. Naeye RL. Standardizing the mortality risk for newborns with very low birth weights. *Am J Dis Child* 1985;139:445–6

16. Grether JK, Nelson KB. Maternal infection and cerebral palsy in infants of normal birth weight. *J Am Med Assoc* 1997;278:207–11

17. Yoon BH, Romero R, Kim JC, *et al.* High expression of tumor necrosis factor-alpha and interleukin-6 in periventricular leukomalacia. *Am J Obstet Gynecol* 1997;177:406–11

18. Hillier SL, Witkin SS, Krohn MA, *et al.* The relationship of amniotic fluid cytokines and preterm delivery, amniotic fluid infection, histologic chorioamnionitis, and chorioamnion infection. *Obstet Gynecol* 1993;81:941–8

19. Silver HM, Sperling RS, St Clair PJ, *et al.* Evidence relating bacterial vaginosis to intraamniotic infection. *Am J Obstet Gynecol* 1989;161:808–12

20. Sperling RS, Newton E, Gibbs RS. Intra-amniotic infection in low-birth-weight infants. *J Infect Dis* 1988;157:113–17

21. Hager WD, Pauly TH. Fetal tachycardia as an indicator of maternal and neonatal morbidity. *Obstet Gynecol* 1985;66:191–4

22. Vintzeleos AM, Tsapanos V. Biophysical assessment of the fetus. *Ultrasound Obstet Gynecol* 1992; 2:133–43

23. Goldstein I, Romero R, Merrill S, *et al.* Fetal body and breathing movements as predictors of intraamniotic infection in preterm premature rupture of membranes. *Am J Obstet Gynecol* 1988; 159:363–8

24. Sampson JE, Theve RP, Blatman RN, *et al.* Fetal origin of amniotic fluid polymorphonuclear leukocytes. *Am J Obstet Gynecol* 1997;176:77–81

25. Markenson GR, Martin RK, Tillotson-Criss M, *et al.* The use of the polymerase chain reaction to detect bacteria in amniotic fluid in pregnancies complicated by preterm labor. *Am J Obstet Gynecol* 1997;177:1471–7

The assessment of fetal lung maturity 32

H. H. de Haan, S. Hundertmark, J. van Eyck and B. Arabin

INTRODUCTION

Neonates born with immature lungs have a high risk of developing respiratory distress syndrome (RDS). To prevent the mortality and morbidity associated with this serious condition when both fetal and maternal condition allow prolongation of pregnancy, assessment of fetal pulmonary maturity may help to optimize the timing of birth. This chapter focuses on the physiology of fetal lung maturation and discusses the available fetal lung maturity tests.

As the fetal lung matures, various elements are secreted into the amniotic fluid. The major component of lung secretion is a group of detergent compounds known as surfactant, consisting of a mixture of phospholipids (90%) and at least three surfactant proteins (SP) (10%), mainly SP-A, SP-B and SP-C. These are all released by the type II pneumocyte (Figure 1). Surfactant reduces surface tension at the air/fluid interface at the alveolar surface. The reduction of surface tension is achieved by forming a stable monolayer of surfactant phospholipids (Figure 1). These phospholipids can be further divided into lecithin (70%), phosphatidylglycerol (15%) and others (15%), whereas the proteins mainly consist of albumin. A crucial compound is dipalmytoyl-phosphatidylcholine (DPPC), the disaturated form of phosphatidylcholine (PC), that forms the stable monolayer at the internal alveolar surface (Figure 1). Lamellar bodies and tubular myelin are two morphological forms of surfactant called *heavy subtype surfactant* and are surface active. Used phospholipids which form small vesicles with reduced amounts of surfactant proteins, also called *light subtype surfactant*, are recycled by the type II pneumocyte (Figure 1)[1].

Surfactant stabilizes the alveoli at end-expiration. This prevents atelectasis and alveolar edema and secures an optimal surface area for gas exchange. Several factors influence the function of surfactant and the associated chance that neonatal respiratory support will be needed. Of these factors gestational age has the main influence. The probability that the neonate will develop respiratory distress decreases dramatically when gestational age increases. Poorly controlled diabetes mellitus has a negative impact on lung maturation. The underlying mechanism is imprecisely understood, but it has been speculated that fetal hyperinsulinemia plays an important role[2]. Although intrauterine infections raise endogenous corticosteroid levels and thus theoretically increase pulmonary maturity, pneumonia may damage lung tissue. In contrast to factors with a negative impact, endogenous stress, such as in severe intrauterine growth restriction, is supposed to have a beneficial effect. There is some evidence that infants born after this type of chronic stress are pulmonarily (and neurologically) more mature than 'unstressed' infants[3].

Liggins' original studies in fetal lambs demonstrated by serendipity that corticosteroid treatment accelerated fetal lung maturity. His group proceeded to perform a randomized controlled trial that proved the effectiveness of antenatal corticosteroid therapy in humans in reducing the incidence of RDS[4]. Extensive meta-analysis of studies reveals that administration of corticosteroids prior to preterm delivery reduces perinatal mortality and morbidity caused by RDS[5].

Additional experimental work in fetal lambs showed synergistic effects of thyro-

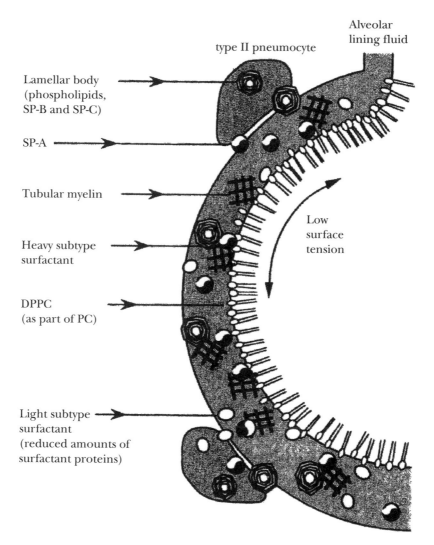

Figure 1 *Schematic model of surfactant production and function in a normal alveolus. DPPC (dipalmytoyl-phosphatidylcholine) is responsible for the reduction of alveolar surface tension. PC, phosphatidylcholine; SP-A, SP-B and SP-C, surfactant protein A, B and C, respectively. Modified according to Erasmus[1]*

tropin releasing hormone in combination with corticosteroids; both lung fluid phospholipid levels and lung distensibility were increased[6]. In clinical trials, however, antenatal administration of thyrotropin releasing hormone in combination with corticosteroids prior to preterm delivery has not shown significant benefit[7]. In fetal rat lungs, thyroid hormones improved morphological lung maturation but had a negative effect on surfactant synthesis. Glucocorticosteroids had the opposite effect; surfactant production was enhanced whereas morphological maturation

was inhibited. The combination of both thyroid hormones and glucocorticoids had the most negative effect on morphogenesis. This suggests that sequential administration of thyrotropin releasing hormone followed by corticosteroids may primarily lead to anatomical maturation, followed by physiological maturation (S. Hundertmark, personal communication).

Since the classic reports of Gluck and colleagues[8] and Clements and colleagues[9] various methods have been developed to evaluate fetal pulmonary maturity. Tests differ with respect to clinical reliability, time and experience required, costs and equipment needed. Accordingly, the clinical usefulness of these tests varies considerably.

TESTING METHODS

Foam test (foam stability index)

The foam stability index (or 'shake test' or 'bubble-stability test') is a cheap and easy method to assess fetal lung maturity and has been advocated as the first in a cascade of measurements. It is based on the tendency of aqueous surfactant to form foam when shaken in the presence of air. Alcohol suppresses this foaming. Larger concentrations of surfactant require larger concentrations of alcohol to suppress the foaming. It has been found that if an amniotic fluid sample continues to foam in the presence of 47.5% (or more) of alcohol, there is a small likelihood of RDS[9]. Therefore, a Foam Stability Index of 47.5 is taken as the cut-off for maturity. The test is subjective, since it involves visual assessment of the state of the foam formed. Vaginal secretions, blood and meconium interfere with the reproducibility of the test[9].

Lecithin/sphingomyelin ratio

The concentration of surfactant in amniotic fluid may vary throughout gestation, owing to differences in amniotic volume production. Measuring surfactant alone may lead to falsely elevated or falsely low levels, incorrectly reflecting fetal lung maturity. Lecithin and sphingomyelin are both phospholipids present in amniotic fluid. The concentration of sphingomyelin stays relatively constant during pregnancy, whereas that of lecithin increases as the lungs mature. The latter may thus serve as a constant internal reference, correcting for uncertainties due to different amniotic fluid volumes. The lecithin/ sphingomyelin ratio is measured after centrifugation, extraction and acetone precipitation of amniotic fluid, followed by tedious thin-layer chromatography, coloring and densitometry[8]. Owing to the multitude

of critical steps, the results of the test may vary from laboratory to laboratory. The test is time consuming and therefore relatively expensive, but it is still regarded as the classic test to detect lung maturity, since it is relatively independent of additional substances in the amniotic fluid.

Phosphatidylglycerol

Phosphatidylglycerol is a minor phospholipid secreted by the lung. It is found in amniotic fluid only after the lungs are fully mature, and even then it is not always detected. Its measurement is useful in diabetic pregnancies, where the lecithin/sphingomyelin ratio may falsely predict fetal lung maturity[10]. It is measured by thin-layer chromatography or by a simple slide (latex) immunoagglutination assay (Amniostat®) and is reported as either 'present' or 'absent'. The immunoagglutination test is quick and easy to perform. In pregnant diabetic patients at term phosphatidylglycerol was reported to be undetectable in 21%[11].

Surfactant/albumin ratio

Instead of determining the lecithin/ sphingomyelin ratio, where only lecithin is measured in surfactant, the commercially available TDx Fetal Lung Maturity II assay measures the entire amount of surfactant (i.e. all phospholipids, including other surface-active compounds which form the surfactant aggregate) by fluorescent polarization. Thereby, the concentration of albumin is used as a constant internal reference. A fluorescent dye is added to amniotic fluid. This dye is structurally similar to lecithin and therefore has binding and solubility characteristics similar to those of surfactant-associated phospholipids in amniotic fluid (i.e. high affinity for hydrophobic regions of liposomal aggregates). However, because the dye also exhibits high affinity for endogenous proteins such as albumin, it is partitioned between phospholipids and endogenous albumin. When the probe is bound to albumin, net polarization values are high, whereas when the

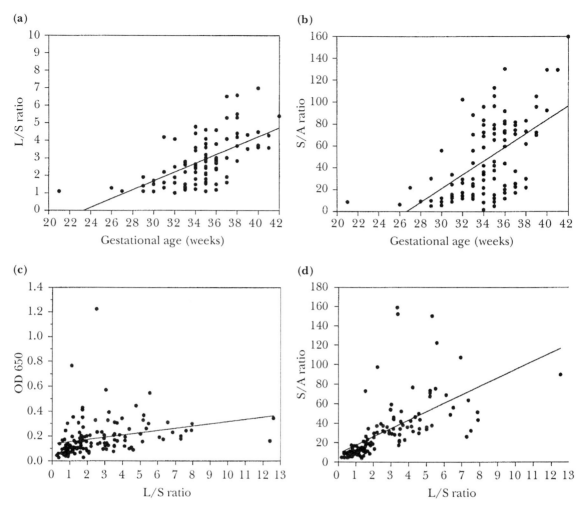

Figure 2 *Distribution of lecithin/sphingomyelin (L/S) ratio (a) determined by thin-layer chromatography and the surfactant/albumin (S/A) ratio (b) determined by TDx, all obtained by amniocentesis at various gestational ages according to Ragosch and colleagues[21,22]. Correlation of values determined by optical density (OD) of amniotic fluid at 650 nm with the L/S ratio (c): y = 0.16 + 0.02 x (r = 0.27) and of the S/A ratio determined by TDx with the L/S ratio (d): y = 8.88 + 8.62 x, (r = 0.61) (own values of the same amniotic fluid samples)*

probe is associated with liposomes, net polarization values are low. Thus, the overall polarization measured by the analyzer reflects the ratio of surfactant to albumin in the sample, which increases with gestational age (Figure 2b). The actual value is established by generating a standard curve, composed of calibrators of known surfactant/albumin ratios. It appears that with a ratio greater than 70 mg surfactant per gram albumin there is little likelihood of RDS, although various authors use different cut-off values[12–15]. The instrumentation required is available in virtually all laboratories, and the test can be performed in less than an hour, with small intra-assay and inter-assay variations[13]. High levels of amniotic fluid albumin may be encountered in fetuses suffering from neural tube defects, leading to a false-negative test result. The surfactant/albumin ratio measured by the TDx Fetal Lung Maturity II assay correlates well with the lecithin/sphingomyelin ratio (Figure 2d) and has few falsely mature results (Table 1). In addition, the test is rapid and easy and therefore excellent for screening.

Table 1 *Characteristics of the various fetal lung maturity tests*

Test	Method	Cut-off value	Variation	Time-lag	Cost	Sensitivity (%)	Specificity (%)	PPV (%)	NPV (%)	Fluid required (ml)	Reference no.
Foam test	alcohol suppresses foaming	47.5 (Foam Stability Index)	large (subjective interpretation)	short	low	?	?	?	?	2.0	9,12
L/S ratio	chromatography	2	complicated process	>3 h	high (tedious, manpower)	48–86	60–89	53	86	5.0	13,14,17
Phosphatidylglycerol	chromatography or immunoagglutination	+ or –		<1 h	depending on reagents	84–92	51–71	40	95	1.5	10,11,13
S/A ratio	fluorescent dye, polarization curve	55–70	small	<1 h	fluorescent polarization	89–96	50–73	47	96	1.0	13,14,15,22
Lamellar body count	platelet counter (/μl)	> 30 000 < 10 000	small (equipment, centrifugation)	<1 h	low	75	95	67	96	1.0	16
OD 650	light absorbance	>0.25	contamination by meconium, blood	<1 h	low	50	94	89	67	1.0	12,17

PPV, positive predictive value; NPV, negative predictive value; L/S, lecithin/sphingomyelin; S/A, surfactant/albumin; OD, optical density

Lamellar body count

Lamellar bodies are concentrically layered structures released by type II pneumocytes. They consist almost entirely of phospholipids and represent the storage form of pulmonary surfactant. As the fetal lung matures, increased lamellar body production is reflected by an increase in amniotic fluid phospholipids and the lecithin/sphingomyelin ratio. Because lamellar bodies and platelets are indistinguishable to cell counters, the lamellar body count is obtained by analysis of the amniotic fluid sample with a cell counter and recorded as platelet count[16]. Advantages of the test include speed, objectivity, small sample volume required and universal availability of the necessary instrumentation. Neither meconium nor autolyzed blood has a significant effect on the lamellar body count. The cut-off value used to predict fetal pulmonary status depends on the type of cell counter and the speed of centrifugation.

Optical density of amniotic fluid at 650 nm

This test measures the turbidity of amniotic fluid. Mainly owing to the presence of lamellar bodies and phosphatidylglycerol, the turbidity increases as pregnancy approaches term. Absorbance at various wavelengths has been proposed, and at 650 nm interference by pigments, meconium, hemolyzed blood or bilirubin seems minimal. A sample is centrifuged at room temperature. The supernatant is placed in a small cuvette and its absorbance is determined, using a spectrophotometer against a control of de-ionized water, within 1 h of obtaining the specimen. Measurement of the optical density of amniotic fluid at 650 nm is simple, fast and inexpensive, and requires only common laboratory instruments[12,17]. Owing to the speed and low volume required, the test acts as a rapid screening test in clinical routine. However, our own data show a poor correlation between values for OD 650 and the lecithin/sphingomyelin ratio within the same specimen (Figure 2c).

Ultrasound

By means of ultrasonography the density of fetal lung tissue was evaluated throughout gestation and compared with the simultaneously calculated liver density[18]. Although this would allow determination of fetal lung maturity non-invasively, the diagnostic value of the method remains to be elucidated.

GENERAL CONSIDERATIONS OF THE DIAGNOSTIC VALUE OF THE VARIOUS TESTS

Determination of fetal lung maturity is clinically of value at a gestational age of approximately 26 to 36 weeks. The diagnostic value depends not only on the method used but more importantly on the gestational age at testing and the associated variation in prevalence. The prevalence for RDS is 60%, 30%, 10% and 1% for a gestational age of 29, 32, 35 and 37 weeks, respectively. For the lecithin/sphingomyelin ratio this means that an absolute value of < 2 is associated with a higher probability of RDS if detected at 27 weeks than at 35 weeks (Figure 3). Since gestational age-dependent differences in the

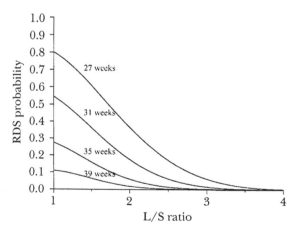

Figure 3 *The probability of developing respiratory distress syndrome (RDS) depends on the gestational age at testing. In the presence of an amniotic fluid lecithin/sphingomyelin ratio of, for example, 2, the chance the newborn will be affected by RDS decreases from 35% at 27 weeks' gestation to 15%, 5% and 2% at 31, 35 and 39 weeks' gestation, respectively. From reference 19*

prevalence of RDS have been considered in only a limited number of publications, there is a large variation in the calculated predictive value of the various tests. Quite often gestational age is not even mentioned in the respective papers, as discussed by a number of authors[13,19,20]. In practice, a positive test result at a gestational age of 29–31 weeks is still associated with a 30% chance that RDS will occur. After 35 weeks' gestation the chance of RDS with a positive test result is less than 10%[19,20]. Given a negative test result the chance that RDS will develop varies from 84% at 29 weeks' gestation, and 60% at 32 weeks' gestation, to 27% at 35 weeks' gestation. Beyond 37 weeks' gestation negative and positive test results have similar chances (around 3%) of predicting eventual RDS. Assessment of fetal pulmonary maturity beyond 37 weeks' gestation therefore has no clinical use.

Determining the diagnostic value of the various tests in predicting RDS also implies that the time interval between test and delivery with subsequent diagnosis or exclusion of RDS is short. In general, an interval of 3 days or less is accepted. Papers need to address this so-called verification bias.

Data from our group show a gradual increase in both the lecithin/sphingomyelin ratio (Figure 2a) and the surfactant/albumin ratio (Figure 2b) when gestational age increases, although there is a considerable variability. The correlation between both ratios is reasonable ($r = 0.60$) (Figure 2d).

There are several statistical methods for comparing the diagnostic value of tests in predicting RDS. Sensitivity and specificity can be used and simple comparisons with standard lecithin/sphingomyelin ratios can be performed. The more advanced receiver operator characteristics consider the variation in both sensitivity and specificity to detect RDS, but also different cut-off levels, and are therefore ideal when new tests are introduced into clinical routine[21].

Table 1 shows the variation in sensitivity, specificity and positive and negative predictive values. Cut-off levels between studies vary. The number of neonates in the reported studies

suffering from well-documented RDS is mostly limited, as is the number of specimens from pregnancies in which delivery occurs within a time interval of less than 3 days.

Chromatographic methods, such as the lecithin/sphingomyelin ratio, are reasonably reliable but labor-intensive, lengthy and technique-dependent. Furthermore, the phospholipid profile, the lecithin/sphingomyelin ratio and the OD 650 may be invalidated by contamination with meconium or blood. Phosphatidylglycerol develops only late in gestation, limiting its value at the (clinically more important) earlier gestational ages.

In conclusion, a large number of techniques are now available to assess fetal pulmonary maturation. Rapid screening tests such as the TDx Fetal Lung Maturity II assay, the lamellar body count, OD 650, or Amniostat appear to be reliable to indicate lung maturity and are therefore ideal screening tests. The determination of a lecithin/sphingomyelin ratio in these cases is not mandatory. Owing to the multitude of etiological factors determining fetal pulmonary maturity, a perfect single test is not available. Therefore, a protocol of testing has been proposed in which a sequence of fetal lung maturity tests is carried out. If one of the rapid tests suggests fetal lung maturity, the sequence is terminated and no further test is done[22,23]. This stepwise approach is time- and cost-effective. However, in cases with negative results from the 'rapid' tests, as well as in complicated pregnancies such as after intrauterine growth restriction, diabetes mellitus, or Rhesus-immunization, the lecithin/sphingomyelin ratio is still the method of choice in most units.

It must be mentioned that lung maturity testing is of limited value in a perinatal unit in many cases. In all pregnancies threatened with early intrauterine demise, the obstetrician is forced to terminate pregnancy regardless of lung maturity testing, resulting in iatrogenic prematurity. In many cases with threatening premature labor the perinatologist would try to prolong pregnancy for as long as possible. Nevertheless, there might be situations in which knowledge of lung maturity would facilitate active termination of pregnancy and thus prevent possible intrauterine damage due to hypoxia or interleukins[24], or long-term sequelae due to intrauterine growth deficiencies[25]. Vice versa, there are situations, such as in questionable lengths of gestation, diabetes and various indications of elective termination, where knowing fetal lung immaturity would prevent untimely delivery, the associated neonatal morbidity and unnecessary separation of mother and child.

ACKNOWLEDGEMENTS

The cooperation and help of Dr J.G.C. van de Meene, Dr J.J.C.M. van de Leur, Dr E. Kuipers and J. Otten from the Department of Clinical Chemistry is greatly appreciated. The Clara Angela Foundation has been very supportive.

References

1. Erasmus ME. *Pulmonary surfactant and lung transplantation.* Thesis, Groningen, the Netherlands 1997:10–14
2. Piper JM, Langer O. Does maternal diabetes delay fetal pulmonary maturity? *Am J Obstet Gynecol* 1993;168:783–6
3. Amiel-Tison C, Pettigrew AG. Adaptive changes in the developing brain during intrauterine stress. *Brain Dev* 1991;13:67–76
4. Liggins GC, Howie RN. A controlled trial of antepartum glucocorticoid treatment for prevention of the respiratory distress syndrome in premature infants. *Pediatrics* 1972;50:515–25
5. Crowley P. Corticosteroids prior to preterm delivery (Cochrane review). *The Cochrane Library,* Issue 2. Oxford: Update Software, 1998
6. Liggins GC, Schellenberg JC, Manzai M, Kitterman JA, Lee CC. Synergisms of cortisol and thyrotropin releasing hormone in lung maturation in fetal sheep. *J Appl Physiol* 1988; 65:1880–4
7. Crowther CA, Alfirevic Z, Haslam RR. Antenatal thyrotropin-releasing hormone (TRH) prior to preterm delivery (Cochrane review). In *The Cochrane Library,* Issue 2. Oxford: Update Software, 1998
8. Gluck L, Kulovich MV, Borer RC, Brenner PH, Anderson GG, Spellacy WN. Diagnosis of the respiratory distress syndrome by amniocentesis. *Am J Obstet Gynecol* 1971;109:440–5
9. Clements JA, Platzker ACG, Tierney DF, *et al.* Assessment of the risk of the respiratory distress syndrome by a rapid test for surfactant in amniotic fluid. *N Engl J Med* 1972;286:1077–81
10. Amon E, Lipshitz J, Sibai BM, Addella TN, Whybrew DW, El-Nazer A. Quantitative analysis of amniotic fluid phospholipids in diabetic women. *Obstet Gynecol* 1986;68:373–8
11. Ojomo EO, Coustan DR. Absence of evidence of pulmonary maturity at amniocentesis in term infants of diabetic mothers. *Am J Obstet Gynecol* 1990;163:954–7
12. Oulton M, Fraser M, Robinson S. Correlation of absorbance at 650 nm with the presence of phosphatidylglycerol in amniotic fluid. *J Reprod Med* 1990;35:402–6
13. Hagen E, Link JC, Arias F. A comparison of the accuracy of the TDx-FLM assay, lecithin–sphingomyelin ratio, and phosphatidylglycerol in the prediction of neonatal respiratory distress syndrome. *Obstet Gynecol* 1993;82:1004–8
14. Herbert WNP, Chapman JF, Schnoor MM. Role of the TDx FLM assay in fetal lung maturity. *Am J Obstet Gynecol* 1993;168:808–12
15. Livingston EG, Herbert WNP, Hage ML, Chapman JF, Stubbs TM. Use of the TDx-FLM assay in evaluating fetal lung maturity in an insulin-dependent diabetic population. *Obstet Gynecol* 1995;86:826–9
16. Dalence CR, Bowie LJ, Dohnal JC, Farrell EE, Neerhof MG. Amniotic fluid lamellar body count: a rapid and reliable fetal lung maturity test. *Obstet Gynecol* 1995;86:235–9
17. Tsai MY, Josephson MW, Knox GE. Absorbance of amniotic fluid at 650 nm as a fetal lung maturity test: a comparison with the lecithin/sphingomyelin ratio and tests for disaturated phosphatidylcholine and phosphatidylglycerol. *Am J Obstet Gynecol* 1983;146:963–6
18. Sohn C, Stolz W, Bastert G. Erste Ergebnisse einer neuen Methode zur sonographischen Lungereifediagnostik. *Untraschall Med* 1992;13:37–40
19. Hunink MG, Richardson DK, Doubilet PM, Begg CB. Testing for pulmonary maturity: ROC analysis involving covariates, verification bias, and combination testing. *Med Decis Making* 1990;10: 201–11
20. Dubin SB. Assessment of fetal lung maturity by laboratory methods. *Clin Lab Med* 1992;12: 603–20

21. Ragosch V, Jurgens S, Lorenz U, Arabin B, Weitzel HK. Prediction of RDS by amniotic fluid analysis: a comparison of the prognostic value of traditional and recent methods. *J Perinat Med* 1992;20:351–60

22. Ragosch V, Hundertmark S, Stolowsky C, Lorenz U, Arabin B, Weitzel HK. Antepartale Lungenreifebestimmung aus dem Fruchtwasser-Indikationen und neue Methoden. *Geburtsh Frauenheilk* 1994; 54:679–84

23. Bender TM, Stone LR, Amenta JS. Diagnostic power of lecithin/sphingomyelin ratio and fluorescence polarization assays for respiratory distress syndrome compared by relative operating characteristic curves. *Clin Chem* 1994;40:541–5

24. Gomez R, Romero R, Ghezzi F, Hyun Yoon B, Mazor M, Berry SM. The fetal inflammatory response syndrome. *Am J Obstet Gynecol* 1998;179: 194–202

25. Barker JDP. *Mothers, Babies and Health in Later Life*. Churchill Livingstone, 1998

Umbilical cord nucleated red cell count as an index of intrauterine hypoxia

33

F. Saraçoğlu

INTRODUCTION

The Apgar score is still the most widely used criterion for defining perinatal asphyxia or hypoxia, although it is poorly correlated with metabolic acidosis at birth and with the risk of long-term neurological damage[1-4]. Neurologic outcome also seems to be correlated poorly with acidosis at birth diagnosed by cord blood pH measurements, still considered the gold standard of obstetric care[4,5].

Because of the close correlation between abnormal umbilical artery blood flow in Doppler studies and fetal acid–base derangement, the need for an evaluation of fetal acid–base status has been disputed. However the absence of end-diastolic velocities may precede fetal death by several weeks, and antepartum improvements of Doppler waveforms may occur in up to 16% of fetuses[5]. Therefore, fetal hypoxemia and/or acidemia are late features of abnormal blood flow. Even if acid–base determination does not discriminate between the fetuses which will die and those which will survive[5], blood pH is still considered the gold standard of indications for delivery.

As demonstrated in previous studies, nucleated red blood cell (NRBC) counts and serum erythropoietin levels in cord blood are closely associated with pH[5]. It has also been noted that the NRBC count may be a better index of hypoxic tissue damage than blood pH[6]. Both NRBC count and erythropoietin levels were elevated in cases complicated by maternal diabetes mellitus, hypertension, red blood cell isoimmunization, prematurity, intrauterine growth restriction (IUGR) and asphyxia[4-7]. The time required to produce a rise in NRBC count is unknown, but appears to be relatively short in light of the rapidity of the response observed in those with uterine rupture[7].

In the absence of an asphyxial event, pre-existing IUGR, maternal diabetes, Rh-isoimmunization or prematurity could produce an elevated NRBC count. This could confuse the clinical picture and make it difficult to determine whether one of these fetuses is affected by asphyxia or not. In these conditions the clearance rate of NRBCs would be helpful.

BACKGROUND

Nucleated red blood cells are immature erythrocytes that were first noted in 1871 to be present in the blood of neonates[8]. Until weeks 6 and 7 of gestation, all fetal red blood cells are nucleated. By the end of the first trimester, NRBC counts decline and are uncommon in the circulation of term newborns.

The incidence and significance at term of NRBCs has been a matter of controversy for 70 years, but authors have written that fetal NRBCs signify fetal hypoxia[9]. In 1924, Lippman[10] stated: 'Geissler and Japha, Hayem and Loos conclude that NRBCs do not occur normally in newborn blood and their presence must be considered a pathological finding'. According to Lippman, no newborn had demonstrable NRBCs on the 5th postnatal day. Green and Mimouni[12] also found that, in the absence of hemolysis or blood loss, a postnatal NRBC count of $> 1 \times 10^9/l$ should be considered as a potential index of intrauterine asphyxia. Many laboratories report NRBCs according to the number of these immature red cells per 100 white blood cells. However, sometimes this does not reflect the newborn's total nucleated red cells. Therefore, Benitz from Stanford Medical Center has provided some formulas for conversion of white blood cell counts to NRBCs per liter. The calculations are based on a NRBC count of 7 per 100 white blood cells, a corrected white blood cell count of 57 500/mm^3 and absolute white blood cell count of 61 500/mm^3 (Table 1)[9].

There is great concern about using the white blood cells as a denominator in determining the significance in counting the NRBCs. Many factors may influence the number of white blood cells, and these might either contribute to or compete with the significance of NRBCs. They include stress factors that might increase NRBCs but at the same time cause the white blood cells to increase[8]. Another important condition, fetal sepsis, might cause the white blood cells to decrease while creating a clinical condition that would enhance the risk of hypoxia.

STUDY OF NUCLEATED RED CELL COUNT AND FETAL HYPOXIA

The NRBC data were calculated in the following manner: a complete blood cell count was performed in the hospital hematology laboratory in the cord blood obtained at delivery or by cordocentesis. The total white blood cell count was initially determined. The number of NRBCs was determined by an examination of the blood smear from the differential white blood cell count. The white

Table 1 *Calculations of nucleated red blood cell (NRBC) counts from accompanying white blood cell count*

Simplest calculation of absolute NRBC count
WBC = CWBC + NRBC
NRBC = WBC − CWBC
$\quad$ = 61 500/μl − 57 500/μl
$\quad$ = 4000/μl

Correction of WBC to CWBC
CWBC = WBC × 100/(100 + NRBC per 100 WBC)
$\quad$ = 61 500/μl × 100/100 + 7
$\quad$ = 57 500/μl
This confirms that relative NRBC count was 7/100 WBC

Alternative calculation of absolute NRBC count
NRBC = WBC × NRBC per 100 WBC
$\quad$ = 57 500/μl × 7/100
$\quad$ = 4000/μl

WBC, absolute, uncorrected white blood cell count; CWBC, corrected white blood cell count after adjustment by technologist who counts the number of NRBCs in a smear of 100 or 200 white blood cells

blood cell count was then corrected for the NRBC count. The number of NRBCs per 100 white blood cells is expressed as the NRBC count.

Normal, non-asphyxiated newborns had a mean ± SD of 3.4 ± 3.9 NRBC with a range of 0–12 NRBCs[7,8,11]. Table 2 shows the normative data for the NRBC counts in healthy term neonates. In the normal newborn the number of NRBCs is dependent on the gestational age of the fetus. With advancing gestational age there is a decline in the NRBC count: 90% of normal term neonates have circulating NRBCs of < 1 × 10^9/l at 12–24 h of age. Studies suggest that a value greater than this number

Table 2 *Reported normative data in term infants for nucleated red blood cells (NRBC) per 100 white blood cells (WBC). Mean ± SD*

Authors	n	NRBC/100 WBC
Sinha *et al.* (1972)[26]	84	2.3 ± 0.6
Shivhare *et al.* (1976)[27]	33	4.1 ± 2.4
Green *et al.* (1990)[12]	102	1.7 ± 6.2
Phelan *et al.* (1995)[7]	83	3.4 ± 3.0
Hanlon-Lundberg *et al.* (1997)[8]	1112	8.5 ± 10.25
Saraçoğlu *et al.* (1998)[11]	45	8.5 ± 10.27

Table 3 *Mean nucleated red blood cell (NRBC) count, pH, po₂ and pco₂ values of the study and the control groups and statistical analysis*

	Control	AFD	CFD	*p* Value Control vs. AFD	*p* Value Control vs. CFD	*p* Value AFD vs. CFD
NRBC (per 100 WBC)	7.56 ± 3.85	11.18 ± 4.92	24.43 ± 20.05	< 0.05	< 0.005	< 0.01
pH	7.28 ± 0.67	7.27 ± 0.82	7.20 ± 0.12	> 0.05	< 0.05	> 0.05
po_2 (mmHg)	25.53 ± 11.71	21.51 ± 5.74	17.85 ± 8.69	> 0.05	< 0.01	> 0.05
pco_2 (mmHg)	47.96 ± 10.07	53.47 ± 8.99	60.54 ± 20.66	> 0.05	< 0.05	> 0.05
Hemoglobin (g/dl)	15.46 ± 1.73	14.05 ± 3.38	16.42 ± 1.39	> 0.05	> 0.05	> 0.05
Leukocytes (× 10³/mm³)	13.04 ± 3.10	16.72 ± 8.84	17.42 ± 10.03	> 0.05	< 0.05	> 0.05

AFD, acute fetal distress; CFD, chronic fetal distress; WBC, white blood cells

in the absence of hemolysis or blood loss, although still possibly seen in 10% of healthy term neonates, should be considered as a potential index of intrauterine hypoxia[12]. We prospectively studied 77 pregnant women delivered at Ankara Numune Research and Training Hospital[11]. The study group was evaluated in two subgroups: acute and chronic fetal distress. The acute fetal distress group (AFD) consisted of 11 women who did not have signs of chronic fetal hypoxia such as abnormal fetal heart rate (FHR) tracings during the antenatal period, IUGR, oligohydramnios or abnormal Doppler findings. Even these women had a normal antenatal period. During delivery, acute fetal distress, determined by FHR tracings (late or deep variable decelerations, prolonged bradycardia), occurred because of various reasons such as cord occlusion, hypertonic uterus, premature rupture of the membranes (PROM), abnormal presentation or prolonged delivery. The chronic fetal distress (CFD) group included 21 women who had disorders of placental perfusion and showed the signs of chronic fetal hypoxia listed above. Mean NRBC counts were found to be 11.18 ± 4.92 per 100 WBC for the AFD group, and 24.43 ± 20.05 for the CFD group (Table 3). Both of the values were significantly higher than that of the control group. In addition, the mean NRBC count was significantly higher in CFD cases than in the AFD group. We also found a significant negative correlation between NRBC counts and umbilical arterial pH. This association implies that NRBC counts may also predict the severity of the condition.

We found that the NRBC count correlated well with pH. The correlation coefficient between NRBC and pH was −0.57 ($p < 0.001$). In order to evaluate whether the number of NRBCs could be a marker of fetal acidosis, a receiver operating characteristics (ROC) graph was drawn (Figure 1). A value of pH lower than 7.20 was accepted as a positive test. The sensitivity and specificity of various levels of NRBC counts were calculated. An ideal curve of a reasonable test should be placed on the upper left triangle of the ROC graph. This presumption was accomplished, as seen

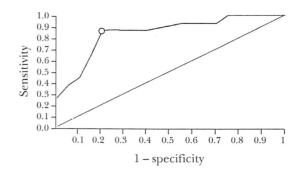

Figure 1 *Receiver operating characteristic (ROC) graph to discriminate the acidotic infants from non-acidotic infants. The circle marks the level of the maximum sensitivity with a minimum false-positive rate, which establishes the cut-off value as 14*

in the figure. The cut-off value for NRBC counts predicting fetal acidosis was established as 14, the value that provided the maximum sensitivity with a minimum false-positive rate. When the NRBC count was > 14 the sensitivity of predicting fetal acidosis was 86.67% and the specificity was 80.65%.

DISCUSSION

Nicolaides and co-workers[13,14] determined the fetal blood NRBC count and reticulocyte counts in umbilical cord samples obtained by cordocentesis at 17–36 weeks' gestation from pregnancies complicated by red blood cell isoimmunization. The reticulocyte counts increased linearly with fetal anemia and the NRBC count increased exponentially. When the hemoglobin deficit was over 7 g/dl, at which tissue hypoxia occurs, the increase in NRBC count was more significant[12].

In pregnancy complicated by red blood cell isoimmunization, the fetus is subjected to varying degrees of anemic hypoxia and compensation with cardiovascular adjustments (increased fetal cardiac output and tissue perfusion) and increased erythropoiesis. The life span of fetal red blood cells is reduced, because antibody-coated red blood cells are destroyed in the reticuloendothelial system[13,14].

The NRBC count is an indirect measure of extramedullary (liver) hematopoiesis, whereas reticulocytes are the product of both medullary and extramedullary erythropoiesis. Reticulocytosis in the absence of an increase in NRBC count indicates that the fetus responds to mild or moderate degrees of anemia by stimulating intramedullary hematopoiesis[13].

Maternal diabetes mellitus is also associated with increased levels of erythropoietin and NRBC count[8,15]. The suggested mechanism is the disturbed metabolic state of diabetes, including hyperglycemia, which produces relative hypoxia, with activation of the erythropoietin–hematopoiesis system (Figure 2).

Growth-restricted fetuses are at increased risk of intrauterine death, premature delivery,

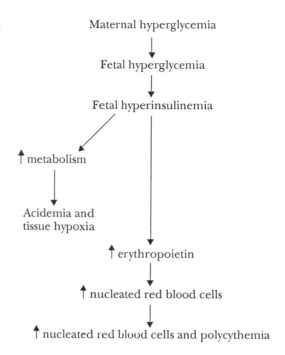

Figure 2 *Suggested mechanism for producing elevated nucleated red blood cell counts and polycythemia in pregnancies complicated by maternal diabetes mellitus*

fetal distress in labor and asphyxia at birth as a result of abnormal gas exchange and decreased transport of nutrients across the maternal–placental interface[16], all of which lead to increased perinatal mortality and long-term morbidity[17]. Several previous studies in growth-restricted infants also showed higher NRBC counts[17–19]. Allstair and co-workers[18] reported that growth-restricted fetuses weighing 500–1500 g and admitted to the neonatal intensive care units in the first 24 h after birth with elevated NRBCs did not return to normal until after 3–12 days. If the growth-restricted fetuses have no continuing postnatal hypoxic stimulus, postnatal decrease of elevated NRBCs is the rule[3]. The explanation for the elevated NRBC counts of small-for-gestational-age fetuses includes erythropoietin-induced premature release of red blood cells from the bone marrow, recruitment of hepatic erythropoiesis or a delay in the switch from hepatic to marrow erythropoiesis[19].

Soothill and co-workers[17] sampled the umbilical venous blood by cordocentesis at 21–36 weeks' gestation in 35 consecutive pregnancies in which intrauterine growth restriction was diagnosed in their hospital. The oxygen tension of the 38 fetuses was significantly lower than that of the controls, and significant positive correlations with NRBC counts was found. The mean NRBC count fell from 72/100 WBC at 16 weeks' gestation to 25 at 23 weeks and remained at a similar value thereafter. There was also evidence of red blood cell destruction and liver damage[20]. Because of the chronic hypoxia, a fetal 'hibernation' state occurs as an adaptation. This concept is supported by biophysical observations (for example, loss of breathing activity, reduced fetal movements and tone). Growth-restricted fetuses are in a low energy state, with low fetal glucose and insulin concentrations, both in basal conditions and after a glucose challenge[5]. Therefore, the fetal response to reduced placental transfer of oxygen is a complex process, which a single determination of acid–base balance is unlikely to be able to express. Indeed, the best prediction of perinatal outcome at one test was achieved by the combination of the degree of growth restriction and the NRBC count[16]. Both these features probably reflect the duration and/ or extent of the reduction in fetal oxygen supply and may better indicate the end stage of fetal adaptation.

Meconium may be a marker of intrauterine stress and it is also associated with higher NRBC counts[8,21]. Erythropoietin levels have been found to be elevated in cases where meconium is present at term[8]. When erythropoietin is elevated, NRBC counts would be expected to rise in response over time. The passage of meconium and rise in erythropoietin with subsequent elevation of NRBCs may be in response to the same stress, intrauterine hypoxia.

Naeye and Localio[22] suggested that the NRBC count in the blood of neonates may identify the time before birth when brain-damaging ischemia or hypoxia occurred. In their data NRBC counts increased to 2000/mm^3 or more within 2 h after brain-damaging ischemia, and normal infants had NRBC counts of $560 \pm 771/mm^3$. Intrauterine hypoxia is a known risk factor for intraventricular hemorrhage[22], injury involving the cerebral cortex and brain stem[24]. Clinical studies of hypoxic-ischemic injuries in the central nervous system (CNS) of neonates have demonstrated sequelae in approximately 30% of the surviving children[24]. Additionally, significant correlations have been demonstrated between CNS signs in neonates and subsequent long-term motor and cognitive handicap[24]. Green and co-workers[23] also showed that an elevated or increasing NRBC count in a preterm newborn might be a marker for intraventricular hemorrhage. NRBC counts were consistent with the finding that 90% of all cases of intraventricular hemorrhage occur in the first 72 h of life[23].

Korst and colleagues[25] compared NRBC counts from 153 term neurologically impaired infants with the counts of 83 term non-asphyxiated infants. They found that the count of the neurologically impaired group was significantly higher. Their data also showed that NRBC levels might assist in determining the timing of fetal neurological injury. The time required to produce the elevation in NRBC count remains unknown, but appears to be relatively short in light of the rapidity of the response observed in the acute groups[25]. However, some studies could not establish the degree and duration of hypoxia that would result in CNS injury[24].

A large body of data suggesting that abnormal umbilical artery Doppler studies are associated with fetal asphyxia and adverse outcome has been accumulated in the 1980s and 1990s. Because of these findings, Bernstein and associates[16] checked the umbilical artery Doppler velocity waveforms of 52 growth-restricted fetuses with elevated NRBC counts. They observed that elevated NRBC counts were associated with abnormal umbilical artery Doppler waveforms. There were no correlations of cord blood gases with the NRBC count, arterial or venous base excess. However, they reported that absent or reversed end-diastolic velocity and birth weight were significant, independent determinants of the NRBC count. Nicolini and colleagues[5] also examined the association between umbilical artery Doppler waveforms and NRBC counts, in 46 growth-restricted fetuses that were structurally and chromosomally normal. They found that those with absent end-diastolic velocity had significantly lower levels of venous pH, po_2 and base excess and higher levels of pco_2 and NRBC counts. They therefore concluded that, among growth-restricted newborns, the response to increased placental impedance includes an elevation in NRBCS. Increased thrombotic events in the placenta as evidenced by decreased platelet counts may be responsible for the increased placental impedance to blood flow demonstrated by Doppler ultrasonography, fetal growth restriction and the failure of asphyxia to affect fetal hemoglobin content. Therefore, they hypothesized that the neonatal complete blood cell count combined with umbilical artery Doppler velocimetry is useful in distinguishing a normally grown small-for-gestational-age neonate from one with placental insufficiency.

CONCLUSIONS

In light of the data reviewed above, it can be concluded that NRBC counts might be a useful marker in determining both the duration and the degree of asphyxial insult. Cord blood NRBC counts may be obtained non-invasively and analyzed by personnel without any requirement for complicated training or equipment. This can be widely used for the purpose of predicting fetal hypoxia, instead of other complicated and relatively expensive tests. If NRBC counts are obtained during the antepartum period by cordo-centesis, they may play a role in deciding the time for delivery.

References

1. Dennis J, Johnson A, Mutch L, Yudkin P, Johnson P. Acid base status at birth and neurodevelopmental outcome at four and one-half years. *Am J Obstet Gynecol* 1989;161:213–20
2. Ruth VJ, Raivo KO. Perinatal brain damage; predictive value of metabolic acidosis and the Apgar score. *Br Ed J* 1988;297:24–7
3. Ruth V, Widness JA, Clemons G, Raivio KO. Postnatal changes in serum immunoreactive erythropoietin in relation to hypoxia before and after birth. *J Pediatr* 1990;116:950–4
4. Maier RF, Böhme K, Dudenhausen JW, Obladen M. Cord blood erythropoietin in relation to different markers of fetal hypoxia. *Obstet Gynecol* 1993;81:575–80
5. Nicolini U, Nicolaides P, Fisk NM, *et al.* Limited role of fetal blood sampling in prediction of outcome in intrauterine growth retardation. *Lancet* 1990;336:768–72
6. Thilaganathan B, Atahanoglu S, Özmen P, Creighton S, Watson NR, Nicolaides KH. Umbilical cord blood erythroblast count as an index of intrauterine hypoxia. *Arch Dis Child* 1994;70:F192–F194
7. Phelan JP, Ahn MO, Korst LM, Martin G. Nucleated red blood cells: a marker for fetal asphyxia? *Am J Obstet Gynecol* 1995;173:1380–4
8. Hanlon-Lundberg KM, Kirby RS, Gandi S, Broekhuizen FF. Nucleated red blood cells in cord blood of singleton term neonates. *Am J Obstet Gynecol* 1997;176:1149–56
9. Altshuler G. Role of the placenta in perinatal pathology. *Ped Path Lab Med* 1996;16:207–33
10. Lippman HS. A morphologic and quantitative study of the blood corpuscles in the newborn period. *Am J Dis Child* 1924;27:473–526
11. Saraçoğlu ÖF, Eser E, Şahin I. Nucleated red blood cells: as a marker in acute and chronic fetal asphyxia. Presented at the *XI International Congress 'Fetus as a Patient'*, Amsterdam, 1998
12. Green DW, Mimouni F. Nucleated erythrocytes in healthy infants and in infants of diabetic mothers. *J Pediatr* 1990;116:129–31
13. Nicolaides KH, Thilaganathan B, Rodeck CH, Mibashan RS. Erythroblastosis and reticulocytosis in anemic fetuses. *Am J Obstet Gynecol* 1988;159:1063–5
14. Thilaganathan B, Salvesen DR, Abbas A, Ireland RM, Nicolaides KH. Fetal plasma erythropoietin concentration in red blood cell-isoimmunized pregnancies. *Am J Obstet Gynecol* 1992;167:1292–7
15. Salvesen DR, Brundenel JM, Snijders JM, Ireland RM, Nicolaides KH. Fetal plasma erythropoietin

in pregnancies complicated by maternal diabetes mellitus. *Am J Obstet Gynecol* 1993;168:88–94

16. Bernstein PS, Minior VK, Divon MY. Neonatal nucleated red blood cell counts in small for gestational age fetuses with abnormal umbilical artery Doppler studies. *Am J Obstet Gynecol* 1997;177:1079–84

17. Soothill PW, Nicolaides KH, Campbell S. Prenatal asphyxia, hyperlacticaemia, hypoglycaemia, and erythroblastosis in growth retarded fetuses. *Br Med J* 1987;294:1051–3

18. Allstair GS, Philip MD, Tito AM. Increased nucleated red blood cell counts in small for gestational age infants with very low birth weight. *Am J Dis Child* 1989;143:164–9

19. Snijders RJM, Abbas A, Melby O, Ireland RM, Nicolaides KH. Fetal plasma erythropoietin concentration in severe growth retardation. *Am J Obstet Gynecol* 1993;168: 615–19

20. Cox WL, Daffos F, Forestier F, *et al.* Physiology and management of intrauterine growth retardation: a biologic approach with fetal blood sampling. *Am J Obstet Gynecol* 1988;159:36–41

21. Richey SD, Ramin SM, Bawdon RE, *et al.* Markers of acute and chronic asphyxia in infants with meconium stained amniotic fluid. *Am J Obstet Gynecol* 1995;172:1212–15

22. Neaye RI, Localio JD. Determining the time before birth when ischemia and hypoxemia initiated cerebral palsy. *Obstet Gynecol* 1995;86: 713–19

23. Green DW, Hendon B, Mimouni FB. Nucleated erythrocytes and intraventricular hemorrhage in preterm neonates. *Pediatrics* 1995;96:475–8

24. Low JA, Galbraith RS, Muir DW, Killen HL, Pater EA, Karchmar EJ. Intrapartum fetal hypoxia: a study of long term morbidity. *Am J Obstet Gynecol* 1983;145:129–34

25. Korst LM, Phelan JP, Ahn MO, Martin G. Nucleated red blood cells: an update on the marker for fetal asphyxia. *Am J Obstet Gynecol* 1996;175:843–6

26. Sinha HB, Mukherjee AK, Bala D. Cord blood haemoglobin (including foetal haemoglobin), and nucleated red blood cells in normal and toxaemic pregnancies. *Indian J Pediatr* 1972;9: 540–3

27. Shivhare K, Chawla, K Khan MA, Mathur PS. Effect of maternal toxaemia on total haemoglobin, foetal haemoglobin and nucleated red blood cells in cord blood. *Indian J Pediatr* 1976; 43:349–56

Modern intrapartum surveillance of the fetus – some problems in its evolution

34

E. Saling

INTRODUCTION

In the history of obstetrics since Hippocrates (i.e. over the past 2400 years), the most important advances with respect to the unborn child are to be seen in the recent four decades. This is also relevant for intrapartum fetal monitoring, which – historically seen – represents the very first developed clinical step in modern obstetrics. Up to 1959 intermittent auscultation using a simple stethoscope was the only way of monitoring the unborn. Nowadays the fetus can be monitored like a patient in intensive care during the most critical recognizable phase of our life – i.e. in all stages of labor – by continuous recording of the fetal heart rate and, if indicated, additionally by fetal scalp blood analysis introduced for clinical use in 1960. Modern intensive supervision of the fetus during labor provides the greatest possible safety for the fetus and the lowest possible frequency of unnecessary operative interventions, provided that the available methods are used in an appropriate way.

Problem

Some colleagues seem to have become so used to this enormous progress and the achievable advantages, that they no longer keep them in mind.

THE MAIN TASK OF INTRAPARTUM SURVEILLANCE OF THE FETUS

The main aim of modern intrapartum fetal monitoring is not so much a further reduction of fetal and infant mortality, which are now relatively low, and not so much the reduction of cases with cerebral palsy (see later), but rather the prevention of all kinds of early and later neonatal morbidity caused by hypoxia and acidemia. There are several reasons for supporting this contention. According to Shankaran and colleagues[1], the following organ systems have been impaired in 28 term infants with clinically diagnosed severe asphyxia: pulmonary in 86%, central nervous system in 79%, renal in 54%, cardiac in 50%, metabolic in 46% and hematological in 36%. According to Sexson and colleagues[2] there is a multisystem involvement in asphyxiated newborns. In 1990, Portman and co-workers[3], also reported multiple asphyxia-associated organ dysfunctions. Perlman and associates[4] pointed out the dependence of single or multiple organ injuries on the duration of hypoxia in asphyxiated term infants and the function of the adaptation of cardiovascular mechanisms, as we described them in the 1970s, the so-called 'oxygen-conserving adaptation of the fetal circulation'[5]. In the Anglo-American literature this adaptation of the fetal circulation has later been erroneously called the 'brain-sparing effect': erroneously, because it is also at least a 'heart-sparing' and often also an 'adrenal-sparing effect'.

Problem

Some authors thought in the past that the main aim of modern monitoring was the prevention of severe neurological impairment – including cerebral palsy. However, particularly the latter is caused by intrapartum asphyxia in less than 10% of cases[6,7]. Logically,

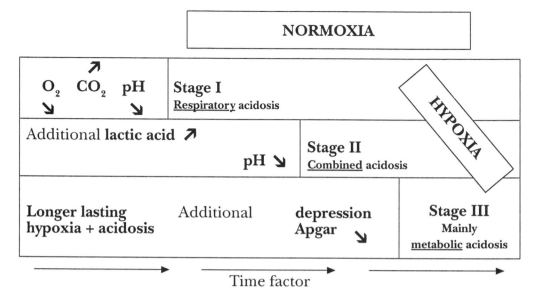

Figure 1 *Important stages of progressive fetal hypoxia*

a renunciation on modern fetal monitoring could be considered, because the frequency of neurological impairment has not been reduced by such surveillance, and intermittent auscultation could be accepted as an equivalent method. Such considerations would ignore the existence of all other organ morbidity in newborn infants, both premature and mature, following hypoxia and acidosis. It is of course important to prevent severe fetal acidosis if possible in each fetus, particularly when it is of longer duration. No neonatologist in an intensive care unit nor an anesthesiologist would accept that their patient could be carelessly exposed to hypoxia and acidosis. It would be ominous if some obstetricians believed that such events are harmless to the fetus.

SOME ESSENTIAL PATHOPHYSIOLOGIC ASPECTS

It is important to understand the relationship between the stages of fetal hypoxia and the clinical state of the neonates. Intrauterine hypoxia leads primarily to an initial decrease in the pH of the fetal blood caused by the accumulation of carbon dioxide and thus to respiratory acidosis; this would be stage I in Figure 1, demonstrating the step-by-step development of hypoxia and acidosis. In stage II there is an additional overloading of organic acids, leading to combined acidosis. Owing to anaerobic glycolysis, this mainly concerns lactic acid; the fetal blood pH levels decrease still further. In stage III, the acidosis which has progressed in the meantime, and which is predominantly of metabolic character, begins to have a negative effect on the whole fetal organism. The central nervous system becomes depressed and so – depending on the duration, which is an important factor – incisive changes occur, having a depressing effect on the muscles, the reflexes, the respiration and the circulation. If the infant is born during this stage (stage III), a reduced Apgar score can often be expected.

Problem

The characteristics and clinical importance of these three pathophysiologic stages are often misunderstood. Situations occurring during labor are described (e.g. a pathological cardiotocogram and decreasing fetal pH, as can be seen in Figure 2 as the dotted line) which are afterwards compared with the Apgar score. 'False-positive' findings during labor are said to have been present in infants whose Apgar score was 'still good'. Bearing

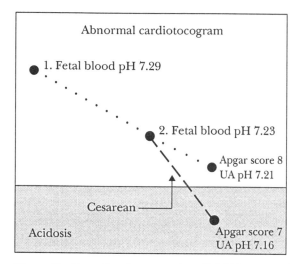

Figure 2 *Example of erroneously called 'false-positive' findings. Operative delivery indicated by real 'fetal distress' because of (apparently) decreasing pH values. UA, umbilical artery*

in mind what has just been said, it must be clear how ill-considered this scientifically untenable conclusion is. Neither a pathological cardiotocogram caused by hypoxia nor decreasing pH levels lead inevitably to a reduced Apgar score. An appropriate long latency period must be taken into consideration. If an infant is born before stage III it will often still be vigorous, with an Apgar score of 8 or 7 (in the shaded part of Figure 2) in slight acidosis. This is certainly not a 'false-positive' finding from the clinical aspect, but rather a 'correct positive' finding, because the decreasing pH values have undoubtedly proved that there is an evident biochemical change caused by hypoxia. To assess the state of the newborn only by using the Apgar score is antiquated and inadequate. Much better postpartum hypoxia diagnostics in the newborn can be achieved by using a combination of the Apgar score and measurements of the pH in the umbilical cord blood, which we introduced into routine clinical practice in 1965, 33 years ago[8]. Contrary to some published opinions concerning the poor relationship between fetal acidosis and the clinical state of the infant, for instance that by Sykes and

co-workers[9], an evaluation of Brandt-Niebelschütz and Saling[10] found that there have of course been apparent connections.

As can be seen in Figure 3, the proportion of infants with acidosis (umbilical artery pH < 7.20) contained the highest number of depressed infants (35.4%). The newborns with preacidotic umbilical artery cord pH levels of 7.20–7.24 included 12.2% of clinically depressed infants, two-thirds lower than in the acidotic group. In the small group of infants who were born with normal pH levels, none was depressed.

SOME COMMENTS ON THE JUDGEMENT OF FETAL MONITORING DURING LABOR

Numerous studies about the value of the different fetal monitoring methods during labor have been published. Most of them illustrate how difficult it is to find realistic clinical conditions for reliable and efficient labor ward routine. It seems that too many researchers have concentrated too much on highly sophisticated statistical methods and have hardly taken established clinical methods into consideration in their randomized controlled studies. This has not been just our opinion for a long time. Gardosi from Nottingham recently published some noteworthy critical comments concerning randomized trials and their synthesis in the form of meta-analyses[11]. Some extracts:

> The studies need to be examined carefully for their suitability for inclusion, taking into account heterogeneity of study design, patient characteristics, treatments and measures of outcome. Apart from statistical heterogeneity, there is also clinical heterogeneity within and, more importantly, between studies. Meta-analyses may incorporate trials with different criteria for defining the condition under study, the method of admitting patients, the selection and administration of treatment and the assessment of outcome, which can preclude them from being combined with any validity. . . . Differing levels of

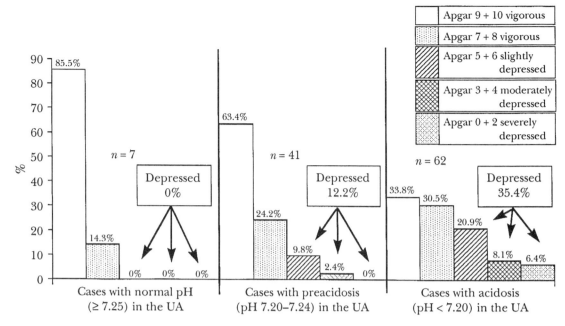

Figure 3 *Clinical condition of 110 newborns immediately after delivery (modified Apgar score), delivered operatively because of fetal pH findings according to the acidity in the umbilical artery (UA)*

risk may also make the results of the analysis not applicable. Due to such heterogeneity, current methods of statistical analysis may be seriously flawed and lead to misleading conclusions.

For our critical appraisal we have chosen as an example a study cited often in the past. In the large prospective Dublin Study[12] there is, apart from some weak critical conditions, an unacceptable result. For the evaluation of newborns with acidosis, only umbilical vein blood samples were used. As is known, these are not nearly as representative of the fetal condition as are umbilical artery blood samples. Moreover, the pH measurement in umbilical blood was performed in only 540 out of 6530 cases in the electronic fetal heart rate monitoring group and in 535 out of 6554 in the intermittent auscultation group. The number of newborns with moderate to severe acidemia (pH < 7.1) in the intermittent auscultation group at 2.1% (11 out of 535) was twice as high as in the electronic fetal monitoring group at 1% (five out of 540). This difference was not significant. The authors

therefore retained the null hypothesis. However, a more detailed analysis of the data indicates that the type II error probability[13] was very high. This addresses the error probability of wrongly retaining the null hypothesis in case of a negative (not significant) test result. In the case of the Dublin trial the probability of a type II error was $\beta = 0.91$[14]. Consequently, owing to the insufficient sample size, the test power of $1 - \beta = 0.09$ was very low. The Dublin question could only be answered by increasing the sample size. For example, if the acidosis risk had been doubled within the whole group of 6530 cases, then the error probability of rejecting the null hypothesis would have been only $p < 0.001$. At the same time, the test power would have been 0.9 (even for a significance level chosen as $p < 0.01$).

Accordingly, in contrast to the former interpretation of the Dublin Study, we propose that a considerable number of seriously acidotic newborns were contained in the group of fetuses monitored by intermittent auscultation. These important results have, as far as we know, neither been stated in the publication concerned nor recognized by any other author who has cited this study. From our point of view the results of the Dublin Study rather confirm that electronic fetal monitoring during labor is more efficient in prevention of critical hypoxia and acidosis than is intermittent auscultation.

For several years attempts have been made to put a number of studies together, with the hope that such a 'conglomerate' of results – a so-called meta-analysis – would provide more reliable evidence. The problem is that a large number of patients, as in the Dublin Study, have a correspondingly high influence on the resulting conclusions. After we found in the Dublin Study that the rate of early morbidity (considerably acidotic infants) in the intermittent auscultation group after a correct statistical evaluation was very probably significantly higher, such meta-analytic considerations were confirmed as questionable.

In 1993 a randomized trial with a more convincing concept was performed in two Greek university hospitals and published by Vintzileos and co-workers[15]. These results showed a significant reduction of hypoxia-related mortality rates in the group of fetuses with electronic monitoring, compared to a group with intermittent auscultation.

Apart from all these results, the decisive question is, on principle, how much progress can be expected for clinical purposes from a comparison of two unsatisfactory methods within prospective randomized studies.

Problem

Oddly enough, most such studies have focused on the question of the reliability of intermittent auscultation and electronic fetal monitoring, bearing in mind all the advantages and disadvantages of the methods concerned. There is an apparent lack of realistic consideration of the fact that there is a decisive difference between the use of intermittent auscultation in a study model compared to its practical use in the daily labor ward routine. We have our relevant experi-

ence in this matter. For about 8 years, namely after fetal blood analysis was introduced into clinical routine in 1960, cardiotocography was not available until 1968. During this long period we depended very much on reliable fetal heart rate auscultation. We tried to motivate our midwives, who in general were co-operative in using lists at the bed of each parturient for recording the counted heart rate, and we installed a gong which produced a noise every 15 min to remind them to auscultate the fetal heart sounds regularly. The results were disappointing to a high degree and did not correspond at all with such theoretical demands as are described in the 'materials and methods' sections the published prospective studies. However, in the literature there are also other negative arguments of why the use of auscultation is nonsensical[16].

Another painful error was that the results that were found with electronic fetal monitoring – such as a high rate of operations – have been uncritically transmitted to modern monitoring in general as its essential properties. This is inexcusable because it is well known that the skilful combined use of electronic fetal monitoring and fetal blood analysis minimizes the disadvantages of electronic fetal monitoring when it is used alone. It is therefore unintelligible why the most suitable and most efficient measures (such as the combined employment of cardiotocography and fetal blood analysis, provided the latter is appropriately applied) are not used in general in most studies as a 'reference standard', as is the case with 'intrapartum surveillance'. Gardosi recently wrote[17]: 'There is wide-spread agreement that the intrapartum CTG requires a second parameter to make it more specific and reduce false-positives, and the current 'gold standard' for this is fetal blood sampling'. In the same way the two great colleges, namely the American College of Obstetricians and Gynecologists[18] and the Royal College of Obstetricians and Gynaecologists[19,20], and the FIGO Study Group on the Assessment of New Technology[21] also recommended using fetal blood analysis in addition to cardiotocography.

Fetal hypoxia is a far-reaching biochemical metabolic event and consequently the most suitable direct diagnostic tool would be the use of examination methods of original biochemical character such as fetal blood analysis to assess the course of such a complication. With all non-biochemical examinations, the users try to draw diagnostic conclusions in an indirect and therefore less reliable way, as to what happens in the center of the events in the biochemical compartment.

It is also an interesting point that, since activities to introduce pulse oximetry as a new method of fetal monitoring were started, fetal blood analysis has been used as a 'gold standard' by most authors to prove the validity and reliability of pulse oximetry. At first sight it seems rather curious that a new method – which we also recommend for intrapartum surveillance[22,23] – actually demonstrates the considerable value of an old method which has been neglected by a number of clinicians.

It would also be advisable to classify the methods of surveillance that have been used mostly for comparative prospective studies, and to put them into a priority system. Then it would not be acceptable to search for the most reliable method of surveillance by using only lower ranged methods for such studies, i.e. methods with misleadingly higher rates of failure, as is the case with intermittent auscultation and electronic fetal monitoring.

For better understanding, let us present an agricultural example (Figure 4). One farmer plows his acre with an old blind horse – this should illustrate intermittent auscultation with its very limited efficiency. Another farmer plows with a nervous racing horse. This illustrates cardiotocography, with its rate of false-positive diagnoses that is too high. The third farmer plows with a suitable multipurpose farming horse. This illustrates combined electronic–biochemical monitoring, the best solution for reliable results.

An argument that demonstrates another weakness of most of the prospective studies is that the often so successful routine use of tocolytics during labor in cases of imminent fetal hypoxia has hardly been employed. We found in a former evaluation in our department[24] that, in about 75% of cases with decreasing fetal pH, acidosis could be prevented by the use of tocolytic treatment. The results of comparative studies might be quite different if tocolytic treatment had been used frequently during labor. The results achieved in such studies can be related only to the level of obstetrics practiced – particularly when that level is not based on the most advanced procedures. Such aspects demonstrate, again, how difficult it seems to be to steer the evolution of a new medical field onto the shortest possible logical and pragmatic course. If one agrees that such modern studies are questionable, and that it is difficult or impossible to perform clinically relevant prospective studies, then retrospective evaluations, now as before, have a realistic importance.

So-called observational studies again find some justification in the recent literature. In 1996, Black, from Health Services Research in London[25], wrote:

The view is widely held that experimental methods (randomised controlled trials) are the 'gold standard' for evaluation and that observational methods (cohort and case control studies) have little or no value. This ignores the limitations of randomised trials, which may prove unnecessary, inappropriate, impossible, or inadequate. . . . The false conflict between those who advocate randomised trials in all situations and those who believe observational data provide sufficient evidence, needs to be replaced with mutual recognition of the complementary roles of the two approaches.

It may therefore be of particular interest to compare the fetal mortality during labor as an easily available statistic for typical periods of different kinds of supervision in our department in the past almost 40 years. Such a review shows the efficacy of the old methods as they were used in those days, and the efficacy of correctly employed modern methods.

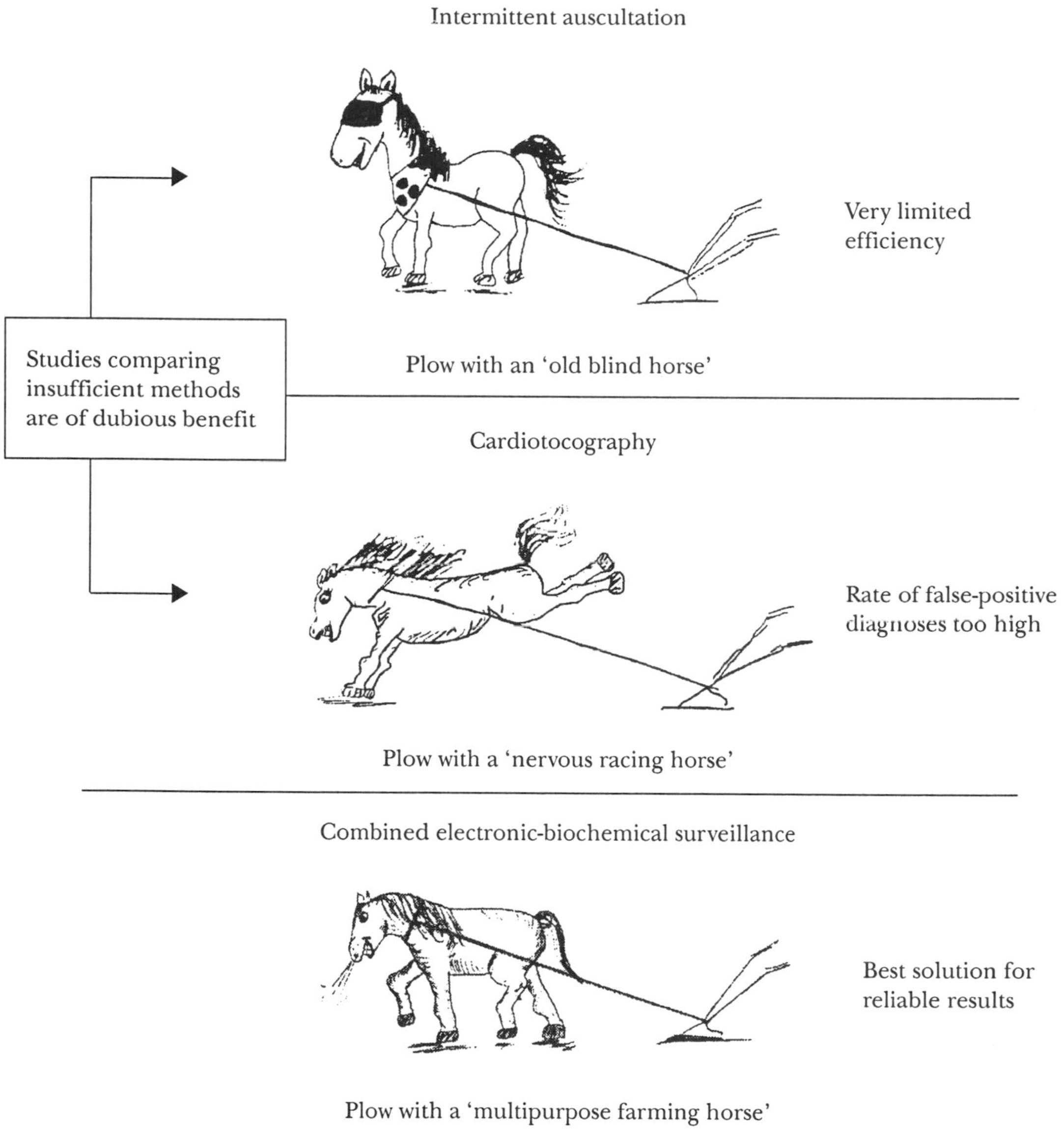

Figure 4 *Symbolic presentation of the three methods of intrapartum surveillance with their typical attributes. (Drawn by our secretary Sabine Al-Mustapha)*

Before any new method had become available, supervision was performed by simple auscultation of the fetal heart sounds. The fetal mortality during labor in this period until 1960 was 0.56%. After fetal blood analysis had been introduced in 1960 and used routinely from 1961 until 1967 – cardiotocography still not being available – the mortality went down to 0.32%. During the first 10 years, between 1968 and 1977, in which fetal blood analysis was combined with cardiotocography, the mortality rate was reduced to 0.17%, and during the next 13 years until 1990, owing to further improvements in labor room management – including intensive fetal monitoring – it was reduced to as low as 0.04%.

THE IMPORTANCE OF COMBINED INTRAPARTUM FETAL MONITORING

With the use of intrapartum fetal monitoring combined with cardiotocography and, if necessary, additional fetal blood analysis, highly remarkable results can be achieved, as we can present from our unit. Such results should preferably be seen in the context of all the important clinical conditions in a perinatal center. They represent the period of the decade of the 1980s when the author was responsible for conducting the obstetric department. The main factors are:

(1) The frequency of higher risk cases. In our obstetric unit, if all cases with any known symptom of increased risk are included, the frequency in the 1970s and 1980s was between 70 and 80%.

(2) The number of infants with low birth weight (< 2500 g) was on average 8.4%.

(3) In spite of the high number of higher risk cases, the frequency of Cesarean sections amounted to only 9–10%.

(4) The frequency of moderately or severely depressed (Apgar score ≤ 4) and simultaneously moderately or severely acidemic infants (umbilical artery pH < 7.1) was only 0.2%.

(5) The perinatal mortality rate, according to the World Health Organization standard was 5.3 per 1000.

Taking into account all the publications which theoretically and statistically seem to be so highly sophisticated, there is hardly any other department that uses combined electronic–biochemical supervision during labor and can present better clinical results within such a mosaic of different important clinical parameters.

LIMITED USE OF FETAL BLOOD ANALYSIS AND THE PROBLEMS CONCERNED

In a publication in 1985, Clarke and Paul[26] reported, amongst other things, that in 25 perinatal centers in the USA fetal blood analysis had been performed on only about 3% of the parturients. They listed six reasons for practical problems and thus explained why the use of fetal blood analysis is not more widespread. There were objections such as unavailability of technical personnel and equipment, technical difficulty in performing the procedure, time delay in obtaining results, misinterpretation of data and insufficient initial training. These problems would also seriously jeopardize any other essential medical procedure. One must be able to solve such basic but typical difficulties of poor organization, inexperience or prejudice. An objective observer will not be convinced by such a weak line of argument, particularly because general costs, staff expenses and expenses incurred later by the higher morbidity of a great number of unnecessary Cesarean sections – which could be prevented by fetal blood analysis – were not considered at all.

In our unit, with about 3000 deliveries per year and the changing rate within the decades of 10–20% of cases with fetal blood analysis, none of the reasons mentioned above creates an essential practical problem which would make performing fetal blood analysis an unreasonably expensive or difficult procedure. In our opinion, the authors of such publications, in the interests of an objective investigation, should previously have visited the place where fetal blood analysis was developed and where practical and clinical experience has been collected on more than 20 000 examined cases, and should then check on the real reasons why there are such different opinions on biochemical monitoring.

In a more recent publication[27] Goodwin and co-workers from Paul's group advocated 'elimination of fetal scalp blood sampling on a large clinical service'. Fetal scalp blood analysis was used during the first 3 years of the study at a frequency of 1.8% and after the 'elimination' in the following 4 years at 0.3%; at such an insignificant frequency, practically no changes could be expected. They also did not measure the umbilical artery pH after delivery; this is more conclusive than Apgar score evaluations alone. Such statements have little value.

We hope that this contribution may give an impetus to more critical and realistic judgement in the future of what are the best solutions for intrapartum monitoring and how we can achieve the safest care of our two patients – the mother and the fetus.

References

1. Shankaran S, Woldt E, Koepke T, Bedard MP, Nandyal R. Acute neonatal morbidity and long-term central nervous system sequelae of perinatal asphyxia in term infants. *Early Hum Dev* 1991;25: 135–48

2. Sexson WR, Sexson SB, Rawson JE, *et al.* The multisystem involvement of the asphyxiated newborn. *Pediatr Res* 1976;10:432

3. Portman RJ, Carter BS, Gaylord MS, Murphy MG, Thieme RE, Merenstein GB. Predicting neonatal morbidity after perinatal asphyxia: a scoring system. *Am J Obstet Gynecol* 1990;162:174

4. Perlman JM, Tack ED, Martin T, Shackleford G, Amon E. Acute systemic organ injury in term infants after asphyxia. *Am J Dis Child* 1989;143:617

5. Saling E. O$_2$-conserving adaptation of the foetal circulation. *Modern Trends Paediatr* 1970;3:51

6. Jaffee N, Attias D, Dar H, Eli J, Judes J. Prevalence of gestational and perinatal insults in brain damaged children. *Isr J Med Sci* 1985;21:940–4

7. Blair E, Stanley FJ. Intrapartum asphyxia: a rare cause of cerebral palsy. *J Pediatr* 1988;122:575–9

8. Saling E. Zustandsdiagnostik beim Neuge-borenen unmittelbar nach der Geburt. *Gynaecologia* 1965;160:133

9. Sykes GS, Molloy PM, Johnson P, *et al.* Fetal distress and the condition of the newborn infant. *Br Med J* 1983;287:943–5

10. Brand-Niebelschütz S, Saling E. Indications for operative termination of labor on cardio-tocography and fetal blood analysis: the reliability of these methods. *J Perinat Med* 1994;22:19–27

11. Gardosi J. Systematic reviews: insufficient evidence on which to base medicine. *Br J Obstet Gynaecol* 1998;105:1–5

12. McDonald D, Grant A, Sheridan-Pereira M, Boylan P, Chalmers I. The Dublin randomised trial of intrapartum fetal heart rate monitoring. *Am J Obstet Gynecol* 1985;152:524–39

13. Spiegel MR. *Theory and Problems of Probability and Statistics: Schaums Outline Series in Mathematics.* New York: McGraw-Hill, 1975:212

14. Heiselbetz C, Ortseifen C. In Weber E, ed. *Technical Report 'Planung'.* Heidelberg: Abt. Biostatistik, Deutsches Krebsforschungszentrum, 1985

15. Vintzileos AM, Antsaklis A, Varvarigos I, *et al.* A randomised trial of intrapartum electronic fetal heart rate monitoring versus intermittent auscultation. *Obstet Gynecol* 1993;81:899–907

16. Morrison JC, Chez BF, Davis ID, *et al.* Intrapartum fetal heart rate assessment: monitoring by auscultation or electronic means. *Am J Obstet Gynecol* 1993;168:63–6

17. Gardosi J. Monitoring technology and the clinical perspective. In Gardosi J, ed. *Intrapartum Surveillance. Baillières Clin Obstet Gynaecol* 1996; 10:2

18. American College of Obstetricians and Gynecologists. *Assessment of Fetal and Newborn Acid–Base Status. Technical Bulletin no. 127.* ACOG, 1989

19. Royal College of Obstetricians and Gynae-cologists. *Intrapartum Fetal Surveillance.* London: RCOG, 1993:387

20. Royal College of Obstetricians and Gynae-cologists. *Minimum Standards of Care in Labour; Report of the Working Party.* London: RCOG, 1994

21. FIGO Study Group on the Assessment of New Technology. Intrapartum surveillance: recom-mendations on current practice and overview of new developments. *Int J Gynecol Obstet* 1995;49: 213–21

22. Saling E. Fetal pulse oximetry during labor: issues and recommendations for clinical use. *J Perinat Med* 1996;24:476–8

23. Saling E. Recommendations for a combined supervision of the fetus during labor by cardiotocography, fetal blood analysis and pulse oximetry. *Fetal Diagn Ther* 1998;13:4–7

24. Zitzelsberger U. *Tokolyse sub partu.* Doctoral Thesis, The Free University of Berlin, 1982

25. Black N. Why we need observational studies to evaluate the effectiveness of health care. *Br Med J* 1996;312:1215–18

26. Clark SL, Paul RH. Intrapartum fetal surveil-lance: the role of fetal scalp blood sampling. *Am J Obstet Gynecol* 1985;153:717

27. Goodwin TM, Milner-Masterson L, Paul RH. Elimination of fetal scalp blood sampling on a large clinical service. *Obstet Gynecol* 1994;83: 971–4

New perspectives in fetal surgery: prenatal repair of myelomeningocele

35

B. Westerburg, R. W. Jennings and M. Harrison

Over the past two decades, sophisticated ultrasonographic imaging and invasive diagnostic procedures have had a tremendous impact on the study of abnormal fetal development. Since the first report of *in utero* ultrasonographic diagnosis of congenital anomalies in the 1970s, increasingly accurate prenatal ultrasonography has identified a growing number of disorders that are amenable to prenatal surgical correction. As a result, the fetus has claimed its role as an independent patient[1].

Although most prenatally diagnosed malformations are best managed by appropriate medical and surgical therapy after planned delivery near term, an increasing number of simple anatomical abnormalities with predictable devastating developmental consequences have been successfully corrected before birth.

In the 1980s, the pathophysiology of several potentially correctable fetal lesions was elucidated, and the feasibility of fetal repair established using a variety of animal models. Concomitantly, the natural history of these abnormalities was determined by serial ultrasonographic observation of human fetuses. Selection criteria for prenatal intervention were developed, and anesthetic, tocolytic and surgical techniques for hysterotomy and fetal surgery were developed and refined[1,2]. Three approaches to the fetus were developed: percutaneous, fetoscopic and open fetal surgery

To date, clinical experience with fetal surgical procedures has been limited to lethal disorders such as severe congenital diaphragmatic hernia or hydropic fetuses with congenital cystic adenomatoid malformation of the lung or sacrococcygeal teratoma. Much like postnatal surgery, minimally invasive surgery is assuming a more prominent role in fetal surgical procedures. The advent of fetoscopic techniques with its decreased maternal morbidity has spawned an interest in the repair of non-lethal defects, namely myelomeningocele.

ASSESSING RISK AND BENEFIT

For both mother and fetus the benefit of any *in utero* procedure must be weighed against the potential risks. For the fetus, the benefit of intervention in the face of certain death clearly outweights the risks of the procedure. For the mother, the risk–benefit assessment is less unambiguous. Maternal safety is paramount since most fetal malformations do not directly threaten the mother's health. However, she must bear the significant risk and discomfort from the surgical procedure and the postoperative tocolytic therapy, its side-effects and prolonged bed-rest. Significant morbidity is related to preterm labor and its treatment[3,4]. Open fetal surgery is associated with a risk of pulmonary edema, most probably due to high-dose tocolytics that are often necessary to control postoperative preterm labor. Although reversible, this complication emphasizes the need for close monitoring in an intensive care setting[5,6]. Since the mid-gestation hysterotomy is not in the lower uterine segment, delivery after fetal surgery and all subsequent deliveries should be by Cesarean section. Finally, the ability to carry and deliver subsequent pregnancies does not appear to be jeopardized by fetal surgery.

INTERVENTION FOR NON-LETHAL FETAL DEFECTS

Fetal surgery for myelomeningocele has recently assumed a position in the spotlight[7,8]. Currently, at least three centers in the USA are attempting to repair myelo-meningoceles prenatally. This presents several new technical and ethical aspects. First, although severely disabling, myelomeningocele is not a lethal malformation. The benefit of fetal intervention has to be weighed against the increased risk of prematurity in a baby that will in all probability be born alive. Second, the natural history and outcome of spina bifida is extremely variable. High (thoracic) lesions are known to have a worse prognosis than low (lumbar) lesions. However, the overlap is considerable and may hinder the assessment of the benefits of prenatal surgery. Most important, the prenatal natural history, i.e. the progression of neurological damage, is not known, and it is difficult to establish, because sonographic observation cannot distinguish between active and passive movement of the lower extremities. The rationale for prenatal intervention is that lower extremity function present in early pregnancy is progressively lost in later gestation. Furthermore, recent animal experiments from our laboratory indicate that the Chiari-II malformation almost always associated with myelomeningocele may be prevented by *in utero* repair. However, although compelling and logical, experimental evidence demonstrating the significant benefit of prenatal intervention is scant. Large animal models and investigations into the pathophysiology of meningomyelocele and the effects and risks of prenatal intervention are still warranted.

MYELOMENINGOCELE: NATURAL HISTORY AND POSTNATAL MANAGEMENT

Myelomeningocele affects about 1 of every 2000 babies born in the world. Between 1500 and 2000 babies are born with this lesion in the USA every year. As much as $200 000 000 in costs is incurred every year[8,9].

Neural tube defects are characterized by a midline vertebral defect (spina bifida), most often in the dorsal portion of the lumbosacral vertebrae. If the meningeal sac protrudes it is called a meningocele; if the sac contains spinal cord it is called a myelomeningocele. Ventral defects are extremely rare and are characterized by a split ventral vertebral body and the creation of a neurenteric cyst.

The etiology of neural tube defects is not completely understood. Isolated neural tube defects are multifactorial in inheritance. A number of gene loci have been identified, but the mechanism of action remains unclear[10]. The basic problem may lie in abnormalities of glycosaminoglycans, which produce defects in the extracellular matrix and structures derived from that matrix[11]. The most commonly held belief is that myelomeningocele is formed as a consequence of lack of fusion of the neural folds over the invaginating neural plate[12]. Recently, however, the theory of reopening of the neural tube has gained emphasis[13]. Myelomeningocele is associated with chromosomal abnormalities, such as trisomies 13 and 18, or may be due to teratogens such as valproic acid, carbamazepine and hyperthermia. Genetically determined defects in embryonic folate metabolism may play an important role in the development of myelomeningocele[14], since maternal folic acid supplementation even in the presence of normal serum folate levels significantly reduces the risk of spina bifida[15].

More than 80% of children with spina bifida may be identified before birth with maternal serum α-fetoprotein (MSAFP) screening and ultrasonography[16-18]. Ultrasonography reveals the characteristic shape of the calvarium and frontal bones, referred to as the 'lemon sign', and a dysplastic cerebellum, called the 'banana sign', in virtually all cases before 24 weeks[19]. Direct visualization of the fetal spine can usually be accomplished by 16 weeks' gestation but is less sensitive for the detection of myelomeningocele. Table 1 summarizes ultrasonographic prognostic indicators and suggested prenatal workup of fetuses with spina bifida.

Table 1 *Evaluation of the fetus with spina bifida*

Ultrasound findings	Favorable prognostic indicators	Unfavorable prognostic indicators	Prenatal workup	Associated anomalies
Arnold–Chiari malformation (most common) Lemon sign (frontal bone scallopment), present in most fetuses before 24 weeks' gestation Banana sign (abnormal curvature of the cerebellum), present in most fetuses before 24 weeks' gestation and may disappear later Cerebral ventriculomegaly Direct visualization of the defect (rare) Paralysis of the lower extremities (rare) Bladder distension Obliteration of the cisterna magna Club foot	late onset of hydrocephalus atria of lateral ventricle < 12 mm cortical brain mantle (ventricle–skull distance > 10 mm) low level of lesion (low lumbar or sacral) no macrocephaly	early onset of hydrocephalus atria > 12 mm cortical brain mantle < 10 mm ventricle–skull distance high level of the lesion (thoracic or high lumbar L1–2 macrocephaly	karyotype level II ultrasound	abnormal karyotype in 17% (trisomy 18, trisomy 13, triploidy and translocation). In 20% of these, spina bifida is an isolated abnormality

Table 2 *Outcome of prenatally diagnosed spina bifida in relation to level of the lesion*

	Thoracolumbar	Lumbar	Sacral
Independent ambulation	0%	7%	57%
Bowel/bladder control	0%	0%	17%
School performance	64% in low grade for age, or special class	40% in age- and grade-appropriate school programs	46% in age- and grade-appropriate school programs

Although not lethal, the spinal cord malformation leads to neurological injury below the lesion with paraplegia, urinary and fecal incontinence, sexual dysfunction and skeletal deformations. The outcome and residual neurological capacity depend largely on the level of the lesions (Table 2). Although seriously debilitating, peripheral neurological dysfunction is rarely lethal. However, 35% of children with myelomeningocele die despite surgical intervention and aggressive medical management[20-22]. The majority of these deaths are due to the Chiari-II malformation that is associated with myelomeningocele in nearly 100% of cases.

First described by Arnold and Chiari in the 19th century[23,24], the Chiari-II malformation is defined as the maldevelopment of a small

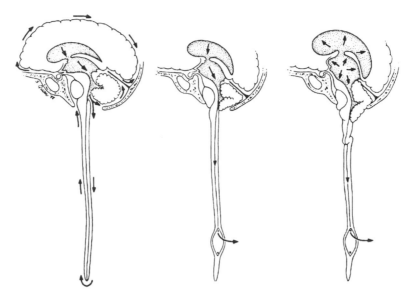

Figure 1 *Development of Chiari-II malformation. Normal development of the brain and the skull, in particular the posterior fossa, is thought to be dependent upon gentle distension of the embryonic ventricles. Decrease of pressure due to loss of spinal fluid through a myelomeningocele lesion induces the development of an abnormally small posterior fossa. This malformation causes the herniation of brainstem and cerebellum through the foramen magnum and tentorium. As the cerebellum herniates through the foramen magnum, the normal circulation of cerebrospinal fluid is obstructed. Hydrocephalus subsequently develops*

posterior fossa and herniation of the cerebellar vermis and brainstem through an enlarged foramen magnum.

The etiology of the Chiari-II malformation is not completely understood. The predominant hypothesis maintains that an imbalance of hydrodynamic forces occurs, owing to loss of cerebrospinal fluid from the lesion (Figure 1). Normal development of the brain and the skull, in particular the posterior fossa, is thought to be dependent upon gentle distension of the embryonic ventricles. Decrease of pressure due to loss of spinal fluid induces the development of an abnormally small posterior fossa, along with other brain abnormalities seen in children with myelomeningocele, such as agenesis of the corpus callosum, enlargement of the massa intermediata, cortical heterotopia and polymicrogyria[25].

This hindbrain deformity leads to hydrocephalus in the vast majority of cases, most probably due to impaired circulation of the cerebrospinal fluid[26]. The development of hydrocephalus as a consequence of the Chiari-II malformation is not well understood.

Oldfield and colleagues[27] make the argument that the herniated tonsillar pillars act as a one-way ball valve. Increases in cerebrospinal fluid pressure below the foramen magnum will allow fluid to cross up into the cranium, while increases in the cerebrospinal fluid pressure above the foramen magnum would cause impaction of the tonsillar pillars and accumulation of fluid. A similar hypothesis is considered by Williams, with the result being a pressure differential across the impacted tonsils in the foramen magnum[28].

Hydrocephalus is the probable cause of the impaired mental development usually seen in these children[20]. Symptoms may develop despite good control of the associated hydrocephalus[29,30]. They may be due to cranial nerve palsies, or direct brainstem compression or distortion. Newborns often present with severe respiratory stridor, apnea, facial nerve palsies, lack of gag reflex and quadriparesis[31]. Respiratory and swallowing difficulties may lead to neonatal death. Often patients who survive infancy will later develop limb weakness, spasticity, nystagmus and opisthotonos[26,32].

In older children the presentation may include nystagmus, weakness or spasticity of the upper limbs, limb or truncal ataxia, as well as neck pain and swallowing difficulties[31]. Scoliosis often develops as the child grows[33,34].

Many patients with myelomeningocele have no intrinsic brain abnormality that mandates mental retardation. Intellectual function does not seem to be dependent on the level of the spinal lesion. The high incidence of observed mental retardation is probably due to the recurrent insults from infection, hypoxia, cerebrospinal fluid shunt malfunction and hydrocephalus – all consequences of the Chiari-II malformation.

Although many authors feel that surgical decompression for infants with the Chiari-II malformation is indicated[35,36], the efficacy of cervical decompression in newborns to alter the course of the disease is still debated[20,27,36,37]. Ventricular cerebrospinal fluid shunting is indicated in most affected infants in order to prevent progression of the hydrocephalus.

THE RATIONALE FOR TREATMENT BEFORE BIRTH

There is a growing body of evidence indicating that major damage to the exposed spinal cord occurs during gestation. Indeed, animal studies from our and other laboratories have demonstrated that prenatal repair of the lesion may preserve peripheral neurological function[38-41].

Fetal movements of the lower extremities may be seen despite the presence of a clinically significant spina bifida earlier in gestation. This suggests that toxic effects of amniotic fluid[38] or direct trauma of the exposed spinal cord[42] may be in part responsible for the neural damage commonly seen. Protection of the exposed spinal cord might therefore prevent secondary neural damage and warrant *in utero* intervention for myelomeningocele.

The etiology of the Chiari-II malformation is thought to be due either to unbalanced pressures in the cerebrospinal fluid, or to a traction injury caused by cranial cervical growth imbalance. Several reports of cerebellar herniation following postnatal lumbosacral spinal fluid shunting have been published[43-46]. In these cases the tonsillar descent was reversible when the shunt was removed. It is therefore our hypothesis that prevention of further leakage of the spinal fluid out of the spinal canal (analogous to the lumbosacral shunt) may reverse the herniation at a time when the brain is still malleable enough to achieve normal development. Indeed, the experimental data from our laboratory presented in this chapter confirm that the Chiari-II malformation can be prevented by prenatal myelomeningocele coverage.

A malformation amenable to prenatal intervention must fulfil a number of conditions. It must be severe enough to warrant the risks associated with *in utero* treatment. Further, it must be reliably detectable before birth. Finally, the pathophysiology must be reversible by fetal intervention, significantly improving the prognosis over postnatal treatment. In the case of lethal anomalies, the calculation is a simple one: the benefits of the operation clearly outweigh the certainty of death without intervention. The benefits of prenatal intervention for non-lethal malformations have not yet been clearly delineated. Human case numbers are small[8,47], and the variable neurological outcome of the unrepaired lesion hinders the assessment of the benefit of prenatal intervention.

The parental choices have so far been confined to pregnancy termination or postnatal closure of the lesion. Postnatal treatment may prevent further degeneration of peripheral neural function, but is not effective in altering prenatal neural damage or the consequences of the Chiari-II malformation.

EXPERIMENTAL PATHOPHYSIOLOGY AND FETOSCOPIC REPAIR

It has been the strategy of the Fetal Treatment Center at the University of California, San Francisco, to refrain from human fetal

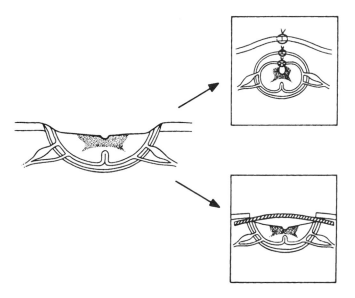

Figure 2 *Creation of a myelomeningocele lesion. An oval skin excision over the lumbar spine and an L1–L4 laminectomy are performed and the dura subsequently excised using microsurgical techniques. To achieve a communication of the central canal with the amniotic space – as is seen in spontaneous myelomeningoceles – the central canal is then exposed by a longitudinal incision in the midline of the spinal cord*

interventions until the benefit was clearly proven in the animals model. Furthermore, since the risks of prematurity associated with open fetal surgery may offset the gain of prenatal intervention in a situation where surgery is elective, it was decided to develop endoscopic techniques before attempting fetal repair. Although the peripheral neurological sequelae due to the spinal lesion may be severe for the child, the parents and siblings, they are rarely life-threatening. However, up to one-third of children with myelomeningocele die as a consequence of the Chiari-II malformation. If not only peripheral neural damage, but also the Chiari-II malformation, could be ameliorated by prenatal surgery, a much stronger case could be made to repair myelomeningoceles *in utero*. We therefore conducted a large animal study designed to create a model not only of spina bifida, but also of Chiari-II malformation development. Subsequently, we tested whether the most severe and lethal consequence of spina bifida – the Chiari-II malformation – would be prevented by prenatal intervention. To maintain our requirement for endoscopic intervention for

non-lethal malformation we developed a novel technique for myelomeningocele coverage that would be amenable to endoscopic intervention.

A surgical myelomeningocele was created in fetal lambs at 75 days of gestation (term equals 150 days), modifying previously described techniques (Figure 2)[42]. After creation of the lesion, the pregnancy was allowed to continue until the fetuses were again exposed at about 100 days' gestation for myelomeningocele repair. Two techniques for coverage of the lesion were employed. One was a formal neurosurgical repair identical to postnatal myelomeningocele repair (Figure 3a). The other technique involved coverage of the myelomeningocele with Alloderm (LifeCell Corporation, The Woodland, TX), which provides an impermeable membrane made of acellular cadaveric skin to protect the spinal cord (Figure 3b). Unrepaired control fetuses were exposed at the same gestational age as the fetuses undergoing myelomeningocele repair to document the presence of a uniform myelomeningocele lesion. Lambs that did not undergo fetal surgery served as normal controls.

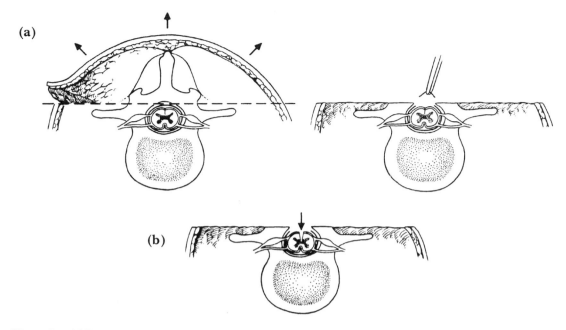

Figure 3 *(a) Primary surgical repair of a myelomeningocele lesion. The open neural placode and its overlying fascia are separated using sharp dissection to create a cord–dural plane. The placode is then reformed into a tube and the dural sheath is reformed around it. The paraspinal muscles are then partially reapproximated and the skin is closed. (b) Coverage of the lesion with Xenoderm. The skin is undermined on each side of the defect and a piece of Alloderm is fitted in the resultant pocket over the defect. The patch is stitched in place. The spinal cord itself is not manipulated*

All pregnancies were allowed to go to term. The neonatal lambs were sacrificed and the head and neck were examined for elements of the Chiari-II malformation and hydrocephalus by a blinded investigator.

EXPERIMENTAL RESULTS

Prenatal repair was shown to prevent development of the Chiari-II malformation. All animals developed remarkably similar myelomeningoceles (Figure 4). There was a flattened area of the spinal cord, partly covered with dura, protruding through the open vertebral defect.

Evaluation of the brain revealed that lambs that had undergone the creation of a myelomeningocele-type lesion and had not undergone subsequent repair demonstrated distinct signs of the Chiari-II malformation. A small posterior fossa was seen along with herniation of the medulla and vermis of the cerebellum through the foramen magnum (Figure 5). All animals that had undergone

repair of the lesion either by coverage with Xenoderm or by primary repair did not show signs of a Chiari-II malformation. The posterior fossa was of normal size and the medulla and vermis of the cerebellum were located well above the foramen magnum (Figure 6).

Magnetic resonance imaging of the brain demonstrated the absence of hydrocephalus in all animals.

'FETENDO' AND THE FUTURE OF FETAL INTERVENTION

Recent experimental and clinical investigations suggest that fetal repair may preserve spinal cord function in myelomeningocele[8,40]. Until now, there has been no investigation into the effects of fetal surgery on the Chiari-II hindbrain malformation. Our animal model of development of the Chiari-II malformation shows that the primary surgical repair of a myelomeningocele allows the fetal brain to develop normally. More importantly, our data indicate that coverage with an

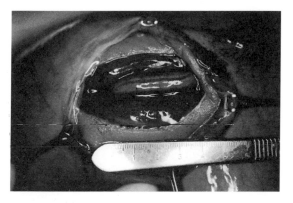

Figure 4 *Development of a myelomeningocele 3 weeks after creation of the lesion in a fetal lamb. All animals developed remarkably similar myelomeningoceles. There was a flattened area of the spinal cord, partly covered with dura, protruding through the open vertebral defect. In some fetuses, clear cerebrospinal fluid was aspirated from a fascia-enclosed space ventral to the spinal cord. Surrounding the vertebral defect was a larger defect in the paraspinal musculature and an equivalent defect in the fetal skin*

impermeable membrane such as Alloderm suffices to prevent fluid leakage and thus the Chiari-II malformation. Formal surgical repair can be postponed until after birth. This is important, because coverage of the lesion with membrane can be performed using minimally invasive fetal endoscopic ('fetendo') techniques. Fetoscopic repair reduces the incidence of preterm labor and maternal morbidity. Maternal hospital stay is reduced in comparison to that for fetal surgery. Fetendo may allow very early repair, positively influencing the child's sensorimotor function.

These findings raise the possibility of preventing the development of the Chiari-II malformation in a human fetus diagnosed with a myelomeningocele at an early gestational age. Owing to screening of maternal serum α-fetoprotein and high-resolution ultrasound a high percentage of these lesions are amenable to early or middle second-trimester diagnosis. The strategy would be to prevent leakage of spinal fluid, thereby inducing higher pressure in the telencephalic ventricles, leading to normal brain development.

Although myelomeningocele is disabling and frequently fatal, it is not a uniformly lethal fetal malformation – cases for which

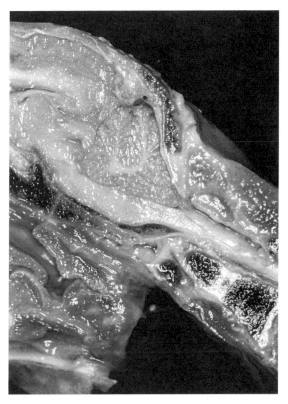

Figure 5 *Development of the Chiari-II malformation in unrepaired myelomeningocele. Evaluation of the sagittal brain sections revealed that lambs that had undergone the creation of a myelomeningocele-type lesion and had not undergone subsequent repair demonstrated distinct signs of the Chiari-II malformation. A small posterior fossa is seen along with herniation of the medulla and vermis of the cerebellum through the foramen magnum*

fetal open surgery has traditionally been reserved. Laparoscopic interventions decrease the incidence of preterm labor and preterm delivery of the fetus and may be warranted in serious but non-lethal fetal malformations.

Several technical obstacles to successful fetoscopic surgery had to be overcome to make this a viable treatment option. Solutions to these technical problems have evolved over 15 years of experimental and clinical work[48–52]. In the operating room, the mother is positioned with left uterine displacement to avoid inferior vena cava compression by the gravid uterus. Anesthesia of mother and fetus is established with a halogenated agent. Maternal monitoring is

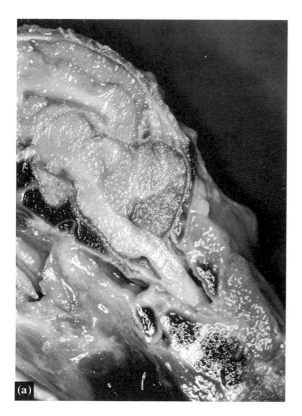

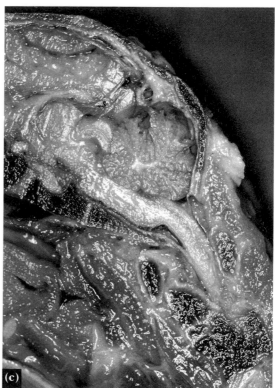

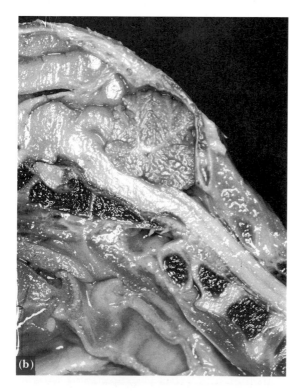

Figure 6 *Absence of Chiari-II malformation in repaired (a) and control lambs (b, c). All animals that had undergone repair of the lesion either by coverage with Alloderm or by primary repair did not show signs of a Chiari-II malformation. The posterior fossa was of normal size and the medulla and vermis of the cerebellum were located well above the foramen magnum.*

accomplished with routine non-invasive monitors plus central venous and arterial catheters.

Intraoperatively, sonography maps the placental position and guides trocar placement. Usually three balloon/compression trocars are used to perform fetal endoscopic procedures. Instruments of 3 and 5 mm are used. The most substantial obstacle that had to be overcome was lack of adequate visualization due to cloudy amniotic fluid or minor bleeding into the amniotic cavity. A refined system of continuous irrigation uses a pump irrigation system via the sheath endoscope. The fetus is monitored by transuterine ultrasonography. A miniaturized telemeter that can be placed into the amniotic cavity via a trocar site has been developed and is currently being tested. Each uterine puncture site is closed with one or two absorbable sutures and a fibrin glue plug.

Further studies need to be performed to define the pressures needed to induce normal brain development as well as the time in gestation when intervention may still reverse signs of the Chiari-II malformation. This is important, to determine whether fetal surgical repair of a myelomeningocele is best performed with or without a spinal drain. If drainage seems advantageous, the required spinal distension pressures will need to be investigated. The development and progression of hydrocephalus with and without repair need to be further studied in the lamb model.

We believe that fetal surgery for myelomeningocele holds great promise for alleviating the consequences of this devastating – if not lethal – malformation.

References

1. Harrison M, Golbus M, Filly R, eds. *The Unborn Patient*. Philadelphia: WB Saunders, 1991
2. Albanese CT, Harrison MR. Surgical treatment for fetal disease. The state of the art. *Ann NY Acad Sci* 1998;847:74–85
3. Longaker MT, Golbus MS, Filly RA, Rosen MA, Chang SW, Harrison MR. Maternal outcome after open fetal surgery. A review of the first 17 human cases. *J Am Med Assoc* 1991;265:737–41
4. Harrison MR. Fetal surgery. *West J Med* 1993;159:341–9
5. DiFederico EM, Burlingame JM, Kilpatrick SJ, Harrison M, Matthay MA. Pulmonary edema in obstetric patients is rapidly resolved except in the presence of infection or of nitroglycerin tocolysis after open fetal surgery. *Am J Obstet Gynecol* 1998;179:925–33
6. DiFederico EM, Harrison M, Matthay MA. Pulmonary edema in a woman following fetal surgery. *Chest* 1996;109:1114–17
7. Adzick NS, Sutton LN, Crombleholme TM, Flake AW. Successful fetal surgery for spina bifida [Letter]. *Lancet* 1998;352:1675–6
8. Tulipan N, Bruner JP. Myelomeningocele repair *in utero*: a report of three cases. *Pediatr Neurosurg* 1998;28:177–80
9. Noetzel MJ. Myelomeningocele: current concepts of management. *Clin Perinatol* 1989;16:311–29
10. Harris MJ, Juriloff DM. Genetic landmarks for defects in mouse neural tube closure. *Teratology* 1997;56:177–87
11. Di Rocco C, Rende M. Neural tube defects. Some remarks on the possible role of glycosaminoglycans in the genesis of the dysraphic state, the anomaly in the configuration of the posterior cranial fossa, and hydrocephalus. *Childs Nerv Syst* 1987;3:334–41
12. French BN. The embryology of spinal dysraphism. *Clin Neurosurg* 1983;30:295–340
13. Campbell LR, Sohal GS. The pattern of neural tube defects created by secondary reopening of the neural tube. *J Child Neurol* 1990;5:336–40
14. Copp AJ. Prevention of neural tube defects: vitamins, enzymes and genes. *Curr Opin Neurol* 1998;11:97–102
15. Czeizel AE, Dudas I. Prevention of the first occurrence of neural-tube defects by periconceptional vitamin supplementation [see comments]. *N Engl J Med* 1992;327:1832–5
16. Brock DJ, Barron L, Raab GM. The potential of mid-trimester maternal plasma alpha-fetoprotein measurement in predicting infants of low birth weight. *Br J Obstet Gynaecol* 1980;87:582–5
17. Purdie DW, Young JL, Guthrie KA, Picton CE. Fetal growth achievement and elevated maternal serum alpha-fetoprotein. *Br J Obstet Gynaecol* 1983;90:433–6
18. Brock DJ, Barron L, Watt M, Scrimgeour JB, Keay AJ. Maternal plasma alpha-fetoprotein and low birthweight: a prospective study throughout pregnancy. *Br J Obstet Gynaecol* 1982;89:348–51
19. Nicolaides KH, Campbell S, Gabbe SG, Guidetti R. Ultrasound screening for spina bifida: cranial and cerebellar signs. *Lancet* 1986;2:72–4
20. McLone DG, Naidich TP. Myelomeningocele: outcome and late complications. In McLaurin RL, Schut L, Venes JL, Epstein F, eds. *Pediatric Neurosurgery*. Philadelphia: Saunders, 1989
21. Hoffman HJ, Neill J, Crone KR, Hendrick EB, Humphreys RP. Hydrosyringomyelia and its management in childhood. *Neurosurgery* 1987;21:347–51
22. Paul KS, Lye RH, Strang FA, Dutton J. Arnold–Chiari malformation. Review of 71 cases. *J Neurosurg* 1983;58:183–7

23. Chiari H. Über Veränderungen des Kleinhirns, der Pons und der Medulla oblongata in folge von congenitaler Hydrocephalie des Grosshirns. *Denschr Akad Wissensch Math-Naturw Kl* 1895;63: 71

24. Arnold J. Transposition von Gewebskeimen und Sympodie. *Beitr path Anat allgem Pathol* 1894;16:1

25. McLone DG, Knepper PA. The cause of Chiari II malformation: a unified theory. *Pediatr Neurosci* 1989;15:1–12

26. Carmel PW. The Chiari malformations and syringomyelia. In Hoffman HJ, Epstein F, eds. *Disorders of the Developing Nervous System: Diagnosis and Treatment.* Boston: Blackwell Scientific, 1986

27. Oldfield EH, Muraszko K, Shawker TH, Patronas NJ. Pathophysiology of syringomyelia associated with Chiari I malformation of the cerebellar tonsils. Implications for diagnosis and treatment [see comments]. *J Neurosurg* 1994;80:3–15

28. Williams B. On the pathogenesis of syringomyelia: a review. *J R Soc Med* 1980;73:798–806

29. Park TS, Hoffman HJ, Hendrick EB, Humphreys RP. Experience with surgical decompression of the Arnold–Chiari malformation in young infants with myelomeningocele. *Neurosurgery* 1983;13:147–52

30. DiRocco C, Rende M. Chiari malformations. In Raimondi AJ, Choux M, DiRocco C, eds. *The Pediatric Spine II: Developmental Anomalies.* New York: Springer-Verlag, 1989

31. Ruge JR, Masciopinto J, Storrs BB, McLone DG. Anatomical progression of the Chiari II malformation. *Childs Nerv Syst* 1992;8:86–91

32. Carmel PW. Management of the Chiari malformations in childhood. *Clin Neurosurg* 1983;30: 385–406

33. Williams B. Orthopaedic features in the presentation of syringomyelia. *J Bone Joint Surg [Br]* 1979;61:314–23

34. Hoffman HJ. Syringomyelia in childhood. In Batzdorf U, ed. *Syringomyelia: Current Concepts in Diagnosis and Treatment.* Baltimore: Williams & Wilkins, 1991

35. Dyste GN, Menezes AH. Presentation and management of pediatric Chiari malformations without myelodysplasia [see comments]. *Neurosurgery* 1988;23:589–97

36. Vandertop WP, Asai A, Hoffman HJ, et al. Surgical decompression for symptomatic Chiari II malformation in neonates with myelomeningocele. *J Neurosurg* 1992;77:541–4

37. Menezes AH, Smoker WRK, Dyste GN. Syringomyelia, Chiari malformations, and hydromyelia. In Youmans J, ed. *Neurological Surgery.* Philadelphia: WB Saunders, 1990

38. Heffez DS, Aryanpur J, Hutchins GM, Freeman JM. The paralysis associated with myelomeningocele: clinical and experimental data implicating a preventable spinal cord injury. *Neurosurgery* 1990;26:987–92

39. Heffez DS, Aryanpur J, Rotellini NA, Hutchins GM, Freeman JM. Intrauterine repair of experimental surgically created dysraphism. *Neurosurgery* 1993;32:1005–10

40. Meuli M, Meuli-Simmen C, Hutchins GM, et al. *In utero* surgery rescues neurological function at birth in sheep with spina bifida. *Nature Med* 1995;1:342–7

41. Michejda M. Intrauterine treatment of spina bifida: primate model. *Z Kinderchir* 1984;39: 259–61

42. Meuli M, Meuli-Simmen C, Yingling CD, et al. Creation of myelomeningocele *in utero*: a model of functional damage from spinal cord exposure in fetal sheep [see comments]. *J Pediatr Surg* 1995;30:1028–32; discussion 1032–3

43. Payner TD, Prenger E, Berger TS, Crone KR. Acquired Chiari malformations: incidence, diagnosis, and management. *Neurosurgery* 1994; 34:429–34; discussion 434

44. Fischer EG, Welch K, Shillito J Jr. Syringomyelia following lumboureteral shunting for communicating hydrocephalus. Report of three cases. *J Neurosurg* 1977;47:96–100

45. Chumas PD, Kulkarni AV, Drake JM, Hoffman HJ, Humphreys RP, Rutka JT. Lumboperitoneal shunting: a retrospective study in the pediatric population [see comments]. *Neurosurgery* 1993; 32:376–83; discussion 383

46. Chumas PD, Armstrong DC, Drake JM, et al. Tonsillar herniation: the rule rather than the exception after lumboperitoneal shunting in the pediatric population [see comments]. *J Neurosurg* 1993;78:568–73

47. Adzick NS, Sutton LN, Crombleholme TM, Flake AW. Successful fetal surgery for spina bifida [Letter]. *Lancet* 1998;352:1675–6

48. Harrison MR. Fetal surgery [see comments]. *Am J Obstet Gynecol* 1996;174:1255–64

49. Harrison MR, Adzick NS. Fetal surgical techniques. *Semin Pediatr Surg* 1993;2:136–42

50. Bond SJ, Harrison MR, Slotnick RN, Anderson J, Flake AW, Adzick NS. Cesarean delivery and hysterotomy using an absorbable stapling device. *Obstet Gynecol* 1989;74:25–8

51. Jennings RW, Adzick NS, Longaker MT, Lorenz HP, Harrison MR. Radiotelemetric fetal monitoring during and after open fetal operation. *Surg Gynecol Obstet* 1993;176:59–64

52. Harrison MR, Mychaliska GB, Albanese CT, et al. Correction of congenital diaphragmatic hernia *in utero*. IX: Fetuses with poor prognosis (liver herniation and low lung-to-head ratio) can be saved by fetoscopic temporary tracheal occlusion. *J Pediatr Surg* 1998;33:1017–22; discussion 1022–3

Section 3

Current perspectives in clinical perinatology

Discrepancy between gestational age and fetal maturity among ethnic groups 36

É. Papiernik and G. R. Alexander

GESTATIONAL DURATION AND MATURATION

Gestational age at birth is principally perceived as the duration of pregnancy and, in this regard, is traditionally measured as the interval from the date of the last menstrual period (LMP) to the date of birth[1-3]. When accurately determined, gestational age is a useful surrogate measure for the extent of fetal maturation, development and readiness for birth and, as such, is an important indicator of fetal and newborn risk status. It is highly correlated with a newborn's chances during its first year of life of being free of serious morbidity and complications, having a normal development and surviving[1,4,5]. However, in spite of the strong association between a fetus's gestational age and its state of maturation and development, these are separate and distinct concepts. It has been emphasized that the association and concordance between gestational duration and fetal maturation may be markedly affected by the presence of morbid stressors that may stem from infectious, nutritional, psychosocial, environmental, substance abuse and other sources[1]. Consequently, both the length of gestation and the degree of fetal development and maturation at birth may tangibly, albeit subtly, vary among risk groupings and populations[1].

ETHNIC VARIATIONS

Ethnic variations in the length of gestation and percentage of preterm delivery have been repeatedly observed in the USA, Europe and other parts of the world[6-13]. The determinants of these ethnic disparities in average and extreme gestational age have yet to be fully explained. Although many precursors of preterm birth have been identified (e.g. smoking, prior preterm birth, use of diethylstilbestrol and low pre-pregnancy weight) the overall contribution or attributable risk of these known risk factors for preterm delivery is small and only a few factors are modifiable[14-17]. Moreover, investigations of the determinants of gestational age and birth weight have explained only a modest proportion of the ethnic disparities in these birth outcomes, when taking into account environmental conditions, lifestyle, social class and economic status, nutritional and anthropometric factors, health-care utilization and maternal demographic, behavioral and medical risk characteristics[18-33].

In addition to repeated observations of ethnic differences in length of gestational age, gestational age-specific mortality has also been reported to vary consistently among ethnic groups[4,8,11,18]. For example, in the USA, African-Americans, as compared with Whites, have a greater chance of survival at gestational ages less than 37 weeks even though they exhibit a greater proportion of preterm deliveries[4,11]. At term and beyond, the reverse is apparent with African-Americans having a greater risk of early mortality. While it is unclear to what extent the factors that increase the risk of preterm delivery also improve the chance of survival, these and other ethnic differences in gestational age- and birth weight-specific mortality are recognized to have a profound impact on ethnic disparities in total infant

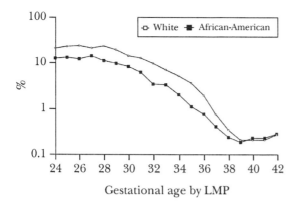

Figure 1 *Percentage with hyaline membrane disease by ethnicity of mother. Single live births in 1995 to mothers resident in the USA. LMP, last menstrual period*

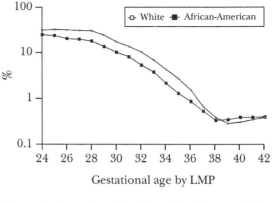

Figure 2 *Percentage of newborns placed on ventilation for more than 30 min by ethnicity of mother. Single live births in 1995 to mothers resident in the USA. LMP, last menstrual period*

mortality. Other ethnic populations in the USA, for example Asian-Indians, also have comparably higher low and very low birth-weight percentages than Whites but lower infant mortality rates, largely suggesting a relatively better gestational age-specific survival rate[33].

FETAL MATURATION FOR GESTATIONAL AGE

The factors underlying the improved survival rates of preterm infants of certain ethnic groups are a subject of increasing research scrutiny. Among the hypotheses for this phenomenon is one suggesting that it reflects differences in the extent and rate of fetal maturation for gestational age. The literature provides several examples of ethnic variations in fetal maturation for gestational age based on investigations of hyaline membrane disease, meconium staining and newborn neurological and physical characteristics[34–43].

Previous research has noted that the gestational age-specific mortality risk from hyaline membrane disease is higher among White preterm infants in contrast to comparable infants of African-American mothers and suggests that this dissimilarity in mortality is a function of ethnic differences in lung maturation at earlier gestational ages[34–36]. For illustration, Figure 1 provides the

percentages of 1995 single live births to mothers resident in the USA with hyaline membrane disease, by ethnicity of the mother. The data for this and the other figures shown in this report were drawn from the 1995 U.S. Perinatal and Natality Data Files, made available on CD-ROM for public use by the National Center for Health Statistics. Prior to 39 weeks' gestation, a higher proportion of White infants in comparison to African-American infants have hyaline membrane disease. Using the same database to examine the proportion of newborns placed on ventilation for more than 30 min, one typical clinical response to hyaline membrane disease, a similar ethnic divergence is apparent, supporting the notion of less fetal lung maturation of White infants at earlier gestational ages (Figure 2).

Meconium stained amniotic fluid is another clinical condition that has been shown to vary with advancing gestational age and has been suggested to be associated with increased fetal maturity[37–39]. Although meconium stained amniotic fluid is found with greater frequency in post-term deliveries, it has been reported to occur in higher levels and at earlier gestational ages in African-American infants, as compared with Whites, even after controlling for clinical and sociodemographic factors[21,37]. These reports suggest that proposed ethnic differences in fetal maturation at earlier gestational ages, as drawn from observations of hyaline membrane disease, continue into the term and post-term periods.

Investigators using pediatric assessments of physical and neurological characteristics at birth have reported that infants of African ancestry present signs of more advanced maturity than White infants of the same gestational age duration[40-44]. These ethnic differences persist after maternal characteristics and pregnancy complications are taken into account[40,43]. Collectively, these data have led to one interpretation that duration of gestational age may not be a valid indicator of fetal maturity, development, readiness for birth and infant risk status across all ethnic groups.

While much of the existing data suggesting ethnic variation in fetal maturity for length of gestation come from dichotomous comparisons of White and African-American populations, there is a growing body of research that suggests that there is considerable diversity in gestational age duration, birth weight and mortality among many ethnic groups[8,12,28,29,33]. The observed disparities in birth outcomes among multi-ethnic populations have been attributed to many factors, such as environmental, social class, health care and maternal socio-demographic, behavioral and medical risk characteristics. Although researchers agree that these factors are involved in the ethnic differences in medical conditions and pregnancy outcomes, appreciable variation in gestational age and other pregnancy outcome measures remains after controlling for these factors[4,12,18,22-29,31,45-50]. Some authors have suggested that the failure of the typically used socioeconomic and related risk indicators to explain ethnic disparities in birth outcomes stems from their inability to obtain valid measurements of the additional effects of racism and classism, but others have expressed doubt that the consideration of yet more highly correlated indicators of poverty and adverse living conditions will markedly increase knowledge of the determinants of ethnic disparity in gestational age and its relationship to the risk of mortality[33,51].

Factors specific to each ethnic group have also been suggested to contribute to observed variations in gestational age duration and maturity at birth[11,24,52,53]. However, some have argued passionately that there is no role for biologically intrinsic, genetic or multi-generational factors in determining ethnic disparities in pregnancy outcomes, perhaps misinterpreting such hypotheses as implying the inferiority of some ethnic groups[51,54,55]. Nevertheless, a careful reading of the literature suggests that in the last few decades these terms have not been used to imply this negative and fallacious connotation but instead have only been employed to refer to the impact of possibly inheritable factors related to maternal anthropometrics, prior preterm and low birth weight delivery and the multigenerational impact of disease and poverty. Granted the political sensitivity of the issue, the unacceptably high preterm delivery and infant mortality rates among some ethnic groups demand that every reasonable avenue of scientific inquiry be explored in pursuit of reducing these adverse disparities.

CLINICAL IMPLICATIONS

While research continues on the underlying determinants of ethnic differences in birth outcomes, an equally critical question emerges: can we apply our present knowledge of ethnic variation in birth weight, gestational age and fetal maturation, along with our understanding of their independent association with subsequent morbid outcomes, to improve care and lower mortality? Fetal mortality may be one area where reducing ethnic disparities may be possible with our present knowledge.

To the degree that fetal maturity may occur faster in some populations, it is unclear whether early maturity is accompanied by an earlier onset of postmaturity-related problems including fetal distress and fetal mortality. Figure 3 presents by gestational age the proportion of 1995 single live births to White and African-American mothers resident in the USA with a report of fetal distress. While for very preterm birth African-Americans have a

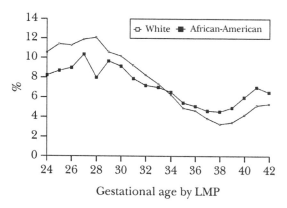

Figure 3 *Percentage with fetal distress by ethnicity of mother. Single live births in 1995 to mothers resident in the USA. LMP, last menstrual period*

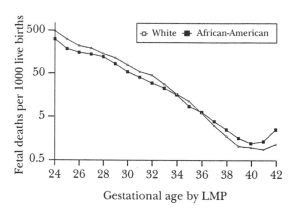

Figure 4 *Fetal mortality ratio by ethnicity of mother. Single live births in 1995 to mothers resident in the USA. LMP, last menstrual period*

lower percentage of fetal distress compared to Whites, the reverse is found above 33 weeks. A similar pattern is observed for fetal mortality. As depicted in Figure 4, African-Americans have an increased risk of fetal death beyond 36 weeks' gestation. At 42 weeks' gestation, the risk of fetal death for African-Americans is approximately double that of Whites.

Forty weeks from the date of LMP has traditionally been used as the approximate normal length of gestation, stemming from observations of White English populations during the last century[2]. Standards of care for all ethnic groups are based on this norm, in spite of the considerable ethnic variation in average gestational age. Post-term pregnancies, which are at increased risk of morbidity and mortality, are accordingly given more intensive clinical evaluation and, as needed, intervention. However, if the extent of fetal maturation at 42 weeks' gestation is not equivalent for all populations, universal application may not be appropriate for the conventional definition of post-term, i.e. 42 weeks' gestation. The increased risk of fetal distress, meconium staining and fetal death exhibited by African-Americans, in contrast to Whites, suggests that they may have an earlier onset of postmaturity-related problems. Instituting routine fetal surveillance at 40 or 41 weeks' gestation for African-American and other populations with earlier

gestational maturation, e.g. twins and hypertensives, may help reduce their disparate risk of fetal death and other postmaturity-related adverse outcomes. Currently, this proposal for redefining post-term has been undertaken for women of African ancestry in the French Caribbean and for women of Asian-Indian ancestry in Singapore[56].

CONCLUSIONS

While no single theory has emerged that fully explains the ongoing ethnic disparities in birth outcomes, the present evidence suggests that the reduction of these disparities will not be achieved solely by medical solutions that focus only on the perinatal period[30]. Eventually, the continued exploration of the antecedents, mediators and markers of the multiple etiological pathways for preterm birth may uncover additional important precursors of small and early birth, which may further increase our understanding of the factors underlying the ethnic disparities in these adverse outcomes[57–59]. However, working towards the elimination of barriers to the provision of quality health care, which includes removing financial barriers as well as barriers in our medical and health-care systems that result from racism and classism, are fundamental activities that should be undertaken while these investigations continue. Concurrently, we need to reassess whether the prevailing use of largely low-risk, White population-based fetal growth and post-term norms may result, for other ethnic or high-risk groups, in the mis-specification of risk status and failure of prompt identification of infants in need of intervention services both during pregnancy and beyond[60]. Moreover, the assumption that all ethnic groups have the same normal rate, extent and duration of fetal development needs to be rigorously and systematically examined in order to assure that current norms are appropriate to support the provision of optimal care that takes diversity into account.

While the long-term goals of addressing any adverse influences that tradition, poverty and racism have had on our health-care practices and systems are laudable, clinicians, faced with the pressing needs of a pregnancy in crisis, need more immediate strategies. Recommendations for earlier fetal surveillance have been made previously[61,62]. Emphasizing these for use in specific ethnic and other high-risk groups with average gestational ages that differ from those used to create reference standards is a prudent proposal for recognizing the diverse needs of each ethnic group. While using ethnicity as a proxy for earlier fetal maturation has problems similar to its use to indicate social class and poverty, i.e. not all members of the ethnic group will have early maturation or be impoverished[30], the recognition of the increased risk of an earlier onset of postmaturity may assist clinicians in the more timely detection of these problems, thereby potentially lowering ethnic disparities in fetal mortality.

ACKNOWLEDGEMENTS

This work was supported in part by DHHS, HRSA, MCHB grants MCJ-9040.

References

1. Alexander GR, Allen MC. Conceptualization, measurement and use of gestational age: I. Clinical and public health practice. *J Perinatol* 1996;16:53–9

2. Reid J. On the duration of pregnancy in the human female. *Lancet* 1850;2:77–81

3. Silverman WA. Nomenclature for duration of gestation, birth weight and intrauterine growth. *Pediatrics* 1967;39:935–9

4. Alexander GR, Tompkins ME, Altekruse JM, Hornung CA. Racial differences in the relation of birth weight and gestational age to neonatal mortality. *Public Health Rep* 1985;100:539–47

5. Allen MC. Developmental outcome and follow-up of the small for gestational age infant. *Semin Perinatol* 1984;8:123–56

6. Meyer AW. *Fields, Graphs and Other Data on Fetal Growth.* Contributions to embryology, No. 4, Pub. No. 222. Washington, DC: Carnegie Institute, 1915

7. Anderson NA, Brown EW, Lyon RA. Causes of prematurity. III Influences of race and sex on duration of gestation and weight at birth. *Am J Dis Child* 1943;65:523–34

8. Papiernik E, Cohen H, Richard A, Montes de Oca M, Feingold J. Ethnic differences in duration of pregnancy. *Ann Hum Biol* 1986;13:259–65

9. Shiono PH, Klebanoff MA, Graubard BI, *et al.* Birth weight among women of different ethnic groups. *J Am Med Assoc* 1986;255:48–52

10. Kessel SS, Kleinman JC, Koontz AM, *et al.* Racial differences in pregnancy outcomes. *Clin Perinatol* 1988;15:745–54

11. Papiernik E, Alexander GR, Paneth N. Racial differences in pregnancy duration and its implications for perinatal care. *Med Hypoth* 1990;33:181–6

12. Baruffi G, Fuddy LJ, Onaka AT, Alexander GR, Mor JM. Temporal trends in maternal characteristics and pregnancy outcomes: their relevance to the provision of health services. *Hawaii Med J* 1997;56:149–53

13. Slugk M, Tripathy K, Arya LS. Birth weight gestational age correlates of neonatal mortality. *Indian J Pediatr* 1982;49:511–17

14. Lumley J. The epidemiology of preterm birth. *Baillière's Clin Obstet Gynaecol* 1993;7:477–98

15. Berkowitz GS, Papiernik E. The epidemiology of preterm birth. *Epidemiol Rev* 1993;15:477–98

16. Kramer MS. Determinants of low birth weight: methodological assessment and meta-analysis. *Bull World Health Org* 1987;65:663–737

17. Berkowitz GS, Lapinski RH. Relative and attributable risk estimates for preterm birth. *Prenat Neonat Med* 1998;3:53–5

18. Alexander GR, Cornely DA. Racial disparities in pregnancy outcomes: the role of prenatal care utilization and maternal risk status. *Am J Prevent Med* 1987;3:254–61

19. Wise PH, First LR, Lamb GA, *et al.* Infant mortality increase despite high access to tertiary care: an evolving relationship among infant mortality, health care, and socioeconomic change. *Pediatrics* 1988;81:542–8

20. Gould JB, Davey B, LeRoy S. Socioeconomic differentials and neonatal mortality: racial comparison of California singletons. *Pediatrics* 1989;83:181–6

21. Langkamp DL, Foye HR, Roghmann KJ. Does limited access to NICU services account for higher neonatal mortality rates among blacks? *Am J Perinatol* 1990;7:227–31

22. Fichtner RR, Sullivan KM, Zyrkowski CL, Trowbridge FL. Racial/ethnic differences in smoking, other risk factors, and low birth weight among low-income pregnant women, 1978–1988. MMWR CDC Survey Summary. *Morbid Mortal Weekly Rep* 1990;39:13–21

23. Hulsey TC, Levkoff A, Alexander GR, Tompkins ME. Differences in black and white infant birth weights: the role of maternal demographic factors and medical complications of pregnancy. *South Med J* 1991;84:443–6

24. Goldenberg RL, Cliver SP, Cutter GR, *et al.* Black–White differences in newborn anthropometric measurements. *Obstet Gynecol* 1991;78:782–8

25. Hulsey TC, Levkoff A, Alexander GR. Birth weights of infants of black and white mothers without pregnancy complications. *Am J Obstet Gynecol* 1991;164:1299–302

26. Kempe A, Wise PH, Barkan SE, *et al.* Clinical determinants of the racial disparity in very low birth weight. *N Engl J Med* 1992;327:969–73

27. McGrady GA, Sung JFC, Rowley DL, Hogue CJR. Preterm delivery and low birth weight among first-born infants of African-American and White college graduates. *Am J Epidemiol* 1992;136:266–76

28. Alexander GR, Baruffi G, Mor JM, Kieffer EC, Hulsey TC. Multi-ethnic variations in the pregnancy outcomes of military dependents. *Am J Public Health* 1993;83:1721–5

29. Shiono PH, Rauh VA, Park M, Lederman SA, Zuskar D. Ethnic differences in birthweight: the role of life style and other factors. *Am J Public Health* 1997;87:787–93

30. Kogan MD, Alexander GR. Social and behavioral factors in preterm birth. *Prenat Neonat Med* 1998;3:29–31

31. Alexander GR, Kogan MD, Himes JH, Mor J, Goldenberg R. Racial differences in birth weight for gestational age and infant mortality in extremely-low-risk U.S. populations. *Paediatr Perinat Epidemiol* 1999: in press

32. Wilcox A, Russell I. Why small black infants have a lower mortality rate than small white infants: the case for population-specific standards for birth weight. *J Pediatr* 1990;116:7–10

33. Alexander GR, Kogan MD. Ethnic differences in birth outcomes: the search for answers continues. *Birth* 1998;23:210–13

34. Hulsey TC, Alexander GR, Robillard P-Y, Annibale DJ, Keenan A. Hyaline membrane disease: the role of ethnicity and maternal characteristics. *Am J Obstet Gynecol* 1993;168:572–6

35. Gould JB, Gluck L, Kulovich MV. The relationship between accelerated pulmonary maturity and accelerated neurological maturity in certain chronically stressed pregnancies. *Am J Obstet Gynecol* 1977;127:181–6

36. Robillard P-Y, Hulsey TC, Alexander GR, Sergent M-P, de Caunes F, Papiernik E. Hyaline membrane disease in black newborns: does fetal lung maturation occur earlier? *Eur J Obstet Gynecol Reprod Biol* 1994;55:157–61

37. Alexander GR, Hulsey TC, Robillard P-Y, de Caunes F, Papiernik E. Determinants of meconium-stained amniotic fluid in term pregnancies. *J Perinatol* 1994;XIV:259–63

38. Wong WS, Wong KS, Chang A. Epidemiology of meconium staining of amniotic fluid in Hong Kong. *Aust NZ J Obstet Gynaecol* 1985;25:9093

39. Dysart M, Graves BW, Sharp ES, Cotsonis G. The incidence of meconium stained amniotic fluid from 1980 through 1986, by year and gestational age. *J Perinatol* 1991;XI:245–8

40. Alexander GR, de Caunes F, Hulsey TC, Tompkins ME, Allen MC. Ethnic variation in postnatal assessments of gestational age: a reappraisal. *Paediatr Perinat Epidemiol* 1992;6:423–33

41. Parkin JM, Hey EN, Clowes JS. Rapid assessment of gestational age at birth. *Arch Dis Child* 1976;51:259–63

42. Brueton MJ, Palit A, Prosser R. Gestational age assessment in Nigerian newborn infants. *Arch Dis Child* 1973;48:318–20

43. Alexander GR, Hulsey TC, Smeriglio VL, *et al.* Factors influencing the relationship between a newborn assessment of gestational maturity and the gestational interval. *Paediatr Perinat Epidemiol* 1990;4:133–46

44. Robillard P-Y, de Caunes F, Alexander GR, Sergent MP, Romano P, Berchel C. Evaluation of the validity of gestational age assessment for low birth weight infants from a Caribbean community. *J Perinatol* 1992;XII:115–19

45. Schoendorf KC, Hogue CJR, Kleinman JC, Rowley D. Mortality among infants of African-American as compared with white college-educated parents. *N Engl J Med* 1992;326:1522–6

46. Kieffer EC, Alexander GR, Kogan MD, *et al.* The

influence of diabetes during pregnancy on gestational age-specific newborn weight among U.S. black and white infants. *Am J Epidemiol* 1998;147:1053–61

47. Leland NL, Petersen DJ, Braddock M, Alexander GR. Ethnic variations in pregnancy outcomes of young adolescent mothers in the United States. *Public Health Rep* 1995;110:53–8

48. Mor JM, Alexander GR, Kogan MD, Kieffer EC, Ichiho HM. Similarities and disparities in maternal risk and birth outcomes of Whites and Japanese-Americans. *Paediatr Perinat Epidemiol* 1995;9:59–73

49. Alexander GR, Baruffi G, Mor JM, Kieffer EC. Pregnancy outcomes among whites and Filipinos: a paradoxical birth weight–neonatal mortality relationship. *Am J Hum Biol* 1993;5:203–9

50. Goldenberg RL, Cliver SP, Mulvihill FX, *et al.* Medical, psychosocial and behavioral risk factors do not explain the increased risk of low birth weight among black women. *Am J Obstet Gynecol* 1996;175:1317–24

51. Krieger N, Rowley DL, Herman AA, Avery B, Phillips MT. Racism, sexism and social class: implications for studies of health, disease and well-being. *Am J Prevent Med* 1993; Suppl 9: 82–122

52. Geronimus AT. The weathering hypothesis and the health of African-American women and infants: evidence and speculation. *Ethnic Dis* 1992;2:207–21

53. Emanuel I, Hale CB, Berg CJ. Poor birth outcomes of American black women: an alternative explanation. *J Public Health Policy* 1989;Autumn:299–308

54. David RJ, Collins JW. Differing birth weight among infants of U.S.-born blacks, African-born blacks, and U.S.-born whites. *N Engl J Med* 1997;337:1209–14

55. Hessol NA, Fuentes-Afflick E, Bacchetti P. Risk of low birth weight infants among black and white parents. *Obstet Gynecol* 1998;92:814–22

56. August M. France birth theory causes stir. New York: Associated Press, Nov. 20, 1998

57. Holzman C, Paneth N, Fisher R. Rethinking the concept of risk factors for preterm birth: antecedents, mediators and markers. *Prenat Neonat Med* 1998;3:47–52

58. Goldenberg RL, Iams JD, Mercer BM, *et al.* The preterm prediction study: the value of new and standard risk factors in predicting early and all spontaneous preterm births. *Am J Public Health* 1998;88:233–8

59. Holzman C, Paneth N. Preterm birth: from prediction to prevention. *Am J Public Health* 1998;88:183–4

60. Allen MC, Alexander GR. Using gross motor milestones to identify very preterm infants at risk of cerebral palsy. *Dev Med Child Neurol* 1992;34:226–32

61. Bochner CJ, Williams J, Castro L, Medearis A, Hobel CJ, Wade M. The efficacy of starting postterm antenatal testing at 41 weeks as compared with 42 weeks of gestational age. *Am J Obstet Gynecol* 1988;159:550–4

62. Guidetti DA, Divon MY, Langer O. Postdate fetal surveillance: is 41 weeks too early? *Am J Obstet Gynecol* 1989;161:91–3

Intrahepatic cholestasis of pregnancy: physiopathology and fetal outcome

37

N. Berkane, J. J. Cocheton, P. Merviel, R. Gaudet, D. Brehier and S. Uzan

INTRODUCTION

Cholestasis of pregnancy occurs during the second half of pregnancy. It generally combines generalized pruritus with abnormal liver function tests. These clinical and liver function disturbances disappear completely several days after delivery. They may recur during future pregnancies or during oral contraceptive use.

The incidence of this disorder among pregnant women varies according to country and ethnic group. It complicates 15% of the pregnancies among Indian women in Chile, 1% of pregnancies in Sweden, only 0.1% in France, and it seems nearly non-existent among Blacks[1-3].

Its cause is not well known, in marked contrast to its complications, in particular for the fetus. These have now been clearly demonstrated; prevention requires close monitoring and active management at the end of pregnancy.

DEFINITION

This disorder is marked by cutaneous pruritus, which is generalized, predominantly nocturnal and often intense, even disabling. Jaundice in varying degrees has been described, but does not appear consistently. This pruritus may be differentiated from itching of a dermatological origin by its association with liver abnormalities. The specific liver function anomalies sought may vary from one study to another. These may be the standard signs of cholestasis: elevated conjugated bilirubinemia, elevated plasma alkaline phosphatases, in particular

the 5' nucleotidase fraction. Markedly elevated transaminase values, indicating cytolytic action, are often observed and are considered by some to signal the gravity of the disease. Moreover, whatever the laboratory anomalies, it appears that pruritus either isolated or associated with moderate liver function anomalies has a better fetal prognosis[4].

The past several years have seen the development of assays for total plasma bile acids, and several authors have begun to develop new definitions[5,6], basing the diagnosis of cholestasis on the association of pruritus and an increase in plasma bile acids, even in the absence of other liver function anomalies. This definition has, however, been criticized. Although Laatikainen and Ikonen[7] found a 92% increase in bile acids among patients with classic signs of cholestasis of pregnancy, Lunzer and colleagues[2] reported only an 80% increase in bile acids when pruritus was present. Moreover, in the latter study, only 48% of the patients with increased plasma bile acids did not have pruritus.

Cholestasis of pregnancy is not the only cause of cholestasis during pregnancy. The other possible causes must therefore be ruled out: virus, drug reactions, lithiasis and primitive bile cirrhosis. Indispensable elements for accepting or ruling out a diagnosis of cholestasis of pregnancy include: the interview, virological testing for hepatitis A, B and C or cytomegalovirus (CMV), testing for anti-mitochondrial antibodies, and an abdominal ultrasound examination.

274

PHYSIOPATHOLOGY

The variable distribution of this disorder by ethnic origin suggests a genetic predisposition. One study found that HLA BW 16 was the group best represented in the population with this disorder[8]. Nonetheless, other studies have not confirmed this hypothesis.

In 1994, Davies and co-workers[9] studied the *in vitro* and *in vivo* effect of estrogens on the sulfation and hepatic glycuronidation capacities in a group of patients with a history of cholestasis of pregnancy and in a control group. Glycuronic acids have the particularity of being hepatotoxic and of thus leading to cholestasis, while sulfated derivatives are not. He concluded that an elevated estrogen level during pregnancy could interfere with sulfation and thereby promote cholestasis. These findings could explain why cholestasis occurs at a higher rate in multiple pregnancies, where the level of circulating steroid hormones is higher than normal.

The seasonal and geographic character of this disorder is surely related to the environmental factors associated with it, one of which may be a selenium deficiency[10]. It appears that an anomaly involving estrogen – its level? its metabolism? its susceptibility? – leads to stagnation of the bile acids in the bile ducts, and their passage into the maternal circulation. These bile acids are toxic to hepatocytes[11]. They also induce a proliferation of cells in the bile ducts, thus promoting an aggravation of the cholestasis[12]. Crossing the placenta, they can affect fetal cells in the same way.

COMPLICATIONS

Maternal

This is essentially a benign disease for the mother, bothersome only by an annoying pruritus that can be the source of cutaneous excoriation. On the other hand, the use of some treatments can promote problems with coagulation, with a diminished prothrombin time and digestive difficulties.

Fetal

An elevated bile acid level in the maternal blood can also be found in the fetus, for bile acids cross the placenta. There is, in fact, a correlation between maternal and fetal bile acid levels[13]. These acids can induce hepatotoxicity in the fetus as they do in the mother. Animal studies have shown an alteration of hepatic function that lasts into the neonatal period (8 weeks in a rat population) and low weight[14].

El Mir and co-workers[15] have shown that the development of cholestasis in the mother promotes changes in the infant's bile lipids and secretion of bile acids. The bile acids are the activators of the various stages that lead to secretion of the bile lipids. One of the consequences is a state of latent, reversible cholestasis in the infant.

In a similar study, Zimber and associates[16] observed histological and biochemical alterations in fetal and neonatal liver sections from rats whose mothers had an excessive oral intake of lithocholic acid, which caused an excess of bile acids. Briukhin and Mikhailova[17] found thymic hypotrophy in rat fetuses with cholestatic mothers. In another study several years later, Briukhin uncovered a simultaneous depression of cellular immunity and increase of humoral immunity[18].

Both retrospective and prospective studies performed in humans to assess the fetal impact of cholestasis of pregnancy have observed an abnormally high rate of *in utero* fetal death, fetal growth restriction, chronic and acute fetal distress and preterm delivery. Acute fetal distress was observed in 22% and meconium staining in 43% of the cases in the series reported by Fisk and Storey[19], a retrospective study of 83 patients and 86 pregnancies complicated by cholestasis of pregnancy. Shaw and colleagues[6] found even higher rates: 33% with acute fetal distress, and 58% with meconium staining. These two outcomes may be related, because meconium discharge may induce an umbilical vein constriction that leads to fetal hypoxia, a cause of acute fetal distress. Reid and co-workers[20] reported that 27% of 56 patients had meconium staining.

Another study[21] compared two groups of patients: 79 women with cholestasis of pregnancy, and 79 others with a history of *in utero* fetal death. It found fetal distress among 25% of the first group and only 6% of the latter, and meconium staining in 44.3% and 7.6%, respectively. There were two *in utero* fetal deaths in the first group and none in the second. In the study by Fisk and Storey[19], two *in utero* fetal deaths occurred in the 86 pregnancies. Reid and associates[20] had an 11% perinatal death rate; only one of the deaths occurred after (very premature) birth. Laatikainen and Ikonen[7] published a series of 86 pregnancies complicated by cholestasis, which they classified into three groups of increasing gravity, according to their liver function values. The fetal death in this study belonged to the most seriously ill group, as did most of the cases with fetal distress and meconium staining.

In a study of 13 patients with cholestasis of pregnancy by Davies and colleagues[22], there were eight *in utero* fetal deaths, one neonatal death, two preterm births and one Cesarean section for acute fetal distress. Twelve of the 13 pregnancies had not received any special management. In looking at these extreme rates, it must be borne in mind that there was a recruitment bias, as only the gravest cases were referred to this center.

Fetal deaths result from complex and poorly understood physiopathological mechanisms. They appear unforeseeable, even with monitoring by umbilical Doppler, which, on the other hand, helps foresee vasculorenal syndromes[23,24]. Similarly, no early warning signs have been seen with fetal heart monitoring[21]. Nonetheless, this monitoring is often carried out only once or twice a week; performed more frequently, its prognostic value might be greater.

The rate of preterm delivery in the study by Fisk and Storey[19] was 44%. Palma and co-workers[25], assessing the efficacy of ursodeoxycholic acid for treating this disorder, observed a preterm delivery rate greater than 50% (4/7) in the placebo group. Reid and colleagues[20] reported 36% preterm deliveries.

This frequency of preterm deliveries may be related to the potentiation of oxytocin by bile acids at the level of the uterine muscle, as demonstrated by Israel and colleagues[26] in a study of six patients with cholestasis of pregnancy and six control patients. Other factors also play a role, including the fact that attending physicians stop all treatment, especially tocolytics, once cholestasis is diagnosed, and that all the preterm deliveries are not spontaneous. That is, clinical aggravation of the mother's or fetus's condition may be an indication for inducing delivery.

SURVEILLANCE

Early studies looked at the prognostic value of such biological markers as urinary estriol, serum placental lactogen and α-fetoprotein, but none of these provided helpful input to patient monitoring[27].

More recent studies are contradictory. Berg and co-workers[4] argued that the prognosis was good when the cholestasis was minimally symptomatic, but Shaw and co-workers[6] found no correlation between liver function and fetal prognosis. Currently, neither threshold values nor specific liver criteria have any prognostic value. Patients with severely impaired liver function must be carefully monitored, without, however, underestimating the possible effect of apparently more moderate disease[6,7].

The value of other paraclinical tests is quite limited, as discussed above for the umbilical artery flow rates and fetal heart rate monitoring. Nonetheless, the value of such monitoring several times daily has not been studied: the fetal deaths reported by Alsulyman and colleagues[21] occurred within 5 days of normal fetal heart rate monitoring, and the *in utero* fetal deaths in the study of Davies and co-workers[22] had no special management at all.

It has also been suggested that amniocentesis could be used to verify the color of the amniotic fluid and thus screen for meconium staining[19]. This test, which would need to be repeated several times to be useful, has not been widely implemented.

MANAGEMENT

The potential gravity of this disorder requires, we believe, a system of clinical and paraclinical surveillance that includes two or three fetal heart rate monitoring daily and one or two laboratory tests weekly. Surveillance of this intensity generally requires that the patient must be hospitalized. Interrupting all tocolysis seems useful to us, for the disease is grave and premature delivery may in the long run be better than continuing the pregnancy at any price, with the associated risk of acute fetal distress. In addition, some tocolytic treatments (progesterone, salbutamol?) may provoke a cholestastic reaction.

The substantial discomfort caused by the mother's pruritus or the severity of the liver function impairment has led some authors to propose various anti-pruritic treatments and bile acid chelators (cholestyramine), but without appreciable success. The prescription of ursodeoxycholic acid, a bile acid less toxic than chenodeoxycholic or lithocholic acids, seems to improve fetal prognosis and maternal itching, without side-effects[25,28,29]. Nonetheless, the small number of patients in these series means that further studies are required before

its use is generalized. In any case, the birth should be induced as soon as pulmonary maturation is attained, most often at 37 weeks' gestation[6,19,21].

Postpartum, normalization of the liver function tests and clinical symptoms must be monitored. After patients have been reassured, they must be warned about the theoretical risk of recurrence while using estrogen–progestogen combined contraception and the much greater risk of recurrence in future pregnancies[30].

CONCLUSION

Cholestasis of pregnancy is a disease of unknown etiology, but probably associated with high levels of steroid hormones during pregnancy, among patients with a genetic predisposition. There is no special maternal risk, but the serious risks to the fetus require that mother and fetus be closely watched. Because the factors most often monitored lack predictive value for the occurrence of serious accidents, physicians should induce labor as soon as the fetal pulmonary maturation is complete.

References

1. Heikkinen J, Maentausta O, Ylostalo P, Janne O. Changes in serum bile acid concentrations during normal pregnancy and in pregnant women with itching. *Br J Obstet Gynaecol* 1981; 88:240–5
2. Lunzer M, Barnes P, Byth K, O-Halloran M. Serum bile acid concentrations during pregnancy and their relationship to obstetric cholestasis. *Gastroenterology* 1986;91:825–9
3. Wilson JA. Intahepatic cholestasis of pregnancy with marked elevation of transaminases in a black American. *Diag Dis Sci* 1987;32:665–8
4. Berg B, Helm G, Petersohn L, Tryding N. Cholestasis of pregnancy. Clinical and laboratories studies. *Acta Obstet Gynecol Scand* 1986;65: 107–13
5. Laatikainen T, Tulenheimo A. Maternal serum bile acid levels and fetal distress in cholestasis of pregnancy. *Int J Gynaecol Obstet* 1984;22:91–4

6. Shaw D, Frolich J, Wittmann BA, Willms M. A prospective study of 18 patients with cholestasis of pregnancy. *Am J Obstet Gynecol* 1982;142:621–5
7. Laatikainen T, Ikonen E. Serum bile acid in cholestasis of pregnancy. *Obstet Gynecol* 1977;50: 313–18
8. Reyes H. The enigma of intrahepatic cholestasis of pregnancy: lessons from Chile. *Hepatology* 1982;2:87–96
9. Davies MH, Ngong JM, Yucesoy M, *et al.* The adverse influence of pregnancy upon sulphatation: a clue to the pathogenesis of intrahepatic cholestasis of pregnancy? *J Hepatology* 1994;21: 1127–34
10. Kauppila A, Korpela H, Makila UM, Yrjanheikki E. Low serum selenium concentration and glutathione peroxidase activity in intrahepatic cholestasis of pregnancy. *Br Med J* 1987;294: 150–2

11. Holsti P. Experimental cirrhosis of the liver in rabbits induced by gastric instillation of desiccated whole bile. *Acta Pathol Microbiol Scand* 1956;112:61–7

12. Larusso NF, Szczepanik PA, Hofmann AF. Effect of deoxycholic acid ingestion on bile acid metabolism and biliary lipid secretion in normal subjects. *Gastroenterology* 1977;72:132–40

13. Watkins JB. Placental transport: bile acid conjugation and sulfation in the fetus. *J Pediatr Gastroenterol Nutr* 1983;2:365–73

14. Monte MJ, Morales AI, Arevalo I, Macias RI, Marin JJ. Reversible impairment of neonatal hepatobiliary function by maternal cholestasis. *Hepatology* 1996;23:1208–17

15. El-Mir MY, Monte MJ, Morales AI, Arevalo M, Serrano MA, Marin JJ. Effect of maternal cholestasis on biliary lipid and bile acid secretion in the infant rat. *Hepatology* 1997;26:527–36

16. Zimber A, Zusman I, Bentor R, Pinus H. Effects of lithocholic acid exposure throughout pregnancy on late prenatal and early postnatal development in rats. *Teratology* 1991;43:355–61

17. Briukhin GV, Mikhailova GI. The structural-functional changes in the thymus of the progeny of female rats with experimental chronic cholestasis. *Morfologia* 1992;102:93–9

18. Briukhin GV. The indices of the physiopathological maturity of the progeny under conditions of chronic cholestatic lesions of the liver in the mother. *Morfologia* 1995;108:35–8

19. Fisk NM, Storey GN. Fetal outcome in obstetric cholestasis. *Br J Obstet Gynaecol* 1988;95:1137–43

20. Reid R, Ivey KJ, Rencret RH, Storey B. Fetal complications of obstetric cholestasis. *Br Med J* 1976;1:870–2

21. Alsulyman O, Ouzounian J, Ames-Castro M, Murphy Goodwin T. Intrahepatic cholestasis of pregnancy: perinatal outcome associated with expectant management. *Am J Obstet Gynecol* 1996;175:957–60

22. Davies M, Da Silva R, Jones S, Weaver J, Elias E. Fetal mortality associated with cholestasis of pregnancy and the potential benefit of therapy with ursodeoxycholic acid. *Gut* 1995;37:580–4

23. Kaar K, Jouppila P, Kuikka J, Luotola H, Toivaen J, Rekonen A. Intervillous blood in normal and complicated late pregnancy measured by means of intravenous ^{133}Xe method. *Acta Obstet Gynecol Scand* 1980;59:7–10

24. Zimmerman P, Koskinen J, Vaalamo P, Ranta T. Doppler umbilical artery velocimetry in pregnancies complicated by intrahepatic cholestasis. *J Perinatol Med* 1991;19:351–5

25. Palma J, Reyes H, Ribalta J, *et al*. Ursodeoxycholic acid in cholestasis of pregnancy: final report of a randomized double blind placebo controlled study. *Hepatology* 1996;24:373–7

26. Israel EJ, Guzman ML, Campos GA. Maximal response to oxytocin of the isolated myometrium from pregnant patients with intra hepatic cholestasis. *Acta Obstet Gynecol Scand* 1986;65:581–2

27. Garoff L. Prediction of fetal outcome by urinary estriol, maternal serum placental lactogen and alpha protein in diabetes and hepatosis of pregnancy. *Obstet Gynecol* 1976;48:659–66

28. Diaferia A, Nicastri PL, Tartagni M, Loizzi P, Iacovizzi C, Di Leo A. Ursodeoxycholic acid therapy in pregnant women with cholestasis. *Int J Gynaecol Obstet* 1996;52:133–40

29. Isla CR, Cappelletti CA, Tielli G, *et al*. Value of ursodeoxycholic acid in the treatment of intrahepatic cholestasis of pregnancy. *Gastroenterology* 1996;110:A1219

30. Gonzalez MC, Reyes H, Arrese M, *et al*. Intrahepatic cholestasis of pregnancy in twin pregnancies. *J Hepatol* 1989;9:84–90

Perinatal Rh hemolytic disease: screening, treatment and personal experience

38

L. S. Voto and M. Margulies

Severe hemolytic disease due to Rh incompatibility is still a source of concern for obstetricians and pediatricians. In Argentina, as in most developing countries, this disease is one of the main causes of fetoneonatal morbidity and mortality, owing to the lack of appropriate prophylaxis with postpartum anti-D γ-globulin and inadequate prenatal control[1]. Perinatal hemolytic disease represents one of the most significant examples in medicine of successful management of a disease and adequate prophylaxis.

By the first half of this century, perinatal hemolytic disease accounted for 45% of all perinatal deaths. Currently, this rate has fallen markedly to 5%, which results from in-depth understanding of the etiology and pathogenesis of the disease, the advances in perinatal technology, the creation of sophisticated centers for high-risk perinatal care and, mainly, from its prophylaxis.

THE Rh BLOOD GROUP ANTIGENS

Biochemistry and molecular genetics

A group of non-glycosylated hydrophobic transmembrane proteins of 30–32 kDa are known to carry the Rh blood antigens (D, Ce and Ee series). These proteins, which are not found in the red cells of rare Rh_{null} individuals with membrane defects, are specific for erythrocytes and have a distinctive sequence homology. The RhD and non-D proteins show 92% sequence identity and a similar predicted membrane topology. The Rh proteins D and Cc/Ee are encoded by the RHD and RHCE genes, respectively; these genes are arranged in tandem on chromosome 1p34–p36 and probably result from the duplication of a common ancestral gene.

The human RH locus is considered to be a two-gene model where all RhD-positive haplotypes have two structural genes (namely, RHD and RHCE) and most RhD-negative ones have only one structural gene (namely, RHCE). D protein is encoded by the RHD gene, whereas the C/c and E/e proteins are encoded by the RHCE gene. The relationship between blood group D epitopes and the amino acid polymorphisms of the Rh proteins still remains unclear, but it has been found that the molecular basis for the C/c (Ser → Pro) and E/e (Pro → Ala) specificities results from amino acid polymorphisms at positions 103 and 226, respectively. In the Rh system, polymorphism and gene diversity seem to be produced mainly by gene conversion. However, cases of gene deletion have also been observed in the Rh system. Rh_{null} phenotypes have been found to be caused by a mechanism of transcriptional regulation that has not yet been clearly described.

In the cells of the Rh_{null} individuals, morphological and functional abnormalities of cation transport as well as phospholipid asymmetry have been observed and are thought to lead to severe clinical conditions. Also, Rh proteins and other glycoproteins (such as Rh50 glycoprotein, CD47, glycophorin B, Duffy, LW) are either not present, or their quantity is markedly lower in the cells of Rh$_{null}$ individuals, which might mean that Rh proteins form a multimeric complex with these glycoproteins[2].

ETIOLOGY AND PATHOGENESIS OF Rh-Hr INCOMPATIBILITY

The antigens of the Rh system are located on the surface of the erythrocyte, although they are also thought to be part of the trophoblast. Anti-D antibodies of the Rh system are responsible for the majority of clinically detectable cases of perinatal hemolytic disease. This situation is observed in Rh-negative mothers whose husbands are Rh-positive, and whose immunization occurred during pregnancy, abortion, postpartum or incompatible transfusion.

There are other Rh-Hr system antibodies that are capable of producing a clinical disease. They are listed here in order of frequency: anti-c (hr'), anti-C (rh'), anti-e (hr''), or the combination of any of these with factor D.

In Argentina 13% of couples are Rh incompatible, and it is estimated that there is one case of perinatal hemolytic disease in every 150 deliveries. On the other hand, according to different statistics, the immunization rate is between 7 and 14%.

Rh SENSITIZATION MECHANISM

The passage of fetal red blood cells to the maternal circulation is considered to be normal during pregnancy. Using the Kleihauer–Betke technique it was established that the passage of fetal red blood cells was not higher than 0.1–0.2 ml. In this case the competent immunological system would not be activated; however, the chances of it being stimulated are much higher if transplacental hemorrhage is greater than the established values.

There are certain obstetric events that can increase the risk, such as placenta previa, abruptio placentae, external version, Cesarean section, manual removal of the placenta and – in the early stages of pregnancy – abortion and ectopic pregnancy. All invasive procedures during pregnancy cause the passage of fetal red blood cells. Chorionic villus sampling performed during the first trimester of pregnancy, frequently used nowadays, has been associated with very severe cases of hemolytic disease, even with hydrops. Amniocentesis causes fetomaternal hemorrhage in 2–3% of cases. Spontaneous or induced abortion is also associated with transplacental hemorrhage.

Antigen D has already developed by days 35–45 of gestation, which explains why 4–5% of post-abortion patients may become sensitized. Intravenous drug abuse can also lead to isoimmunization. When an Rh-negative person receives Rh-positive blood, an immunological response takes place in 50% or more of the cases.

The primary immunological response is usually weak. The initial antibodies are of the IgM class, with a high molecular weight, and are unlikely to cross the placenta. As a result, they do not produce fetal hemolysis. Later in pregnancy, IgG antibodies cross the placenta and produce hemolysis. The IgG antibodies involved in the etiology and pathogenesis of perinatal hemolytic disease due to anti-D are mainly subtypes IgG I and IgG III. The former cross the placenta early in pregnancy, and therefore have a role in the most severe cases of disease.

In our experience, the frequency of immunization in Rh-negative patients during their second pregnancy with compatible Rh-positive fetuses is 12–15%.

ABO incompatibility in an Rh-negative patient provides partial protection against primary anti-Rh isoimmunization, but not against a secondary immunological response. In the former, the anti-A or anti-B incompatible immunized blood cells are captured by the liver, which is not an immunologically active organ and does not produce anti-Rh antibodies. On the other hand, in a secondary immunological response, the spleen receives the blood cell stroma and produces anti-Rh antibodies. Therefore, there is a higher incidence of Rh hemolytic disease in children whose parents are ABO compatible.

PATHOGENESIS AND PHYSIOPATHOLOGY OF PERINATAL HEMOLYTIC DISEASE

According to different studies, the rate of active transport of human IgG varies in the course of normal gestation; before 12 weeks of pregnancy this transfer is very low; but it has been demonstrated that, in severe Rh disease, the direct antiglobulin test on the fetal (Rh-positive) red cells may be positive as early as 6–10 weeks. The IgG antibodies rise exponentially until term. Sometimes, IgG levels in infants can be higher than in the mother.

The pathogenesis of perinatal hemolytic disease lies in the hemolysis of fetal erythrocytes caused by maternal antibodies. Hemolysis then results in fetal anemia. According to the severity of hemolysis, the disease will be anemic, icteroanemic or hydropic. In hydropic hemolytic disease the hepatic parenchyma is replaced partially with secondary erythropoietic tissue, which causes a portal and umbilical venous hypertension syndrome, as well as alterations in the metabolism of proteins, and decreased albumin. Both clinical conditions cause edema and ascites, which are characteristic of hydrops.

Frequently, fetal cardiac failure secondary to severe anemia is observed. Both other forms of perinatal hemolytic disease, anemic and icteroanemic, are the result of a less severe hemolysis that does not compromise either the cardiocirculatory system or protein metabolism.

FOLLOW-UP OF THE Rh-NEGATIVE PATIENT

The anamnesis will focus on relevant data such as: number of previous deliveries, history of anti-D prophylaxis, history of perinatal morbidity and mortality attributable to hemolysis, history of previous transfusions and history of neonatal exchange transfusions or luminotherapy in previous deliveries.

If an indirect Coombs' test does not detect anti-D antibodies, it should be repeated every 4 weeks until immediate puerperium. If the test is positive, we proceed as follows:

(1) Study of husband's zygosity. If he is heterozygous, the fetus might not be Rh-positive;

(2) Serial titration of anti-D antibodies every 3 weeks with the purpose of drawing a curve;

(3) Amniotic fluid spectrophotometry, in accordance with previous history of Rh disease and levels of anti-D antibodies in relation to the patient's gestational age;

(4) Serial ultrasonographic follow-up to evaluate fetal growth or detect characteristic signs of the disease: polyhydramnios, hepatomegaly, ascites, soft tissue edema;

(5) Antenatal fetal monitoring as soon as it is reliable, to assess fetal vitality and especially sinusoid patterns.

Figures 1 and 2 show the steps to follow.

TREATMENT OF SEVERE MATERNAL–FETAL Rh-INCOMPATIBILITY

In 1963, Liley[3] described intrauterine transfusion as the only possible way to prevent intrauterine fetal death of severely affected Rh-positive fetuses. When pregnancy interruption is indicated, fetal prematurity becomes an aggravating factor which conspires against successful results. The purpose of all the procedures described below is to allow the fetus to reach viability.

Intrauterine fetal transfusion

Intraperitoneal route

It is estimated that the total amount of blood transfused into the peritoneal cavity flows into the fetal bloodstream within 7 to 10 days after being injected. This technique relies on the absorption capability of the fetal peritoneum and subdiaphragmatic lymphatic, and it is not usually indicated before the 24th week of gestation. Ultrasound plays an essential role

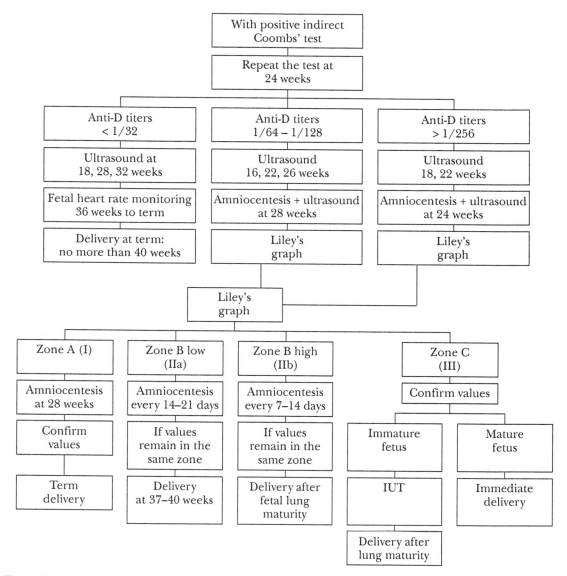

Figure 1 *Steps to follow with Rh-isoimmunization in patients with no maternal or perinatal history of the disease*

in this procedure: it locates the fetal abdomen and shows the precise point of entry. The inferior portion of the peritoneal cavity is accessed, with the bladder used as a reference point to prevent injury to the liver or spleen. Ascites, if present, should be evacuated before the procedure, although in this case the intravascular route is always preferred.

Type O, Rh-negative blood – compatible with maternal blood – with a hematocrit of not less than 75% should be transfused. Blood should have been recently extracted (not more than 48 h before the procedure). The use of uterine inhibitors is recommended; the administration of antibiotics in order to prevent possible infection is controversial. The procedure should be repeated, according to the development of the patient's condition, every 14 days or more, until fetal viability is achieved.

The amount of blood to be transfused should be estimated as follows: gestational age in weeks minus 20, multiplied by 10. For example, in a 28-week pregnancy, $(28 - 20) \times 10 = 80$, therefore a total of 80 ml of erythrocytes should be transfused.

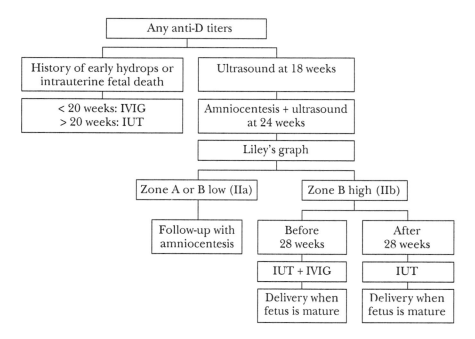

Figure 2 *Steps to follow with Rh-isoimmunization in patients with maternal and/or perinatal history of the disease. IVIG, intravenous immunoglobulin; IUT, intrauterine transfusion*

Intravascular fetal transfusion

This approach is indicated especially in cases of fetal hydrops or very severe fetal anemia. The technique, which may be used from 18 weeks of pregnancy, involves access to an umbilical vessel near its placental insertion, in the intrahepatic portion of the umbilical vein, or in the fetal heart (fetal rescue operation). This procedure is currently regarded as superior to intrauterine transfusion, because it allows the immediate reversal of fetal anemia, by enabling a sample of fetal blood to be obtained for determination of its hematocrit and hemoglobin values. Also, a faster remission of fetal hydrops is observed in most cases.

The amount of blood to be transfused depends on the patient's gestational age and the hematocrit of the blood of the donor and fetus. The procedure should be repeated according to post-transfusion hematocrit values, until fetal extraction is indicated. If no complications occur, this technique allows the lengthening of intrauterine fetal life until the fetus is viable, which results in a marked decrease in perinatal mortality rates.

High-dose intravenous IgG

Intrauterine fetal transfusion, by either the intraperitoneal or the intravascular route, has been shown to be an effective treatment of Rh hemolytic disease. However, some fetuses are already severely compromised at an early stage, when it is technically impossible to indicate the procedure.

In agreement with other authors, we have found that repeated invasive techniques result in an important increase in anti-D titers, owing to the variable amounts of fetomaternal bleeding inevitably caused by the procedure itself. As a result of this, moderate Rh disease in a present pregnancy can often become a severe disease in the subsequent gestation.

The use of high doses of intravenous immunoglobulin (IVIG) in the treatment of immunological diseases in both children and adults because of recurrent intrauterine fetal loss has frequently been reported in the literature, with varying degrees of effectiveness. Although the mechanisms of action of IVIG during pregnancy remain unclear, several explanations have been proposed: feedback inhibition of antibody synthesis, competition for macrophage or Fc receptors of target cells and blockade of Fc-mediated antibody placental transport. We have used IVIG therapy in a prospective study in order to analyze its effectiveness in the antenatal treatment of severe Rh hemolytic disease.

The only immunoglobulin that is transferred into the fetal circulation is IgG; the other classes of maternal immunoglobulins either are not transferred or only cross the placenta in small quantities. The mechanisms involved in the active transfer of IgG across the human placenta are not yet known. The studies of Brambell and colleagues[4] in rabbits suggest that the transport of IgG molecules across the placenta is mediated through a receptor for the Fc part of the molecule. Further studies have clarified the role of a placental Fc receptor for IgG; this receptor has been demonstrated on the surface of the trophoblast at 10 weeks and at term.

The mechanisms of placental transfer of exogenous IgG infused into the mother are still to be elucidated. It must be emphasized that transplacental IgG transfer is a slow process and requires an intact Fc portion of the IgG molecule. The studies of Gitlin and co-workers[5] demonstrated that, when labelled IgG was injected into pregnant women at various intervals before delivery, even after 12 days, the concentration in the infant's serum was only about 40% of that in the mother. Studies performed by Contractor and associates[6] about IgG transport in perfused placentas suggest that the trophoblast absorbs a substantial amount of human IgG and all bovine IgG, both broken down in small fractions by a mechanism of non-specific endocytosis, and transmits these fragments to the fetal circulation. A small amount of human IgG, however, would escape this process of lysosomal destruction by diverse protective mechanisms, and would be released intact on the fetal side.

There are very few cases in the literature reporting the treatment of severe Rh hemolytic disease with high doses of IVIG and the findings are too dissimilar to allow for conclusive generalizations to be drawn.

Rewald and Berlin obtained satisfactory results with the combined use of plasmapheresis and IVIG in four cases of severe Rh hemolytic disease. De la Cámara and colleagues reported the successful treatment of two cases with repeated doses of IVIG throughout gestation. Scott and co-workers, on the other hand, used a combined protocol of IVIG and repeated intrauterine transfusions in one case of hemolytic disease.

We have administered IVIG as the only treatment in 24 severely Rh-sensitized patients with a previous history of affected fetuses and/or neonates, with elevated anti-D titers, and a high degree of intrauterine hemolysis. Patients in group 1 (< 20 weeks; $n = 8$) fulfilled the first two of these inclusion criteria, whereas in groups 2 (20–28 weeks; $n = 7$) and 3 (> 28 weeks; $n = 9$), IVIG treatment was indicated on the basis of intrauterine hemolysis. IVIG was infused at a daily dose of 0.4 g/kg maternal body weight for 4–5 consecutive days, and repeated every 21 days until delivery.

Group 3 also included those patients who attended the antenatal clinic very late in pregnancy; as a consequence of this delay, the fetuses in these cases were highly compromised because of the advanced stage of the hemolytic disease, and they evidenced major neonatal depression and severe fetal anemia at birth, requiring – in almost all cases – exchange transfusions.

In group 1 patients, as the indication for IVIG had been a previous history of severe fetal/neonatal hemolytic disease and high maternal anti-D titers, all the fetuses showed good intrauterine recovery and only half of the neonates required transfusional therapy at birth.

Group 2 patients responded more satisfactorily to IVIG treatment, as evidenced by the hematological condition of the neonates and the low degree of postnatal hemolysis.

Three fetuses were hydropic at the onset of treatment (two from group 1 and one from group 2). IVIG administration, which is used to reduce intrauterine hemolysis by preventing the development of severe fetal anemia, was clearly not the appropriate therapeutic indication in these cases.

In view of the advanced gestational age at delivery and the fairly high mean birth weight (2500 g) in all the groups, neonates did not require mechanical ventilation and responded more satisfactorily to therapy in the immediate neonatal period. The decrease in pre- versus post-treatment anti-D antibody quantification, the reduction in intrauterine hemolysis and the strongly positive direct antiglobulin test in all neonates may indicate that the mode of action of high doses of IVIG in Rh hemolytic disease is first, feedback inhibition of antibody synthesis; and second, partial blockade of Fc-mediated antibody transport across the placenta. No adverse effects from the drug were observed in the mothers or neonates.

Our findings showed that IVIG treatment was effective in both groups 1 and 2, where IVIG was administered before the 28th week of gestation and the fetuses were not hydropic at the onset of therapy. In group 3, however, where fetal anemia was already advanced at the time of treatment, intrauterine transfusions and prompt fetal extraction should have been the treatment of choice.

The analysis of the series, including only the 13 most severely affected patients as judged by their history of fetal/neonatal death, demonstrated again the effectiveness of IVIG treatment. It can be inferred from the results in this particular group of patients that first, after 28 weeks' gestation the administration of IVIG does not elicit significant reductions in anti-D titers and intrauterine hemolysis, thus intrauterine transfusion is the therapy of choice; and second, that IVIG treatment is not indicated in case of hydrops fetalis. Excepting these two indications, it is in this series, with the poorest history, the highest antibody level and failure of transfusional therapy in previous gestations, where we find the most encouraging therapeutic results of IVIG treatment.

The high cost of IVIG therapy is immediately outweighed by the highly satisfactory perinatal results obtained in our population of extremely severe Rh-sensitized patients. Moreover, babies born after treatment with intrauterine transfusions, as well as those prematurely delivered because of their severe disease, require a prolonged stay in the neonatal intensive care unit (a mean of 60 days in the latter case), the cost of which greatly exceeds that of IVIG therapy.

In conclusion, the results of our study, which to our knowledge is the largest reported in the literature, show the value of high doses of IVIG in the treatment of severe Rh incompatibility when administered repeatedly before 28 weeks' gestation and in the absence of hydrops fetalis[1].

High-dose intravenous IgG followed by intrauterine transfusions

Intrauterine fetal transfusion is currently the therapy of choice in cases of severe anti-D isoimmunization. However, its efficacy is reduced in patients with early severe hydrops fetalis, owing to the technical difficulties in performing this procedure before 20 weeks' gestation and because the fetuses are already anemic at that time. The purpose of this study was to determine whether the early onset of high-dose immunoglobulin therapy followed by intrauterine transfusions is more effective than intrauterine transfusions alone in the treatment of very severe isoimmunized fetuses.

The population studied in this retrospective clinical research was assigned to one of the following two groups: the Gamma group comprised 30 patients receiving immuno-globulin therapy before 21 weeks' gestation and intrauterine transfusions after 20 weeks; the IUT group comprised 39 patients receiving intrauterine transfusion treatment starting at a gestational age of 20–25 weeks. Both groups were statistically similar regarding history of perinatal deaths and anti-D antibody titers.

The number of hydropic fetuses at the first intrauterine transfusion and the number of fetal deaths were significantly higher in the IUT than in the Gamma group. No significant differences were observed between the groups in fetal hematocrit at the time of first transfusion or at birth. However, the percentage of severely anemic fetuses was higher in the IUT group. The fetal mortality rate was 36% less in the Gamma group.

In very severe cases of Rh isoimmunization, the following are found:

(1) The development of fetal hemolysis in the first 20 weeks of gestation increases the risk of fetal death;

(2) The early onset of invasive fetal therapy is only partially effective and potentially harmful;

(3) According to the present study, those patients who received high-dose IVIG in the first 20 weeks of pregnancy seemed to have a better fetal outcome.

In summary, therefore, our results suggest that high-dose immunoglobulin therapy followed by intrauterine transfusions may improve fetal survival in these severe cases. Further randomized clinical trials are needed to confirm these results[7].

PROPHYLAXIS

In 40–50% of pregnancies the passage of fetal red blood cells to the maternal circulation usually takes place during the last trimester. In the majority of cases the amount of blood transferred is less than 0.1 ml[8].

In 1977 there were 110 cases of stillbirth or postnatal death due to anti-D hemolytic disease in the UK. In 1992, the figure decreased to only nine cases. This decrease came as a result of the introduction in 1969 of anti-D immunoglobulin prophylaxis. In 1969 the prophylaxis protocol consisted of anti-D immunoglobulin administration only after the birth of an Rh-positive child, or after certain pregnancy events such as antepartum hemorrhage. Most of the deaths resulted from maternal sensitization between 28 and 40 weeks of the first pregnancy (third trimester) and during the postpartum.

Further studies have determined that the percentage of sensitization decreased from 1.2 to 0.28% if antenatal prophylaxis was carried out[9]. In practice, the combination of antenatal and postnatal prophylaxis will prevent immunization in 96% of the high-risk cases. The remaining 4% corresponds to the absence or inappropriate administration of immunoglobulin when it is indicated.

Owing to the fact that isoimmunization during pregnancy is caused by transplacental hemorrhage, the risk of immunization increases after the following procedures[10]:

(1) Spontaneous or induced abortion;

(2) Amniocentesis;

(3) Chorionic villus sampling;

(4) Cordocentesis;

(5) Ectopic pregnancy;

(6) Fetal manipulation: external version;

(7) Antepartum hemorrhage;

(8) Antepartum fetal death;

(9) Positive blood transfusion.

The standard postpartum dose of 300 µg contains enough anti-D to neutralize at least 15 ml of fetal red blood cells.

There are different methods to detect excessive fetomaternal hemorrhage: the Kleihauer–Betke test is, if carried out correctly, a very sensitive and specific method, but it is subject to laboratory and technological errors. Flow cytometry is also a very sensitive method, but it is difficult to perform and expensive. The rosette method is easy to carry out and very sensitive, but it has low specificity and its results must be confirmed by the Kleihauer–Betke test or flow cytometry.

Anti-D immunoglobulin has very few adverse effects. Some fetuses yield a slightly positive direct Coombs' test at birth after antenatal administration. The presence of anemia or hyperbilirubinemia is very rare. All plasma involved in the production of anti-D immunoglobulin is carefully checked for infectious diseases. There have not been any HIV cases due to contaminated plasma.

The American College of Obstetricians and Gynecologists recommends both typifying the pregnant patient and looking for antibodies at her first visit and again at 24–28 weeks, and offering anti-D immunoglobulin to all Rh-negative, non-sensitized patients. It has been found that transplacental hemorrhage occurs in 3, 12 and 45% of cases during the first, second and third trimesters, respectively. The capacity of an antibody to eliminate D-red cells *in vivo* depends both on its avidity and, to a lesser degree, on its affinity for the D-antigen. Absorption is also a limiting factor.

Even though antepartum immunoglobulin administration offers many additional benefits, some authors argue that, as the incidence of isoimmunization is relatively small, it makes medication 16 times less cost-effective than postpartum prevention programs.

Pharmaceutical preparations

Anti-D Polyclonal is produced from male donors and highly sensitized females. The quality control shows biosafety. *Anti-D Monoclonal* is in phase 1 of experimentation. It has unknown safety, efficiency, dependability and cost. The unit equivalents are shown in Table 1.

The intramuscular route is used, via the deltoides muscle. In the gluteal area, the

Table 1 *Unit equivalents of immunoglobulins*

Micrograms (µg)	International units (IU)
50	250
100	500
225	1250
300	1500

preparation penetrates to only the subcutaneous tissue, thus absorption is prolonged. The recommended dose is 500 IU or 100 µg for every 4 ml of fetal red blood cells in the maternal circulation. Indications are: postpartum, within the first 72 h, 300 µg; prenatal, as follows:

(1) First trimester: abortion, ectopic pregnancy, chorionic villus sampling or amniocentesis;

(2) Second trimester: suspected fetomaternal hemorrhage, or invasive procedures;

(3) Third trimester: prophylactic. 500 IU at 28 and 34 weeks, or only one dose of 300 µg between the above-mentioned weeks.

References

1. Margulies M, Voto LS, Mathet ER, *et al.* High-dose intravenous IgG for the treatment of severe rhesus alloimmunization. *Vox Sang* 1991;61: 181–9
2. Carton JP. Defining the Rh blood group antigens. Biochemistry and molecular genetics. *Blood Rev* 1994;8:199–212
3. Liley AW. Intrauterine transfusion of fetus in haemolytic disease. *Br Med J* 1963;2:1107–9
4. Brambell FWR, Hemmings WA, Oakley CL, Porter RR. The relative transmission of the fractions of papain hydrolized homologous gammaglobulin from the uterine cavity to the fetal circulation in the rabbit. *Proc R Soc Ser B* 1960;151:478–82
5. Gitlin D, Kumate J, Urrusti J, Morales C. The selectivity of the human placenta in the transfer of plasma proteins from mother to fetus. *J Reprod Immunol* 1983;5:265–73

6. Contractor SF, Eaton BM, Stannard PJ. Uptake and fate of exogenous immunoglobulin G in the perfused human placenta. *J Reprod Immunol* 1983; 5:265–73
7. Voto LS, Mathet ER, Zapaterio JL, Orti J, Lede RL, Margulies M. High-dose gammaglobulin (IVIG) followed by intrauterine transfusions (IUTs): a new alternative for the treatment of severe fetal hemolytic disease. *J Perinat Med* 1997; 25:85–8
8. Jorgensen J. Foetal–maternal bleeding during pregnancy and delivery. *Acta Obstet Gynecol Scand* 1977;56:487–90
9. Nusbacher J, Bove JR. Immunoprophylaxis: is antepartum therapy desirable? *N Engl J Med* 1980;303:935–7
10. Urbamak SJ. Rh (D) hemolytic disease of the newborn. *The Changing Scene Borns* 1985;291: 4–6

Fetal consequences of maternal inherited hypercoagulable states (thrombophilia) 39

D. Blickstein and I. Blickstein

INTRODUCTION

Spontaneous or minimal-stimulus thrombosis does not occur in the normal circulation since inhibitors present in the plasma control the extent and speed of blood coagulation and fibrinolysis. The quantitative and/or qualitative dysfunction of these inhibitors is associated with hyperactivity of the coagulation system and substantive risk for thromboembolic events. The increased tendency for thrombosis, known as thrombophilia (thrombo- + G. philos, fond), may be inherited or acquired (Table 1). Inherited thrombophilia is defined as a genetically determined tendency for increased risk of thrombo-embolic disease[1].

An efficient uteroplacental unit associated with optimal fetal growth and development may be compromised by states related to maternal thrombophilia. This association was suggested in the 1960s; however, only in the past two decades did several publications specifically address these conditions. In this chapter we discuss the influence of maternal inherited thrombophilia on fetal outcome.

ANTITHROMBIN III

Antithrombin III (ATIII) is a naturally occurring anticoagulant, which inactivates thrombin and other coagulation enzymes. Its deficiency, an autosomal dominant disorder, may be caused by one of more than 80 different gene mutations (chromosome 1q 23-25). The normal limitation of the coagulation cascade is impaired in both types of ATIII deficiency (i.e. in combinations of qualitative and/or quantitative reductions) and, as in many other autosomal dominant traits, the

Table 1 *Inherited and acquired thrombophilia*

Inherited disorders	Acquired disorders
Antithrombin III deficiency	Antiphospholipid syndrome
Protein C deficiency	Myeloproliferative disorders
Protein S deficiency	Paroxismal nocturnal hemoglobinuria
Activated protein C resistance	Malignancy
Hyperhomocysteinemia	Cancer chemotherapy
Prothrombin gene mutation	Nephrotic syndrome
Rare conditions	Estrogen-containing medication
Dysfibrinogenemia	
Factor XII deficiency	
Factor XIII deficiency	
Hypo-dysplasminogenemia	
Heparin cofactor II deficiency	
High plasminogen activator inhibitor	
Abnormal thrombomodulin	

deficiency is usually encountered in hetero-zygotic individuals.

Sanson and co-workers[2] found 27.8% abortions and stillbirths occurring in 36 pregnancies in women with ATIII deficiency. In the European Prospective Cohort On Thrombophilia (EPCOT) study[3], ATIII deficiency was associated with a significantly increased risk of miscarriage (OR 1.7, 95% CI 1.0–2.8) and stillbirth (OR 5.2, 95% CI 1.5–18.1). These figures represent the highest risk of all isolated thrombophilic states and emphasize the importance of anticoagulation in these patients.

Since inhibition of coagulation factors by ATIII is markedly accelerated by heparin, these patients should receive prophylactic anticoagulation by heparin or low molecular weight heparin[4]. ATIII concentrate may be added in acute thromboembolic events, as an alternative anticoagulant, or when lower doses of heparin may be required (e.g. during labor and delivery)[5]. Neonates with ATIII levels < 30% of the normal may require fresh frozen plasma or ATIII concentrate[5].

PROTEIN C AND PROTEIN S DEFICIENCIES

Inactivation of factors Va and VIIIa by the naturally occurring protein C is greatly enhanced by its cofactor protein S. The combined activity of protein C and protein S interferes with coagulation and fibrin formation, whereas hypercoagulability is produced in quantitative and/or qualitative deficiency states. At least 160 and 30 gene mutations are involved in the autosomal dominant protein C and protein S deficiencies, respectively[5]. The protein C gene is located on chromosome 2q13-14 and the active α gene is located on the region 3p11.1-3q11.2 in protein S.

Sanson and colleagues[2] found a fetal loss rate of 27.9% and 16.5% in pregnancies occurring in patients deficient in protein C and protein S, respectively. In the EPCOT study[3] the odds ratio for miscarriage was 1.4 (95% CI 0.9–2.2) and that for stillbirth was 2.3 (95% CI 0.6–8.3) in protein C deficiency and the respective risks

for protein S deficiency were 1.2 (95% CI 0.7–1.9) and 3.3 (95% CI 1.0–11.3). The authors concluded that the risk for miscarriage and stillbirth was greatly increased for isolated protein C and protein S deficiencies, although the confidence intervals do not support the conclusion.

ACTIVATED PROTEIN C RESISTANCE

In most cases, activated protein C resistance (APCR) results from a point mutation in the factor V gene, the so-called factor V Leiden mutation (FV Q506) located on chromosome 1q 21-25. This gene defect prevents protein C from inactivating active factor V. The mutation has been traced to a single common origin in Caucasians, in whom this defect is found in approximately 10%, whereas the mutation is rarely found in African and Asian populations. APCR is the most common heritable thrombophilia in Caucasians[1,4,6]. As opposed to ATIII, protein S and protein C deficiencies, APCR may be 'acquired' during pregnancy, and therefore the diagnosis should be confirmed by DNA analysis for factor V Leiden mutation[1]. 'Acquired' APCR is also found in association with the antiphospholipid syndrome[6], a known risk for placental thrombosis and fetal loss.

The fetal consequences of APCR have been extensively studied. Rai and associates[7] screened 120 women attending a recurrent miscarriage clinic for APCR. The prevalence of APCR was significantly higher among women who had experienced at least one second-trimester abortion (20%) as compared with those who had experienced only first-trimester miscarriage (5.7%, $p < 0.02$) and with parous controls (4.3%, $p < 0.02$).

In a case–control study conducted by Grandone and colleagues[8], APCR was found in seven of 43 Caucasian women with a history of recurrent abortions (16.3%) as compared to five of 118 parous women without fetal loss (4.2%, $p = 0.01$). APCR was significantly more common in women who experienced late abortions (31.2% vs. 7.4%, $p = 0.04$).

Dizon-Townson and co-workers evaluated the fetal APCR status[9]. In a case–control comparison, they observed a two-fold increase in the fetal factor V Leiden mutation carrier frequency in 12 of 139 (8.6%) abortuses compared with 17 of 403 (4.2%, $p < 0.05$) unselected pregnant women at labor (OR 2.15, 95% CI 0.9–4.9). It should be mentioned that the 95% confidence interval of the case–control study does not support significant statistics. In addition, they found a significant increase in the fetal factor V Leiden mutation carrier frequency in placentas with more than 10% infarction as compared to placentas with less than 10% infarction (42% vs. 1.9%, $p < 0.0001$, OR 37.2, 95% CI 11.0–130.4). It should be mentioned that only five of the 17 fetuses carrying the mutation were from normal pregnancies, whereas eight of the 17 pregnancies were complicated by hypertension. Thus, the interesting suggestion of a prenatal phenotype and effects of the Leiden mutation at the fetoplacental interface should await confirmation.

Ridker and colleagues[10] compared 113 consecutive patients referred to a recurrent abortion clinic with 437 postmenopausal women with at least one successful pregnancy and no pregnancy loss and with 387 postmenopausal women with at least one pregnancy loss. The prevalence of APCR was greater among cases (8.0%) than among controls (3.7%, OR 2.3, 95% CI 1.0–5.2, $p = 0.05$). The prevalence was somewhat greater in the subgroup of patients with three or more pregnancy losses (9.0%, OR 2.6, 95% CI 1.0–6.7, $p = 0.048$). The comparison to postmenopausal women with at least one pregnancy loss showed an almost identical prevalence to the cases (7.5%). The authors were cautious in stating that the data were compatible with the hypothesis that factor V Leiden mutation may play a role in some cases of recurrent pregnancy loss.

The EPCOT study[3] also failed to reveal an increased incidence of miscarriage (OR 0.9, 95% CI 0.5–1.5) and stillbirth (OR 2.0, 95% CI 0.5–7.7). By contrast, a study conducted by Brenner and colleagues[6] found that 48% of 39 patients with recurrent fetal loss had APCR. Of the 128 pregnancies in these patients, only 25% ended as live births, more

than half ended as early spontaneous abortions and 15% as second-trimester abortions. Nine of the 39 patients did not have the factor V Leiden mutation, but an 'acquired' APCR.

Differences between observations may be due to ascertainment. For example, the EPCOT study was conducted on unselected patients with the mutation, whereas other studies considered cases with recurrent pregnancy loss. In any case, the results seem to suggest that APCR is at least not uncommon in patients with adverse fetal outcome.

In addition to fetal loss, APCR has been associated with severe, early-onset, pre-eclampsia. Dizon-Townson and co-workers[11] reported that 8.9% of 158 women with severe pre-eclampsia were heterozygous for factor V Leiden mutation as compared with 4.2% of 403 normotensive controls ($p = 0.03$). A potential association of APCR with the HELLP syndrome has also been suggested[12].

HYPERHOMOCYSTEINEMIA

Inherited hyperhomocysteinemia results from several genetic defects in the methionine–homocysteine metabolic enzymatic pathways in which folate, cobalamine and pyridoxine act as co-factors[4]. A common defect of the remethylation pathway is a thermolabile mutant (C 677T substitution) of methylene tetrahydrofolate reductase (MTHFR), which has about 50% of the normal enzyme activity. The homozygous state of this MTHFR is found in about 5–10% of the general population, and leads to mild (16–24 µmol/l) and moderate (25–100 µmol/l) fasting hyperhomocysteinemia[1,4]. The thrombophylic properties of hyperhomocysteinemia are poorly understood and both vessel wall damage and interference with activation of coagulation factors and/or the natural inhibitors have been proposed[4].

The association of hyperhomocysteinemia and neural tube defects (NTD) is well documented and represents a neat explanation of how folate supplementation may reduce the risk of NTD[1]. It has also been observed that recurrent abortions before 17 weeks' gestation are 2–3 times more frequent in women with the MTHFR gene mutation[13]. Some forms of hyperhomocysteinemia were found in 18% of patients with early onset pre-eclampsia[14], in 26% with placental abruption, in 11% with fetal demise and in 38% of those delivering growth-restricted neonates[15].

COMBINED DEFICIENCIES

A significant proportion of patients with manifest thrombophilia have a condition with a multifactorial background. The concept of interaction suggests that patients with combined gene deficiencies, or those with gene–environment interaction, have an increased expression of thrombosis. Of particular interest are the combinations of factor V Leiden mutation and hyperhomocysteinemia and the combined effects of factor V Leiden mutation and familial antiphospholipid syndrome. The EPCOT study found that combined defects had an increased risk of stillbirth (OR 14.3, 95% CI 2.4–86.0) but a decreased risk for miscarriage (OR 0.8, 95% CI 0.2–3.6)[3]. Others have found that 13 of 85 women (15.3%) with severe early onset pre-eclampsia had combinations of thrombophilic defects[14].

RARE OBSERVATIONS

Thrombophilic factors are intensively studied. Thus, we witness a plethora of small series and case reports associating a rare deficiency with adverse fetal outcome. An incomplete list of these factors includes: familial dysfibrinogenemia[16], congenital absence of prothrombin activity[17], factor XII deficiency[18] and factor XIII deficiency[19]. Other thrombophilic disorders such as prothrombin gene mutation, thrombomodulin gene mutation, elevated factor VIII and heparin co-factor II deficiency have not yet been studied in relation to pregnancy outcome.

The complex of thrombin–antithrombin (TAT) is a marker of thrombin generation. It has been observed that women with pregnancies complicated by intrauterine growth restriction had higher levels of the TAT complex[20]. In addition, Vincent and co-

Table 2 *Important selection criteria to evaluate healthy women for inherited thrombophilia*

Familial history (including gynecological) of thromboembolism occurring in young first-degree relatives

Unexplained episodes of venous and/or arterial thromboembolism in patients aged less than 45 years

Recurrent thrombosis

Thromboembolic phenomena during pregnancy, the puerperium and hormonal contraception

Recurrent miscarriages, stillbirth, or intrauterine growth restriction

Early onset severe pre-eclampsia with or without the HELLP syndrome

Thrombosis in unusual venous sites

Thrombosis during the neonatal period

workers found raised TAT values in women with recurrent miscarriage[21].

DIAGNOSIS

Since screening the general population for inherited thrombophilia is currently not cost-effective, the first step in diagnosis is appropriate selection of patients[1,4]. Table 2 lists important selection criteria in healthy women without acquired causes for performing the relatively complex and expensive assays for thrombophilia. Since combined defects are quite common, a thrombophilia survey should include the whole battery of tests. Care should be taken in interpreting the results (Table 3).

THERAPY

Patients with major thromboembolic events (e.g. pulmonary embolism, visceral or cerebral vein thrombosis, recurrent deep vein thrombosis) should have been evaluated for inherited thrombophilia before pregnancy, and obviously should be maintained on anticoagulants and/or antiplatelet agents throughout gestation.

Patients in whom the diagnosis has been reached following an unfavorable obstetric

Table 3 *Interpretation of laboratory values*

Factor	Levels during normal pregnancy	Comment
Antithrombin III	no change	—
Protein C	no change	use functional (protein C activity) assays oral anticoagulants decrease levels
Protein S	free protein S levels may decrease during second trimester	use free protein S values (higher sensitivity and specificity) oral anticoagulants decrease levels
Activated protein C resistance (APCR)	acquired APCR may be seen with advancing normal pregnancy	use DNA analysis of FVQ506 for definite diagnosis
Hyperhomocysteinemia	no change	changes with dietary intake of folate, vitamin B_6 and vitamin B_{12} in high levels look for the MTHFR gene mutation

MTHFR, methyl tetrahydrofolate reductase

history should be maintained on anti-thrombotic therapy primarily as a prophylactic measure against thromboembolism during pregnancy. Although the literature has abundant proofs for maternal indications, thromboprophylaxis during pregnancy for fetal indications has been only extrapolated. The EPCOT study provided only recently a rationale for clinical trials of prophylactic anticoagulation for affected women with recurrent fetal loss[3].

For the time being, the clinician is faced with two options: either to await evidence-based recommendations[3] or to consider adverse fetal outcome as a thrombotic phenomenon that justifies anticoagulation (heparin or low molecular weight heparin)[6] for both maternal and fetal indications. Patients with hyperhomocysteinemia should receive supplemental vitamins, in particular folic acid, but also pyridoxine and cobalamine[4]. Finally, replacement therapy with ATIII and protein C concentrates may be used to reduce the risks of peripartum bleeding and as an alternative to conventional anticoagulation.

SUMMARY

The cause and effect relationship of inherited hypercoagulable states and poor pregnancy outcome is being extensively studied. Although observations are not unanimous, adverse pregnancy events such as unexplained fetal loss and recurrent miscarriages are customarily regarded as thrombotic events that indicate diagnosis and prophylactic therapy. Adequate prospective clinical trials are expected to show whether thromboprophylaxis in patients with inherited thrombophilia will also improve pregnancy outcome.

References

1. Girling J, de Swiet M. Inherited thrombophilia and pregnancy. *Curr Opin Obstet Gynecol* 1998;10: 135–44
2. Sanson BJ, Friederich PW, Simioni P, *et al.* The risk of abortion and stillbirth in antithrombin-, protein C-, and protein S-deficient women. *Thromb Haemost* 1996;75:387–8
3. Preston FE, Rosendaal FR, Walker ID, *et al.* Increased fetal loss in women with heritable thrombophilia. *Lancet* 1996;348:913–16

4. De Stefano V, Finazzi G, Mannucci PM. Inherited thrombophilia: pathogenesis, clinical syndromes, and management. *Blood* 1996;87:3531–44

5. Barbour LA, Pickard J. Controversies in thromboembolic disease during pregnancy: a critical review. *Obstet Gynecol* 1995;86:621–33

6. Brenner B, Blumenfeld Z. Thrombophilia and fetal loss. *Blood Rev* 1997;11:72–9

7. Rai R, Regan L, Hadley E, Dave M, Cohen H. Second-trimester pregnancy loss is associated with activated protein C resistance. *Br J Haematol* 1996;92:489–90

8. Grandone E, Margaglione M, Colaizzo D, *et al.* Factor V Leiden is associated with repeated and recurrent unexplained fetal losses. *Thromb Haemost* 1997;77:822–4

9. Dizon-Townson DS, Meline L, Nelson LM, Varner M, Ward K. Fetal carriers of the factor V Leiden mutation are prone to miscarriage and placental infarction. *Am J Obstet Gynecol* 1997;177:402–5

10. Ridker PM, Miletich JP, Buring JE, *et al.* Factor V Leiden mutation as a risk factor for recurrent pregnancy loss. *Ann Intern Med* 1998;128:1000–3

11. Dizon-Townson DS, Nelson L, Katrina Easton BS, Ward K. The factor V Leiden mutation may predispose women to severe preeclampsia. *Am J Obstet Gynecol* 1996;175:902–5

12. Brenner B, Lanir N, Thaler I. HELLP syndrome associated with factor V R506Q mutation. *Br J Haematol* 1996;92:999–1001

13. Nelen WLDM, Steegers EAP, Eskes TKAB, Blom HJ. Genetic risk factor for unexplained recurrent early pregnancy loss. *Lancet* 1997;350:861

14. Dekker GA, de Vries JIP, Doelitzsch PM, *et al.* Underlying disorders associated with severe early onset preeclampsia. *Am J Obstet Gynecol* 1995;173:1042–8

15. de Vries JIP, Dekker GA, Huijgens PC, Jacobs C, Blomberg BME, van Geijn HP. Hyperhomocysteinemia and protein S deficiency in complicated pregnancies. *Br J Obstet Gynaecol* 1997;104:1248–54

16. Haverkate F, Samama M. Familial dysfibrogenemia and thrombophilia. *Thromb Haemost* 1995;73:151–61

17. Catanzarite VA, Novotny WF, Cousins LM, Schneider JM. Pregnancies in a patient with congenital absence of prothrombin activity: case report. *Am J Perinatol* 1997;14:135–8

18. Gris JC, Ripart-Neveu S, Maugard C, *et al.* Prospective evaluation of the prevalence of haemostasis abnormalities in unexplained primary recurrent miscarriages. *Thromb Haemost* 1997;77:1096–103

19. Egbring R, Kroniger A, Seitz R. Factor XIII deficiency: pathogenetic mechanisms and clinical significance. *Sem Thromb Haemost* 1996;22:419–25

20. Bellart J, Gilabert R, Fontcuberta J, Carreras E, Miralles RM, Cabero L. Coagulation and fibrinolytic parameters in normal pregnancy and in pregnancy complicated by intrauterine growth retardation. *Am J Perinatol* 1998;15:81–5

21. Vincent T, Rai R, Regan L, Cohen H. Increased thrombin generation in women with recurrent miscarriage. *Lancet* 1998;352:116

Pregnancy outcome and obstetric complications following hysteroscopic metroplasty

40

S. Kupesic, A. Kurjak and D. Đulepa

INTRODUCTION

Congenital uterine malformations vary in frequency and are usually estimated to represent 3–4% of the general population, although less than half have clinical symptoms[1–3]. The most frequent symptomatic malformation is the septate uterus (close to 50%)[3,4].

During the first trimester of pregnancy, the risk of spontaneous abortion in patients with a septate uterus is between 28 and 45%, whereas the frequency of late spontaneous abortions during the second trimester is approximately 5%[3]. Premature deliveries, abnormal fetal presentations, irregular uterine activity and dystocia at delivery are likely in cases of septate uterus[5]. Poor vascularization of the septum was proposed as a potential cause of miscarriage[4]. An electron microscopy study by Fedele and colleagues indicated a decrease in the sensitivity of the endometrium covering the septa of malformed uteri to preovulatory changes[6]. This could play a role in the pathogenesis of primary infertility in patients with a septate uterus.

An unfavorable obstetric prognosis can be transformed by surgical correction of the intrauterine septum. Formerly, removal of the septum was performed by transabdominal metroplasty[7]. Hysteroscopic treatment is currently proposed as the procedure of choice for the management of these disorders. This simple and effective treatment has an obvious advantage in that the uterus is not weakened by a myometrial scar. Cararach and co-workers[8] and Goldenberg and co-workers[9]

reported pregnancy rates of 75% and 88.7%, respectively, after operative hysteroscopy.

The simplicity and effectiveness of hysteroscopy have faced the clinician with the need for an early and correct diagnosis of the uterine anomalies. When used as a screening test for detection of congenital uterine anomalies, transvaginal ultrasound had a sensitivity of almost 100%[10,11]. However, drawing a clear distinction between different types of abnormalities was impossible and operator-dependent[12,13].

X-ray hysterosalpingography (HSG) is an invasive test that requires the use of contrast medium and exposure to radiation. Although HSG provides a good outline of the uterine cavity, the visualization of minor anomalies and a clear distinction between different types of lateral fusion disorders is sometimes impossible. More recently hysterosonography has been introduced for detection of uterine cavitary abnormalities[14]. Transvaginal ultrasound is carried out after distension of the uterine cavity by instillation of a saline solution. This produces anatomical images of the endometrium and myometrium, and allows accurate depiction of the septate uterus, and even the measurement of the thickness and height of the septum[15].

Although some reports have indicated a high diagnostic accuracy of magnetic resonance imaging[16,17] in the diagnosis of congenital uterine anomalies, this technique is rarely routinely used for this indication. In patients scheduled for corrective surgery, the evaluation is usually completed by another invasive procedure – diagnostic hysteroscopy[18]. Three-dimensional ultrasound has been reported to be very efficient in detection of the septate uterus[19], and can stand in place of invasive diagnostic procedures.

ULTRASOUND IMAGING IN DIAGNOSIS AND TREATMENT OF THE SEPTATE UTERUS

Our study attempted to evaluate the combined use of transvaginal ultrasound, transvaginal color and pulsed Doppler sonography, hysterosonography and three-dimensional ultrasound in the preoperative diagnosis of the septate uterus[20]. The second part of the study analyzed obstetric and perinatal complications of the septate uterus, and assessed the reproductive outcome after hysteroscopic treatment.

A total of 420 infertile patients undergoing operative hysteroscopy were included in this study. Table 1 summarizes the intraoperative findings. The final diagnosis of the uterine disorder was confirmed by hysteroscopy, and 278 patients had an intrauterine septum corrected surgically. Forty-three of the patients with septate uteri had a history of repeated spontaneous abortion, 71 had one spontaneous abortion (56 in the first trimester, whereas 15 reported spontaneous abortion during the second trimester), 82 had primary sterility and 20 had premature delivery, including six with breech and two with transverse presentation. A positive history of ectopic pregnancy was noted in 76 patients.

Each patient underwent transvaginal ultrasound and transvaginal color Doppler examination during the luteal phase of their cycle. A systematic examination of the uterine position, size and morphological characteristics was performed. With the use of B-mode transvaginal sonography, the morphology of the uterus was carefully explored with the emphasis on the endometrial lining in both sagittal and transverse sections. The septum was visualized as an echogenic portion separating the uterine cavity into two parts (Figure 1). Once B-mode examination was completed by an experienced sonographer, transvaginal

Table 1 Intraoperative findings in 420 infertile patients undergoing hysteroscopy

Hysteroscopic finding	n	%
Submucous leiomyoma	46	10.9
Endometrial polyp	35*	8.3
Intrauterine synechiae	19*	4.5
Septate uterus	278	65.9
Arcuate uterus	28	6.6
Bicornuate uterus	16†	3.8
Total	422	100.0

*One patient with endometrial polyp and one with intrauterine synechiae had an intrauterine septum; †diagnosis made by combined use of laparoscopy and hysteroscopy

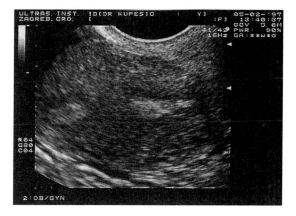

Figure 1 Septate uterus as demonstrated by transvaginal ultrasound: echogenic portion representing septum separates the uterine cavity into two parts

color Doppler examination was performed by another skilled operator who was unaware of the previous finding.

Color and pulsed Doppler were superimposed to visualize intraseptal and myometrial vascularity. Flow velocity waveforms were obtained from all the interrogated vessels (Color Plate O). For each recording, at least five waveform signals of good quality were obtained. During each procedure the resistance index (RI) was automatically calculated (Color Plate P). The RI was calculated from the maximum frequency envelope by the formula: peak systolic velocity minus end-diastolic velocity divided by peak systolic velocity. Instillation of isotonic saline (hysterosonography) was carried out on a gynecological examination table. In 76 patients the uterine cervix was exposed with a speculum disinfected with iodine solution. A catheter with external diameter of 1.6 mm and internal diameter of 1.1 mm was slowly introduced into the cervix. The balloon was insufflated with 1.5–2 ml of sterile saline solution to avoid outflow of the fluid. A syringe containing 20 ml isotonic saline solution was attached to the catheter and fluid was slowly injected. For distension of the uterine cavity about 10–20 ml of the contrast was required. The speculum was then withdrawn and the endovaginal probe introduced. Transverse and sagittal sections were carefully explored, and the septum was visualized as an echogenic portion separating the uterine cavity into two parts.

Eighty-six women undergoing hysteroscopy were examined by three-dimensional ultrasound. They all had a transvaginal scan and color and pulsed Doppler evaluation performed prior to three-dimensional examination. Twelve of these patients underwent additional examination: instillation of the isotonic saline solution into the uterine cavity. The results of the previous diagnostic tests were not available to the ultrasonographer performing the three-dimensional ultrasound. Three perpendicular planes of the uterus were simultaneously displayed on the screen, allowing a detailed analysis of the uterine morphology to be made. Frontal reformatted sections were particularly useful for detection of the uterine abnormalities (Figure 2).

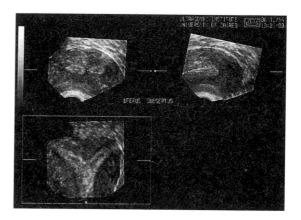

Figure 2 *Examination of the uterus using planar reformatted sections. Conventional transverse and longitudinal sections are displayed in planes A (upper left) and B (upper right). The third plane (lower left) is a frontal section through the uterus which is difficult to visualize on conventional scan. Note the clear separation of the endometrial lining on a frontal reformatted section suggestive of a septate uterus*

Table 2 summarizes the sensitivity, specificity and positive and negative predictive values of transvaginal sonography, transvaginal color and pulsed Doppler ultrasound, hysterosalpingography and three-dimensional ultrasound for the diagnosis of the septate uterus. In 264 cases a septate uterus was suspected by transvaginal ultrasound, while a normal finding was reported in 14 patients. The sensitivity of transvaginal sonography in the diagnosis of septate uterus was 94.96%.

Transvaginal color and pulsed Doppler enabled the diagnosis of septate uterus to be made in 276 cases, reaching a sensitivity of 99.28%. In one patient with an endometrial

Table 2 *Sensitivity, specificity, positive predictive value (PPV) and negative predictive value (NPV) of transvaginal ultrasound, transvaginal color Doppler, hysterosonography and three-dimensional ultrasound for the diagnosis of septate uterus in 420 patients with a history of infertility and recurrent abortion*

Imaging modality	True positives (n)	True negatives (n)	False positives (n)	False negative (n)	Sensitivity (%)	Specificity (%)	PPV (%)	NPV (%)
Transvaginal sonography	264	134	10	14	95.0	93.1	96.4	90.5
Transvaginal color Doppler	275	144	1	2	99.3	99.3	99.6	98.6
Hysterosonography	54	21	1	0	100.0	95.5	98.2	100.0
Three-dimensional ultrasound	58	23	1	4	93.6	95.9	98.3	85.2

polyp and one with intrauterine synechiae, a septate uterus was not correctly diagnosed. Therefore, the reliability of color and pulsed Doppler examination was reduced if other intracavitary structures (such as an endometrial polyp or submucous leiomyoma) were present. Color and pulsed Doppler studies of the septal area revealed vascularity in 198 (71.22%) patients (Color Plate O). The RI values obtained from the septum ranged from 0.68 to 1.0 (mean RI = 0.84 ± 0.16) (Color Plate P). Eighteen patients demonstrated absence of diastolic blood flow, while in the rest a continuous diastolic flow was present.

In 76 patients, intrauterine injection of an isotonic saline solution was advised before the hysteroscopic procedure was started. In 54 (71.05%) patients a septate uterus was clearly identified. The sensitivity and negative predictive value of hysterosonography following transvaginal color Doppler examination reached 100%. However, in one patient with an extensive intrauterine synechia, hysterosonography did not detect an intrauterine septum.

Good-quality three-dimensional images were obtained in 86 patients (Figures 2 and 3). Three-dimensional ultrasound agreed with hysteroscopy in 58 patients with septate uteri. However, in four patients with a septate uterus, three-dimensional ultrasound indicated the arcuate uterus. Distortion of the uterine cavity by a fundal fibroid was shown in these four patients. One false-positive diagnosis of septate uterus with three-dimensional ultrasound was obtained in a patient with intrauterine synechiae.

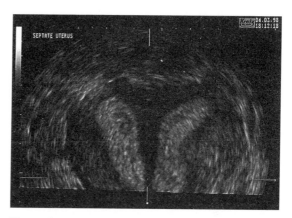

Figure 3 *Another three-dimensional scan of a septate uterus. Thick septum divides the uterine cavity. The extent of the defect is clearly measured*

The second part of our study attempted to evaluate the obstetric complications in a population of 278 patients with septate uterus and to compare these with the general population, represented by a control group during the 5-year period 1992–96 (Table 3)[20]. Early abortions appeared at a rate of 114/278 (41.01%) as compared to a rate of 15% for controls. Late abortions and premature deliveries appeared at a rate of 35/278 (12.59%) as compared to a rate of 7% for normal pregnancies. Intrauterine growth restriction appeared in two (8.7%) pregnancies with septate uterus as compared to 6% among the general population. Intrauterine fetal death occurred in one (4.35%) patient as compared to 0.5% in our control population. Abruptio placentae was found in one (4.35%) patient with septate uterus, as well as placenta praevia (4.35%). Breech presentation was found in six

Table 3 *Obstetric complications in patients with septate uterus and in controls*

Obstetric complication	Septate uterus (%)	Controls (%)	Significance (%)
Early abortion	41.0	15.0	$p < 0.001$
Late abortion	12.6	7.0	$p < 0.05$
Intrauterine growth restriction	8.7	6.0	$p < 0.05$
Breech presentation	26.1	3.7	$p < 0.001$
Transverse presentation	8.7	0.5	$p < 0.001$
Cervical incompetence	25.7	5.8	$p < 0.001$
Ectopic pregnancy	27.3	13.3	$p < 0.001$

(26.09%) pregnancies complicated by intrauterine septum, while transverse presentation occurred in two (8.70%) patients. Since abnormal fetal presentation was significantly more frequent in patients with septate uterus, a remarkably higher rate of Cesarean section (34.78%) occurred. Cervical incompetence during pregnancy appeared in nine (25.71%) women with intrauterine septum.

Extrauterine pregnancy appeared in 76 patients at a rate of 27.34%, which was 2 times higher than in our control group (13.3%). Bilateral ectopic pregnancy was noted in seven patients with septate uterus.

We assessed the reproductive outcome in 116 patients (32 with primary sterility, 16 with one spontaneous abortion, 12 with premature deliveries, 26 with recurrent abortion and 30 undergoing medically assisted reproduction) following operative hysteroscopy for an intrauterine septum. The prospective follow-up period was 24 months for each patient. The pregnancy rate in the studied group was 50.86%: 44 patients (74.58%) had term deliveries, 11 (18.64%) had first-trimester abortion and four (6.78%) reported preterm delivery. Other patients (n = 162) are followed in the same manner, but the follow-up period is less than 24 months and is therefore not reported in this study.

CAN ULTRASOUND PREDICT PREGNANCY OUTCOME IN PATIENTS WITH SEPTATE UTERUS?

Until now at least two procedures have been used for detection of congenital uterine anomalies. Gynecologists should be aware that long diagnostic evaluation delays the treatment and increases the cost, patient's discomfort and risk associated with each of the diagnostic procedures[15]. Therefore, quick and reliable diagnosis is important in patients with septate uterus, since surgical correction should be recommended. Fedele and colleagues[6] recently indicated that intra-uterine septum may be a cause of primary infertility. They demonstrated significant ultrastructural alterations in septal endometrium compared with endometrium from the lateral uterine wall in samples obtained during the preovulatory phase. The ultrastructural alterations included a reduced number of glandular ostia distributed irregularly, ciliated cells with incomplete ciliogenesis and a reduced ciliated : non-ciliated ratio. The ultrastructural morpho-logical alterations were indicative of irregular differentiation and estrogenic maturation of septal endometrial mucosa. Since the hormonal levels of the patients enrolled in this study were normal for the cycle phase, the most convincing hypothesis was that endometrial mucosa covering the septum was poorly responsive to estrogens, probably owing to scanty vascularization of septal connective tissue.

March[21] stated that the septum is built of fibroelastic tissue, whereas Fayez[22] believed that in the septum there are fewer muscle fibers and more connective tissue. However, our study did not confirm this. Color and pulsed Doppler revealed septal vascularity in 71.22% of the patients, indicating that most of the septa comprised myometrial vessels.

Dabrashrafi and co-workers[23] performed a histological study of the uterine septa in 16 patients undergoing abdominal metroplasty. Four biopsy specimens were taken from the uterus in each case: from the septum near the serosal layer, at the midpoint of the septum, at the level of the tip of the septum and from the left posterior aspect of the uterus away from the septum. The analysis confirmed that most of the uterine septa were composed of muscle tissue, interlacing muscle and vessels with muscle wall, which is contradictory to the classic view on the histological features of the uterine septum.

Less connective tissue in the septum can be the reason for poor decidualization and placentation in the area of implantation[22,23]. Increased amounts of muscle tissue and muscle interlacing in the septum can cause an abortion by the higher and uncoordinated contractility of these muscles (Color Plate Q).

A recent study from our department[24] found no correlation between septal height and occurrence of obstetric complications

($p > 0.05$). Abortions and late pregnancy complications occurred with the same rate in patients with small septa that were dividing less than one-third of the uterine cavity, and those with division of more than two-thirds of the uterine cavity. The same was related to septal thickness: obstetric complications were found in the same proportion of patients with thin and those with thick septa ($p > 0.05$). Indeed, pregnancy loss correlated significantly with septal vascularity (Color Plate R). Patients with vascularized septa had significantly higher incidence of early pregnancy failure and late pregnancy complications than those with avascularized septa ($p < 0.05$) (Color Plate S).

By using transvaginal ultrasound it is possible to perform a precise assessment of the uterine morphology, including the endometrial lining and outer shape of the uterine muscle. The color Doppler technique allows simultaneous visualization of morphology and the vascular network, giving full information on the type of anomaly and the extent of the defect. The visualization of the myometrial portion is further enhanced by detection of myometrial vessels by the color Doppler technique. Furthermore, Doppler imaging can detect deficient intraseptal vascularity and/or inadequate endometrial development in patients with septate uteri[24,25].

Three-dimensional ultrasound enables planar reformatted sections to be obtained through the uterus, allowing precise evaluation of the fundal indentation and the length of the septum (Figure 3). Although having very high sensitivity and specificity, this technique may give a wrong impression of an arcuate uterus in patients with fundal location of the leiomyoma. In these cases the uterine cavity has a concave shape, and fundal indentation is shallower. Furthermore, shadowing caused by the uterine fibroids, irregular endometrial lining and decreased volume of the uterine cavity (in cases of intrauterine adhesions) are obvious limitations of three-dimensional ultrasound.

Kupesic and Kurjak[20] clearly showed that obstetric complications were more frequent among patients with septate uterus than among other women. Furthermore, they demonstrated that ectopic pregnancy occurred at double the rate (27.34%) in these patients, compared to controls (13.3%). A possible etiology for this finding is the menstrual reflux, commonly present in patients with uterine anomalies, with sequelae that may interfere with the passage of the fertilized egg into the uterine cavity. The benefit of removing the intrauterine septum in patients suffering from infertility and recurrent pregnancy wastage is obvious, and has been reported widely[8,9,20]. It is expected that the cumulative pregnancy rate will be even higher than the reported 51%, since some of the patients with primary infertility who are involved in the *in vitro* fertilization program because of male factor await the procedure[20].

Conventionally it has been agreed not to intervene until the first obstetric accidents have occurred, because a large proportion of septate uteri have no obstetric pathology[26]. However, hypofecundity of the patients with septate uterus and good results achieved by endoscopic surgical treatment oblige us to propose hysteroscopy as soon as we diagnose septate uterus even prior to any pregnancy[20,24,27]. It seems that septal incision eliminates an unsuitable site of implantation, through revascularization of the connective uterine fundal tissue and/or elimination of the unfavorable uterine contractions[6]. Since both of these events can be detected by color and pulsed Doppler ultrasound, this technique can be efficiently used for detection of the congenital uterine malformations and follow-up of the patients undergoing hysteroscopy.

References

1. Ashton D, Amin HK, Richart RM, Neuwirth RS. The incidence of asmyptomatic uterine anomalies in women undergoing transcervical tubal sterilization. *Obstet Gynecol* 1988;72:28–30

2. Sorensen S. Estimated prevalence of mulerian anomalies. *Acta Obstet Gynecol Scand* 1988;67:441–5

3. Gaucherand P, Awada A, Rudigoz RC, Dargent D. Obstetrical prognosis of septate uterus: a plea for treatment of the septum. *Eur J Obstet Gynecol Reprod Biol* 1994;54:109–12

4. Fedele L, Arcaini L, Parazzini F, Vercellini P, Nola GD. Metroplastic hysteroscopy and fertility. *Fertil Steril* 1993;59:768–70

5. Heinonen PK, Saarikoski S, Pystynen P. Reproductive performance of women with uterine anomalies. An evaluation of 182 cases. *Acta Obstet Gynecol Scand* 1982;61:157–62

6. Fedele L, Bianchi S, Marchini M, Franchi D, Tozzi L, Dorta M. Ultrastructural aspects of endometrium in infertile women with septate uterus. *Fertil Steril* 1996;65:750–2

7. McShane PM, Reilly RJ, Schiff L. Pregnancy outcome following Tompkins metroplasty. *Fertil Steril* 1983;40:190–4

8. Cararach M, Penella J, Ubeda J, Iabastida R. Hysteroscopic incision of the septate uterus: scissors versus resectoscope. *Hum Reprod* 1994;9:87–9

9. Goldenberg M, Sivan E, Sharabi Z. Reproductive outcome following hysteroscopic management of intrauterine septum and adhesions. *Hum Reprod* 1995;10:2663–5

10. Valdes C, Malini S, Malinak LR. Ultrasound evaluation of female genital tract anomalies: a review of 64 cases. *Am J Obstet Gynecol* 1984;149:285–90

11. Nicolini U, Bellotti B, Bonazzi D, Zamberleti G, Battista C. Can ultrasound be used to screen uterine malformation? *Fertil Steril* 1987;47:89–93

12. Reuter KL, Daly DC, Cohen SM. Septate versus bicornuate uteri: errors in imaging diagnosis. *Radiology* 1989;172:749–52

13. Randolph J, Ying Y, Maier D, Schmidt C, Riddick D. Comparison of real time ultrasonography, hysterosalpingography, and laparoscopy/hysteroscopy in the evaluation of uterine abnormalities and tubal patency. *Fertil Steril* 1986;5:828–32

14. Richman TS, Viscomi GN, Cherney AD, Polan A. Fallopian tubal patency assessment by ultrasound following fluid injection. *Radiology* 1984;152:507–10

15. Salle B, Sergeant P, Galcherand P, Guimont I, De Saint Hilaire P, Rudigoz RC. Transvaginal hysterosonographic evaluation of septate uteri: a preliminary report. *Hum Reprod* 1996;11:1004–7

16. Marshall C, Mintz DI, Thickman D, Gussman H, Kressel Y. MR evaluation of uterine anomalies. *Radiology* 1987;148:287–9

17. Carrington BM, Hricak M, Naruddin RN. Mullerian duct anomalies: MR evaluation. *Radiology* 1990;170:715–20

18. Taylor PJ, Cumming DC. Hysteroscopy in 100 patients. *Fertil Steril* 1979;31:301–4

19. Jurkovic D, Giepel, A, Gurboeck K, Jauniaux E, Natucci M, Campbell S. Three dimensional ultrasound for the assessment of uterine anatomy and detection of congenital anomalies: a comparison with hysterosalpingography and two-dimensional sonography. *Ultrasound Obstet Gynecol* 1995;5:233–7

20. Kupesic S, Kurjak A. Pregnancy after diagnosis and treatment of uterine anomalies. *Croatian Med J* 1998;39:185–90

21. March CM. Hysteroscopy as an aid to diagnosis in female infertility. *Clin Obstet Gynecol* 1983;26:302–12

22. Fayez JA. Comparison between abdominal and hysteroscopic metroplasty. *Obstet Gynecol* 1986;68:399–403

23. Dabrashrafi H, Bahadori M, Mohammad K, Alavi M, Moghadami-Tabrizi N, Zandinejad R. Septate uterus: new idea on the histologic features of the septum in this abnormal uterus. *Am J Obstet Gynecol* 1995;172:105–7

24. Kupesic S, Kurjak A. Septate uterus: detection and prediction of obstetrical complications by different forms of ultrasonography. *J Ultrasound Med* 1998;17:631–6

25. Kupesic S, Kurjak A. Uterine and ovarian perfusion during the periovulatory period assessed by transvaginal color Doppler. *Fertil Steril* 1993;3:439–43

26. Gaucherand P, Awada A, Rudigoz RC, Dargent D. Obstetrical prognosis of septate uterus: a plea for treatment of the septum. *Eur J. Obstet Gynecol Reprod Biol* 1994;54:109–12

27. Keltz MD, Olive DL, Kim AH, Arici A. Sonohysterography for screening in recurrent pregnancy loss. *Fertil Steril* 1997;67:670–4

Fetal oxygenation and vasoactive agents 41

E. V. Cosmi and E. Cosmi, Jr

INTRODUCTION

An adequate supply of oxygen to the fetus is of paramount importance for its normal homeostasis, for its growth and development, for cellular function and for the birth of a healthy newborn infant. Under normal conditions, despite the lower arterial pao_2 of the fetus as compared to that of the mother, the amount of oxygen transferred from the mother is sufficient to meet the metabolic requirement of the fetus which, in terms of oxygen consumption, has been estimated to be about 8 ml/kg/per min, i.e. twice that of the adult[1-4]. Most of the pioneer studies performed in the 1960s, such as the one in which the similarity between po_2 from the fetal scalp capillaries and arterial blood from the carotid artery was demonstrated in monkeys[5], have been useful for the understanding of current methods for the assessment of fetal well-being in obstetrics. In the human fetus, these methods have included fetal pulse oximetry[6] (Figure 1) and computerized cardiotocography, and in neonatology the assessment of neonatal acid–base status and differentiation of central from obstructive apnea in the preterm newborn infant.

PHYSIOLOGICAL CONSIDERATIONS

There are many factors that may affect the oxygen supply to the fetus (Table 1). The most important factor is the uterine–placental–fetal blood flow. At term, the uterine blood flow accounts for 20–25% of maternal cardiac output; approximately 80–90% passes through the intervillous space, the remainder largely supplying the myometrium. Uterine blood flow varies directly with perfusion pressure (i.e. uterine arterial minus uterine venous pressure) and inversely with uterine vascular resistance. Under normal conditions,

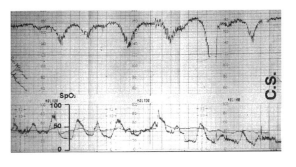

Figure 1 *Pulse oximetry chart, also showing the fetal heart rate recording and tocographic activity, from a pregnancy at 38 weeks, presenting premature rupture of the membranes. The neonate was born uneventfully after Cesarean section. Umbilical artery pH, 7.28; pco_2, 53.2; HCO^-_3, 24.8; po_2, 12.2; O_2 saturation, 6.3%. Female; birth weight 2970 g, Apgar scores 9/10 at 1 and 3 min after birth*

Table 1 *Factors affecting the oxygen supply to the fetus*

Rates of maternal and fetal blood flow

Oxygen capacity (hemoglobin concentration and oxygen affinity) of maternal blood

Oxygen capacity (hemoglobin concentration and oxygen affinity) of fetal blood

po_2 in fetal and maternal arterial blood

Maternal and fetal blood pH and pco_2

Ratio of maternal to fetal blood flow in exchanging areas, shunting around exchange sites

Maternal and fetal blood volume

Placental O_2 consumption (10 ml/kg/per min)

Fetal O_2 consumption (7–8 ml/kg/per min)

Placental diffusing capacity

the uterine vascular bed is almost maximally dilated, with little, if any, capacity to dilate further, whereas it responds to α-adrenergic stimulation with marked vasoconstriction. In the past 10 years, other substances such as endothelin have been shown to act as potent vasoconstrictors at the uterine blood flow site (see below).

Umbilical blood flow is regulated primarily by fetal cardiovascular dynamics and the autonomic nervous system through chemo-receptors and baroreceptors. At term it represents 40–50% of fetal cardiac output[1-4]. According to Rudolph[7], the Frank–Starling mechanism is essentially inoperative in the fetal myocardium because of the large shunts between the left and right sides of the heart, and because of the fact that the two ventricles work in parallel by virtue of the presence of the foramen ovale and the ductus arteriosus[8]. Thus, in contrast to the adult, the fetus has only a limited ability to increase cardiac output by increasing stroke volume. The increase in cardiac output is accomplished primarily by increasing the heart rate. Therefore, baroreflex-induced bradycardia would cause a reduction of cardiac output and hence of umbilical blood flow, with impairment of placental gas exchange[5,6]. Ventricular cardiac output is influenced by heart rate, pre-load, after-load and intrinsic myocardial contractility. We have found that the injection of prostaglandin E_2 into the umbilical vein of the human fetus undergoing therapeutic abortion causes vasoconstriction and a decrease of umbilical blood flow, which returns to pre-injection levels if fetal tachycardia is induced with the intravenous administration of aminophylline to the mother[4].

Near term, human fetal blood has a greater oxygen capacity than does maternal blood (about 50% greater)[2]. (Oxygen capacity is the product of the hemoglobin concentration and the moles of O_2 that may be bound by each mole of hemoglobin. Each mole of hemoglobin can combine with 4 moles of O_2 for a normal O_2 capacity of about 8 mmol/l or 1.368 ml/g.) Erythrocyte count and fetal hemoglobin concentration increase with advancing gestational age, reaching levels significantly greater than those in the mother (the mean fetal hemoglobin concentration is about 17 g/dl at term). The higher concentration of hemoglobin in the fetus is possibly the result of stimulation of erythropoiesis by erythropoietin[9,10]. In contrast, the mean corpuscular volume (i.e. packed cell volume/erythrocyte count) and erythrocyte hemoglobin content (i.e hemoglobin concentration/erythrocyte count) decrease[2]. Maternal erythropoiesis also increases in response to enhanced erythropoietin production; therefore, the maternal cell mass is greater than in non-pregnant states[9]. Thus, during gestation, the erythrocyte mass increases by 25–30%, whereas the plasma volume increases by 40–50%. As a result of the hemodilution, the mean maternal hemoglobin concentration progressively decreases to 12 g/dl with an O_2 capacity of 16.4 ml/dl[1-4]. It has been calculated that 1 g of hemoglobin can bind 1.36 ml of O_2; however, the exact value varies slightly depending on the amount of methemoglobin and carboxyhemoglobin present.

The maternal–fetal blood flow is analogous to ventilation-perfusion within the lung; the exchange of oxygen will be optimal if the flows are evenly matched, whereas inequalities in the ratio and shunting around exchange sites will decrease the efficiency of oxygen transfer[1-4]. Normally, the po_2 of fetal blood (carotid artery, scalp sample or umbilical artery following cordocentesis) is around 30 mmHg. Several factors are responsible for the large maternal–fetal gradient for pao_2, including the functional heterogeneity of the placenta due to the uneven distribution of maternal and fetal blood flows, vascular shunts, non-uniform distribution of placental diffusing capacity to blood flow, and the oxygen consumption of the placenta, which averages 10 ml O_2/kg wet weight per min (thus at term 20–50% of the O_2 derived from maternal blood is consumed by the placenta)[1-4]. Fetal blood has greater affinity than does adult blood. Under normal conditions, the hemoglobin–O_2 dissociation curve of fetal blood is displaced to the left of that for maternal blood (Figure 2). Thus, at a given po_2, and under identical conditions of temperature and pH, fetal hemoglobin has a greater oxygen affinity than does maternal hemoglobin[1,4,11]. This permits a relatively higher oxygen saturation of fetal hemoglobin at relatively low po_2 values than maternal hemoglobin, whereas the acute slope of fetal hemoglobin causes a major decrement in O_2 content for a small po_2 decrease. The higher affinity of fetal hemoglobin for oxygen is mainly the result of its failure to bind 2,3-diphosphoglycerate (DPG) to the same degree as does adult hemoglobin[9,12,13]. Fetal hemoglobin is a tetramer of two alpha chains and two gamma chains; adult hemoglobin is a tetramer of two alpha chains and two beta chains. The interaction of heat-stable phosphate intermediates (2,3-DPG and ATP) occurs primarily with beta chains of the hemoglobin molecule. However, this is not the predominant factor in the placental transfer of oxygen[9,13]. It has also been found that the concentration of 2,3-DPG in maternal erythrocytes increases during gestation and that this could account for the shift to the right of the maternal hemoglobin–O_2 dissociation curve[14]. The concentration of ATP in maternal and fetal erythrocytes could also play a role in the rightward and leftward displacement of the hemoglobin–oxygen dissociation curve, i.e. an increased concentration of ATP in maternal erythrocytes would reduce the affinity of hemoglobin for oxygen, whereas a low concentration in fetal erythrocytes would increase the affinity[9].

Towards the end of gestation, the amount of adult hemoglobin in fetal blood increases by up to 20–25%, thereby reducing its oxygen affinity, independently of changes in pH and 2,3-DPG levels. However, the decreased oxygen affinity of fetal blood has little effect on placental diffusing capacity[1-4]. During its passage through the intervillous space, maternal blood receives carbon dioxide and acid products of metabolism from the fetus and the placenta. This increases the release of O_2 from maternal hemoglobin by displacement to the right of the oxygen

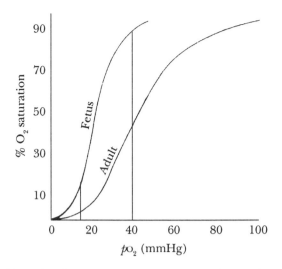

Figure 2 *Oxyhemoglobin dissociation curves for lamb fetus and adult pregnant sheep at pH 7.4 and body temperature. In the 15–40 mmHg range (the area enclosed by the two vertical lines), fetal erythrocytes bind much more oxygen than adult erythrocytes. From reference 1*

dissociation curve (positive Bohr effect). At the same time, the loss of these acids causes a displacement of the fetal hemoglobin–oxygen dissociation curve to the left (negative Bohr effect), which thereby increases oxygen release from maternal blood. A similar mechanism operates at the tissue level for the release of oxygen from blood to fetal tissues. The role of the double (maternal and fetal) Bohr effect on oxygen transfer across the placenta is still controversial. Some have estimated that the double Bohr effect accounts for about 8–20% of the total O_2 exchanged under normal conditions. In contrast, the placental double (maternal and fetal) Haldane effect (formation of carboxyhemoglobin following O_2 dissociation from hemoglobin) accounts for about 46% of the total CO_2 exchange[2].

The term 'diffusing capacity' has been used in reference to the lung although it may be confusing, since what is being measured is not necessarily the maximum exchange possible. In a steady state, the amount of gas exchanged by simple diffusion per unit time through the placenta is related to Fick's diffusion equation. For respiratory gases (the partial pressure of which is closely related to concentration), the partial pressure multiplied by the Bunsen solubility coefficient is substituted for concentration (Henry's law). The diffusing capacity for gas (the volume of gas in millileters which diffuses across the placenta each minute per unit of partial pressure gradient between the maternal and the fetal blood) depends, among other factors, on the solubility and temperature of the gas and on the chemical properties of the gas and of the placenta. An increase in the diffusing capacity effected by opening the villous capillaries or by reducing the thickness of the membrane will augment the transfer of gases. When the diffusing capacity remains fixed, such transfer can be increased up to a finite limit by an increase in maternal or fetal–placental blood flow[1,7]. Moderate changes in diffusing capacity would not appreciably affect the oxygen transfer from mother to fetus, because the placenta is very permeable to oxygen and consumes significant amounts. Recent studies have shown that the placental diffusing capacity for O_2 is about 3 ml/min/mmHg/ per kg; thus it constitutes a relatively minor factor in determining oxygen transfer from the mother to the fetus. Other factors that may regulate fetal oxygenation include maternal and fetal blood viscosity (the latter is about 50% greater than that of the adult per kilogram of body mass under normal conditions), tissue capillarity and diffusion distance from capillaries into the tissues[1,7].

In conclusion, despite the lower po_2 (30 mmHg) and oxyhemoglobin or O_2 saturation of the fetus than that of the mother (75% vs. 98%), the O_2 concentration of arterial blood flowing to the fetal brain and heart is greater than that of maternal arterial blood (16.5 vs. 15.4 ml/dl). The rate of O_2 consumption of the fetus is twice that of the adult per unit weight (8 vs. 4 ml /min/per kg); at term its O_2 reserve is approximately 42 ml and therefore only enough to meet its metabolic needs for 1–2 min. Therefore, in theory, in case of acute oxygen deprivation, the fetus has less than a 2-min supply of oxygen. On the other hand, fetal blood oxygen affinity and capacity are greater than those of the mother. Nevertheless, the fetus has important compensatory mechanisms that may permit it to survive hypoxic situations. These mechanisms include:

(1) Redistribution of blood flow to vital organs, including the heart, brain and adrenal glands;

(2) Decreased total oxygen consumption;

(3) Anaerobic metabolism in certain organs, particularly non-vital organs[1–4,15].

These defence mechanisms, however, are limited, for although cardiac output remains virtually constant, the blood redistribution to vital organs may be diverted away from the placenta, thereby further reducing the oxygen supply from the mother.

FACTORS CAUSING FETAL HYPOXIA

There are many factors that may reduce oxygen transfer from the mother to the fetus, leading to fetal hypoxemia; the most important are listed in Table 2. Uterine blood flow may decrease in the presence of maternal hypotension from any cause, maternal hypertension, marked maternal hypovolemia, increased blood viscosity, uterine hyper-

Table 2 *Causes of fetal hypoxemia*

Decreased uterine blood flow

Maternal hypotension (aortocaval compression, anesthesia, hemorrhagic and septic shock)

Maternal hypertension and pre-eclampsia

Increased blood viscosity (active sickling, hypergammaglobulinemia, maternal hypertension and pre-eclampsia)

Uterine hypertonus

Vasoconstrictors

Decreased umbilical blood flow

Placental insufficiency

Maternal hypoxemia (< 50 mmHg), hypoventilation, pulmonary and heart diseases, anesthetic mishaps

Maternal hyperventilation

Carbon monoxide (CO) poisoning

Maternal methemoglobinemia (cytochrome-b_5 reductase deficiency, prilocaine)

activity, endogenous and exogenous vaso-constrictors and synthetic progestagens[1-4,16]. Normally, posture-related compression of the inferior vena cava by the gravid uterus can occur in almost all pregnant women from 28 weeks to term gestation, when they lie supine. Significant maternal hypotension occurs in only about 15%. Depending on the degree of obstruction to the vena cava, uterine blood flow and fetal oxygenation may decrease substantially as a result of reduction of venous return of blood to the heart and therefore of stroke volume and cardiac output, without marked changes in maternal blood pressure and heart rate[17-19]. With compression of the aortoiliac vessels, maternal blood pressure may remain normal, but uterine blood flow is severely reduced[16,17]. Animal studies have shown that, under normal conditions, uterine blood flow can drop to approximately half its normal values before severe fetal hypoxemia and acidosis develop[15,17]. Tolerance to this asphyxial insult is decreased when fetal homeostasis is already compromised, e.g. in the presence of placental insufficiency.

Many drugs, including hypnotics, analgesics and inhalation agents, and sympathetic blockade during regional anesthesia may increase the hemodynamic disturbances produced by aortocaval compression by interfering with compensatory mechanisms so that significant hypotension and a reduction of uterine blood flow occur. Maternal hypotension is the most frequent complication of improperly performed regional blocks, the degree of hypotension depending on the level of sympathetic blockade. The effects are more pronounced with maternal hypovolemia. Barbiturates and certain inhalation agents (halothane, enflurane, isoflurane) can also reduce maternal blood pressure and uterine–placental–fetal blood flow, particularly when they are administered at high doses[1-4,20].

The generalized vasoconstrictive response to maternal hemorrhage and hypovolemia involves the uterine circulation. Continued hemorrhage and hypovolemia may cause a significant reduction of uterine blood flow as a result of both decreased systemic perfusion

and vasoconstriction. The fetus is further compromised by maternal hemorrhage, owing to the decreased oxygen-carrying capacity of maternal blood. The coexistence of fetal anemia (as in erythroblastosis), or maternal or fetal hemoglobinopathies will further impair fetal oxygenation[1,7]. Maternal oxygen-carrying capacity can vary from profound anemia to polycythemia under a wide variety of conditions; these changes are associated with alterations in oxygen affinity, because the intra-erythrocyte concentration of 2,3-DPG varies inversely with hemoglobin concentration. With polycythemia, uterine blood flow may decrease as a result of increased blood viscosity; maternal hypertension affects uterine blood flow as a result of both increased vascular resistance and blood viscosity due to changes in the erythrocyte membrane composition (increased cholesterol/phospholipid ratio)[21]; placental function is further compromised by maternal hypovolemia, hypoproteinemia, relative anemia and ultrastructural alterations in the placenta. A decrease of uterine blood flow may indirectly cause a variable and delayed fall in umbilical blood flow as a result of fetal hypoxemia and baroreflex-induced bradycardia. Fetal acidosis and some transplacentally acquired drugs and anesthetics may indirectly decrease umbilical blood flow by altering fetal myocardial performance[20]. Cord compression affects umbilical blood flow directly, causing an immediate fall. If the compression preferentially obstructs the umbilical vein, the venous return to the fetal heart will be reduced, and cardiac output and umbilical arterial blood flow will fall[1-7].

Compression of the umbilical arteries would raise aortic pressure, thereby causing baroreflex-induced fetal bradycardia and hence a fall in umbilical blood flow. Abnormal insertion of the umbilical cord may also directly alter the umbilical circulation and severely compromise oxygen delivery to the fetus[1-7]. Other clinical situations in which there is a cessation of oxygen delivery to the fetus include sudden total placental abruption and prolapse of the cord. There are various conditions that may induce ultrastructural alterations in the placenta, producing a state of insufficiency; these include maternal hypertension and pre-eclampsia, diabetes, malnutrition, Rhesus alloimmunization, intrauterine infections, cigarette smoking and prolonged gestation.

Maternal hypoxia has been extensively studied. Its impact on fetal oxygenation varies, depending on the degree, duration and mechanism, and also on fetal condition and compensatory mechanisms. It has been calculated that fetal oxygenation is normally impaired at a maternal arterial po_2 of 50 mmHg or less. Maternal hypoxemia is a frequent complication of pulmonary hypoventilation, secondary to exaggerated upper airways and laryngeal edema, with pre-eclampsia, pre-existing pulmonary or heart diseases such as asthma and cyanotic heart diseases, and depression of respiratory centers from the administration of narcotics, sedatives or magnesium, or from passive regurgitation and aspiration of gastric contents, or from various anesthetic mishaps. Contrary to earlier beliefs, moderate maternal hypoxia and hypercapnia do not affect uterine blood flow and fetal oxygenation, whereas marked degrees of maternal hypoxia (for example, administration of less than 15% of inspired oxygen) and hypercapnia decrease uterine–placental–fetal blood flow and fetal oxygenation[1,4,15,20]. Thus, there are two important factors that contribute to decreased oxygen transfer to the fetus during maternal hypoxia. The first is the diminished oxygen content and tension in the maternal blood, and the second is the decrease in uterine–placental–fetal blood flow. It should be noted that because of the reduced functional residual capacity (20%) and higher oxygen consumption (20%) compared with the non-pregnant state, the expectant mother is more likely to became hypoxic during induction of general anesthesia than is the non-pregnant woman; also, there is quicker induction and recovery from general anesthesia. Another often overlooked cause of reduced uterine blood flow and fetal oxygenation is forced maternal hyperventilation by the overzealous anesthetist during general anesthesia. This has a number of harmful effects on normal fetal oxygenation. The mechanical effects of marked hyperventilation significantly reduce uterine blood flow, by impeding the venous return to the heart; the resultant hypocapnia causes constriction of uteroplacental vessels and a reduction of intervillous space perfusion; the alkalosis will move the oxygen dissociation curve of maternal hemoglobin to the left, thereby impeding the release of oxygen to maternal tissues and fetal blood. Furthermore, if the fetus becomes acidotic, oxygen diffusion across the placenta may be severely compromised, as maternal and fetal hemoglobin saturation curves become nearly superimposed[1,2,20].

The oxygen supply to the fetus is greatly impaired in case of carbon monoxide poisoning or methemoglobinemia. The adverse effects of carbon monoxide result from the decrease in both oxygen release to the tissues, because the affinity of adult hemoglobin for carbon monoxide is 230 times greater than the affinity for oxygen, and uptake by the tissues[2]. Carbon monoxide combines with other heme pigments, including myoglobin, Barkans' pseudo-hemoglobin and the cytochromes. Carbon monoxide intoxication is encountered in pregnant women exposed to air pollution or those who are heavy smokers[2]. Increasing carbon monoxide levels in maternal blood reduce its oxygen capacity and content and shift the oxygen dissociation curve to the left. These changes are more pronounced in anemic patients. Similar changes occur in fetal blood following a rapid or substantial transfer of carbon monoxide. Fetal pao_2 decreases in proportion to carboxy-hemoglobin concentrations in fetal and maternal blood, thereby leading to tissue hypoxia and anoxia[2,22]. Methemoglobinemia also reduces the oxygen-carrying capacity of blood and moves the oxygen dissociation curve to the left, so reducing O_2 release to the tissues. This disorder may be hereditary, due to cytochrome b_5 reductase deficiency, or it may be caused by a local anesthetic prilocaine[1-4], which is no longer commercially available.

PROPHYLATIC ADMINISTRATION OF OXYGEN TO THE MOTHER

Various reports indicate that, by increasing the maternal concentration of inspired oxygen, there is a progressive, although not proportional, increase in fetal pao_2, and babies are born in better condition[22,23]. It has been shown in several studies that raising maternal pao_2 from 100 mmHg (breathing air) to 600 mmHg (breathing 100% O_2) increases maternal O_2 concentration by 1.5 ml/dl/per min, from 16 to 17.5 ml/dl/per min. The administration of high concentrations of O_2 to the mother to improve her supply to the fetus should not be considered a panacea for the treatment of fetal hypoxia, because conflicting results have been reported for this practice. In general, it has been found that fetal pao_2 increases, although not in proportion to the maternal increase[1–4,24].

Since the human placenta stimulates a concurrent exchange, the fetal umbilical vein follows the uterine vein po_2; therefore any increase in maternal po_2 will be associated with a smaller increase in uterine venous po_2 which in turn leads to a small increase in umbilical venous po_2. Fetal arterial po_2 may or may not increase, depending on fetal oxygen consumption and cardiac output[25]. The amount of additional physically dissolved O_2 in maternal blood would be only 1–2 ml/dl. In case of fetal hypoxia secondary to impaired uterine–placental–fetal blood flow, it is unlikely that fetal pao_2 would rise, despite a marked increase in maternal pao_2. However, the administration of high concentrations of oxygen to the mother may be a temporary supportive measure for the treatment of fetal hypoxemia. Also, it is worth remembering that maintenance of the blood pressure in the systemic circulation, or more specifically in the brachial artery, is not synonymous with normal uteroplacental perfusion.

VASOACTIVE AGENTS

Uteroplacental blood flow is mainly regulated through the release of several mediators, vasodilators and vasoconstrictors, produced by vascular endothelium and by vasoactive agents, both endogenous and exogenous, e.g. catecholamines, bradykinins, vasoactive intestinal polypeptide, betastimulants, aminophylline, narcotics including cocaine, analgesics and anesthetics and certain hormones, including estrogens and corticosteroids. In fact, because of the lack of nervous innervation, the placental circulation is mainly regulated by the action of vasoactive substances. Among these vasoactive agents, endothelin, the most potent vasoconstrictor yet discovered, has been found to play a significant role in the regulation of fetoplacental hemodynamics in physiological and pathological states such as pre-eclampsia and intrauterine growth restriction. Perfusion studies on the placenta have demonstrated that endothelin-induced pressor responses are of long duration and are associated with an involvement of other vasoactive substances, suggesting that endothelin may act as an endogenous modulator of the fetoplacental circulation in an autocrine/paracrine fashion. Vasoconstriction of the uteroplacental circulation is responsible for chronic fetal hypoxia, a potent stimulus for endothelin secretion[26]. Increased concentrations of endothelin in the amniotic compartment from patients with pre-eclampsia and intrauterine growth restriction suggests that local release of this peptide from fetoplacental structures may be of importance for the impairment of the uteroplacental circulation in these conditions. Fetoplacental tissues also release nitric oxide, a potent vasodilator synthesized from L-arginine, that plays a key role in the control of vascular tone in several vascular beds[27]. Nitric oxide synthase is present in the human fetoplacental tissues and endothelial nitric oxide synthase mRNA has been detected in placental villi. Adrenomedullin, a novel peptide, was found to be involved in the regulation of blood pressure through different mechanisms[28]. Unpublished data from our group (R. Di Iorio and colleagues) show that the concentrations of nitric oxide metabolites and adrenomedullin in amniotic fluid from pregnant women who delivered neonates affected by respiratory distress syndrome were lower than in normal pregnancies. These findings suggest that nitric oxide and adrenomedullin may play a significant role in the distribution and absorption of fetal pulmonary fluid and possibly in surfactant production.

hypertension, uterine hyperactivity and placental insufficiency. During Cesarean section, added complications such as anesthetic overdose and prolonged uterine incision-to-delivery interval may further compromise fetal oxygenation.

CONCLUSIONS

If fetal hypoxia, complicated by acidosis, is found at birth, a number of etiological factors may exist. The most common are marked maternal hypotension, hypoxia, hyperventilation, hypovolemia and anemia,

ACKNOWLEDGEMENTS

This work was supported by the Consiglio Nazionale delle Ricerche (CNR), the Ministry of Research and Technology (MURST) and the Italian Section of the MCI-IAMANEH, Rome, Italy.

References

1. Cosmi EV, Caldeyro-Barcia R. Fetal homeostasis. In Cosmi EV, ed. *Obstetric Anesthesia and Perinatology.* New York: Appleton-Century-Crofts, 1981:103–317
2. Longo LD. Respiratory gas exchange in the placenta. In Fishman AP, Farhi LE, Tenney SM, *et al.*, eds. *Handbook of Physiology, The Respiratory System IV.* Bethesda, MA: American Physiological Society 1987:351–401
3. Cosmi EV, Torregrossa G, Collini P, Pieretti M, Anceschi MM. Optimum oxygenation during cesarean section. In Belfort P, Pinotti JA, Eskes TKAB, eds. *Advances in Gynecology and Obstetrics.* Vol. 5 Pregnancy and Labor. Carnforth, UK: Parthenon Publishing, 1988:251–63
4. Cosmi EV, Mazzocco M, Cosmi E Jr. Fetal oxygenation. In Hawkins M, Di Renzo G, Cosmi EV, eds. *Proceedings of the International Course on Recent Advances in Perinatal Medicine,* Erice, Italy 1996. Singapore: World Scientific Publishing, 1996
5. Adamsons K, Beard R, Cosmi EV, Myers R. The validity of capillary blood in the assessment of the acid–base state of the fetus. In Adamsons K, ed. *Diagnosis and Treatment of Fetal Disorders.* New York: Springer-Verlag, 1969:175–7
6. Dildy GA, Clark CL, Loucks CA. Intrapartum fetal pulse oximetry: past, present and future. *Am J Obstet Gynecol* 1996;175:1–9
7. Rudolph AM. *Congenital Disease of the Heart.* Chicago: Year Book Medical Publishers, 1974
8. Rudolph AM, Heymann MA. Cardiac output in the fetal lamb. The effects of spontaneous and induced changes of heart rate on right and left ventricular output. *Am J Obstet Gynecol* 1976; 124:183–92
9. Jepson JH. Factors influencing oxygenation in mother and fetus. *Obstet Gynecol* 1974;44:906–14
10. Zanjani ED, Petersen EN, Gordon GS, Wasserman LR. Erythropoietin production in the fetus: role of the kidney and maternal anaemia. *J Lab Clin Med* 1974;83:281–7
11. Meschia G. Evolution of thinking in fetal respiratory physiology. *Am J Obstet Gynecol* 1978;132:806
12. Novy MJ. Alteration in blood oxygen affinity during fetal and neonatal life. In Astrup P, Rorth M, eds. *Oxygen Affinity of Haemoglobin and Red Cell Acid Base Status.* Copenhagen: Munksgaard, 1972:696
13. Orzalesi MM, Hay WW. The regulation of oxygen affinity of fetal blood. 1. *In vitro* experiments and results in normal infants. *Pediatrics* 1971;48:857–64
14. Rørth M, Bille-Brahe NE. 2,3-DPG in human pregnancy. In Astrup P, Rørth M, eds. *Oxygen Affinity of Haemoglobin and Red Cell Acid Base Status.* Copenhagen: Munksgaard, 1972:692
15. Parer JT. Uteroplacental circulation and respiratory gas exchange. In Shnider SM, Levinson G, eds. *Anesthesia for Obstetrics.* Baltimore: Williams and Wilkins, 1987:13–28
16. Bassell GM. Anesthesia for caesarean section. *Clin Obstet Gynecol* 1985;28:722–34
17. Lotgering FK, Wallenburg HCS. Haemodynamic effects of caval and uterine venous occlusion in pregnant sheep. *Am J Obstet Gynecol* 1986;155:1164–70
18. Calvin S, Jones OW III, Knieriern K, Weinstein L. Oxygen saturation in supine hypotensive syndrome. *Obstet Gynecol* 1988;71:872–7
19. Eastman NJ. Fetal blood studies. V. The role of

anesthesia in the production of asphyxia neonatorum. *Am J Obstet Gynecol* 1936;31:563–72

20. Cosmi EV. Effects of anesthesia on the uteroplacental blood flow and the fetus. In Cosmi, EV, ed. *Obstetric Anesthesia and Perinatology.* New York: Appleton-Century-Crofts, 1981:401–50

21. Piazze Garnica JJ, Pierucci F, Vozzi G, Cosmi EV, Anceschi MM. The cholesterol to phospholipid ratio (C/PL) of the erythrocyte membrane in normotensive, hypertensive pregnant women and in cord blood as assessed by a simple enzymatic method. *Scand J Clin Lab Invest* 1994;54:631–5

22. Cosmi EV. Fetal oxygenation. In Genazzani AR, Petraglia F, Genazzani AD, *et al.*, eds. *Current Research in Gynecology and Obstetrics.* Carnforth, UK: Parthenon Publishing, 1991:231–48

23. Romanathan S, Gandhi S, Arismendy J, Chalon J, Turndorf H. Oxygen transfer from mother to fetus during caesarean section under epidural anesthesia. *Anesth Analg* 1982;61:576–81

24. Cosmi EV, Joelsson I. Effects of volatile anesthetics on the cardiovascular system maternal and acid base equilibrium of the fetus. *Riv Ost Ginecol It* 1968;23:177–86

25. Battaglia F. Metabolism of the placenta: its physiologic implications. *Mead Johnson Perinat Dev Med* 1981;18:9–13

26. Isozaki-Fukuda Y, Kojima T, Hirata H, *et al.* Plasma immunoreactive endothelin-1 concentration in human fetal blood: its relation to asphyxia. *Pediatr Res* 1991;30:244–7

27. Palmer RMJ, Ashton DS, Moncada S. Vascular endothelial cells synthesize nitric oxide from L-arginine. *Nature (London)* 1988;333:664–6

28. Di Iorio R, Marinoni E, Scavo D, Letizia C, Cosmi EV. Adrenomedullin in pregnancy. *Lancet* 1997;349:328

Fetal effects of maternally administered hypotensive drugs: fact and fiction?

42

L. S. Voto, A. Lapidus and M. Margulies

INTRODUCTION

The unknown etiology of pregnancy-induced hypertension has not allowed us to find a unique therapy to treat women affected with this serious disease; moreover, it has brought about a great deal of controversy over the different treatments available.

It is a fact that all current therapies are symptomatic and controversial. They do not cure the disease; they are simply aimed at preventing or reducing the risks for the mother and fetus. In the literature, there are numerous clinical studies describing the use of several drugs that have been used to prolong gestation and improve perinatal results in hypertensive pregnancies[1-6]. Some of these drugs have been used in pregnancy very frequently, others very rarely, and still others are currently on trial. In addition, it is very difficult to evaluate or compare the results of these studies, owing to the heterogeneity of the populations studied (different types of hypertension, gestational age at the onset of medication, length of treatment). Most of these studies were retrospective, very few were controlled and the size of the population was usually very small[7].

In a thorough review of published papers on antihypertensive drugs and pregnancy, carried out in 1991, Redman[8] found that the design of the studies varied a great deal, and that definite conclusions could not be drawn because of the small groups of patients analyzed. As regards maternal effects, the only consistent characteristic found in all the groups was the reduction of maternal blood pressure[9,10]. This, however, simply shows that the drugs used had the intended effect, but by no means does reduced blood pressure imply a totally beneficial effect on pregnancy. An important finding in these studies was that early treatment of chronic hypertension does not necessarily prevent the later development of superimposed pre-eclampsia.

The pharmacological management of hypertension in pregnancy has reduced maternal and perinatal mortality significantly, causing at the same time deleterious side-effects on both the mother and, in particular, the fetus. Most drugs bring about unwanted effects; therefore, physicians should have a clear idea of what to expect from a drug and weigh up the potential benefits and risks of a given therapy[11,12].

Accordingly, the ideal antihypertensive drug to be used in pregnancy should meet the following basic requirements: it should be harmless to the mother and fetus; it should not have side effects; it should reduce blood pressure effectively; and should be inexpensive and easily affordable. Unfortunately, to this day there is no such ideal drug. Therefore, obstetricians, physicians, internists, cardiologists and clinicians are forced to resort to that medication which most closely fulfils the ideal requirements listed above. Once the drug has been chosen, it should be considered whether the benefits it will bring to the mother and her child will outweigh the unwanted side-effects inherent in any medication.

The treatment of hypertension in pregnancy raises three basic questions: why, when and how to treat?

WHY TREAT HYPERTENSION IN PREGNANCY?

Although it is well known that pregnancy-induced hypertension manifests itself basically in elevated blood pressure, its physio-pathology still remains a mystery. Consequently, any therapy resulting in a decrease in blood pressure will not improve the underlying pathology. Then why treat?

(1) To lower the risk of maternal encephalopathy;

(2) To reach fetal viability and achieve neonatal survival.

The decision to start medicating should be considered carefully, always bearing in mind that our ultimate aim is the well-being of both mother and child.

WHEN SHOULD HYPERTENSION IN PREGNANCY BE TREATED?

The decision to begin treatment is made according to the maximum blood pressure measurements recorded twice, 24 h apart, with the patient at bedrest.

Absolute indications are: early severe hypertension in pregnancy; pre-existing cardiovascular disease; pre-existing renal disease; hypertension of $\geq 170/110$ mmHg; and hypertension in pregnant women with diabetic nephropathy.

A relative indication is moderate hypertension (140–160/90–109 mmHg). Antihypertensive therapy in patients with diastolic blood pressure higher than 110 mmHg has been found to lower the incidence of cerebrovascular and cardiovascular accidents[13]. In moderate hypertension, however, this relationship is not so clearly established.

As can be inferred, we do not make any distincion between women with essential hypertension and those with gestational hypertension, because we consider that, in clinical practice, the origin of the hypertensive disorder is very difficult to determine on the patient's first visit, unless the patient was diagnosed with hypertension before becoming pregnant.

In patients with essential hypertension, the early administration of hypotensive drugs does not necessarily preclude the later development of superimposed pre-eclampsia or the worsening of their hypertensive condition. Consequently, a careful assessment of risks and benefits should be carried out before any medication is indicated.

HOW SHOULD A HYPERTENSIVE PREGNANT PATIENT BE TREATED?

The treatment of the hypertensive pregnant woman resembles a scale on which the benefits of a drug and its potential risks should be perfectly balanced.

Pharmacokinetics of antihypertensive drugs in pregnancy

The changes in maternal physiology that accompany hormonal modifications during pregnancy can alter the absorption, distribution, protein binding and hepatic and renal drug clearance.

The fetoplacental unit is especially vulnerable to the effects of drug administration, owing to the placental transfer that follows maternal treatment. During intrauterine life and the first days of extrauterine life, the hepatic enzyme systems – responsible for the metabolism of many drugs – are immature. The fetal kidneys receive only 2% of cardiac output, whereas in adults they receive ten times that amount. Thus, the drugs that cross the placenta – and all antihypertensive drugs do – could have a longer half-life and a more prolonged effect on the fetal circulation. Therefore, in terms of drug activity, the pregnant patient is considered a special case in which all pharmacological treatments have both therapeutic and adverse effects[14].

Many drugs have been and are being used to treat this condition. They are divided below according to their mechanism of action.

Central action drugs

α-Methyldopa

This is rarely used in non-pregnant patients,

since it causes pronounced sedation, orthostatic hypotension, depression, excessive liquid retention, hepatic (function) disorders and hemolytic anemia, with a positive Coombs' test[15]. However, it has been and still is frequently used in pregnancy. Sixty per cent of the drug is excreted without modifications. The rest is metabolized into α-methyl-repinephrine, an α_2 agonist, which is a sympatholytic agent that acts upon the central nervous system, stimulating central α post-synaptic receptors, which causes a decrease in peripheral sympathetic activity that translates into a decreased peripheral resistance, without affecting cardiac output, renal plasma flow, or heart rate. It is well known that α-methyldopa crosses the placenta and, when it is administered until delivery, a decreased systolic blood pressure is observed in the newborn during the first days of life, owing to its slow clearance. On the other hand, Cockburn and co-workers[16] conducted a 7-year study on children born to mothers who received antihypertensive treatment during pregnancy, and they did not find any development or growth anomalies. The administration of α-methyldopa during pregnancy has become increasingly popular, mainly because of the absence of harmful effects on the fetus[8], rather than because of its antihypertensive effectiveness.

Clonidine

This is a central action α_2 agonist. Its effect is related to local norepinephrine (nor-adrenaline) concentration. Heart rate and systolic volume decrease after its oral administration; the reduction of heart rate, however, is seldom severe. Clonidine is well absorbed, and reaches its maximum concentration 1–3 h after its oral administration. The acute clonidine administration during pregnancy leads to an initial blood pressure increment that lasts only a few minutes, and is followed by moderate hypotension, increased peripheral resistance and a minute volume drop, which indicates that, in the presence of severe pre-eclampsia, this drug would not achieve a desirable effect.

Clonidine has been successfully used to treat hypertension in pregnancy; however, little is known about its effects on the fetus. Thus, it offers few advantages over α-methyldopa[17].

Drugs that act upon minute volume

β-blocking agents

β-blockers compete with the normal β-adrenergic agonists at bronchial, cardiac, arterial and uterine levels. Their anti-hypertensive effect is due to a decrease in both cardiac output and plasma volume, and to renin release inhibition. β-blocking agents are indicated for treatment of idiopathic hypertension as well as gestational hyper-tension, the latter being associated with increased vascular reactivity.

One of the most important side-effects is hypoglycemia due to glucogenesis decrease. Some authors believe that this drug causes fetal and neonatal bradycardia and hypo-glycemia, as well as low birth weight for gestational age[9,18] and smaller placentas[19].

The β-blockers that have been used during pregnancy are atenonol, labetalol, oxprenolol and metoprolol. Propranolol causes fetal bradycardia.

Drugs that act upon peripheral resistance

Hydralazine

Hydralazine is an arterial vasodilating agent that blocks calcium access to the cell, causing relaxation of the smooth muscle of the medial arterial layer. Although it reduces peripheral resistance, the sympathetic nervous system is activated as a result of baroreceptor stimu-lation, and compensatory increases in heart rate and cardiac output take place, which makes hydralazine relatively ineffective when used alone. Owing to the activation of the renin–angiotensin system, there is water retention which, along with cardiac stimulation, neutralizes the long-term antihypertensive effect of this drug. Therefore, hydralazine is indicated to treat only short-term hypertensive emer-gencies[20].

Cephaleas, nausea, anorexia, palpitations, sweating and a reversible systemic lupus erythematosus-like syndrome have been reported among its side-effects.

Hydralazine does not reduce utero-placental blood flow, and it is known to cross the placenta, where inactive metabolites can accumulate. This can cause fetal thrombo-cytopenia that can take up to 3 weeks to revert[21]. Small concentrations of hydralazine can also be found in maternal breast milk[22].

Diazoxide

Diazoxide is another drug that has been used intravenously when blood pressure is extremely and persistently high. It has a powerful vasodilating effect, it decreases peripheral resistance and increases cardiac output.

It can reduce glomerular filtration and cause significant sodium and water retention; therefore, it is usually administered along with a diuretic. Cerebral ischemia and maternal death have been reported in connection with this drug[23]. Hyperglycemia is another adverse effect of this drug, and comes as a result of inhibited pancreatic insulin release. Diazoxide crosses the placenta, and, as a consequence, fetal tachycardia and fetal or neonatal thrombocytopenia and hyper-bilirubinemia have also been reported. Its use is not currently recommended.

Nitrates

Sodium nitroprusside is a powerful, antihypertensive agent of rapid action. It directly and specifically acts upon the arterial smooth muscle layer and it does not affect uterine muscle. Its action is quick and short. It begins to act within 2 min of its administration and its effects last for 5 min. Sodium nitroprusside is not lipid-soluble, and crosses the placenta freely and rapidly after its intravenous administration. The possible advantages of sodium nitropusside should be balanced against its potential toxicity. Sodium nitropusside combines with sulfhydryls in erythrocytes and tissues, releasing cyanhydric

acid, and inhibiting aerobic metabolism. In the kidneys and liver it turns into thiocyanates, which are cleared through urine. There is very little information about the use of this drug during pregnancy, but it is believed to affect both maternal and fetal circulation, possibly leading to fetal cyanhydric poisoning[24].

This drug should be used only for short periods of time, by emergency-trained personnel and with adequate patient monitoring.

Calcium channel-blocking agents

Nifedipine, isradipine and nitrendipine are powerful coronary and arteriolar dilating agents[25], but they can cause peripheral edema. Like β-blocking agents, these drugs undergo extensive presystemic clearance and have an average life of 1–4 h. Among their side-effects, edema, dizziness, nausea and vomiting, hypotension and skin rash have been reported. The cerebral vasodilating effect of nimodipine has been extensively studied. Nimodipine has been found to have a beneficial effect on vasospasms associated with eclampsia[26].

Amlodipine also belongs to this group and causes vasodilatation in the renal artery. In our experience this drug has been both effective and safe in the treatment of hypertension in pregnancy.

Nifedipine

Nifedipine is an arterial vasodilating agent that inhibits slow calcium channels, thus relaxing the smooth muscle. Its average life is prolonged in those patients presenting with renal disorders, as are found in pre-eclamptic patients. It is important to note that the effects of this drug will differ according to whether it is administered orally or sublingually. When given sublingually, its effects are observed immediately: a sudden drop in blood pressure and uteroplacental flow, which is usually uncontrollable. The simultaneous use of nifedipine and magnesium has been contraindicated, as there have been reports of severe hypotension when both drugs are administered together[27].

Converting enzyme inhibitors

Captopril, enalapril and lisinopril are included in this group. During pregnancy an increase in plasma renin activity, angiotensin II and renin substrate is observed. These drugs prevent the production of angiotensin II, a powerful vasoconstrictor; therefore, they are particularly useful in the treatment of renovascular hypertension. Cases of acute renal failure in newborns born to mothers who received treatment with converting enzyme inhibitors during the last trimester of pregnancy have been reported in the literature[28]. A review of 12 pregnancies[29], in which the mothers received captopril, alone or combined with other medication, showed one intrauterine death, four cases of oligohydramnios and/or neonatal anuria, and three fetal–neonatal deaths. Intrauterine growth restriction during captopril therapy was reported in four cases. It is important to point out that these are not teratogenic drugs; consequently, no risk is run by a woman who becomes pregnant and is under converting enzyme inhibitor treatment during the embryogenic period. However, it is necessary to change the medication and adopt a more suitable one for pregnancy.

Probable fetal renal damage results from the fact that the fetal kidney is a low-pressure perfusion system. Glomerular filtration improves with the vasoconstriction of the efferent glomerular arteriole, mediated by angiotensin II[30] (Figure 1).

Enalapril

Enalapril is usually indicated during the puerperium. It acts on essential and reno-vascular hypertension. It is a very effective and well-tolerated drug.

Angiotensin II A_{T1} receptor agonist: losartan

To date, only experimental trials in animals are available with this drug. The first studies indicate that losartan might cause hypotension, renal dysplasia, anuria/oliguria, oligohydramnios, intrauterine growth restric-

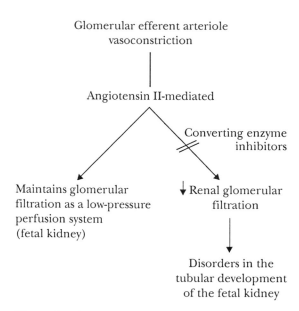

Figure 1 *Converting enzyme inhibitor in pregnancy. Probable mechanism of fetal renal damage*

tion, pulmonary hypoplasia, incomplete craneal ossification and perinatal death[31].

FINAL THOUGHTS

In spite of extensive research done on hypotensive drugs, it is very difficult to determine whether their fetal–neonatal impact is a consequence of the effects of the drugs *per se*, and to what extent it is the result of the pre-eclamptic syndrome itself. The natural consequence of the latter, which is an endothelial disease, is intrauterine growth restriction and oligohydramnios.

We evaluated 554 pregnant patients at the Hypertension in Pregnancy Office, Obstetric Department, Hospital J. A. Fernandez. The incidence of low birth weight was 5.3% ($n = 7$) for normotensive patients, and 24.5% for hypertensives. At the same time, out of the total number of cases with low birth weight ($n = 51$), 53% involved pure or superimposed pre-eclampsia. Thirty-one per cent of very low birth weight newborns were born to non-proteinuric hypertensive patients, and 69% to pre-eclamptic patients.

Oligohydramnios occurred in 55% of the cases. Different types of drugs were used to treat both hypertensive groups. Eighteen hypertensive patients presenting with intrauterine growth restriction did not receive any hypotensive drugs. There was no evidence of any relationship between medication and low birth weight or oligohydramnios. This situation makes it even more difficult for the doctors to decide when and how to medicate. There are no 'good' or 'bad' drugs for the fetus. Indeed, it is a fact that the hypertensive disease acts upon the fetus, even if the mother has not been medicated. The best option is the physician's good judgement as to why, when and how to medicate.

References

1. Rubin P. Hypertension in pregnancy. *J Hypertens* 1987;5 (Suppl 3): S57–60
2. Rubin PC. Beta-blockers in pregnancy. *N Engl J Med* 1981;305:1323–6
3. Gallery EDM. Chronic hypertension in pregnancy. *Aust NZ J Obstet Gynaecol* 1984;24:76–9
4. Gallery EDM, Saunders DM, Hunyor SN, Gyory AZ. Improvement in foetal growth with treatment of maternal hypertension in pregnancy. *Obstet Gynecol Surv* 1979;34:584
5. DeSwiet M. Antihypertensive drugs in pregnancy. *Br Med J* 1985;291:365–6
6. Voto LS, Lapidus AM, Salgueiro A, Uranga Imaz F, Margulies M. Analisis comparativo del uso de drogas hipotensoras en el tratamiento de la hipertensión en el embarazo. *Rev Arg Card* 1987;55 (Suppl):S44
7. Sibai B. Preeclampsia–eclampsia. *Curr Probl Obstet Gynecol Fertil* 1990;XIII: Jan–Feb
8. Redman CWG. Controlled trials of antihypertensive drugs in pregnancy. *Am J Kidney Dis* 1991;XVII:149–53
9. Sibai BM, Gonzalez AR, Mabie WC, *et al.* A comparison of labetalol plus hospitalization versus hospitalization alone in the management of preeclampsia remote from term. *Obstet Gynecol* 1987;70:323–7
10. Plouin P-F, Breart G, LLado J. A randomized comparison of early with conservative use of antihypertensive drugs in the management of pregnancy-induced hypertension. *Br J Obstet Gynecol* 1990;97:134–41
11. Voto LS, Quiroga CA, Lapidus AM, Catuzzi P, Uranga Imaz F, Margulies M. Effectiveness of antihypertensive drugs in the treatment of hypertension in pregnancy. *Clin Exp Hypertens* 1990;B9: 339–48
12. Margulies M, Voto L, Lapidus A, Neira J, Sánchez R. Treatment of hypertension. Perinatal results. *Clin Exp Hypertens* 1984;B3:410
13. Sibai BM, Anderson GD. Pregnancy outcome of intensive therapy in severe hypertension in first trimester. *Obstet Gynecol* 1986;67:517–22
14. Shoenfeld A, Segal J, Friedman S, Hirsch M, Ovadia J. Adverse reactions to antihypertensive drugs in pregnancy. *Obstet Gynecol Surv* 1986;41:67–71
15. Rud P, Blaschke TF. Agentes antihipertensivos y farmacoterapia de la hipertensión. In Gilman AG, Goodman LS, Rall TW, Murad F, eds. *Las bases farmacológicas de la terapéutica*, 7th edn. Buenos Aires: Panamericana 1986:747–67
16. Cockburn J, Moar V, Ounsted M. Final report of study on hypertension during pregnancy: the effects of specific treatment on the growth and development of the children. *Lancet* 1982;1:647–9
17. Horvath JS, Phippard A, Korda A, Henderson-Smart DJ, Child A, Tiller DJ. Clonidine hydrochloride – a safe and effective antihypertensive agent in pregnancy. *Obstet Gynaecol* 1985;66:634–8
18. Butters L, Kennedy S, Rubin PC. Atenolol in the treatment of essential hypertension during pregnancy. *Br Med J* 1990;301:587–9
19. Thorley KJ. Randomized trial of atenolol and methyl dopa in pregnancy related hypertension. *Clin Exp Hypertens* 1984;B3:168
20. Less KR, Rubin PC. Treatment of cardiovascular diseases. *Br Med J* 1987;294:358–60
21. Widerlov E, Karlman I, Storsater J. Hydralazine-induced neonatal thrombocytopenia [letter]. *N Engl J Med* 1980;301:1235
22. Liedholm H, Wahlin-Boll E, Hanson A, Ingermarsson I, Melander A. Transplacental passage and breast milk concentrations of hydralazine. *Eur J Clin Pharmacol* 1982;21:417–19
23. Pritchard JA. Management of preeclampsia and eclampsia. *Kidney Int* 1980;18:259–66
24. Lindheimer MD, Katz AI. Preeclampsia pathophysiology, diagnosis, and management. *Ann Rev Med* 1989;40:233–50
25. Rubin PC, McCabe R, Low RAL. Calcium channel blockade with nifedipine combined with atenolol in the management of severe pre-eclampsia. *Clin Res* 1985;33:21A

26. Belfort MA, Carpenter RJ, Kirshon B, *et al.* The use of nimodipine in a patient with eclampsia: color flow Doppler demonstration of retinal artery relaxation. *Am J Obstet Gynecol* 1993;169:204

27. Waisman GD, Mayorga LM, Camera Mi, Vignolo CA, Martinotti A. Magnesium plus nifedipine: potentiation of hypotensive effect in pre-eclampsia. *Am J Obstet Gynecol* 1988;159:308–9

28. Knott PD, Thorpe SS, Lamont CAR. Congenital dysgenesis possibly due to captopril. *Lancet* 1989;1:451

29. Plouin PE, Tchobroutsky C. Inhibition de l'enzyme de conversion de l'angiotensine au cours de la grossesse humaine. *Presse Med* 1985;14: 2175–8

30. Mastrobattista JM. Angiotensin converting enzyme inhibitors in pregnancy. *Semin Perinatol* 1997;21:124–34

31. Sorensen AM, Christensen S, Jonassen TE, Andersen D, Petersen JS. Teratogenic effects of ACE-inhibitors and angiotensin II receptor antagonists. *Ugeskr Laeger* 1998;160:1460–4

Management of HIV in pregnancy

43

S. R. Inglis

INTRODUCTION

Deaths from AIDS have been declining in the USA, but the infection is continuing to spread. In the USA. women are the group with the greatest increase in the rate of HIV infection. The spread of infection from men to women is most concerning. In other countries the spread of infection is still reaching epidemic proportions. As success in the management of the infection continues and life spans are increased, vertical transmission to offspring will take on increasing importance. Management of HIV infection has changed tremendously. Treatment of non-pregnant patients had a therapeutic revolution with the advent of highly active antiretroviral therapy (HAART), which consists of a protease inhibitor and two nucleoside analogs. Not long ago HIV treatment was limited to sequential use of nucleoside analogs or nucleoside analog combinations – so mediocre that it took years to show that they were superior to zidovudine (AZT). The proliferation of medications and lack of research in pregnancy make recommendations for antiretroviral therapy during pregnancy increasingly complex. Management of HIV disease in pregnancy begins with prevention of vertical transmission and stabilization of HIV disease. Prevention of opportunistic diseases and assessment of social and medical risk factors in pregnancy are also important. These are the cornerstones of successful pregnancy outcome when complicated by serious medical illness. This chapter begins with a discussion of the current status of HIV treatment in general and in pregnancy. This is followed by our current protocol for the management of HIV in pregnancy.

IS HIV DISEASE THE SAME IN MEN AND WOMEN?

It was on 28 February 1998 that the Centers for Disease Control (CDC) first released statistics for HIV and AIDS for the USA showing that AIDS deaths had decreased[1]. New York State had previously reported the same, but the finding was thought to be a statistical aberration. In this report the CDC reported that the number of AIDS deaths had decreased by 14% for the first half of 1996. This was hailed as the first proof of improved therapy and outcome for patients with HIV infection. Hidden in this report and perhaps more importantly, the data showed much less improvement for women. In fact, AIDS deaths increased by 4% for the same period for women. Why would women not be benefiting from the new therapies so successful in men? Possible explanations include differences in the method and therefore timing of discovery of infection, or that women are treated differently from men. Possibly women are treated differently because of intervening pregnancies, or women have an inherently different response to this infection. Very recently, a study was released on this question of gender difference[2]. The Johns Hopkins School of Public Health studied 650 patients who had participated in research studies since 1988. These patients all had frozen samples of blood that were available for study and the long-term outcome of these patients was available. The investigators found that those women with the same viral load as a man had a 60% higher risk of developing AIDS. At a given stage of disease, a woman's viral load was lower than a man's, even though her immune system had sustained similar damage. These researchers warned that those who use

Table 1 *Risks and benefits of early treatment of HIV*

Potential benefits of early intervention with antiretroviral therapy
Control of viral replication and mutation, reduction of viral burden
Prevention of progressive immune system injury
Delay of progression to AIDS and prolongation of life
Decreased risk of selection of resistant virus
Decreased risk of drug toxicity

Potential risks of early intervention with antiretroviral therapy
Reduction in quality of life from adverse drug effects and the inconvenience of taking medications
Earlier development of drug resistance
Limitation in future choices of antiretroviral agent due to development of resistance
Unknown long-term toxicity of antiretroviral drugs
Unknown duration of effectiveness of current antiretroviral therapies

the viral load as a benchmark may be misled into thinking that a woman is healthier than she really is. This difference is likely to be confirmed as others are reporting similar findings. These findings will add fuel to the debate regarding the best time for patients with HIV infection to initiate antiretroviral therapy. Most importantly, such findings bring into question whether guidelines for the general population are appropriate for women or their pregnancies.

TO TREAT OR NOT TO TREAT?

During pregnancy, fortunately, we know that treatment has a defined benefit for the unborn fetus by reducing the risk of vertical transmission. All patients are offered AZT at 12 weeks' gestation. For the general population the debate surrounds whether people with CD4 counts of > 500 and viral load of < 10 000 (bDNA) or < 20 000 (reverse transcriptase-polymerase chain reaction (RT-PCR)) are better served by starting therapy or by observing. Essentially, the question is whether one feels it is acceptable for a patient to have detectable virus in the circulation and not treat it. Treatment can be early, before the immune system undergoes injury, but there is a risk of running out of medications later because of viral resistance. Experts in the field differ widely on this question. Some would even observe people with CD4 counts of 350–500 as long as the viral load remains < 10 000 (bDNA) or < 20 000 (RT-PCR). Table

1 summarizes the essential points of the debate on the risks versus potential benefits of early intervention with antiretroviral therapy.

WHEN TO INITIATE ANTIRETROVIRAL THERAPY IN PREGNANCY?

For pregnant women with HIV infection, management has been based on the ACTG O76 trial. In this trial patients were randomized to oral zidovudine or placebo starting at 14 weeks in the antepartum period, intravenous zidovudine in the intrapartum period and oral zidovudine syrup for the neonate. The risk of vertical transmission may be reduced to as low as 8% with the use of zidovudine[3]. In most institutions a documented reduction in vertical transmission has been seen. The Jersey City Medical Center in Jersey City, New Jersey, serving an indigent population, documented a drop in vertical transmission from 33 to 11% with the use of zidovudine during pregnancy and the postnatal period. Oral zidovudine is now recommended for all patients at 14 weeks of gestation; intravenous zidovudine is recommended with a 2 mg/kg load and 1 mg/kg per hour continuous intravenous infusion during labor and has become standard in the USA. The author uses 12 weeks' gestation as the starting point for antiretroviral medications. The selection of 14 weeks is arbitrary and not based on any specific knowledge. Our current understanding of embryology,

Table 2 *Food and Drug Administration use-in-pregnancy ratings of antiretroviral agents*

Category	Interpretation	Antiretroviral agent
A	Controlled studies show no risk. Adequate, well controlled studies of pregnant women have failed to demonstrate risk to the fetus	
B	No evidence of risk in humans. Either animal findings show risk, but human findings do not, or, if no adequate human studies have been done, animal findings are negative	didanosine Saquinavir ritonavir Nelfinavir
C	Risk cannot be ruled out. Human studies are lacking, and animal studies are either positive for fetal risk, or lacking as well. However, potential benefit may justify potential risk and animal studies lacking	zidovudine Lamivudine zalcitabine Stavudine Nevirapine Delavirdine Indinivir
D	Positive evidence of risk. Investigational or postmarketing data show risk to fetus. Nevertheless, potential benefits may outweigh potential risk	
X	Contraindicated in pregnancy. Studies in animals or humans or investigational or postmarketing reports have shown fetal risk that clearly outweighs any possible benefit to the patient	

organogenesis, general knowledge and common clinical practice allows us to use a more convenient time, such as the end of the first trimester or 12 weeks' gestation. Standard therapy also dictates that the neonate be treated with zidovudine syrup in the postnatal period.

The prevailing wisdom for women already on antiretroviral drugs is that therapy during early pregnancy should continue if their disease is controlled. Others prefer to stop all medications for the first 12 weeks of pregnancy and then re-start the medications.

SELECTION OF ANTIRETROVIRAL AGENTS DURING PREGNANCY

At present there are three main classes of antiretroviral medications available. Nucleoside analogs were the first to be discovered. They are similar to the nucleosides that make up DNA. Cells infected with the HIV virus will use these analogs when the virus' reverse transcriptase is activated to make DNA. Once the nucleoside analog is bound by reverse

transcriptase, the enzyme is blocked and unable to continue taking up nucleosides, hence the name chain terminator. In this way, viral information is never copied and never enters the cell nucleus. Production of new virus is blocked at an early stage of the reproductive cycle. Non-nucleoside reverse transcriptase inhibitors are the second class of drug that also work at the level of reverse transcriptase. They bind near the catalytic site of reverse transcriptase and inhibit the enzyme. A new class of antiretroviral drugs called protease inhibitors has been developed. Protease inhibitors work later in the viral reproductive cycle. They work by preventing protease enzymes in the cell from cutting newly produced viral proteins into the smaller pieces used to make the viral capsule. The new viral particles cannot be released because of a lack of viral proteins to make the viral capsule. The use of these newer medications in pregnancy has been sporadic and studies are even rarer, because of concerns regarding fetal effects. Table 2 gives the use-in-pregnancy categories of the Food and Drug Admini-

Table 3 *Antiretroviral classification and side-effects*

Antiretroviral agent	Toxicity/side-effects
Nucleoside analogs	
Zidovudine	anemia, neutropenia, gastrointestinal upset, headache, myopathy
Lamivudine	minimal toxicity
Didanosine	pancreatitis, diarrhea, peripheral neuropathy
Zalcitabine	peripheral neuropathy, pancreatitis, diarrhea
Stavudine	peripheral neuropathy, pancreatitis
Non-nucloside reverse transcriptase inhibitors	
Nevirapine	numerous drug interactions, severe rash
Delavirdine	numerous drug interactions, severe rash
Protease inhibitors	
Indinavir	nephrolithiasis, numerous drug interactions, hyperbilirubinemia, metabolic abnormalities
Saquinavir	numerous drug interactions, gastrointestinal disturbances, metabolic abnormalities
Nelfinavir	numerous drug interactions, severe diarrhea, metabolic abnormalities
Ritonavir	numerous drug interactions, gastrointestinal disturbances, metabolic abnormalities, paresthesias

stration (FDA) for the more commonly used antiretroviral agents. Table 3 has the common side-effects of these medications listed.

Development of resistant strains of HIV virus to antiretroviral medications has been an obstacle to effective control of the virus. The virus recognizes obstacles to its replication and over time develops changes in structure and function to overcome these medications. Eventually, for example, the viral reverse transcriptase no longer recognizes zidovudine as a nucleoside. From then on zidovudine does not block viral replication. Viral mutation results in the development of drug resistance. Finding differences in the viral RNA from the wild-type virus at specific locations can identify mutations in the virus.

It is clear that combination therapy in non-pregnant patients leads to prolonged effectiveness as measured by lower viral loads and non-progression to AIDS[4-6]. It is likely that combination therapy is successful because it more effectively shuts down viral turnover and therefore the development of mutations. Therefore, the International AIDS Society has recommended that combination therapy be used as initial therapy in all cases. The future of triple therapy including a protease inhibitor looks promising but needs further long-term study.

For pregnant women, antiretroviral therapy has historically centered on zidovudine. This therapy is largely based on the outcome of the ACTG O76 trial that employed zidovudine during pregnancy and the postnatal period. The long-term effects of this therapy are still unknown. Monotherapy with zidovudine causes concern, because of the risk of development of resistant virus. For women, the issue of initial antiretroviral therapy is of particular importance, because all women are offered HIV screening during pregnancy and HIV infection is frequently first treated during pregnancy. New data showing that outcome was worse with monotherapy have brought into question the use of monotherapy during pregnancy. In pregnant women initial therapy should take into account the goal of decreased vertical transmission, prolonged maternal survival and non-progression to AIDS. In our

Table 4 *Antiretroviral therapy in pregnancy to patients naive to such agents. Current protocol of the author*

	Viral load	Recommended therapy
Symptomatic (AIDS, thrush, unexplained fever), any value for tests		immediate AZT + 3TC, re-evaluate viral load, consider adding protease inhibitor
CD4 count		
< 500	any	immediate AZT + 3TC, re-evaluate viral load, consider adding protease inhibitor
> 500	> 10 000 (bDNA) or > 20 000 (RT-PCR)	immediate AZT + 3TC, re-evaluate viral load
	< 10 000 (bDNA) or < 20 000 (RT-PCR)	AZT after 12 weeks

AZT, zidovudine; 3TC, Lamivudine; RT-PCR, reverse transcriptase-polymerase chain reaction

opinion these therapies should be discussed with all pregnant women. Recently Minkoff and Augenbraun also stated that we must consider the use of combination therapy in pregnant women[7]. The FDA categorization for each of the antiretroviral agents in Table 2 does not suggest undue risk from these medications.

The selection of which combination therapy to employ is complex in any patient and no less so for a pregnant woman. Once again, the goal of antiretroviral therapy in pregnant women is not only decreased perinatal transmission, but also prolonged maternal survival and non-progression to AIDS. Table 4 contains our protocol for initiation during pregnancy of antiretroviral agents to women naive to antiretroviral agents. It was formulated using outcome data from non-pregnant women[8]. Zidovudine remains the primary antiretroviral agent because of its significant effects on perinatal transmission of the virus. Lamivudine is the second agent because of its excellent safety, side-effect profile and proven efficacy in combination with zidovudine[5,6]. We find that this simple combination is well tolerated by the majority of HIV-positive pregnant women. Commonly, a profound drop in the viral load to none detected and an improved CD4 count is seen. We believe that the main benefit of adding lamivudine during pregnancy is providing a long interval until development of resistance and sustained complete suppression of the virus. Development of viral resistance to AZT

with monotherapy after 6 months is a cause of great concern and a major problem documented by numerous investigators. Furthermore, the advent of viral load testing to assess the efficacy of therapy has pointed out that monotherapy with AZT is not adequate to achieve a sustained decrease in viral load. AZT resistance mutations have now been found during primary infection in 8–26% of cases. In the New York metropolitan area the incidence of AZT resistance is very high. Other nucleoside analogs such as didanosine may be used as needed. Triple combination therapies employing protease inhibitors should be employed if there is failure of the initial antiretroviral regimen. Of the protease inhibitors available, ritonavir appears to have the best safety and side-effect profile.

Zidovudine should be used in any combination therapy during pregnancy. This includes women with a virus known to be resistant to AZT. If the patient has been on another nucleoside analog, it can be interchanged with zidovudine, or zidovudine can be added to the regimen. If the patient has failed to respond to a combination of medications, two other medications should be added and the zidovudine continued. The dosage would optimally replicate the ACTG O76 trial of 500 mg five times per day. In the real world this dosage schedule is close to impossible to maintain. We suggest using 200 mg three times a day or 300 mg twice a day. There is evidence that serum levels are sustained with the twice daily dosing.

Why not just use the 'cocktail' of two nucleoside analogs and a protease inhibitor in everyone? We try to keep the regimens as simple as possible during pregnancy. These pregnant women have numerous other health and family concerns, problems and symptomatology that make using complex regimens very burdensome. If one can prove that the therapy is effective with 'none detected' viral loads sustained throughout pregnancy, we see no benefit from additional medications and their complications. Also, we have no outcome studies in pregnancy with these complex regimens. There is concern regarding the side-effects on the developing fetus. Use of unproven regimens should be in research trial settings where the benefit of experimentation can be defined for future generations of pregnancies and women. Specifically, we have concerns regarding drug interactions, drug intolerance, poor nutrition and severe diarrhea during pregnancy inherent in the triple medication 'cocktail' regimens. Most of these agents, in particular the protease inhibitors, were granted accelerated approval after being studied in only a small number of subjects and even fewer who were pregnant. Reports are surfacing of troubling changes in metabolism, body composition, diabetes and severe coronary artery disease. We know even less about the risks of these drugs to neonates in the short and long term. It is clear that the drug combinations with the best virological responses in terms of viral load generally have the most durable responses. The lower the viral load the lower the risk of development of resistance to medications. It is clear that we are able to document a rapid decrease in the viral load to 'none detected' without the use of protease inhibitors or non-nucleoside reverse transcriptase inhibitors. We feel that, until it is shown that patients with a documented response to AZT and lamivudine are responding poorly in the long term, we would rather avoid the complex, poorly tolerated and unstudied regimens during pregnancy. We reserve triple combination

therapies employing protease inhibitors for failures of the initial antiretroviral regimen. Of the protease inhibitors available, ritonavir appears to have the best safety and side-effect profile. For the pregnant women experienced with antiretroviral agents, the decision of the combination to be used is individualized. Generally, we utilize the same regimen if it was well tolerated and effective in terms of viral suppression.

The viral load measurement during pregnancy may be one of our most important new tools. Viral load assay allows us to determine the risk of progression to AIDS and when to start treatment. The assay can document therapeutic success or failure well in advance of clinical progression with a declining CD4 count. We expect a significant decrease in viral load after 3–4 months of combination antiretroviral therapy. Whenever no such change occurs, a change in therapy is considered. Usually two different agents are started. The goal of this therapy is to achieve a 'none detected' viral load[9-11].

A special circumstance that deserves mention is hyperemesis gravidarum. In HIV-positive women this problem is especially troublesome, because of drug intolerance, low serum drug levels and the development of viral resistance. In severe cases it is better to stop all drugs until the patient has recovered from this complication at 18–20 weeks' gestation.

MANAGEMENT OF THE PERIPARTUM AND POSTPARTUM PATIENT

Intrapartum antiretroviral therapy centers on intravenous zidovudine therapy. Continuation of other antiretroviral agents is of unclear benefit. Management of the neonate consists of oral zidovudine syrup and very careful follow-up. The benefit of other antiretroviral prophylactic therapies for the neonate is unknown at present.

Amniocentesis, prolonged rupture of the membranes, long labor, fetal scalp sampling, internal scalp electrodes, intrauterine pressure monitors, instrumental delivery and episiotomy appear to increase vertical transmission of the virus. Changes in the rate of vertical transmission of virus from Cesarean delivery have been inadequately studied to date. The possibility of reducing the risk of vertical transmission does not justify exposing the mother to unnecessary surgery, health-care providers to large amounts of blood during surgery and complications such as inadvertent laceration of the baby's scalp or buttock at the time of uterine incision. Cesarean section is used for routine obstetric purposes with an eye towards achieving the goals outlined above.

It must always be borne in mind that these pregnant patients have a life-threatening illness. They deserve our very best efforts to optimize therapy for the best possible outcome. Our aim is to minimize perinatal transmission and at the same time ensure the mother of the best long-term outcome. We need to evaluate the response to our therapy with viral load measurements and then look for non-progression to AIDS as the final outcome parameter.

PROTOCOL FOR MANAGEMENT OF HIV IN PREGNANCY

The goals of management are:

(1) Prevention of vertical transmission of the infection;

(2) Stabilization of HIV disease;

(3) Prevention of opportunistic diseases;

(4) Assessment of social and medical risk factors for poor outcome.

Assessment in pregnancy

A comprehensive history should include the following:

(1) *HIV history:* duration, symptomatology, CD4 count, viral load, current medications, current care (where and by whom), risk behaviors;

(2) *Sexual history:* type of activity, number of partners, partners' HIV status, partner contact notification, use of condoms, use of other contraceptives, knowledge of safer sex, history of sexually transmitted diseases (STDs);

(3) *Substance abuse history:* types of drug(s), route(s), frequency, amount and needle-sharing practices;

(4) *Psychosocial status/support systems:* partner support, others with knowledge of serostatus, support from family and friends, history of physical/sexual abuse, coping skills, stage of acceptance of HIV infection, evidence of depression, suicidal ideation/attempts, history of psychiatric illness, history and risk assessment for physical and mental abuse, financial resources, health and life insurance.

A review of systems and physical examination should include the following:

(1) *Constitutional:* fatigue, malaise, anorexia, weight loss, fever and night sweats;

(2) *Dermatological:* rash, sores (skin or mucosal), lesions (molluscum, Kaposi's sarcoma), herpes, shingles and pruritus;

(3) *Lymph node* enlargement;

(4) *Ophthalmological:* decreases in vision, photophobia, pain and retinitis;

(5) *Ear, nose and throat:* sinusitis, oral lesions (thrush, oral hairy leukoplakia), gingivitis, bleeding, dentition and dysphagia/odynophagia;

(6) *Respiratory:* cough, discolored sputum, shortness of breath and pain;

(7) *Gastrointestinal:* diarrhea, nausea/vomiting, pain and hepatosplenomegaly;

(8) *Genitourinary:* vaginal/vulvar irritation, genital lesions (ulcers, blisters, warts), abnormal vaginal discharge, pelvic pain and bleeding;

(9) *Musculoskeletal:* myalgia, weakness and arthralgia;

(10) *Neurological:* memory impairment, cognitive changes, difficulty sleeping, headache, neuropathy (sensory/motor), balance and gait.

Consultants available should be those in maternal–fetal medicine, infectious disease, addiction medicine, hematology, ophthalmology, neurology, social work and nutrition/diet, as needed.

Management in pregnancy

Initial laboratory screening

(1) If no documentation, repeat HIV serology testing;

(2) Viral load assessment and CD4 count;

(3) Complete blood count with differential and platelet counts;

(4) RPR, hepatitis B surface antigen and antibody, hepatitis C antibody;

(5) Cytomegalovirus titer, *Toxoplasma* titer, liver and renal profiles, drug screen;

(6) Cultures for *Chlamydia*, *Neisseria gonorrhoeae*;

(7) Wet mount for *Trichomonas* ± bacterial vaginosis;

(8) Pap smear.

Repeat laboratory screening

(1) Drug screens monthly in those with a history of substance abuse or currently on a treatment program;

(2) Comlete blood count with platelets and liver profile monthly, to monitor effects of antiretroviral therapy;

(3) Viral load assessment and CD4 count every 2–3 months;

(4) Monitoring of HIV-positive women in pregnancy (Tables 5 and 6 have laboratory flow sheets);

(5) Repeat urine drug screens monthly in those with history of substance abuse or in a treatment program.

Tuberculosis screening

Purified protein derivative (tuberculin; PPD) intradermal screening is used unless the patient is known to be PPD-positive. Routine anergy testing is no longer recommended, since false-positive anergy tests occur in patients with known tuberculosis infection and negative PPD skin tests.

The test is read in 48–72 h. Induration of > 5 mm is positive, showing that the patient is symptomatic or has been exposed to active tuberculosis. If the CXR is negative, most elect to postpone treatment until the postpartum. It is advised to consider consultation with an infectious disease consultant if concerns arise. Alternatively, after the first trimester, patients may be treated with INH, 300 mg orally every day and pyridoxine 50 mg orally every day for 12 months or INH 900 mg + pyridoxine 50 mg twice a week for 12 months (directly observed therapy).

Active tuberculosis requires consultation with a specialist, as isolation may be required.

Preventive therapy

(1) Immunizations and behavioral modification;

(2) Counselling regarding avoidance of undercooked meat, cat feces and gardens with cats is especially advised for patients with negative *Toxoplasma* titers;

(3) Counselling regarding nurseries and preschool children, kissing of such children, careful hand washing and pneumococcal vaccine for patients who have never received the vaccine;

(4) Influenza vaccine when appropriate;

(5) Hepatitis B vaccine (if injection drug use, STDs or multiple partners).

We routinely obtain the CD4 count and viral load and then administer the pneumococcal and flu vaccines in pregnancy. Currently we are not routinely using the hepatitis vaccine and tetanus vaccines. There are data suggesting that the viral load assessment will show a rise in viral burden for a few weeks after vaccination. From our perspective, these data have not been shown to be a problem and therefore we prefer to use the vaccines. We would rather avoid any lung infections during pregnancy.

Table 5 *Maternal–fetal medicine in HIV-positive pregnancy: flow sheet*

Allergies:			
LMP:	EDD:		
Gravida:	Para:	Abortion:	Miscarriage:

Test	Date done	Results	Treatment date
RPR	_____	_____	_____
GC	_____	_____	_____
Hepatitis	_____	_____	_____
WBC	_____	_____	_____
HGB	_____	_____	_____
HCRIT	_____	_____	_____
RH	_____	_____	_____
Blood type	_____	_____	_____
UA	_____	_____	_____
Rubella	_____	_____	_____
Glucose	_____	_____	_____
Other	_____	_____	_____

Sonogram date	Weeks' gestation:

Medication Hx: _____

Obstetric Hx: _____

Comments: _____

LMP, last menstrual period, EDD, expected day of delivery; WBC, white blood cell count; HGB, hemoglobin; HCRIT, hematocrit; RH, rhesus; UA, urinalysis

Risk behaviors such as unprotected intercourse, smoking, substance abuse and stress all should be avoided because of the likelihood of increasing the viral load and speeding the disease process.

Nutrition is a variable that may be used to advantage. Nutrition counselling and consultation may offer suggestions regarding ways to enhance adequate weight gain and oral intake.

Prophylaxis for opportunistic infections

Decisions regarding prophylaxis are based upon the lowest value obtained (i.e. even if the CD4 count improves with antiretroviral therapy, prophylaxis should be continued). For *Pneumocystis carinii* pneumonia, prophylaxis is initiated when the CD4 count is < 200, there is a previous history of *P. carinii* pneumonia, unexplained fever (> 100 °F; 37 °C for more than 2 weeks) or oral candidiasis. Treatment consists of TMP-SMX, 1 DS tablet orally qod (Monday, Wednesday and Friday). Alternative treatments are:

(1) TMP-SMX, 1 SS tablet orally every day;

(2) Dapsone, 50 mg orally twice a day or 100 mg orally every day;

Table 6   *Maternal–fetal medicine in HIV-positive pregnancy: flow sheet*

Patient baseline data		
Name:		Date:

Finding	YES / NO	Finding	YES / NO	Finding
Thrush	Y N	Crypto	Y N	CD4 by Hx _____
Esophagitis	Y N	Toxoplasma	Y N	Toxo/CMV Titer _____
TB	Y N	CMV	Y N	Hep B Ag _____
Pneumonia	Y N	Hepatitis	Y N	Hep B Ab _____
PCP	Y N	Anergic	Y N	Hep C Ab _____
ITP	Y N	G6PD NL	Y N	Year Dx _____
Syphilis	Y N	PPD_____		Year first Rx _____
Zoster	Y N	CXR_____		Pneumovax _____

OTHER: MEDS:

DATE	MEDS	HGB HCT	WBC GRAN	PLT CT	AST ALT	BILI	BUN CR	CD4	VL	COMMENT

Medication abbreviations:

A: Retrovir   F: Fluconazole   V: Invirase   X: Crixivan
B: Bactrim   P: Pentamidine   S: Dapsone   Z: Zerit
C: DDC   N: Norvir   T: Epivir (3TC)   M: Zithromax
D: DDI

(3) Dapsone 50 mg orally every day + pyrimethamine 50 mg orally evey week + leucovorin 25 mg orally every week;

(4) Aerosolized pentamidine 300 mg every month via nebulizer.

As prophylaxis for *Toxoplasma* infection, counsel regarding preventive measures. The patient should avoid undercooked meat, working in gardens with cats in the vicinity and changing cat litter. Work areas and fomites should always be cleaned when cutting raw meats or raw vegetables.

Prophylaxis is initiated when the CD4 count is < 100. Use of TMP-SMZ DS, 1 tablet orally every day should be continued until delivery. Concerns regarding bilirubin and kernicterus in the neonate are unwarranted.

For *Mycobacterium avium* complex, prophylaxis is initiated when the CD4 count is < 50. Use of zithromax 1200 mg orally once a week is recommended.

For cytomegalovirus, the patient should be counselled regarding preventive measures. The woman should avoid young children and nurseries, and especially close contact with such children.

Counselling for treatment-naive women in pregnancy

AZT is indicated for all women, regardless of disease status and regardless of resistance, for the prevention of vertical transmission.

Triple therapy is now commonly used as initial therapy and, as such, it is discussed with patients. There is no documented efficacy for this treatment in pregnancy. Our first line is AZT and lamivudine for most patients. Occasional patients warrant triple therapy if the immune system shows severe dysfunction or the maternal status suggests deterioration. Drug adherence is essential for all antiretroviral therapies.

Counselling for antiretroviral treatment-experienced women in pregnancy

The previous regimen is continued in pregnancy. If medications are stopped in early pregnancy, the practitioner should be sure that all antiretrovirals are stopped; the previous regimen is re-started at 12 weeks' gestation.

AZT is indicated for all women, regardless of disease status and regardless of resistance, for the prevention of vertical transmission. AZT should be added if it is not part of the previous regimen. If previously on D4T, this should be switched to AZT. Drug adherence is essential for all antiretroviral therapies.

Guidelines for zidovudine monotherapy

(1) Start at 12 weeks' gestation;

(2) All patients, regardless of CD4 count or viral load, are candidates for AZT therapy;

(3) Document informed consent;

(4) Zidovudine given 100 mg orally every 4 h while awake (five doses per day) or 200 mg orally three times per day or 300 mg orally twice per day (efficacy for prevent-ing perinatal transmission unproven for these last two regimens);

(5) Monthly complete blood count with differential to assess bone marrow suppression (macrocytosis is an indication of compliance);

(6) Discontinue AZT for hemoglobin of < 8 g/dl or absolute neutrophil count of < 750 cells/μl;.

(7) Liver profile for the 1st month and every 3 months thereafter;

(8) CD4 count and viral load assessment every 2–4 months. Tables 5 and 6 have laboratory flow sheets for monitoring HIV-positive women in pregnancy.

Therapy options for AZT-induced anemia include:

(1) Await bone marrow recovery, then reinstate AZT therapy;

(2) Start erythropoietin 100–200 μg/kg three times per week subcutaneously and continue AZT;

(3) Transfuse and continue AZT;

(4) Switch to alternative antiretroviral therapy.

Guidelines for combination antiretroviral therapy

Therapy may be initiated at any time during pregnancy, with acute HIV infection or within 6 months of seroconversion; with CD4 count of < 500 and viral load of > 10 000 copies/ml. The goal of therapy is no detectable virus at 3–4 months using an assay with a threshold of < 500 copies/ml.

Monitoring is by liver profile and complete blood count with platelet count monthly; and with CD4 count and viral load assessment every 2–4 months. Tables 5 and 6 have laboratory flow sheets for monitoring HIV-positive women in pregnancy.

AZT monotherapy usually results in a 0.5–0.7 log decrease in titer. Combination nucleoside analogs lead to a 0.5–1.4 log decrease in titer. Protease inhibitors lead to a 2 log decrease. A 1 log decrease correlates with an increase in the CD4 cell count of approximately 85.

Changing an antiretroviral regimen for suspected drug failure in pregnancy

Criteria for a change in therapy include: detectable viral load after 3–4 months of therapy; reappearance of viremia after suppression to undetectable; and significant increases in plasma viremia from the nadir of suppression.

When the decision to change therapy is based on viral load determination, it is preferable to confirm the viral load with a second specimen. Distinction must be made in the need to change a regimen between drug intolerance or inability to comply with the regimen and drug failure. In the event of drug failure, at least two new agents should be used.

There are no data regarding the use of protease inhibitors in pregnancy and therefore they should be used only in patients with very high viral loads, those with low CD4 counts or those who were previously on them. Protease inhibitors should be used only in combination therapy, in full dose and with good drug compliance.

Changing from ritonavir to indinivir or vice versa for drug failure should be avoided, since high-level cross-resistance is likely. Likewise, changing from nevirapine to delavirdine or vice versa for drug failure should be avoided, since high-level cross-resistance is likely.

Declining CD4 counts by more than 20%. Viral load should not be measured within 1 month of an acute illness or immunization. There is no level below which vertical transmission cannot occur.

Possible alternative regimens, if warranted by maternal status, include:

(1) AZT + ddI;

(2) AZT + lamivudine;

(3) ddI + d4T;

(4) AZT + lamivudine + nevirapine;

(5) AZT + lamivudine + protease inhibitor.

Peripartum and postpartum management

Oral antiretrovirals are discontinued and intravenous AZT is started during labor. The following should be avoided: rupture of membranes, long labor, fetal scalp electrode, fetal scalp sampling, instrumental deliveries and episiotomy.

Cesarean delivery is inadequately studied to be offered as a means of reducing the risk of vertical transmission. Cesarean delivery is used for routine obstetric purposes with an eye towards achieving the goals outlined above. Wall suction is used for meconium. Cord blood samples are obtained by draining the cord. Zidovudine Infusion Protocol for Pregnant Women in Labor

Intrapartum zidovudine

The patient weight in kilograms or pounds should be included for the pharmacy. Zidovudine 1 g/500 ml D5W intravenous infusion via pump. A loading dose of x mg or x ml is administered over 1 h, then the rate is reduced to continuous infusion of x ml/hour until delivery. The infusion guidelines contained in Table 7 should be used to determine the loading dose and flow rates. These guidelines were developed to simplify and expedite the ordering and administration of zidovudine in labor. Additionally, they may avoid medication errors by avoiding all the calculations.

The pharmacy prepares zidovudine infusions immediately prior to use. The entire dose is placed in a single bag. The standard concentration of zidovudine is 1 g/500 ml = 2 mg/ml. Use five vials of zidovudine 10 mg/ml, 20 ml single-dose vial, each vial has 200 mg, totalling 1 g in 100 ml. Add zidovudine 100 ml to D5W 400 ml bag to create a final volume of 500 ml. Label with concentration, loading dose and rate and continuous infusion rate. Protect from light.

Table 7 *Zidovudine infusion guidelines (1 g zidovudine in 500 ml, concentration = 2 mg/ml)*

Patient weight (lb)	Patient weight (kg)	Zidovudine bolus dosage (mg)	Infusion rate for the first hour (ml/h)	Infusion rate for the remainder of labor (ml/h)
110	50	100	50	25
114	52	104	52	26
119	54	108	54	27
123	56	112	56	28
128	58	116	58	29
132	60	120	60	30
136	62	124	62	31
141	64	128	64	32
145	66	132	66	33
150	68	136	68	34
154	70	140	70	35
158	72	144	72	36
163	74	148	74	37
167	76	152	76	38
172	78	156	78	39
176	80	160	80	40
180	82	164	82	41
185	84	168	84	42
189	86	172	86	43
194	88	176	88	44
198	90	180	90	45
202	92	184	92	46
207	94	188	94	47
211	96	192	96	48
216	98	196	98	49
220	100	200	100	50
224	102	204	102	51
229	104	208	104	52
233	106	212	106	53
238	108	216	108	54
240	109	218	109	55
245	111	223	111	56
250	114	227	114	57
255	116	232	116	58
260	118	236	118	59
265	120	241	120	60
270	123	245	123	61
275	125	250	125	63
280	127	255	127	64
285	130	259	130	65
290	132	264	132	66
295	134	268	134	67
300	136	273	136	68

The stability is 8 days at room temperature. A volume of 500 ml of standard drip lasts 8–12 h.

The nurse checks the label and hangs the pharmacy-prepared zidovudine infusion. The dose and rate are checked against the infusion guideline chart in Table 7. The nurse sets the infusion pump so that the loading dose is administered over 1 h.

After 1 h, the nurse resets the infusion pump so that the continuous infusion runs at a reduced rate throughout labor until delivery. The nurse notifies the pharmacy if labor is prolonged and a replacement infusion is needed.

Postpartum management

Breast feeding is contraindicated. Rubella vaccine is administered if indicated. Sterilization is provided if requested.

For contraception counselling, the use of latex condoms, Norplant and Depo-Provera are encouraged. No alterations in standard recommendations for contraception are necessary. An intrauterine device is best avoided. Some protease inhibitors may reduce the efficacy of oral contraceptives.

Arrangements should be made for ongoing maternal and pediatric medical care and social services. Arrangements should also be made for ongoing infectious disease management of HIV disease.

References

1. Centers for Disease Control and Prevention. Update: trends in AIDS incidence, deaths, prevalence – United States, 1996. *Morbid Mortal Weekly Rep* 1996;46:165–73
2. Farzadegan H, Hoover DR, Astemborski J, *et al.* Sex differences in HIV-1 viral load and progression to AIDS. *Lancet* 1998:352:1510–14
3. Connor EM, Sperling RS, Gelber R, *et al.* Reduction of maternal–infant transmission of human immunodeficiency virus type 1 with zidovudine treatment. *N Engl J Med* 1994;331:1173–80
4. Delta Coordinating Committee. A randomized double-blind controlled trial comparing combinations of zidovudine plus didanosine or zalcitabine with zidovudine alone in HIV infected individuals. *Lancet* 1996;348:283–91
5. Eron JJ, Benoit SI, Jemsek J, *et al.* Treatment with lamivudine, zidovudine or both in HIV-positive patients 200–500 per cubic millimeter: North America HIV Working Party. *N Engl J Med* 1995;333:1662–9
6. Hammer SM, Katzenstein DA, Hughes MD, *et al.* A trial comparing nucleoside monotherapy with combination therapy in HIV-infected adults with CD4 cell counts from 200–500 per cubic millimeter: AIDS Clinical Trials Group Study 175 Study Team. *N Engl J Med* 1996;335:1081–90
7. Minkoff H, Augenbraun M. Antiretroviral therapy for pregnant women. *Am J Obstet Gynecol* 1997;176:478–89
8. Carpenter CC, Fischl MA, Hammer SM, *et al.* Antiretroviral therapy for HIV infection in 1997: updated recommendations of the International AIDS Society – USA panel. *J Am Med Assoc* 1997;277:1962–9
9. O'Brien WA, Hartigan PM, Martin D, *et al.* Changes in plasma HIV-1 RNA and CD4+ lymphocyte counts and the risk of progression to AIDS: Veterans Affairs Cooperative Study Group. *N Engl J Med* 1996;334:426–31
10. Mellors JW, Kingsley LA, Rinaldo CR Jr, *et al.* Quantitation of HIV-1 RNA in plasma predicts outcome after seroconversion. *Ann Intern Med* 1995;122:573–9
11. Saksela K, Stevens CE, Rubinstein P, Taylor PW, Baltimore D. HIV-1 messenger RNA in peripheral blood mononuclear cells as an early marker of risk for progression to AIDS. *Ann Intern Med* 1995;123:641–8

Ethical dimensions of HIV infection in pregnancy

44

F. A. Chervenak, L. B. McCullough and W. J. Ledger

INTRODUCTION

In this chapter we present and justify a clinical ethical framework for the management of pregnant women and newborns infected with the human immunodeficiency virus (HIV). First, we identify an ethical framework for the public health dimensions of care for these two patient populations. Second, we develop an ethical framework for the clinical issues that arise in the care of these patients[1].

PUBLIC HEALTH ETHICS FOR HIV INFECTION

The ethics of public health management of these patients begins with securing their right to reliable and adequate clinical management of their problems[2]. Given that the USA, unlike many other developed countries, does not have a centrally organized health-care system, meeting the requirements of such a right falls to state and local government institutions and health-care professionals. In countries with national health systems this is a responsibility of the central government. Physicians should be in the forefront of advocacy for the funds required to meet the clinical needs of these patients, no matter what the national health system or lack thereof. This advocacy should be directed towards government, institutions, oneself and one's colleagues.

Many pregnant women with HIV and their infected newborns come from the lower socioeconomic groups in various societies[1]. Because these patients are often politically and socially marginalized, physicians and health-care institutions must advocate further, especially when no one else appears willing to do so. This leads to the second ethical principle of the public health ethics of HIV infection: justice. In the present context justice involves the obligation to meet the needs of those who are among the least well-off and most vulnerable members of our society[3,4].

CLINICAL ETHICS FOR HIV INFECTION

The clinical ethics of HIV infection appeals to two well-known principles of clinical ethics. The first of these ethical principles is beneficence. This principle obliges the physician to seek for the patient a greater balance of goods over harms as those goods and harms are understood and balanced from a rigorous clinical perspective[5]. In the case of HIV infection, beneficence creates a set of related obligations: to prevent the transmission of HIV when there are safe and effective means for doing so; to undertake vigorous measures of secondary and tertiary prevention for patients with HIV infection; and to meet the needs of patients dying from end-stage HIV infections. The physician has inescapable beneficence-based obligations to newborns, as well as to pregnant women and, in a pregnancy being taken to term, to the fetal patient. Pregnant women also have parallel beneficence-based obligations to the fetal patient and the future newborn that it will become[5].

The second ethical principle of the clinical ethics of HIV infection is respect for autonomy. This principle is required because, in addition to a rigorous clinical perspective on any patient's interests, adult patients have their own perspective on their own interests. This perspective must be respected and taken into account by the physician. Thus, the principle of respect for autonomy obliges the physician to seek for the patient a greater balance of goods over harms for the patient, as those goods and harms are understood and balanced by the patient[5].

The autonomy of the pregnant woman when the pregnancy is going to term is not absolute. Instead, her autonomy is appropriately subject to limitations. Because such pregnancies involve a fetal patient, the woman has beneficence-based obligations to the fetal patient and the newborn and child that it will become. Thus, the autonomy of a pregnant woman whose pregnancy involves a fetal patient is already limited by such beneficence-based obligations. Her primary moral relationship to her physicians, therefore, is not that of a rights bearer – as the civil rights model of HIV would have it. This model applies, if at all, only to non-pregnant individuals. Instead, the pregnant woman is both a rights *and* an obligations bearer. This makes for a more complicated and nuanced moral relationship between physician and patient.

The physician caring for an HIV-infected pregnant woman when the pregnancy is going to term therefore must manage a complex set of ethical obligations:

(1) Beneficence-based obligations to the pregnant woman (the three described above);

(2) Beneficence-based obligations to the fetal patient (the same three described above);

(3) Autonomy-based obligations to the pregnant woman.

The woman's autonomy and therefore the physician's autonomy-based obligations to her are limited by her beneficence-based obligations to the fetal patient, which are precisely the same as the physician's three beneficence-based obligations. Whether and when the physician should in clinical practice invoke and, if necessary, enforce the pregnant woman's beneficence-based obligations becomes a central question in the clinical ethics of HIV infection.

We turn now to the clinical application of this framework. We consider ethical issues that arise in the management of HIV-infected pregnant women.

ETHICAL ISSUES THAT ARISE IN THE MANAGEMENT OF THE HIV-INFECTED PREGNANT WOMAN

Termination of pregnancy and contraception

The authors have argued elsewhere that the decision to terminate a pregnancy before viability is a function of the pregnant woman's autonomy[4], a view held commonly in the literature on the ethics of abortion. It follows, as a matter of strict ethical obligation, that the physician's counselling of the pregnant woman about the alternative of abortion should be non-directive. The physician's own personal views – whether to end the pregnancy because an HIV-infected child will have serious diseases followed by early death or to continue the pregnancy out of pro-life or other personal convictions – should not be allowed to influence the counselling process in any conscious fashion. The physician should also discipline himself or herself to minimize subtle, unconscious bias in the counselling process.

During pregnancy the options of contraception and sterilization for future pregnancies should be offered to the pregnant woman. Counselling about these matters should be non-directive. An essential aspect of this counselling is providing unbiased information about the patient's present life expectancy, rates of vertical transmission, reduction of those rates by zidovudine, the course and premature mortality resulting from HIV infection in newborns and the psychosocial dimensions of rearing a possibly infected child when the woman herself is infected and will become ill[6]. We believe that it is possible for the conscientious physician to raise these ethically relevant matters in a sensitive and honest fashion and to help the woman, in non-directive counselling, to reflect on them carefully and thus reach an informed decision about them.

Partner notification

A pregnant woman who is HIV-infected has the same beneficence-based obligations to others that anyone with a serious infectious disease has, obligations that have become obscured in the civil rights model of the ethics of HIV infection. Her obligations include engaging in primary prevention of the transmission of the disease to immediate partners. This is especially urgent, because her sexual partners and needle sharers may engage in these behaviors with others, further spreading the disease before they themselves learn that they are infected. Thus, anyone with HIV infection has both individual and public health obligations to prevent transmission of HIV.

These beneficence-based obligations of the pregnant woman are buttressed by her autonomy-based obligations to prevent HIV infection. Consider the following line of reasoning. Part of the mechanism of transmission of HIV involves the decisions of individuals to engage in behaviors that are known to transmit HIV. Moreover, despite widespread educational efforts, not everyone engaging in needle sharing or sexual intercourse understands HIV and its modes of transmission. Thus, those with HIV infection cannot assume that those with whom they share needles or have sexual intercourse already know and have consented to the health risks of such behaviors *vis-à-vis* HIV infection. Such consent must be explicit, a requirement of the ethical principle of respect for autonomy that governs all human behavior.

These beneficence-based and autonomy-based analyses combine to create a very strong ethical obligation on the part of anyone with HIV infection to notify sexual partners and needle sharers of that status. Neither men nor pregnant women are exceptions. When the patient refuses to notify others, when she is placing at risk without consent and does not have convincing reasons for doing so, the physician should make another rigorous effort to persuade the patient, by pointing out that this really is a matter of serious, urgent obligation and that she therefore owes it to her sexual partners or needle sharers to notify them. If she agrees to do so, the physician should consider a follow-up mechanism, e.g. telephoning the partner within a very limited time period, e.g. 24 h. If she does not agree to do so, the physician has a public health obligation and an individual beneficence-based obligation to notify partners. There has always existed a physician privilege to violate confidentiality when there is sufficient reason to do so[7] and protecting innocent others from a serious, ultimately life-taking infection surely counts as such a reason. Some states permit such disclosure to the patient's spouse. The reader should familiarize himself or herself with relevant state law and be willing to work to change laws that prohibit disclosure. These laws reflect an excessive emphasis on the civil rights approach to HIV infection.

Disclosure by patient to team

It is surely in the interest of every patient that his or her providers have a complete medical and social history. This is all the more the case for HIV infection, because HIV infection changes the patient's risk profile and response to medical interventions. Moreover, new treatments offer the promise of extended life with a chronic, not immediately fatal, illness. These matters should be explained to all patients, so that HIV-infected patients will not feel singled out for different management.

Patients should also be able to be confident that their serostatus will have no adverse effects on the care that they will receive or behavior of those who care for them. Actual practice and policy should be such as to make this confidence warranted. It is therefore the responsibility of every institution to make sure that policies and procedures support this assumption on each patient's part.

Disclosure to other health-care professionals

Every health-care professional has the same obligations of confidentiality towards patients. This applies to the primary care providers and to all consultants, including consultants who may not see the patient, e.g. in informal or 'curbside' consultation. Again, patients should be able to assume this and institutional policies and practices should ensure that confidentiality is appropriately maintained.

Prevention of vertical transmission

Clinical trials of zidovudine for vertical transmission of HIV have produced the impressive conclusion that the rate of vertical transmission can be reduced by as much as 75%[8]. The pregnant woman has a beneficence-based obligation to accept medical interventions that produce significant benefit for the fetal patient and child it will become when such interventions are on balance either not significantly harmful to her or may even benefit her. Studies of zidovudine have raised questions about its efficacy in changing the course of HIV infection[9]. If clinical judgement follows such trial results, then, at worst, zidovudine is of manageable risk to the pregnant woman and of very significant benefit to the fetal patient and child it will become. In a pregnancy going to term, therefore, the pregnant woman is ethically obliged to accept this preventive measure.

It follows from this that, as a matter of strict ethical obligation, every pregnant woman should be offered HIV testing, and zidovudine should be available to every pregnant woman found to be HIV-infected, consistent with national health policy and funding. If the second condition is not met, offering testing is meaningless in terms of preventing vertical transmission. Thus, policy matters directly affect clinical ethics, adding yet another advocacy obligation to the physician's agenda.

The physician's response to women who refuse to be tested for HIV should be repeated and rigorous efforts aimed at the woman's reconsidering and changing her decision on the assumption that the woman wants a good outcome for her baby. The physician should underscore the woman's obligation to prevent vertical transmission and the importance to her own care of documented serostatus.

Pregnant women taking their pregnancies to term who refuse zidovudine should be vigorously persuaded to change their decisions. Counselling should be directive and vigorous. The physician should revisit the issue throughout pregnancy, since zidovudine may have its preventive effect in the birth canal rather than earlier in pregnancy. Family members may be enlisted to help the pregnant woman think matters through and to help to persuade her of the wisdom of this course. Directive counselling rejects the ethical assumption that the pregnant woman has a right to refuse zidovudine; rather, directive counselling is justified on the assumption that she has a beneficence-based obligation to accept it and that her freedom to refuse is therefore restricted by this obligation.

CONCLUSION

Appropriate clinical management of the HIV-infected pregnant woman involves multi-faceted ethical challenges. We have argued for a balanced and clinically relevant ethical framework that emphasizes the beneficence-based and autonomy-based obligations of the physician of the pregnant woman, as well as the beneficence-based obligations of the pregnant woman to the fetal patient. The ethical principle of respect for autonomy, in particular, shapes the counselling process about termination of pregnancy, contraception and partner notification.

References

1. Chervenak FA, McCullough LB, Ledger WJ. Ethical dimensions of human immunodeficiency virus infection during pregnancy. *Infectious Dis Obstet Gynecol* 1997;5:192–8

2. Minkoff HL, De Hovitz JA. Care of women infected with the human immunodeficiency virus. *J Am Med Assoc* 1991;266:2253–8

3. Rawls J. *A Theory of Justice*. Cambridge: Harvard University Press, 1971

4. Daniels N. *Just Health Care*. Cambridge: Harvard University Press, 1989

5. McCullough LB, Chervenak FA. *Ethics in Obstetrics and Gynecology*. New York: Oxford University Press, 1994

6. Kass NE. Policy, ethics, and reproductive choice: pregnancy and childrearing among HIV-infected women. *Acta Pediatr* 1994;400(Suppl):95–8

7. Beauchamp TL, Childress JF. *Principles of Biomedical Ethics*, 4th edn. New York: Oxford University Press, 1994

8. Conner EM, Sperling RS, Gelber R, Kisilev P, Scott G, O'Sullivan MJ. Reduction of maternal–infant transmission of human immunodeficiency virus type I with zidovudine treatment. *N Engl J Med* 1994;331:1173–80

9. Volberding PA, Lagakos SW, Grimes JM, *et al.* A comparison of immediate with deferred zidovudine therapy for asymptomatic HIV-infected adults with CD4 cell counts of 500 or more per cubic millimeter. *N Engl J Med* 1995; 333:401–7

Maternal death during pregnancy: management and ethical aspects

45

E. Gdansky and J. G. Schenker

INTRODUCTION

The World Health Organization (WHO) estimates that approximately 500 000 maternal deaths occur each year around the world. Over 99% of these cases are in the developing countries. Although impressive, these numbers may not represent the whole truth, since maternal death is seriously underestimated all over the world[1-3]. Two major factors contribute to this underestimation:

(1) Not all countries possess a national register of maternal death cases;

(2) Different countries use different classifications for these cases.

In general, maternal death is divided into direct, indirect and fortuitous causes according to the contribution of the pregnancy to the event of death; it can occur either during pregnancy or thereafter. Because most of the cases of death are related to pregnancy, adequate antepartum and postpartum care is the key for reducing maternal death worldwide and, especially, in the developing countries.

In the past, the fetus had an ominous fate if medical help was not promptly given. A postmortem Cesarean section was the only chance for the fetus to survive. Stories on fetuses who were born from the womb of their dead mother are as old as Greek mythology (around 1000 BC). Dionysus, the god of wine, was delivered by his father, the chief of the Olympian gods, Zeus, after his mother was burned. The second story tells about Apollo, the god of poetry and music, who had mercy on the mortal and beautiful Koronis and delivered her son, Asklepios, after her death.

Asklepios was then given for custody to the wise centaur, Cheiron, who educated him to become a physician. Postmortem Cesarean section was further mentioned in Roman laws, the Babylonian Talmud and laws based on Christianity[4]. The history of this issue is beyond the scope of this chapter. Nevertheless, the history of postmortem Cesarean section demonstrates that since antiquity the fetus has been a patient, in the sense of having the right to be treated, in cases of maternal death.

In the past decades, sophisticated medical technologies and organ transplantation programs have changed our view on death. These advances offered new options of treatment also for cases of maternal death during pregnancy. Perimortem, and not postmortem, Cesarean section was introduced for the sake of the dying mother as well as her fetus. Vital organs of pregnant brain-dead women are sustained artificially for the sake of their developing fetuses. These changes created debates on ethical, legal, societal and religious grounds which are far from being resolved. Our modest scope in writing this chapter is to expose the reader to the present knowledge on the management of pregnancy complicated by maternal death and to raise some of the ethical considerations.

DEFINITION OF DEATH

An interesting philosophical approach to death suggests that the best way to deal with death is to accept it as a series of distinct but related deaths[5]. The basis of this approach is that a human being should not be seen only as a biological organism but also as a person, having cognitive abilities, esthetic sensibilities, emotions, capacity for social interactions and spiritual capacities. Likewise, the death of a human being can appear in more than one form. According to this multiple-deaths approach the *biological death* and the *death of a person* are intimately related but conceptually distinguishable components of death.

Biological death can be defined as a permanent cessation of function of a distinct biological entity. Because different organs and systems may cease to function at different times, a further division of biological death into local death (death of parts of the body), molecular death (death of all tissues) and somatic death (death of the organism as a whole) is sometimes used. According to this definition, death of the human body is to be declared with somatic death.

Since death of some organs or systems is more important than death of others in provoking death of the organism as a whole, it is important to determine which are the organs whose death signifies somatic death. For this purpose, the President's Commission for the Study of Ethical Problems in Medicine and Biomedical and Behavioral Research[6] proposed guidelines for the determination of death which were accepted almost worldwide. According to these guidelines, death of an individual is determined by one of the following criteria:

(1) Irreversible cessation of circulatory and respiratory functions;

(2) Brain death.

CARDIORESPIRATORY DEATH IN PREGNANCY

A pregnant woman does not differ from any other human being regarding the definition of death. Yet, pregnancy involves two patients: the pregnant woman and her fetus. The obstetrician being educated to care for both patients shifts attention towards the fetus in the case of maternal death. The fetus, being totally dependent on the maternal blood supply, cannot suffer prolonged maternal cardiocirculatory arrest, and will die if medical intervention is not immediately offered. Since any intervention will be futile for a non-viable fetus, the issue of fetal viability is of the utmost importance.

Fetal viability

To deliver a fetus of 32 weeks' gestation or more is reasonably safe, since most centers report close to 100% survival and low morbidity. Newborns delivered at 27 completed weeks or more have more than a 60% chance of surviving, but still have the non-negligible misfortune of morbidity. Extremely premature fetuses of less than 27 weeks of gestation are those at major risk regarding viability, and also of short- and long-term morbidity. Survival data of extremely premature newborns differ worldwide and even between different neonatal units in the same country. Combining the results from a number of studies that were carried out in developed countries, it is estimated that the survival rate is around 61% at 26 weeks, 50% at 25 weeks, 39% at 24 weeks and 17% at 23 weeks[7]. The lower limit of fetal viability should be drawn by every medical institution according to the intensive care facilities and survival rate of these infants. Interestingly, the relationship between gestational age and mortality is not linear but exponential, suggesting that the biological barrier to survival lies somewhere between 23 and 25 weeks of gestation[8].

Major morbidity, such as septicemia, chronic lung disease, severe intraventricular hemorrhage and necrotizing enterocolitis, increases with decreasing gestational age. Neurodevelopmental disability is the worst outcome for extremely premature newborns who survive. Moderate to severe neurological disability occurs in more than 50% of newborns born before 25 weeks of gestation. This includes significant motor disorders, a low IQ necessitating special education, or an important deficit in hearing or vision. Unfortunately, many of these infants have more than one disability.

According to the outcome of these extremely premature newborns, the

American College of Obstetricians and Gynecologists[9] stated that 'currently, the birth at or before 25 weeks of gestation or weighing less than 750 g presents a variety of complex medical, social, and ethical decisions'. Counselling of possible outcomes of these extremely premature newborns is warranted to the family, encouraging them to participate actively in the decision-making process. Since in a stressful situation such as extremely preterm labor, it is not always possible to talk about fetal outcome and likely course in any detail with the frightened and overwhelmed family, Rutter[8] has suggested a middle-of-the-road approach: 'full resuscitation and intensive care should be given at 26 weeks of gestation, probably be given at 25 weeks, possibly be given at 24 weeks, but not at 23 weeks or earlier'. This situation is even more complex when maternal death is in concern and decisions of whether to deliver an extremely premature fetus have to be reached. It would be medically and ethically improper to delineate strict guidelines of management of extremely preterm pregnancies complicated by maternal death, but it seems that efforts to save the fetus may begin at 24 completed weeks of gestation.

Postmortem and perimortem Cesarean section

The best way to deliver a viable fetus in pregnancy complicated by cardiorespiratory death is to perform a postmortem Cesarean section. Katz and co-workers[10] summarized the fetal outcome of 61 infants delivered by postmortem Cesarean section. Forty-two infants were delivered within 0–5 min after maternal death and were all neurologically normal; eight infants were delivered after 6–10 min with one reported mild neurological disability; seven infants were delivered after 11–15 min with one case of severe neurological disability; and four infants were delivered after 16 min with three cases of severe neurological disability. Although reports of normal infants, who were delivered after longer periods of cardiac arrest, have been published[11-13], it seems that the sooner the fetus is delivered after maternal cardiac arrest, the better his or her prognosis.

The declaration of maternal death after cardiocirculatory arrest is often made following unsuccessful cardiopulmonary resuscitation (CPR). After the arrest, maternal ventilation and cardiac massage should be immediately initiated. Physiological changes during pregnancy can impede a successful CPR[14]. The growing uterus causes mechanical obstruction of the great abdominal vessels and, therefore, interferes with venous return and cardiac output. Hence, displacement of the uterus toward the maternal left prior to 24 weeks of gestation, and left lateral tilt (15–30°) of the body after 24 weeks of gestation, are of paramount importance for an effective CPR. Furthermore, an increase in oxygen requirements and a reduction in functional residual capacity in the lungs make the pregnant woman more vulnerable to hypoxia and brain damage. Decreased cardiac output and increased risk of brain damage have brought several authors to recommend that, if CPR has not been successful within the first 5 min, a perimortem Cesarean section has to be performed for maternal reasons during advanced pregnancy[10,11,13].

The Four-Minute Rule, suggesting that a Cesarean section should be begun within 4 min and the infant delivered within 5 min after maternal cardiac arrest, seems to be in the interest of both the pregnant woman and the viable fetus. Under these circumstances, aseptic techniques are of limited value. A vertical midline incision on the skin and a classical incision on the uterus are made to deliver the fetus as quickly as possible. CPR should continue during and after the surgery; others recommend a thoracotomy and open chest massage if there is no response to CPR within 15 min[14].

BRAIN DEATH IN PREGNANCY

The diagnosis of brain death, defined as a permanent cessation of functioning of the whole brain, determines human death. The vital organs of the body can function and be sustained artificially for days, or more, after the diagnosis of brain death[15,16]. These bodies may therefore serve, with permission, as a source for organ transplantation. The technological and medical ability to preserve the body of a brain-dead human being 'alive' for a period of time, although limited, created the ground for the use of brain-dead pregnant women as biological incubators of their developing fetuses.

The principles of the management of a brain-dead woman in pregnancy are derived from the growing experience on the management of donors. The aim of appropriate donor management is to optimize the condition of potential transplants and reduce the loss of donors, currently 25%, owing to the lack of suitable management. Likewise, the less damage done to the vital organs of a pregnant brain-dead woman, the better the chances for the fetus.

Pathophysiology of brain death

The pathophysiology of brain death consists of two major events: 'autonomic storm' and endocrine dysfunction. The 'autonomic storm' results from the release of huge amounts of catecholamines to the circulation by the adrenergic nervous system. The duration of this phase is short (10–15 min), but the impact of catecholamines on vital organs is detrimental. Heart injury can be detected by electrocardiogram, demonstrating ischemic changes, ST-T wave abnormalities and pseudo-acute myocardial infarction. Arterial vasoconstriction induces an increase in systemic vascular resistance and hypertension. These changes can provoke left ventricular insufficiency, causing low cardiac output and mitral regurgitation. At this point, high pulmonary capillary pressure develops and capillary integrity is disrupted. The end of this process may eventually result in pulmonary edema.

On light and electron microscopy, tissues and cells demonstrate damage typical to catecholamine–calcium-induced injury[17]. Focal myocyte necrosis in the form of contraction bands and coagulative necrosis or myocytolysis is frequently observed in the heart. The lungs demonstrate alveolar wall edema and hemorrhage and alveolar space edema, while marked reduction of the capillary vascular spaces is seen in the kidneys. In the liver, there is loss of glycogen. Cellular damage is characterized as mitochondrial injury consisting of disruption of the membrane, christi and matrix and accumulation of electron-dense material. According to the degree of injury, the effect on aerobic production of ATP ranges from minimal to total loss.

Endocrine dysfunction occurs as a consequence of disintegration of the hypothalamic–pituitary axis. Changes in the level of circulating hormones are seen within a few hours from the event of brain death. Low levels of thyroxin, cortisol, insulin and antidiuretic hormone (ADH) lead to a reduction in energy stores, a shift from aerobic to anaerobic metabolism and the development of diabetes insipidus. The effects on cellular metabolism and electrolytes further cause deterioration of the circulatory control and tissue damage to the vital organs[17].

Management of brain death in pregnancy

It is obvious that appropriate supportive measures to brain-dead humans include all those directed towards replacing the normal physiology of the living body[17,18]. In case of maternal brain death, the physiological changes of pregnancy should be taken into account, in order to maintain an optimal environment for the developing fetus. Mechanical ventilation is given in order to mimic the mild respiratory alkalosis of pregnancy. Hypotension is first managed with crystalloid and colloid infusions, and anemia should be corrected. To maintain the uteroplacental blood flow in fluid-resistant hypotension, the use of pressor drugs is not contraindicated and dopamine is the drug of choice. Hormone replacement therapy of thyroxin, ADH and cortisol are mandatory for optimal circulatory control. Hyperglycemia is treated with adequate doses of insulin. Warm gases, fluids and blankets are used to overcome the loss of the hypothalamic thermoregulatory mechanism. An adequate amount of calories is supplied by gastric tube or total parenteral nutrition. The immobilized body and the presence of multiple catheters and vascular lines require respiratory physiotherapy, aseptic suction of secretions, heparin prophylaxis and aggressive surveillance for and treatment of infections. These meticulous and time-consuming treatments are all directed to providing the fetus with the optimal environment for development in this situation. Therefore, the fetus needs to be monitored by frequent cardiotocography and ultrasound to detect signs of distress. Finally, the importance of a team of experts from different disciplines and dedicated critical-care nurses in the overall management cannot be overemphasized.

Dillon and colleagues[19] were the first to publish a case of intensive care support to a brain-dead woman during pregnancy. She was a 24-year-old woman at 25 weeks of gestation, who was diagnosed as brain dead owing to meningoencephalitis. Six days after the diagnosis a female infant, weighing 930 g, was delivered by Cesarean section. The infant was discharged from the intensive care nursery at 3 months of age. A management plan for these cases, based on neonatal survival statistics and the lack of evidence that support could prolong somatic life for more than a couple of weeks after brain death, was advanced by the authors of that publication. According to their plan, when brain death occurs after 28 weeks of gestation, delivery by Cesarean section should be executed as soon as possible; when brain death occurs before 24 weeks of gestation, no treatment should be given; and if brain death occurs between 24 and 27 weeks of gestation, treatment should be started, with immediate delivery reserved for instances of fetal distress or significant deterioration of the mother's condition.

Three case reports, published in the English-language literature, challenged Dillon's plan and described successful treatment of brain-dead women for 9, 10 and even 15 weeks[20–22]. They delivered the infants at 31–32 weeks' gestation. In two, more recent, reports of brain death during pregnancy the authors failed to sustain the vital functions of the women for more than 48 hours[23,24]. In these last cases, the etiology of brain death was cocaine abuse with intraventricular hemorrhage, and acute pneumococcal meningitis. Because of the scarce number of case reports, the role of the etiology of brain death to the success or failure of the treatment is unknown. Furthermore, it is possible that the scarcity of published reports merely reflects the many unpublished cases in which prolonged support and fetal survival were not possible. Therefore, although some can argue that no clear lower limit of gestational age exists for the support of the brain-dead pregnant woman, treatment for more than a few weeks should be regarded as experimental, since the possibility of reaching fetal viability is low or at least unknown.

ETHICAL CONSIDERATIONS OF BRAIN DEATH IN PREGNANCY

The four principles of beneficence, non-maleficence, respect for autonomy and justice cover most ethical considerations which are relevant to the practice and science of medicine[25]. If pregnancy is considered as the center of a circle that closely involves the pregnant woman and her fetus, then the husband, the children and the close family form an intermediate circle while society forms the outer circle. The interest of so many participants during pregnancy may create complex situations and ethical dilemmas which are not easy to resolve. The application of the four ethical principles on the different participants is even more difficult in cases of maternal death. The principle of autonomy of the pregnant woman ceases with her death, but the autonomy of the fetus and the rights of, for example, the father are unclear.

Maternal loss of autonomy

Maintaining brain-dead women on life-support systems for the sake of their fetuses presents them as biological incubators. For the mean time, this possibility is limited for a few weeks to months, but it is possible that the understanding of the physiology of these 'neomorts' will improve therapy and lead to longer periods of treatment. Objection to this new treatment was raised because of the fear that women would be viewed as mere fetus containers. In this respect, it is important to distinguish between the respect for autonomy of a living woman and the loss of autonomy with her death. The matter here is not of creating new incubators from women who were not pregnant but prolonging the vital functions of an already pregnant woman. If we consider that the dead pregnant woman has no interests other than fulfilment of prior requests, putting her on treatment gives her child the possibility of developing, while she suffers little (if any) harm[5,26].

In the absence of the woman's advanced consent, who should decide about treating a brain-dead woman in pregnancy? In situations not complicated by pregnancy the next of kin has the authority to make decisions about the disposition of the body after death. In pregnancy, these decisions can sometimes be in conflict with the interest of the fetus. Do the wishes of the next of kin have a priority over the needs of the fetus? Since most cases do not have the woman's consent to being maintained on a life-support system, it seems that, in the absence of other juridical precedents, it is ethically appropriate to respect the wishes of the husband.

The patient–physician relationship

The obligation of the physician to treat a pregnant woman ceases with her death. The fetus is the only patient to be considered in pregnancy complicated by maternal brain death. But is the fetus a patient at all stages of the pregnancy? Those who say yes probably base their answer on the fact that today, we perform *in utero* procedures on fetuses at all stages of gestation. These procedures can be divided into those aimed to inform the future parents on fetal health, and others aimed to treat the endangered developing fetus. The second kind of procedure is a pure example of treating a patient and is done to bring the fetus to a better quality of 'life' *in utero* and

after it is born. On the other hand, those who do not see the fetus as a patient, at all stages of pregnancy, base their argument on the fact that a non-viable fetus will not benefit from its rescue from a dead pregnant woman. Indeed, a third option can bridge the gap between the apparent contradiction of these views. Both see the fetus as a patient according to the results of the treatment after the fetus is born. After birth, every person at need is a patient whether treatment is given or not. Before birth, being a patient depends on the ability to survive after birth. The fact that the potentially viable fetus cannot actively ask for help does not alleviate the physician's responsibility to offer treatment.

The obligation to accept or be given treatment is derived from the ability to offer benefits which are viewed as proportionate to its burdens[27]. The medical issue of fetal viability and neonatal morbidity was discussed earlier. Therefore, a fetus at term or near term should be delivered after maternal brain death, when fetal life is in danger. Our possibilities make no sense in treating fetuses during first and early second trimesters of pregnancy. The ethical dilemmas are therefore the result of uncertainties concerning the outcome of the fetuses around the limits of viability.

The fetus–family relationship

After birth, the child is considered the property of his parents. Benefits and risks of every medical intervention for the child are discussed and the autonomy of the parents to decide is maintained. Since maternal autonomy ceases with her death, should the next of kin be involved in the decision of whether or not to treat the unborn? When the fetus is near term, or the chances of mortality and morbidity are low, it seems ethically and legally justified to deliver the fetus in order to save its life. But when fetal age is at the limits of viability, there is a real possibility that the treatment will not result in a healthy child. The fact that the family will have to deal with rearing this child supports the primary role of the family in the decision-making process.

The management of maternal death during pregnancy is complex and includes various medical and ethical aspects. Making the distinction between maternal cardiocirculatory arrest and brain death is mandatory for the management. The issue of fetal viability is of paramount importance in making decisions of whether to treat and how to treat these cases. Strict criteria for management of these tragic cases cannot be set, since medical, ethical, religious and legal aspects all play a part in creating decisions.

References

1. Atrash HK, Alexander S, Berg CJ. Maternal mortality in developed countries: not just a concern of the past. *Obstet Gynecol* 1995;86:700–5

2. Gissler M, Kauppila R, Merilainen J, Toukomaa H, Hemminki E. Pregnancy-associated deaths in Finland 1987–1994 – definition problems and benefits of record linkage. *Acta Obstet Gynecol Scand* 1997;76: 651–7

3. Fikree FF, Midhet F, Sandruddin S, Berendes HW. Maternal mortality in different Pakistani sites: ratios, clinical causes and determinants. *Acta Obstet Gynecol Scand* 1997;76:637–45

4. Loewy EH. The pregnant brain dead and the fetus: must we always try to wrest life from death? *Am J Obstet Gynecol* 1987;157:1097–101

5. Shrader D. On dying more than one death. *Hastings Cent Rep* 1986;16:12–17

6. Medical Consults on the Diagnosis of Death. Guidelines for the determination of death. Report to the President's Commission for the Study of Ethical Problems in Medicine and Biomedical and Behavioral Research. *J Am Med Assoc* 1981;246:2184–6

7. Morrison JJ, Rennie JM. Clinical, scientific and ethical aspects of fetal and neonatal care at extremely preterm periods of gestation. *Br J Obstet Gynaecol* 1997;104:1341–50

8. Rutter N. The extremely preterm infant. *Br J Obstet Gynaecol* 1995;102:682–7

9. American College of Obstetricians and Gynecologists. Committee opinion. Perinatal and infant mortality statistics. Number 167, December 1995. Committee on Obstetric Practice. *Int J Gynaecol Obstet* 1996;53:86–8

10. Katz VL, Dotters DJ, Droegemueller W. Perimortem cesarean delivery. *Obstet Gynecol* 1986;68:571–6

11. Oates S, Williams GL, Rees GA. Cardiopulmonary resuscitation in late pregnancy. *Br Med J* 1988;297:404–5

12. Lopez-Zeno JA, Carlo WA, O'Grady JP, Fanaroff AA. Infant survival following delayed postmortem cesarean delivery. *Obstet Gynecol* 1990;76:991–2

13. Chen HF, Lee CN, Huang GD, Hsieh FJ, Huang SC, Chen HY. Delayed maternal death after perimortem cesarean section. *Acta Obstet Gynecol Scand* 1994;73:839–41

14. Lee RV, Rodgers BD, White LM, Harvey RC. Cardiopulmonary resuscitation of pregnant women. *Am J Med* 1989;81:311–18

15. Jennett B, Gleave J, Wilson P. Brain death in three neurosurgical units. *Br Med J* 1981;282:533–9

16. Parisi JE, Kim RC, Collins GH, Hilfinger MF. Brain death with prolonged somatic survival. *N Engl J Med* 1982;306:14–16

17. Novitzky D. Donor management: state of the art. *Transplant Proc* 1997;29:3773–5

18. Pagano D, Bonser RS, Graham TR. Optimal management of the heart–lung donor. *Br J Hosp Med* 1995;53:522–5

19. Dillon WP, Lee RV, Tronolone MJ, Buckwald S, Foote RJ. Life support and maternal death during pregnancy. *J Am Med Assoc* 1982;248:1089–91

20. Field DR, Gates EA, Creasy RK, Jonsen AR, Laros RK Jr. Maternal brain death during pregnancy. Medical and ethical issues. *J Am Med Assoc* 1988;260:816–22

21. Heikkinen JE, Rinne RI, Alahuhta SM, *et al.* Life support of 10 weeks with successful fetal outcome after fatal maternal brain damage. *Br Med J Clin Res Ed* 1985;290:1237–8

22. Bernstein IM, Watson M, Simmons GM, Catalano PM, Davis G, Collins R. Maternal brain death and prolonged fetal survival. *Obstet Gynecol* 1989;74:434–7

23. Iriye BK, Asrat T, Adashek JA, Carr MH. Intraventricular haemorrhage and maternal brain death associated with antepartum cocaine abuse. *Br J Obstet Gynaecol* 1995;102:68–9

24. Vives A, Carmona F, Zabala E, Fernandez C, Cararach V, Iglesias X. Maternal brain death during pregnancy. *Int J Gynaecol Obstet* 1996;52: 67–9

25. Hayry M. Ethics committees, principles and consequences. *J Med Ethics* 1998;24:81–5

26. Fost N. The baby in the body. *Hastings Cent Rep* 1994;24:31–2

27. Tuohey JF. Terminal care and the pregnant woman: ethical reflections. *Pediatrics* 1991;88: 1268–73

Epidemiology of pre-eclampsia in The Netherlands

46

J. van Eyck, W. F. de Boer, W. B. Grol and B. Arabin

INTRODUCTION

Hypertensive disorder is reported to occur in almost 10% of all pregnancies[1]. Between 1988 and 1992 hypertensive disorder was responsible for 13 of a total of 66 maternal deaths in The Netherlands, corresponding to 1.7 maternal deaths per 100 000 live births[2]. Despite the fact that, in The Netherlands, pre-eclampsia is considered to be a major cause of maternal and neonatal mortality and morbidity, national epidemiological data are lacking. Therefore, the objective of this study was to collect and analyze national and regional epidemiological data on pre-eclampsia in The Netherlands. Furthermore, we have analyzed for our unit the associated underlying disorders and maternal and perinatal outcome parameters.

MATERIALS AND METHODS

National data

National data were collected from the Central Bureau of Statistics (CBS) over the period 1995 and 1996. The CBS is a national institute responsible for the collection and analysis of epidemiological data of the Dutch population. National data were also obtained from the LVR-2, which is the national obstetric registration system for all hospital deliveries under supervision of a gynecologist. In The Netherlands about 50% of all deliveries take place at home under supervision of a midwife or a house doctor. However, women with pre-eclampsia are always referred to a gynecologist. Only since 1995 has the presence or absence of pre-eclampsia had to be registered.

In this study, we analyzed the incidence of pre-eclampsia, maternal mortality, intra-uterine deaths, gestational age at delivery, birth weight, mode of delivery, perinatal outcome, ethnic origin and seasonal influence. By linking the data to the postal code of all women who delivered in 1995 and 1996, it became possible to study the regional distribution of pre-eclampsia and its relationship with urbanization grade. Thereby, 27 health-care regions were used, according to the Institute of Dutch Hospitals.

Regional data

Regional data from our own center were retrospectively studied for the period from 1989 to 1996. Over the last 2 years of this period, all women with early-onset pre-eclampsia were tested for underlying disorders at around 3 months after delivery. Analysis consisted of tests for anticardiolipin antibodies, hyperhomocysteinemia (with a methionine-loading test), protein S deficiency and activated protein C (APC) resistance (factor V Leiden).

For both the national and the regional studies, pre-eclampsia was defined as the combined presence of a diastolic blood pressure of > 90 mmHg and proteinuria of > 300 mg/l. HELLP syndrome was defined as the combined presence of a platelet count of $< 100 \times 10^9$/l, raised liver enzymes of > 50 IU/l and a haptoglobin count of < 0.3 g/l.

RESULTS

In The Netherlands, a total of 375 700 women were delivered in 1995 and 1996. From this population, 3934 women developed pre-eclampsia, resulting in an overall incidence of 1.05%. In our hospital, 10 452 women were delivered between 1989 and 1996. In this period, 406 women developed pre-eclampsia, resulting in a local incidence of 3.8%.

The national maternal mortality rate, analyzed to date only for 1995, was 7.3 per 100 000 live births; maternal mortality due to hypertensive disorder was 1.5 per 100 000 live births. This is comparable with the mortality rate of the period between 1988 and 1992 inclusive[2]. In our center, the overall maternal mortality was 0.2 per 1000 live births for the observation period from 1989 to 1996 inclusive. The two cases with maternal death were due to pre-eclampsia and maternal cerebral hemorrhage, resulting in a maternal mortality rate of 0.5% in all women with pre-eclampsia. Further severe complications were found in 11 patients with eclamptic insults and one patient with liver rupture out of the 120 patients with HELLP syndrome.

The overall intrauterine death rate in The Netherlands between 1995 and 1996 was 0.7%; in women with pre-eclampsia this was not increased (0.6%). Perinatal mortality (defined as the combined intrauterine deaths after 24 weeks' gestation and neonatal deaths within 1 week after birth) could not be evaluated in the whole population. In our referral center, perinatal mortality among the patients with pre-eclampsia was 5.7%.

The mode of delivery also reflects the increased maternal and fetal risks at early gestational ages. In the national population, 28% of women with pre-eclampsia were delivered by Cesarean section. In our department, this percentage was as high as 55%.

Within the national population, an increased incidence of pre-eclampsia was observed in Black compared to other ethnic groups, such as White, Mediterranean, Hindu and Asiatic mothers. In contrast to studies in Zimbabwe[3], no seasonal influences were demonstrated. With respect to the geographic distribution, the incidence of pre-eclampsia was significantly raised in the regions of Amsterdam, South Limburg and Twente

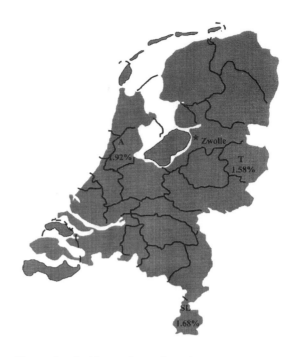

Figure 1 *Incidence of pre-eclampsia in regions of The Netherlands: A, Amsterdam; T, Twente; SL, South Limburg; Zwolle, site of perinatal center*

(Figure 1). Furthermore, pre-eclampsia was associated with a high urbanization grade.

In our center, 87 women who were admitted because of severe early-onset pre-eclampsia and/or HELLP syndrome were tested for underlying disorders, such as anticardiolipin antibodies, hyperhomocysteinemia, protein S deficiency and APC resistance (factor V Leiden). All these disorders have pre-existing endothelial dysfunction in common, and this facilitates the development of pre-eclampsia[4]. The incidence of all these disorders was significantly increased, compared to the incidence in the general Dutch population[4] (Table 1). In the population originating from the eastern province Twente (n = 27), the incidence of hyperhomocysteinemia and protein S deficiency was significantly increased as compared to the population originating from other parts of The Netherlands (n = 60). The incidence of APC resistance in this population, however, was comparable to that of the general Dutch population.

Table 1 *Underlying disorders of patients with early-onset pre-eclampsia referred to our hospital, according to regional differences*

	Study population (n = 87)		Twente (n = 27)		Other regions (n = 60)		National prevalance (%)
	n	%	n	%	n	%	
Anticardiolipin antibodies	15	17*	4	15	11	18	1–3
Hyperhomocysteinemia	18	21*	10	37*	8	13	2–3
Protein S deficiency	11	13*	6	22*	5	8	0.2–2
APC resistance	10	12*	1	4	9	15	3–7
At least one disorder	46	53	18	67	28	47	–

APC, activated protein C; *$p < 0.05$ (χ^2 test)

DISCUSSION

In The Netherlands, it has become possible to study the epidemiology of pre-eclampsia only since 1995. Therefore, this is the first study relating to the epidemiology of pre-eclampsia in The Netherlands. More specific data were obtained from our own referral center.

The Netherlands has about 16 million inhabitants with around 190 000 deliveries per year. The overall incidence of pre-eclampsia in The Netherlands was 1.05% for 1995–96. Within this period, the incidence of pre-eclampsia in our center was 3.8%, with a high percentage of early-onset pre-eclampsia and transfer of pregnant women to our unit, which serves as a tertiary referral center for a region of more than 1 million people in the north-eastern part of The Netherlands. Therefore, the increased rate of maternal mortality and Cesarean section in our center compared to the national data is not surprising.

In Twente, a region from which women with early-onset pre-eclampsia are preferably referred to our hospital, the incidence of pre-eclampsia was 1.58, which is significantly increased compared to that of the overall Dutch population (1.05%). The high incidence of pre-eclampsia in Twente is associated with an increased prevalence of underlying disorders such as hyperhomocysteinemia and protein S deficiency, as compared to other parts of The Netherlands according to our local data. Both disorders are associated with an increased risk of developing pre-eclampsia[5]. The hereditary character of these disorders suggests a genetic basis for the increased incidence of pre-eclampsia in Twente. The suggestion of a genetic basis is supported by the poor 'genetic import' in many parts of this somewhat closed society. At present, studies are being undertaken to treat the underlying disorders in the subsequent pregnancy by preventive measures.

Which environmental or life-style factors contribute to an increased rate of pre-eclampsia in our cities must be the concern of future research.

CONCLUSION

Epidemiological studies of pre-eclampsia provide valuable information for a better understanding of the disease, for strategies of the national and regional obstetric and health-care systems and for the susceptibility in further pregnancies of the individual patient and of groups in a comparable environment. In The Netherlands, there are regional differences in the incidence of pre-eclampsia suggesting underlying hereditary disorders. This observation may offer the possibility of taking preventive measures in order to improve maternal and neonatal outcome and to prevent unnecessary maternal and fetal disease, not only in the individual mothers but also in future generations. This is even more important, since there is an increasing body of evidence that the environment and life style of pregnant mothers influence not only the quality of life *in utero* but also many diseases we might develop later in life[6].

References

1. National High Blood Pressure Education Program Working Group. Report on high blood pressure in pregnancy. *Am J Obstet Gynecol* 1900; 163:1691–712

2. Schuitemaker NWE, Bennebroek Gravenhorst J, Dekker GA, *et al.* Moedersterfte in Nederland 1988–1992. *Ned Tijdsch Obstet Gynaecol* 1996;106: 270–1

3. Wacker J, Schulz M, Fruhauf J, *et al.* Season change in the incidence of preeclampsia in Zimbabwe. *Acta Obstet Gynecol Scand* 1998;77: 712–16

4. Dekker GA, de Vries JIP, Doelizsch PM, *et al.* Underlying disorders associated with severe early-onset preeclampsia. *Am J Obstet Gynecol* 1995;173: 1042–8

5. de Vries JIP, Dekker GA, Huijgens PC, Jakobs C, Blomberg BME, van Geijn HP. Hyperhomo-cysteinaemia and protein S deficiency in complicated pregnancies. *Br J Obstet Gynaecol* 1997;104:1248–54

6. Barker DJP. *Mothers, Babies and Health in Later Life.* Edinburgh: Churchill Livingstone, 1998

Physiopathology of pre-eclampsia and intrauterine growth restriction

47

P. Merviel, M. Beaufils, N. Berkane, A. Dumont, J. C. Challier and S. Uzan

INTRODUCTION

Hypertension during pregnancy, which complicates 10–15% of all pregnancies, is characterized by values of at least 140 mmHg for systolic blood pressure, or at least 90 mmHg for diastolic pressure, or both. When it is associated with significant proteinuria (more than 0.5 g/24 h), as it is in 1–3% of all pregnancies, the patient is diagnosed with pre-eclampsia. The only really effective treatment for pre-eclampsia is terminating the pregnancy, but postponing this action is often essential to avoid the perinatal mortality and morbidity that accompany very preterm delivery. Intra-uterine growth restriction (IUGR) is a frequent disorder (3% of births) and remains, despite the progress of medical imaging, a difficult obstetric problem. During the neonatal period, low-weight or small-for-term babies are exposed to increased risk of hypoglycemia and infection. Moreover, recent epidemiological studies[1] have revealed that subjects born with IUGR are more likely to develop metabolic and cardiovascular diseases in adulthood. IUGR can be linked to a maternal cause (e.g. hypertension, alcoholism, smoking) in nearly 40% of cases and to a fetal chromosomal anomaly in roughly 30%; the other cases remain unexplained. In pre-eclampsia and IUGR, placental development and vascularization are abnormal.

REVIEW OF PHYSIOPATHOLOGICAL ASPECTS OF PLACENTATION

Two phenomena combine to permit the implantation and maintenance of the pregnancy and the growth of the fetus through the hemochorial placenta:

(1) An endometrial vascular structure develops, favorable to implantation from the proliferative stage onward, under the influence of angiogenic and vasomotor factors;

(2) The uterine spiral arteries undergo a vascular transformation, invaded by extravillous cytotrophoblastic cells; the insufficiency of this invasion is considered to be the principal mechanism responsible for pre-eclampsia and IUGR.

Table 1 summarizes these two stages and the interactions between the various molecules.

Vascular invasion by extravillous cytotrophoblastic cells

Placentation begins by the proliferation of extravillous cytotrophoblastic cells at the base of villous columns[2–5]. A change in their pattern of integrin expression at the membrane surface (from $\alpha6\beta4$ to $\alpha5\beta1$ to $\alpha1\beta1$)[6] helps them to migrate and thus interact with various components of the decidual extracellular matrix.

A first invasion towards the internal wall of the intramucous spiral arteries of the endometrium begins in the 6th week of pregnancy. Trophoblast plugs block the opening of these arteries in the intervillous space, and from there, the extravillous cytotrophoblastic cells move backwards into the vascular lumen and then invade the arterial wall, aided by proteolytic enzymes. This phenomenon is accompanied by lesions of the endothelial cells, the reshaping of the internal vessel walls, the disappearance of

Table 1 *Stages in the development of the uterine vascular system at the beginning of pregnancy and the interaction of the relevant molecules*

Stage of uterine vascular system development	Molecules involved	Biological effects
Angiogenesis	FGF b	angiogenesis
	VEGF	mitogenesis of endothelial cells
	(PlGF)	increases vascular permeability
		growth and migration of EVCT
	PDGF	angiogenesis
		growth of vascular smooth muscle cells
Vascular tone	endothelin	vasoconstriction
	nitric oxide	vasodilatation
	prostaglandins	vasoconstriction or vasodilatation
		hormone modulation
		(renin/angiotensin II)
	neuropeptides	vasomotor effects
EVCT invasion of spiral arteries		integrin expression
		role of the metalloproteases and their inhibitors
		increased PGI_2/TXA_2 ratio
		diminution of arterial wall resistance
		increased blood flow in the intervillous space

FGF b, basic fibroblast growth factor; VEGF, vascular endothelial growth factor; PlGF, placenta-like growth factor; EVCT, extravillous cytotrophoblast cell; PDGF, platelet-derived growth factor; PGI_2, prostaglandin I_2, (so-called prostacyclin); TXA_2, thromboxane A_2

smooth muscle cells and the replacement of the collagen–elastin structure by a fibrinoid deposit. Cytotrophoblast cells express E-cadherin, an adhesion molecule. Invasion of the spiral arteries, however, requires a switch to VE-cadherin, and the newly intravascular trophoblastic cells must also acquire molecules specific to endothelial cells, such as VCAM-1 and PECAM-1[7,8]. In placentas of women with pre-eclampsia or IUGR, E-cadherin expression does not switch to VE-cadherin, and VCAM-1 and PECAM-1 do not appear. Moreover, there is a reduction in the expression of MMP9, HLA G, hPL, placental GH and $\alpha1\beta1$, while that of integrin $\alpha6\beta4$ is maintained and that of $\alpha5\beta1$ increases[9].

At the beginning of the second trimester, a second migratory wave affects the intra-myometrial segment of these arteries[10]. In consequence, the resistance of the artery wall to blood drops and the spiral arteries thus escape the normal vasomotor mechanisms (prostaglandins, endothelins, nitric oxide, etc). The invasion of the spiral arteries is complete by the 18th week of pregnancy. The muscular lining of the spiral arteries is replaced by fibrous tissue, a change that can be identified by the disappearance of the protodiastolic notch during a uterine artery Doppler examination. The role of natural killer (NK) cells, the decidual reconnaissance system, might explain the facilitation of this second wave of extravillous cytotrophoblastic intrusion. That is, pre-eclampsia or IUGR may occur more often among primiparas (75% of all cases) precisely because arteries colonized during a first pregnancy may be easier to invade during subsequent pregnancies (this may be a disorder of primipaternity rather than primiparity: cases of pre-eclampsia and IUGR have been observed at higher rates after remarriage).

Two principal factors accompany this invasive phenomenon: tissue factor, or thromboplastin, to prevent extravasation after the extravillous cytotrophoblastic invasion; and thrombomodulin, to ensure blood flow through the uterine spiral arteries. Tissue factor, a substance necessary for coagulation, is located at the membrane of the perivascular decidual cells. Stimulated by progesterone, it contributes to the endometrial perivascular hemostasis necessary after extravillous cytotrophoblastic invasion. Thrombomodulin is secreted by endothelial cells and activates protein C. Its anticoagulant action prevents the formation of intravascular thromboses[11].

Vasoconstricting and vasodilating agents

Uterine vascular tone is primarily regulated by two opposing vasomotor systems: a vasoconstrictor system (endothelin/enkephalinase) and a vasodilator system (nitric oxide). Some disorders, such as vascular hypertensive complications, may be due to deregulation of these systems[12]. Endothelin, which is one of the most powerful vasoconstrictors of the fetoplacental circulation, targets the endothelial cells of the spiral arteries. It is degraded by enkephalinase, an enzyme whose production is induced by progesterone. During the luteal phase, when progesterone levels peak, the endothelin/enkephalinase ratio favors the degradation of endothelin, thereby helping to prevent vasoconstriction of the blood vessels at the implantation site. Moreover, confirmation of the hypothesis that endothelin 1 (ET-1) is involved in disorders such as IUGR and pre-eclampsia appears from the increased concentration of immuno-reactive endothelin observed in the umbilical vessels and maternal blood in these cases[13] and from the increased expression of the ET-1 gene in the placental villi of patients with pre-eclampsia.

When it remains whole, the endothelium produces a highly labile vasodilator that regulates blood flow locally. This factor, initially called endothelium-derived relaxing factor (EDRF) has now been identified as nitric oxide[14]. This gas, which can diffuse across cell membranes, penetrates the smooth muscle cells surrounding blood vessels, where it reaches its target, guanylate cyclase. This enzyme allows the formation of cGMP, which activates the intracellular protein kinases and keeps the smooth muscle cells relaxed[15]. Nitric

oxide is synthesized from L-arginine, by any of three isoforms of nitric oxide synthase (NOS). Two of these – endothelial (eNOS) and nervous – are constitutive and require calcium to act. Several stimuli (acetylcholine, bradykinin, serotonin, ATP, vascular shearing forces) increase eNOS activity and thus provide for autoregulation of the blood flow. The presence of eNOS has been observed in umbilical arteries, chorial vessels and placental villi. During normal pregnancies, urinary excretion of cGMP, NO_2 and NO_3 (metabolites of nitric oxide) increases. Gude and colleagues[16] have shown that the administration of either NOS inhibitors or guanylate cyclase amplifies the vasoconstriction observed with ET-1 and thromboxane A_2 (TXA$_2$). Other substances also participate in the regulation of vascular tone. These include prostaglandins, adrenocorticotropic hormone (ACTH), corticotropin releasing hormone (CRH) and vasomotor peptides.

Prostaglandins are molecules with an activity that can be paracrine or autocrine, activating, constrictive or both (prostaglandin (PG)F$_{2\alpha}$, TXA$_2$), inhibitory, relaxing, or both (PGE$_2$, PGD$_2$, PGI$_2$) and whose action is mediated by adenylate cyclase and cAMP formation. What prostaglandins do, in fact, is modify the action of hormones, amplifying or inhibiting their effects. In particular, prostacyclin (PGI$_2$) diminishes the sensitivity of maternal vessels to angiotensin II (AII), thus producing the blocking of its vasoconstrictive action during normal pregnancy. Prostacyclin is produced by vascular endothelium and trophoblast cells. Its action is vasodilating (relaxing vessels contracted by AII), muscle relaxant and antiagglutinative. Thromboxane A_2, which is synthesized by platelets, is a powerful vasoconstrictive agent that promotes both platelet agglutination and uterine contractility. During a normal pregnancy, intravascular plugs formed by extravillous cytotrophoblastic cells at the junction between the spiral arteries and the intervillous space play a role in inhibiting lipid membrane peroxidation and diminishing TXA$_2$. Thus when PGI$_2$ action predominates over TXA$_2$ action (when the PGI$_2$/TXA$_2$ ratio increases), vasodilatation occurs and vascular resistance is reduced. These plugs are absent in pre-eclampsia because of the inadequate vascular invasion by extravillous cytotrophoblastic cells. This absence reduces PGI_2 synthesis and elevates TXA_2 levels, thereby reducing their ratio. Consequently, maternal vessels become more sensitive to AII, vascular resistance increases, vasodilatation is decreased and localized microthromboses form. Moreover, the vasomotor action of prostaglandins can be modified by vascular changes (fibrin deposits, endothelial lesions, etc.). Such lesions have been found in the placentas of infants with IUGR and of women with hypertension. Their consequence is a supplemental diminution of intervillous perfusion.

ACTH is present in both maternal and fetal circulations during pregnancy, deriving from either the fetal hypophysis or the syncytiotrophoblast. Its vasodilating action may be mediated by the degranulation of mast cells or by release of either histamine or (vasodilating) progesterone[17]. Compared with PGI_2, ACTH is a more powerful vasodilator (187 times), and its action is not mediated by nitric oxide, cGMP or prostaglandins, but rather by a specific receptor. In pregnancies complicated by IUGR, ACTH is elevated in the umbilical artery as a response to stress and to the hypoxemia secondary to diminished blood flow.

CRH, a powerful vasodilator (50 times the strength of PGI_2) whose effect on vascular muscles is mediated jointly during pregnancy by nitric oxide and cGMP[18], increases regularly in the fetal–maternal circulation until term. Its receptor has been found on syncytiotrophoblast and endothelial cells (eNOS has also been localized in the latter). During pregnancies complicated by hypertension or IUGR, the CRH level is higher than normal, in response to the diminished placental vascular flow, but its vasodilating action is reduced because of endothelial changes.

The vasomotor peptides such as vasoactive intestinal polypeptide (VIP), substance P and calcitonin gene-related peptide (CGRP), which are synthetized from nerve fibers near the uterine blood vessels, also participate in the regulation of uteroplacental blood flow[19]. Their action may be mediated by nitric oxide and cGMP. In humans, CGRP appears to be a growth factor for endothelial cells of the umbilical vein and an angiogenic factor in ischemic conditions. During pregnancy, CGRPi (immunoreactive) increases in the circulation through term, then drops dramatically postpartum. Uterine arteries also appear to be more sensitive to CGRP during pregnancy. Experiments with rats have shown that CGRP can inhibit the hypertension induced by L-N^G-nitro-arginine methyl ester (L-NAME) administration, but does not improve birth weight[20].

In addition, chronic hypoxia, a consequence of defective placentation, can also induce the transcription of genes such as ET-1 (vasoconstrictive), angiotensin converting enzyme (hypertensive), plasminogen activator (stimulating the formation of active TGFβ, which inhibits extravillous cytotrophoblastic invasion), and cyclo-oxygenase-1 (COX-1, an enzyme involved in prostaglandin production).

THERAPEUTIC IMPLICATIONS

Role of aspirin

When the extravillous cytotrophoblastic cell invasion of the spiral arteries is incomplete or even absent, the accompanying lack of vasodilatation and the ensuing microthromboses associated with lesions lead to anomalies in prostaglandin regulation and synthesis, in particular for PGI_2 and TXA_2. These prostaglandins are metabolites of arachidonic acid, by the intermediary action of cyclo-oxygenase. Aspirin is a cyclo-oxygenase inhibitor that, by diminishing TXA_2, modifies the PGI_2/TXA_2 ratio and thus tends to re-establish the physiological equilibrium disturbed by the incomplete extravillous cytotrophoblastic invasion[21]. Administration of aspirin in doses from 0.3 mg/kg/per day to 1.5 mg/kg/per day seems to inhibit platelet cyclo-oxygenase activity more than endothelial cell cyclo-oxygenase activity. Endothelial cells, unlike

Table 2 *Principal studies about the effect of the prescription of low doses of aspirin during pregnancy on the prevention of pre-eclampsia and intrauterine growth restriction (IUGR) (in reference 21)*

First author	Reference	Design	Effect on pre-eclampsia	Effect on IUGR	Other effects
Beaufils	*Lancet* 1985;1:840–2	past history 150 mg/day	+	+	
Wallenburg	*Am J Obstet Gynecol* 1987;157:1230–5	past history 1.6 mg/kg/per day		+	
Trudinger	*Am J Obstet Gynecol* 1988;159:681–5	uterine artery Doppler 150 mg/day		+	
Schiff	*Obstet Gynecol* 1990;76:742–4	roll-over test 100 mg/day	+		
Mac Parland	*Lancet* 1990;335: 1552–5	uterine artery Doppler 75 mg/day	+		
Wallenburg	*Am J Obstet Gynecol* 1991;164:1169–73	angiotensin II test anomaly 60 mg/day	+		
Uzan	*Lancet* 1991;337: 1427–31	past history 150 mg/day		+	
Collins	*Cockrane Updates* 1994	meta-analysis	+	+	prematurity
Wenstrom	*Am J Obstet Gynecol* 1995;173:1292–6	high hCG > 2 MoM, 60 mg/day	+	+	

+, significant effect ($p < 0.05$) of preventive aspirin treatment on pre-eclampsia or IUGR; hCG, human chorionic gonadotropin; MoM, multiple of median

platelets, are nucleated; the former can thus resynthesize cyclo-oxygenase, but the latter are permanently inactivated. Only new platelets, formed from megakaryocytes, can then produce TXA_2, but the repeated administration of aspirin prevents any such renewed production. PGI_2, on the other hand, can be renewed rapidly by endothelial cells.

Thus, it is appropriate to prescribe aspirin treatment because of the observed or possible imbalance of the PGI_2/TXA_2 ratio in the following situations: history of pre-eclampsia or IUGR of vascular origin, uterine artery Doppler anomaly (showing increased vascular resistance), an AII test anomaly (dose of intravenously-administred angiotensin necessary to increase diastolic pressure by 20 mmHg, test anomaly if dose < 10 ng/kg per min), antiphospholipid syndrome (in which anticardiolipin antibodies could interfere with endothelial synthesis of PGI_2) (Table 2). Similarly, aspirin should be prescribed for disorders accompanied by endothelial lesions,

such as a past kidney transplant, chronic hypertension, chronic nephropathy, diabetes with vascular compli-cations and systemic lupus erythematosus.

Because the essential phenomenon appears to be the prostaglandin imbalance resulting from the defective extravillous cytotrophoblastic invasion and because this occurs early in pregnancy, aspirin treatment, if indicated by the patient's history, should begin around 14–15 weeks or even earlier, or as soon as a uterine artery Doppler anomaly has been observed (generally around 22 weeks). It should continue through 35 weeks. This early prescription is intended to limit, but not prevent, the cascade of events (increase of renin, angiotensin, aldosterone) that follow the increase of vascular resistance and the obstetric complications that can arise from them.

Nitric oxide and nitric oxide sources

In pre-eclampsia and IUGR of vascular origin,

NOS activity in the placenta diminishes (causing disruption in the L-arginine–nitric oxide–cGMP pathway), even though the basic nitric oxide activity is increased in the umbilical vessels. The placenta's capacity to respond to stimulation by bradykinin (a substance emitted during platelet agglutination) is similarly diminished. Therapeutic applications may flow from the effect of nitric oxide on the perivascular musculature (Table 3)[22]. Inducing nitric oxide production may therefore be a useful treatment that reduces blood pressure, inhibits platelet activation and improves uterine and fetal hemodynamics. Nonetheless, other randomized clinical trials must support the findings so far reported.

Corticosteroids and anticoagulants

Antiphospholipid antibodies are auto-antibodies capable of pathogenic effects by interfering with the lipid membranes of endothelial cells (causing lesions) or intervening in the coagulation cascade (thrombopenia). They also interact with coagulation factors V and X (in the presence of platelet phospholipids and Ca^{++}), prolonging bleeding time. In addition, antiphospholipid antibodies may be responsible for inhibiting the activation of protein C by endothelial cells, thereby increasing the risk of local thrombogenesis[23]. Protein C is usually activated by the thrombin–thrombomodulin pair; it then interacts with protein S in the degradation of the activated forms of coagulation factors V and VIII. Antiphospholipd antibodies also inhibit endothelial biosynthesis of PGI_2, which is vasodilating and antiagglutinative. The PGI_2/TXA_2 ratio is thus lowered and can cause obstetric accidents. These antibodies have been found in patients with and without systemic lupus erythematosus. An increase in the number of abortions, vascular complications (pre-eclampsia, IUGR: 11.7% compared with 1.9% in pregnancies without anticardiolipins) and in utero fetal deaths is associated with antiphospholipid antibodies, including anticardiolipin antibodies and circulating anticoagulants[24]. Study of placentas has revealed extensive infarcts, obliterative vascular lesions and the premature aging of villi. To prevent these obstetric complications, some have suggested corticosteroid therapy, with or without low-dose aspirin treatment. Others have suggested subcutaneous heparin, as in the prevention of venal thromboses. Our team considers this antiphospholipid syndrome to be an indication for preventive aspirin treatment, which we prescribe at its discovery during

Table 3 *Principal studies about the effect of the prescription of nitric oxide sources during pregnancy on the prevention of pre-eclampsia and intrauterine growth restriction (IUGR) (studies cited in reference 21)*

First author	Reference	Design	Effects
Ramsay	*Eur J Clin Invest* 1994;24:76–8	GTN	reduction of pheripheral resistance and uterine artery resistance index
Grunewald	*Obstet Gynecol* 1995;86:600–4	intravenous GTN	reduction of systolic and diastolic blood pressure, and umbilical artery resistance index
Thaler	*Obstet Gynecol* 1996;88:838–43	isosorbide dinitrate	reduction of mean blood pressure, uterine and umbilical artery resistance indices
Lees	*Obstet Gynecol* 1996;88:14–19	GSNO	reduction of mean blood pressure, platelet activity and uterine artery resistance index

GTN, glyceryl trinitrate; GSNO, S-nitrosoglutathione

pregnancy, or at conception, together with corticosteroids, when the syndrome predates the pregnancy. In this case, aspirin treatment is stopped at 36 weeks, replaced by a treatment of heparin calcium in low doses through delivery and during the postpartum period, with the aim of avoiding possible thrombo-embolic accidents, described earlier.

Neuromodulators, calcium, vitamins C and E and polyunsaturated lipids

It has been reported that hypertension during pregnancy can be reduced by calcium supplements. Thus, among women with a positive roll-over test, those who received 2 g/day of calcium had a significantly ($p = 0.01$) lower rate of pre-eclampsia or pregnancy-induced hypertension. It appears that the reduction in blood pressure associated with oral calcium administration is related to the synthesis and circulation of CGRP[25]. To date, no study has confirmed the usefulness of vitamins E and C or polyunsaturated lipids in the prevention of IUGR. Neuromodulators are not currently available.

CONCLUSIONS

Pre-eclampsia and IUGR are disorders with multiple causes, among the most important of which are vascular problems. Aspirin checks the imbalance between PGI_2 and TXA_2, treating thus only a portion of the mechanisms that cause uteroplacental ischemia; nitric oxide sources may be tomorrow's preventive treatment for IUGR, alone or combined with aspirin.

References

1. Barker DJP, Gluckman PD, Godfrey KM. Fetal nutrition and cardiovascular disease in adult life. *Lancet* 1993;341:938–41
2. Aplin JD. Implantation, trophoblast differentiation and haemochorial placentation: mechanistic *in vivo* and *in vitro*. *J Cell Sci* 1991;99:681–92
3. Cross JC, Werb Z, Fisher SJ. Implantation and placenta: key pieces of the development puzzle. *Science* 1994;166:1508–18
4. Pijnenborg R. Establishment of uteroplacental circulation. *Reprod Nutr Dev* 1988;28:1581–6
5. Strickland S, Richards WG. Invasion of the trophoblast. *Cell* 1992;71:355–7
6. Damsky CH, Librach C, Lim KH, *et al.* Integrin switching regulates normal trophoblast invasion. *Development* 1994;120:3657–66
7. Zhou Y, Fisher SJ, Janatpour M, *et al.* Human cytotrophoblasts adopt a vascular phenotype as they differentiate: a strategy for successful endovascular invasion? *J Clin Invest* 1997;99:2139–51
8. Vicovac L, Aplin JD. Epithelial–mesenchymal transition during trophoblast differentiation. *Acta Anat* 1996;156:202–16
9. Zhou Y, Damsky CH, Chiu K. Preeclampsia is associated with abnormal expression of adhesion molecules by invasive cytotrophoblasts. *J Clin Invest* 1993;91:950–60
10. Redman CWG. Cytotrophoblasts: masters of disguise. *Nature Med* 1997;3:610–11
11. Fazel A, Vincenot A, Malassine A, *et al.* Increase in expression and activity of thrombomodulin in term human cytotrophoblast microvilli. *Placenta* 1998;19:261–8
12. Myatt L. Current topic: control of vascular resistance in the human placenta. *Placenta* 1992;13:329–41
13. MacMahon LP, Redman CWG, Firth JD. Expression of the three endothelin genes and plasma levels of endothelin in pre-eclamptic and normal gestations. *Clin Sci* 1993;85:417–24
14. Palmer RMJ, Ferrige AG, Moncada S. Nitric oxide release accounts for the biological activity of endothelium-derived relaxing factor. *Nature (London)* 1987;327:524–6
15. Rees DD, Palmer RMJ, Moncada S. Role of endothelium-derived nitric oxide in the regulation of blood pressure. *Proc Natl Acad Sci USA* 1989;86:3375–8
16. Gude NM, Xie CY, King RG. Effects of eicosanoid and endothelial cell derived relaxing factor inhibition on fetal vascular tone and responsiveness in the human perfused placenta. *Trophoblast Res* 1993;7:133–45
17. Clifton VL, Read MA, Boura ALA, Robinson PJ, Smith R. Adrenocorticotropin causes vasodilatation in the human fetal–placenta circulation. *J Clin Endocrinol Metab* 1996;81:1406–10
18. Clifton VL, Read MA, Leitch IM, *et al.* Corticotropin-releasing hormone-induced vasodilatation in the human fetal–placenta

circulation: involvement of the nitric oxide–cyclic guanosine 3'-5'-monophosphate-mediated pathway. *J Clin Endocrinol Metab* 1995;80:2888–93

19. Graf AH, Hutter W, Hacker GW, *et al.* Localization and distribution of vasoactive neuropeptides in the human placenta. *Placenta* 1996;17:413–21

20. Yallampalli C, Dong YL, Wimalawansa SJ. Calcitonin gene-related peptide reverses the hypertension and significantly decreases the fetal mortality in preeclampsia rats induced by N^G-nitro-L-arginine methyl ester. *Hum Reprod* 1996;11:895–9

21. Merviel P, Beaufils M, Breart G, Uzan S. The indications, ways and means of aspirin during pregnancy. In Weinstein D, Chervenak F, eds. *The First World Congress on Maternal Mortality.* Bologna: Monduzzi Editore, 1997:33–7

22. Moncada S, Higgs EA. Molecular mechanisms and therapeutic strategies related to nitric oxide. *Faseb J* 1995;9:1319–30

23. Carriou R, Tobelem G, Soria C, Caen J. Inhibition of protein C activation by endothelial cells in the presence of lupus anticoagulant. *N Engl J Med* 1986;314:1193–4

24. Yasuda M, Takakuwa K, Tokunaga A, Tanaka K. Prospective studies of the association between anticardiolipin antibody and outcome of pregnancy. *Obstet Gynecol* 1995;86:555–9

25. Wimalawansa SJ. Anti-hypertensive effect of oral calcium supplementation is mediated through the potent vasodilatator CGRP. *Am J Hypertens* 1993;6:996–1002

Induction of labor

48

K. Vairojanavong

INTRODUCTION

The aim of inducing labor is to deliver a healthy newborn vaginally. The method should be safe to both mother and neonate, simple, effective and preferably non-invasive. Stripping membranes and amniotomy have been accepted as the mechanical methods of choice for many years in pregnancies with a favorable cervix.

In medical methods, various kinds of drugs have been used successfully for inducing labor. Oxytocin has been used for nearly half a century, since 1953, as the principle drug of choice for the induction and augmentation of labor. It is synthesized in the hypothalamus and released by the posterior pituitary gland. Prostaglandins and their analogs are used more often among those with an unfavorable cervix, or a low Bishop score, when induction of labor is indicated. Several types of application are used, namely, intravenous, intra-amniotic, intravaginal, intracervical, extra-amniotic and oral.

The subject of this chapter deals with two main products, oxytocin and prostaglandins, which are used for induction of labor in both term and preterm pregnancies. Administration of oxytocin by intravenous infusion pump and continuous monitoring by cardiotocograph are applied to observe the vital signs and changes while patients obtain the infusion. Nursing staff must pay close and careful attention, preferably staying with the patient at all times while oxytocin is given.

Indications for induction of labor, recommended by the American College of Obstetricians and Gynecologists[1] (ACOG) are:

(1) Pregnancy-associated hypertensive diseases;

(2) Premature rupture of membranes;

(3) Chorioamnionitis;

(4) Suspected fetal jeopardy, e.g. fetal growth restriction, isoimmunization;

(5) Maternal medical problems, e.g. diabetes mellitus, renal disease, chronic hypertension, chronic obstructive pulmonary disease;

(6) Fetal demise;

(7) Logistic factors, e.g. risk of rapid labor, distance from hospital;

(8) Post term gestation.

Contraindications are:

(1) Placenta or vasa previa;

(2) Abnormal fetal lie;

Table 1 *Bishop score for determining cervical ripening*

	0	1	2	3
Cervical effacement (%)	0–30	40–50	60–70	> 80
Cervical dilatation (cm)	finger tip	1–2	3–4	5–6
Station (cm)	−3	−2	−1, 0	+1, +2
Position	posterior	middle	anterior	
Consistency	firm	medium	soft	

(3) Cord presentation;

(4) Presenting part above the pelvic inlet;

(5) Prior classical uterine incision;

(6) Active genital herpes infection;

(7) Pelvic structural deformities;

(8) Invasive cervical carcinoma.

The state of the cervix is related to the success of labor induction. Bishop[2] reported a high success rate in induction of labor when a score of 9 or greater was noted (Table 1). The ACOG con-sidered a score of 6 or more to be favorable. Induction of labor in cases of unfavorable cervix will normally need a longer induction–delivery interval. The terms cervical ripening, cervical priming, ripe cervix and favorable cervix are synonyms. This condition is associated with shortening of the induction–delivery interval and reducing the Cesarean section rate when labor is induced.

OXYTOCIN

Throughout pregnancy, the uterine myometrium becomes gradually sensitive to oxytocin; uterine contractions can be induced, and lead to expulsion of the conceptus[3]. Many oxytocin protocols are in use. Routinely, 10 units of oxytocin in a liter of physiological saline solution or in a 5% dextrose in Ringer's lactate solution is used, yielding a concentration of 10 mU/ml. After infusion of a constant dose, a stable uterine response is obtained in 30–60 min. Doses of oxytocin can be gradually increased every 15–30 min until three contractions per 10-min interval are obtained, as recommended by the ACOG[1]. Dosage of oxytocin administration varies widely, as numerous combinations of infusion rates and concentrations can be used safely and effectively. Some authors[4,5] have stressed using the lowest possible total dose, resulting in a low incidence of uterine hyperstimulation. An initial dose of 0.5–3.3 mU/min with incremental doses of up to 7 mU/min every 15–60 min with the maximum of 40 mU/min for a viable fetus are commonly used.

Oxytocin has also been used for ripening of the cervix, utilizing a low-dose oxytocin regimen with a maximum of 8 mU/min infused for up to 24 h before induction of labor is started. A randomized trial was conducted using continuous low-dose oxytocin for the induction of labor[4]. Oxytocin was increased at intervals of not less than 60 min. This is in contrast to the traditional protocol which involves an increase in oxytocin every 30 min, as required. This study demonstrates that a continuous low-dose protocol for oxytocin induction of labor is effective in establishing active labor and achieving vaginal delivery in women both with ripe and with unripe cervices. It is also associated with fewer episodes of uterine hyperstimulation, requiring fewer adjustments of oxytocin infusion than is the traditional protocol.

In case of an unfavorable cervix, which is often found with fetal death *in utero* or where induction of labor is required during the late second or early third trimester, the dosage can be increased and adjusted, starting with 20–40 U in one liter of fluid. In case of augmentation, 5 U (or half the total dose for induction) is usually adequate.

Three categories – low, intermediate and high doses – have been advocated[5]. The low-dose oxytocin infusion is one of the original regimens, starting with 0.5–1.0 mU/min. The infusion is increased every 20–30 min, in increments of 1–2 mU/min, until uterine contractions are adequate – shown by three contractions per 10-min interval. The low-dose regimen may result in a higher Cesarean rate from dystocia[6].

The intermediate-dose regimen is initiated at 1 mU/min, then increased to 2, 4, 8, 12, 16, 20 and 24 mU/min respectively at 20–30-min intervals to a maximum rate of 36 mU/min.

High-dose oxytocin, used in active management of labor, starts with 6 mU/min, increased by 6 mU/min every 20–40 min. The infusion, ranging from 36 to 42 mU/min, requires close and intensive monitoring, since hyperstimulation, perinatal morbidity and mortality[7] can occur more frequently than in the case of low- and intermediate-dose regimens.

The report of the trial of the trial[4] showed no significant increase in time to delivery with low-dose oxytocin, but Cesarean delivery and Cesarean delivery for fetal distress were more frequent in the traditional protocol group, as were the episodes of uterine hyperstimulation. The traditional protocol is to start with 0.5 mU/min of oxytocin and increase to 1, 2, 4, 8, 12, 16, 20 and 24 mU/min as needed. A retrospective and non-randomized study of 1200 cases examining the efficacy of inducing labor using 2, 5 or 10 U of oxytocin per liter of fluid[8], showed that using higher initial concentrations of oxytocin resulted in no differences as measured by the induction – delivery interval or by the rate of vaginal delivery. Higher pre-induction Bishop scores were associated with shorter labor and more vaginal deliveries. It was concluded that low-dose oxytocin infusion is effective for the induction of labor and may be associated with fewer hazards than are higher doses[8].

Vaginal birth after Cesarean section has been accepted for clinical trial if there is no indication for repeat Cesarean section or contraindications for vaginal birth. Successful trial of labor[9] occurred in 68% in the oxytocin group compared with 89% in the no-oxytocin group. This showed that success in trial of labor may be enhanced by waiting for spontaneous labor or, in the case of a favorable cervix, by induction. Summary data from ten studies involving almost 4000 labors[10] showed that the oxytocin group experienced a 66% successful trial-of-labor rate, compared with 79% when oxytocin was not used. Of 115 pregnancies, when the patient had had two Cesarean sections and a vaginal delivery was planned[11], 103 (89%) were in fact delivered vaginally. Spontaneous labor started in 78 (68%) cases and was induced with prostaglandin (PG)E_2 0.5 mg in the remaining 37 cases. There was only one scar dehiscence and this was comparable to the occurrence in women who did not have a trial of labor. Another paper[12] reported a case of uterine rupture with the use of a 1.5 mg PGE_2 tablet, intravaginally.

Adverse effects are rare, when appropriate dosage of oxytocin is infused. Overdose of oxytocin can lead to uterine hyperstimulation, hypertonicity, tetany and uterine rupture. Its weak antidiuretic property may cause a serious problem, if the drug has been administered for a long period. Symptomatic hyponatremia may also occur. In using a very high dose of oxytocin where delivery is needed in cases of fetal death in utero, preterm membrane leakage and cases with unfavorable cervix, water intoxication with convulsion can occur. At a dose of 40 mU/min, oxytocin decreases urine production dramatically, particularly when it is administered in a large volume of electrolyte-free solution.

One of the leading causes of fetal distress is uterine hyperstimulation, which may occur during normal labor. In such a case, discontinuing oxytocin infusion or reducing the infusion rate is urgently needed. Tocolytic agents such as terbutaline and salbutamol will reduce the uterine hyperstimulation.

MIFEPRISTONE (RU486)

This is a steroid compound that antagonizes progesterone at the receptor level. It has been shown to increase uterine activity and to mature and dilate the pregnant cervix[13]. Several conditions such as early pregnancy termination, fetal death and therapeutic pregnancy termination in the second and third trimesters can benefit from this drug. In a double-blind, randomized, placebo-controlled study[13], 120 patients were given either mifepristone (RU486) 200 mg orally for 2 consecutive days or a placebo. In the same procedure, women who did not enter labor spontaneously underwent induction of labor, which was planned for day 4. In unfavorable cervices, PGE_2 2.5 mg intravaginally, repeated every 6 h, was given until cervical softening was obtained, whereas those with favorable cervical conditions received artificial rupture of membranes and oxytocin infusion. More spontaneous labor (18 to 4%), and a smaller mean interval between day 1 and the start of labor (51 h 45 min vs. 74 h 30 min) were noted with mifepristone than with oxytocin.

PROSTAGLANDINS

Prostaglandins are released endogenously from the myometrium at term, as well as by the amniotic membranes and decidua. Vaginal examinations, membrane stripping and rupture of membranes all cause a rapid rise in amniotic fluid prostaglandin levels. Prostaglandins stimulate cervical fibroblast activity, which causes a release of proteolytic enzymes that loosen cervical collagen and cause the cervix to become hydrated. For this reason, prostaglandins are frequently used during the preinduction phase to help ripen the cervix.

The efficacy of various types of prostaglandin used for induction of labor and their routes of administration varies markedly. Clinical trials have shown a wide range of outcomes. Numerous approaches to pregnancy termination, cervical ripening and induction of labor have been studied using $PGF_{2\alpha}$, PGE_2, PGE_1 and its analog, as well as progesterone antagonist (RU486) and relaxin, a polypeptide hormone that is produced in the human corpus luteum, decidua and chorion. They all show potency in accelerating the ripening process rapidly.

PROSTAGLANDIN $F_{2\alpha}$

$PGF_{2\alpha}$ was successfully used to induce labor via the intravenous route in 1968, as were subsequently PGE_2, PGE_1 and its analog. Many routes of administration can be used: intravenous, intravaginal, intracervical, intra- and extra-amniotic and oral. Adverse effects, the potency of drugs when applied by different routes, the cost of the drug, storage, ease of application and the Bishop score have to be assessed very carefully prior to deciding upon the route. At present, usage of $PGF_{2\alpha}$ is rare, as new products are safer and have fewer adverse effects, and the cost is much lower.

PROSTAGLANDIN E_2 (DINOPROSTONE)

Following the successful use of $PGF_{2\alpha}$ by intravenous infusion for the induction of labor, PGE_2 (dinoprostone) has been used for both cervical ripening and induction of labor. An oral dinoprostone tablet of 1 mg hourly for ten doses was not as effective as locally applied prostaglandins. It was found, in comparing the intermediate-dose regimen of oxytocin to dinoprostone 4 mg given intravaginally, that the Cesarean section rate was lower in the dinoprostone group. Oral prostaglandins were well tolerated and induction was successful in two-thirds of patients[5]. For cervical priming and induction of labor in patients with an unfavorable cervix, intravaginal and intracervical applications of PGE_2 were administered, utilizing random doses of 0.5 mg in 2 ml of gel for the intracervical route, or 4 mg in 3 ml of gel for the intravaginal route. In patients with a relatively ripe cervix, small differences in effacing between the two routes were observed. However, in the case of a highly unfavorable cervix, the intracervical application was significantly more effective than the intravaginal method[14]. Three patients out of 15 had gastrointestinal discomfort and several complained of intense uterine contractions; a Cesarean rate of 8% was observed. In a randomized trial of patients with a favorable cervix and a Bishop score of 5 or higher, the mean duration of the first stage of labor was shorter in parous patients (194 min vs. 319 min) as was the mean induction–delivery interval in primigravidas. Oxytocin was used in 75% of primiparas and 40% of multiparas in the PGE_2 group, compared with 100% and 80%, respectively, in the group induced by artificial rupture of membranes[15]. In contrast, a meta-analysis of several clinical trials[15,16], comparing prostaglandins and oxytocin for induction of labor with gross diversity in the methods and patients involved (e.g. type and dosage of prostaglandins, route of administration, parity of participating women, degree of cervical ripening at time of induction of labor) was inconclusive. There was also a report[17] showing that the induction–delivery interval as well as failure to delivery after 12 h of induction was significantly longer in the PGE_2 group.

In using a single dose of PGE_2 intracervically, 40% of the patients did not go into labor, and a significant proportion of these did not achieve cervical ripeness during the 12-h observation period[18]. A further trial for unfavorable cervix, using multiple-dose administration of PGE_2 gel intracervically every 6 h, was performed. In this trial, 47 cases (94%) achieved vaginal delivery. No significant change in the Cesarean section rate or newborn Apgar scores was observed. This confirmed that repeated application of PGE_2 gel intracervically at 6-h intervals in patients with an unfavorable cervix was useful in achieving a successful induction of labor.

A comparison of intravenous oxytocin with and without vaginal PGE_2 gel in term pregnancy with premature rupture of membranes and unfavorable cervix[19] was conducted. It was found that, in two groups, group A (left alone for 4 h) and group B (given PGE_2 3 mg gel vaginally after the initial examination), at the end of 4 h there was no statistical difference in Bishop score; however, several previous investigations reported that PGE_2 applied vaginally had been found effective for cervical priming and induction of term labor in women with intact membranes. Various factors must be considered, e.g. method of gel preparation, dose of PGE_2, interval from premature rupture of membranes to drug administration, leakage of amniotic fluid and amount of bloody mucus discharge. All these factors may influence the efficacy of PGE_2 application.

PROSTAGLANDIN E₁ ANALOG (MISOPROSTOL)

During the past decade, misoprostol, an oral active PGE_1 analog, a product for prevention of peptic ulcer in those who are taking non-steroidal anti-inflammatory drugs has been used. Various routes of administration are available and, lately, the oral route has also proved effective for cervical priming and induction of labor.

Several double-blind clinical trials have been conducted. In one randomized trial[20] comparing the administration of intravaginal misoprostol or a placebo, misoprostol was superior to the placebo in ripening the cervix

and inducing labor. The difference in the Bishop score was 5.3 in the misoprostol group compared with 1.5 in the placebo group. Another trial[21] on intravaginal misoprostol compared with PGE_2 (dinoprostone), as a cervical ripening agent, revealed that the PGE_1 analog was superior to dinoprostone in ripening the cervix and in the induction of labor. The increase in the Bishop score of 5.3 in the misoprostol group compared with 2.3 in the dinoprostone group was observed at 6 h after medication ($p < 0.001$). The mean time from insertion to delivery was 15.6 h in the former, and 22.4 h in the latter group. The need for oxytocin was also significantly lower in the misoprostol group (three compared to 17 cases). No different delivery outcomes in term of complications, Apgar scores and mode of delivery were noted. Tachysystole was found more often in the misoprostol group (55%) than in the dinoprostone group (26%). This finding is compatible with the results from the meta-analysis of misoprostol for cervical ripening and labor induction[22]. Many clinical trials have been conducted using misoprostol in oral form for an unfavorable cervix when induction of labor is needed. One report[23] showed that the Bishop score was significantly improved and the induction rate was also reduced in the misoprostol group as compared with the control group (placebo). The misoprostol group also showed a significantly smaller interval of induction to onset of labor, duration of labor and the interval from induction to delivery.

CONCLUSIONS

In the preterm, when induction of labor has to be started, selection of drugs will depend upon the Bishop score. A low score or unfavorable cervix will need cervical ripening or priming, prior to induction of labor. All prostaglandins have the power to soften the unripe cervix, progressing to effacement, dilatation and descent of the presenting part. Oral PGE_1 analog, the least expensive drug, requires continuous maternal and fetal monitoring; careful attention by the nursing staff is vital. Amniotomy should be delayed until labor comes to the active phase.

Uterine rupture, one of the most serious complications, was reported following the administration of oxytocin or prostaglandins, leading to high maternal and fetal morbidity and mortality. Early detection prior to rupture is life-saving to both mother and neonate.

In conclusion, the selection of the proper method for the induction of labor requires the consideration of safety, simplicity of use, effectiveness, cost and a preference for a non-invasive approach, with the objective of delivering a healthy newborn with no risk of maternal and fetal morbidity or mortality.

Oxytocin continues to be a very useful drug for the induction of labor when the condition of the cervix is favorable. In cases with an unfavorable cervix, several forms and routes of prostaglandin administration are available and have been successfully used. Their efficacy in intravaginal and intracervical application is beneficial, and safe for clinical usage. Their disadvantage is the relatively high cost of the drugs and the fact that the preparation has to be kept in a low-temperature environment. PGE_1 analog has proven its usefulness in cervical priming and induction of labor, but more clinical trials are needed for definition of the appropriate dosage.

References

1. American College of Obstetricians and Gynecologists. *Induction and Augmentation of Labor.* Technical bulletin 157. Washington DC: American College of Obstetricians and Gynecologists, 1991
2. Bishop EH. Pelvic scoring for elective induction. *Obstet Gynecol* 1964;24:266–8
3. Caldeyro-Barcia R, Sereno JA. The response of human uterus to oxytocin throughout pregnancy. In Caldeyro-Barcia R, Heller H, eds. *Oxytocin.* London: Pergamon Press, 1959:177
4. Mercer B, Pilgrim P, Sibai B. Labor induction with continuous low-dose oxytocin infusion: a randomized trial. *Obstet Gynecol* 1991;77:659–63
5. Kelsey JJ, Prevost RR. Drug therapy during labor and delivery. *Am J Hosp Pharm* 1994;51:2394–402
6. O'Driscoll K, Foley M, MacDonald D. Active management of labor as an alternative to cesarean section for dystocia. *Obstet Gynecol* 1984;63:485–90
7. Satin AJ, Leveno KJ, Sherman MI, *et al.* High versus low-dose oxytocin for labor stimulation. *Obstet Gynecol* 1992;80:111–16
8. Wein P. Efficacy of different starting doses of oxytocin for induction of labor. *Obstet Gynecol* 1989;74:863–8
9. Sakala EP, Kaye S, Murray RD, Munson LJ. Oxytocin use after previous cesarean section: why a higher rate of failed labor trial. *Obstet Gynecol* 1990;75:356–9
10. Flamm BJ, Goings JR, Fuelberth NJ, Fishermann E, Jones C, Hersh E. Oxytocin during labor after previous cesarean: results of a multicenter study. *Obstet Gynecol* 1987;70:709–12
11. Chattopadhyay SK, Sherbeeni MM, Anokute CC. Planned vaginal delivery after two previous cesarean sections. *Br J Obstet Gynaecol* 1994;101:498–500
12. Azem F, Jaffa A, Lessing JB, Peyser MR. Uterine rupture with the use of a low-dose vaginal PGE_2 tablet. *Acta Obstet Gynecol Scand* 1993;72:316–17
13. Frydman R, Lelaidier C, Baton-Saint-Mleux C, Fernandez H, Vial M, Bourget P. Labor induction in women at term with mifepristone (RU 486): a double blind, randomized, placebo-controlled study. *Obstet Gynecol* 1992;80:972–5
14. Ekman-Ordeberg G, Uldbjerg N, Ulmsten U. Comparison of intravenous oxytocin and vaginal prostaglandin E_2 gel in women with unripe cervices and premature rupture of membranes. *Obstet Gynecol* 1985;66:307–10
15. Lo L, Ho MW, Leung P. Comparison of prostaglandin E_2 vaginal tablet with amniotomy and intravenous oxytocin for induction of labor. *Aust NZ J Obstet Gynaecol* 1994;34:149–53
16. Kelse M, Van Oppen A. Comparison of prostaglandins and oxytocin for inducing labor. In Chalmers I, Enkin M, eds. *Effective Case in Pregnancy and Childbirth.* Oxford: Oxford University Press, 1989:1080–111
17. Casey CM, Kehoe J, Mylotte MJ. Vaginal prostaglandins for the ripe cervix. *Int J Gynecol Obstet* 1993;44:21–6
18. Nimrod C, Currie J, Yee J, Dodd G, Persaud D. Cervical ripening and labor induction with intracervical triacetin base prostaglandin E_2 gel: a placebo controlled study. *Obstet Gynecol* 1984;64:476
19. Herabutya Y, Suchatwatnachai C, O-prasertsawat P. Comparison of intravenous oxytocin with and

without vaginal prostaglandin E_2 gel in term pregnancy with premature rupture of membranes and unfavorable cervix. *J Med Assoc Thai* 1991;74:92–6

20. Fletcher HM, Mitchell S, Simeon D, Frederick J, Brown D. Intravaginal misoprostol as a cervical ripening agent. *Br J Obstet Gynaecol* 1993;100: 641–4

21. Kovavisarach E, Wattanasiri S. Comparison of intravaginal misoprostol and dinoprotone for cervical ripening and labor induction at term with unfavorable cervix: a randomized controlled trial. *Thai J Obstet Gynecol* 1997;9:175–81

22. Sanchez-Ramos L, Kaunitz AM, Wears RL, Delke I, Gaudier FL. Misoprostol for cervical ripening agent. *Br J Obstet Gynaecol* 1997;89:633–42

23. Ngai SW, To WK, Lao T, Ho PC. Cervical priming with oral misoprostol in pre-labor rupture of membranes at term. *Obstet Gynecol* 1996;87: 923–6

Post-term pregnancies: evaluation, management and outcome

49

Y. J. Meir, G. P. Mandruzzato, G. D'Ottavio, F. Buonomo and G. Conoscenti

INTRODUCTION

Since the introduction of routine ultrasonographic biometry in the first half of pregnancy, the evaluation of the true length of human gestation has dramatically changed. Studies based on ultrasonographic assessment of gestation have found that gestational age derived from menstrual data has a marked tendency to overestimate the length of pregnancy[1,2]. Moreover, there is good evidence in the literature that from the mid-1980s to the mid 1990s, a period in which routine ultrasound scanning in pregnancy was performed in most developed countries, the incidence of prolonged pregnancy significantly decreased[1,3].

In modern obstetrics, prolonged pregnancy is defined as a gestation of 42 weeks or more (294 days or more from the first day of the last menstrual period (LMP)), but this statement refers only to those patients with regular menses and known LMP; for all those patients with irregular menses or with an uncertain LMP, sonographic dating early in pregnancy appears to be mandatory. Moreover, several recent studies have shown that, even in cases of apparently well-known LMP and regular menses, ultrasound is more accurate in dating the gestation[1,2].

In the first half of this century, studies on prolonged pregnancy found a correlation between post-term births and those of infants that exhibited dysmaturity. As a consequence, prolonged pregnancy appeared to be associated with a significant increase in perinatal morbidity and mortality. Figures such as three-fold to five-fold perinatal mortality and morbidity were reported[4,5]. Without the aid of ultrasound, in those years,

many term pregnancies and many with misdiagnosed late intrauterine growth restriction (IUGR) were included among postdates. Attributing increased complications to a heterogeneous group of patients seems, today, at least inadequate.

Recent studies based on nationwide registers have largely redefined the risk of adverse fetal or neonatal outcome in prolonged pregnancies. While some studies deny a significantly increased perinatal risk in uncomplicated post-term pregnancies, other authors still claim an increased relative risk. However, in these studies, the increased risk seems to be more related to IUGR than to gestational age in itself[6-8].

Since the 1970s, new techniques for fetal surveillance have been introduced, and advances in technology keep improving our ability to manage high-risk conditions. Experience with ultrasound, fetal electronic monitoring, Doppler velocimetry and other antenatal monitoring methods has been achieved, and we are certainly more accurate today in recognizing the compromised fetus in stages of adaptation to an adverse condition than we were in the past[9-11]. On the other hand, since the early 1990s, knowledge concerning the physiology of cervical ripening[12], and the availability of new drugs (prostaglandin (PG)E_2 gel) supposed to promote cervical changes before oxytocin administration, have facilitated induction of labor and made it safer. Hence, the management of uncomplicated prolonged pregnancy appears to be controversial. Studies confirm that both expectant management and immediate induction are associated with very low complication rates and good outcomes[13-15]. The outcome parameters are so similar for both approaches that, in many health systems, in cases of low-risk prolonged pregnancy and after giving exhaustive information, the decision on whether to wait for spontaneous onset of labor or proceed with immediate induction is left to the patient.

ASSESSMENT OF GESTATIONAL AGE

The feasibility of accurate estimation of the date of confinement depends on education, social conditions and resources. If all patients undergo a serum β-human chorionic gonadotropin (β-hCG) assay between 2 and 4 weeks after conception, and all have an ultrasound scan performed between 7 and 13 weeks' gestation, the chance of error in the estimation of gestational age is very low. Several methods are in use to adjust to ultrasound dates: the 7-day rule (when there is disagreement equal to or more than 7 days between scan date and menstrual history); the 10-day rule; and the 14-day rule. Recent reports, however, have demonstrated that predicting the date of birth by the dating scan alone is more accurate than any method that also takes the LMP into account[1,2]. The crown–rump length (CRL) is the single most accurate biometric parameter for assessment of gestational age in the first trimester, and if performed between 7 and 13 weeks of gestation it can predict gestational age within ± 3 days. In the mid-trimester, up to 25 weeks, the best ultrasound parameters are the biparietal diameter (BPD) and femur length (FL). Both parameters become insufficiently accurate for dating purposes in the third trimester (error of up to ± 3 weeks).

INCIDENCE OF POST-TERM PREGNANCY

The reported frequency of post-term pregnancy varies from 3 to 13% of all pregnancies. The wide range of variation is comprehensible if we consider that the occurrence is influenced by the definition, the clinical management of complications during gestation and the clinical approach to prolonged pregnancy. If the definition of prolonged pregnancy is based on menstrual history and induction is not performed before 42 completed weeks, prolonged pregnancy will occur in about 10% of all pregnancies. On the other hand, if routine induction at 41 weeks is adopted, no pregnancy will last more than 42 weeks. A factor that reduces the incidence is routine early-pregnancy ultrasound examination with eventual correction of the estimated date of birth. Confounding factors are termination of pregnancy in cases of fetal malformation and elective anticipated delivery, as for example in cases of IUGR, pregnancy-induced hypertension and gestational diabetes.

In the Department of Obstetrics and Gynecology of the Burlo Garofolo Hospital in Trieste, Italy, we have always adopted expectant management of uncomplicated post-term pregnancies. Virtually all patients are offered, as part of our prenatal care program, a routine first-trimester or an early mid-trimester (14 weeks) ultrasound scan, a 20–22-weeks ultrasound screening for fetal abnormalities, a 30–32-weeks ultrasound scan for late-onset fetal anomalies and fetal growth assessment, and a 34–36-weeks scan mainly aimed to detect late-onset IUGR. Gestational age is determined from the LMP and confirmed or re-established by first- or second trimester fetal ultrasound examination. From January 1990 to December 1997, 7320 women delivered their babies in our department. Of all pregnancies, 17.5% (1282/7320) continued beyond 41 weeks, 7% (511/7320) continued beyond 42 weeks and 1.4% (103/7320) lasted 43 weeks or more. The incidence of prolonged pregnancies did not show a significant trend during the years 1990–97 and the range varied from a minimum of 5.8% in 1990 to a maximum of 8.5% in 1996. In our population, with expectant management, only 40% of the pregnancies that lasted 41 weeks continued beyond 42 weeks, and only 20% of these continued beyond 43 weeks.

IMPACT OF PROLONGED PREGNANCY

Before the introduction of antepartum fetal surveillance the perinatal mortality rate

Table 1 *Mode of delivery and principal indications of Cesarean section in term and post-term pregnancies in 1990–97*

	Overall		≥ 42 weeks		37–41 weeks	
	n	*%*	*n*	*%*	*n*	*%*
Deliveries	7320		511		6171	
spontaneous	5747	78.51	365	71.43	5070	82.16
vacuum*	169	2.31	24	4.70	139	2.25
forceps*	45	0.61	7	1.37	34	0.55
Cesarean section*	1359	18.56	115	22.50	928	15.04
fetal distress*			50	43.48	225	24.25
labor progress failure*			47	40.87	242	26.08

*$p < 0.01$

attributed to post-term pregnancies was high. Stillborn fetuses usually demonstrated signs of chronic hypoxemia and starvation. Moreover, congenital malformations were almost doubled in prolonged pregnancies and accounted for a significant portion of the referred mortality[16].

With the advent of antepartum testing, ultrasound screening for fetal malformations, intrapartum electronic monitoring and improved neonatal care, the perinatal mortality has been considerably reduced. While mortality has decreased significantly, the associated morbidity continues to affect neonates and mothers.

In view of these observations we retrospectively analyzed our data regarding all term and post-term uncomplicated pregnancies occurring in the Department of Obstetrics and Gynecology of the Burlo Garofolo Hospital in the period 1990–97. As mentioned above, in this period, all uncomplicated post-term pregnancies with unfavorable cervix were managed expectantly. The purpose of this analysis was to establish the impact of this policy on perinatal mortality, gross perinatal morbidity and obstetric interventions.

As far as delivery is concerned, a significant difference in Cesarean section rate was found between term and post-term pregnancies, whereas the difference between post-term and overall Cesarean section rate was not statistically significant. Although our overall vaginal operative rate is very low, this rose significantly in post-term deliveries. In post-term pregnancies, fetal distress (antepartum and intrapartum) together with failure of labor to progress accounted for almost 85% of all indications for Cesarean section and were found to be 1.8 and 1.6 times higher than in term pregnancies, respectively (Table 1).

There were no fetal or neonatal deaths in the group of post-term pregnancies. Infants weighing ≥ 4000 g accounted for 22% of all babies in the post-term group compared with 8.5% of babies in the term group. Of post-term babies, 4% (21/511) weighed ≥ 4500 g compared with 1% (67/6171) of the term group. Apgar score of ≤ 7 at 5 min accounted for 1% (5/511) and 0.5% (33/6171) of all cases of post-term and term infants, respectively (Table 2).

Further investigation concerning 103 (1.7%) cases of pregnancies that continued beyond 43 completed weeks of gestation (300 days) showed that the Cesarean section rate and the vaginal operative delivery in this group was 32% and 7%, respectively. No perinatal deaths occurred in this group. Birth weight was found to be ≥ 4000 g in 29% of infants, and Apgar score of < 7 at 5 min was found in 2.2% of cases. The presence of thick meconium was found in 11% of cases. One neonate presented meconium aspiration syndrome. Three neonates needed intensive care because of neonatal hypoxia and acidosis. One baby had long-term neurological sequelae.

Our data indicate that good antenatal care clearly selects pregnancies that continue to

Table 2 *Perinatal mortality and neonatal features in term and post-term infants. Number of fetal malformations given in parentheses*

	≥ 42 weeks		37–41 weeks	
	n	%	n	%
Deliveries	511		6171	
Males	280	54.79	3133	50.77
Females	231	45.21	3038	49.23
≥ 4000 g*	115	22.50	527	8.54
≥ 4500 g*	21	4.11	67	1.09
Apgar score at 1 min < 7	44	8.61	372	6.03
Apgar score at 5 min < 7	5	0.98	33	0.53
Stillbirth	0	0	5 (1)	0.08
Intrapartum	0	0	1 (1)	0.016
Neonatal death	0	0	4 (3)	0.065
Perinatal mortality	0	0	10	0.16
corrected	0	0	5	0.08

*$p < 0.01$

develop beyond 42 verified weeks of gestation, confining perinatal mortality and morbidity within acceptable limits. On the other hand, there is an evident increase in Cesarean section rate and the main cause appears to be fetal distress.

SURVEILLANCE METHODS IN POST-TERM PREGNANCIES

Expectant management of post-term pregnancies can be proposed only if fetal well-being can be assured. Although the methods of fetal surveillance usually utilized in uncomplicated post-term pregnancies are the same as those used in high-risk preterm and term pregnancies, there are some conceptual and physiological differences that have to be kept in mind. Fetal well-being is relative, and has different implications that depend on the adversity of the situation. In high-risk preterm and term pregnancies the purpose of fetal surveillance is to watch for the presence of a clinically *acceptable* fetal condition until objective circumstances improve or delivery becomes feasible. In post-term uncomplicated pregnancies delivery is virtually always practicable. Therefore, if the policy is to wait for spontaneous delivery, it is mandatory to assure that fetal condition is good. After

defining the biophysical peculiarities of the normal post-term fetus, we should have the means to identify at-risk fetuses in otherwise low-risk pregnancies.

The principal methods that have been proposed for antepartum objective fetal surveillance are cardiotocography, ultrasound and Doppler velocimetry[17]. Cardiotocography is used in the non-stress test (NST)[11], in the contraction stress test (CST)[18] and as part of the biophysical profile[19]. With ultrasound it is possible to assess fetal growth[10], amniotic fluid volume[20] and part of the biophysical profile. Doppler flowmetry may be used to evaluate maternal, fetal and fetoplacental hemodynamics[9]. Although there is an abundance of studies dealing with each method, there are only a few, controversial, prospective randomized controlled trials comparing one method with another. Each one of these methods alone is associated with a relatively low positive predictive value. The most practical method is still cardiotocography. Great efforts have been made to increase the reliability of the antepartum NST in order to detect fetal deterioration early. However, visual interpretation of fetal heart rate (FHR) records is associated with high inter- and intraobserver variability that greatly reduces its accuracy. Therefore, alternative methods have been developed. Among these, computerized analysis of FHR patterns has gained popularity during the last decade. Since the mid-1980s computerized systems for FHR analysis have been introduced into clinical practice in many maternal–fetal medicine units. Numerical evaluation of FHR patterns eliminates observer variability and supplies measurements that can be followed longitudinally and compared with other numerical variables used in the assessment of fetal conditions. A computerized cardiotocographic system was introduced into the Burlo Garofolo Hospital of Trieste in 1986.

A study that aimed to establish the characteristics of post-term FHR variation was conducted in our department[21]. Between January 1987 and December 1993, a total of 1502 valid computerized FHR patterns were registered in 567 eligible singleton uncomplicated pregnancies that continued beyond 287 days. Comparison was made between outcome of pregnancies, and between FHR variation patterns at 41, 42 and 43 weeks' gestation.

While there were no perinatal deaths in the study group and the outcome of pregnancy was very similar between the three groups, at 41 or 42 weeks or more, the long-term fetal pulse interval variation overall (the mean range) decreased significantly from a mean value of 48.5 ms at 41 weeks to 46.4 ms at 42 weeks and to 44.7 ms at 43 weeks (Figure 1). Episodes of high variation and pulse interval variation in periods of high variation also decreased progressively from 41 to 43 weeks. Hence there is a reduction in pulse interval variation in post-term fetuses.

The long-term fetal pulse interval variation overall (i.e. mean range over a whole record) increased from a mean value of 42.3 ms at 28 weeks to 50.5 ms at term (Figure 1). However, after 40 weeks, it decreased, reaching average values of 44.7 ms at 43 completed weeks. A decreasing trend in FHR variation before or at term usually suggests developing fetal hypoxemia. This precipitates a decision on delivery when the fetus is mature, resulting in either induction of labor or Cesarean delivery. However, according to our results,

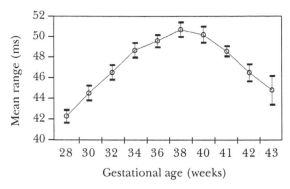

Figure 1 *Mean minute range of the fetal heart rate in uncomplicated pregnancies*

the decreasing trend in fetal pulse interval variation with time in post-term pregnancies was not associated with an increase in perinatal mortality or a significant increase in perinatal morbidity. Although prospective studies are necessary to confirm this conclusion, we presume that the changes in the pattern of FHR variation post-term are physiological. Recognition of this may reduce obstetric intervention.

DISCUSSION

The most recent randomized controlled trials dealing with routine induction versus expectant management in post-term pregnancies have failed to demonstrate an effective improvement in terms of perinatal outcome in the induced group[14,15]. Those most propitious to induction demonstrated only a 15% reduction in Cesarean section rate in the induced group. Hence, the management debate is still open[13]. If we had adopted routine induction of labor at 41 completed weeks in our department during the years 1990–97 we would have induced labor in more than 1000 pregnancies. The only hypothetical advantage would have been prevention of Cesarean section in 17 cases. On the other hand, adopting expectant management, great efforts and resources are consumed in frequent monitoring of fetal well-being.

In summary, post-term pregnancy still represents an important clinical issue with potential and actual risks for the baby and the mother. In the otherwise uncomplicated post-term pregnancy there is little difference in perinatal outcome with expectant management or with immediate induction. Any surveillance policy should include a correct assessment of gestational age in early stages of pregnancy, frequent and integrated fetal surveillance after 41 weeks and eventual anticipation of delivery in cases in which fetal well-being cannot be assured. Finally, continuous efforts should be made in order to increase the accuracy of existing antepartum testing and to find new techniques capable of predicting fetal distress.

References

1. Tunón K, Eik Nes SH, Grøttum P. A comparison between ultrasound and a reliable last menstrual period as predictors of the day of delivery in 15 000 examinations. *Ultrasound Obstet Gynecol* 1996;8:178–85
2. Mongelli M, Wilcox M, Gardosi J. Estimating the date of confinement: ultrasonographic biometry versus certain menstrual dates. *Am J Obstet Gynecol* 1996;174:278–81
3. Fabre E, Gonzales de Aguero R, de Agustin JL, *et al.* Perinatal mortality in term and post-term births. *J Perinat Med* 1996;24:163–9
4. Ballantyne JW, Brown FJ. The problems of postmaturity and prolongation of pregnancy. *J Obstet Gynaecol Br Emp* 1922;29:177–238
5. Walker J. Fetal anoxia. *J Obstet Gynaecol Br Emp* 1954;61:162–6
6. Campbell MK, Ostbye T, Irgens LM. Post-term birth: risk factors and outcomes in a 10-year cohort of Norwegian births. *Obstet Gynecol* 1997;89:543–8
7. Divon MY, Haglund B, Nisell H, *et al.* Fetal and neonatal mortality in the postterm pregnancy: the impact of gestational age and fetal growth restriction. *Am J Obstet Gynecol* 1998;178:726–31
8. Ingemarsson I, Källén K. Stillbirths and rate of neonatal deaths in 76 761 postterm pregnancies in Sweden, 1982–1991: a register study. *Acta Obstet Gynecol Scand* 1997;76:658–62
9. Pearce JM, McParland PJ. A comparison of Doppler flow velocity waveforms, amniotic fluid columns, and the nonstress test as a means of monitoring post-dates pregnancies. *Obstet Gynecol* 1991;77:204–8
10. O'Reilly Green CP, Divon MY. Receiver operating characteristic curves of sonographic estimated fetal weight for prediction of macrosomia in prolonged pregnancies. *Ultrasound Obstet Gynecol* 1997;9:403–8
11. Sherer DM, Onyeije CI, Binder D, Bernstein PS, Divon MY. Uncomplicated baseline fetal tachycardia or bradycardia in postterm pregnancies and perinatal outcome. *Am J Perinatol* 1998;15:335–8
12. Leppert PC. Anatomy and physiology of cervical ripening. *Clin Obstet Gynecol* 1995;38:267–79
13. Cardozo L, Fysh J, Pearce JM. Prolonged pregnancy: the management debate. *Br Med J* 1986;293:1059–63
14. The National Institute of Child Health and Human Development Network of Maternal–Fetal Medicine Units. A clinical trial of induction of labor versus expectant management in postterm pregnancy. *Am J Obstet Gynecol* 1994;170:716–23
15. Hannah ME, Hannah WJ, Hellmann J, *et al.* Induction of labor as compared with serial antenatal monitoring in post-term pregnancy. A randomized controlled trial. The Canadian Multicenter Post-term Pregnancy Trial Group. *N Engl J Med* 1992;326:1587–92
16. Vorherr H. Placental insufficiency in relation to posterm pregnancy and fetal postmaturity. *Am J Obstet Gynecol* 1975;123:67
17. Alfirevic Z, Walkinshaw SA. A randomised controlled trial of simple compared with complex antenatal fetal monitoring after 42 weeks of gestation. *Br J Obstet Gynaecol* 1995;102:638–43
18. Freeman RK, Garite TJ, Modanon H, *et al.* Postdate pregnancy: utilization of contraction stress testing for primary fetal surveillance. *Am J Obstet Gynecol* 1981;140:128
19. Manning FA, Morrison I, Harman CR, *et al.* Fetal assessment based on fetal biophysical profile scoring: experience in 19 221 referred high risk pregnancies. II. An analysis of false negative fetal deaths. *Am J Obstet Gynecol* 1987;157:880–4
20. Divon MY, Marks AD, Henderson CE. Longitudinal measurement of amniotic fluid index in postterm pregnancies and its association with fetal outcome. *Am J Obstet Gynecol* 1995;172:142–6
21. Mandruzzato GP, Meir YJ, D'Ottavio G, *et al.* Computerised evaluation of fetal heart rate in post-term fetuses: long term variation. *Br J Obstet Gynaecol* 1998;105:356–9

Cerebral palsy in multifetal pregnancies: facts and hypotheses

50

I. Blickstein

INTRODUCTION

Congenital cerebral palsy includes a wide range of lifetime physical disabilities caused by damage to the brain during intrauterine and early neonatal life. In most cases the cause is unknown. The long-held belief that intrapartum asphyxia is the most prevalent cause of cerebral palsy has been challenged, and it is now believed that this might be the case in no more than 8–9%[1]. The risk of cerebral palsy is increased among survivors of premature birth and in infants of low birth weight (LBW). However, it is unknown whether the putative injury occurs before or after the premature birth. Plagued by increased prematurity and LBW rates, multifetal pregnancies have been notoriously associated with increased rates of cerebral palsy as well. In light of the epidemic dimensions of current multiple birth rates, this chapter discusses recent epidemiological research and contemporary hypotheses related to cerebral palsy in multifetal gestations (Table 1).

PREVALENCE OF CEREBRAL PALSY

Using compiled data from 11 cerebral palsy series, Javier Laplaza and colleagues have shown a 7.4% average prevalence of twins among cerebral palsy cases[2]. The most relevant question, however, is whether the increased rate of cerebral palsy among multiple pregnancies stands for a true association or is an over-representation of multiple pregnancies among LBW and premature babies. In the past decade, results of various population-based registries suggested several lines of evidence to support the former assumption.

The prevalence of cerebral palsy increases with plurality. Different studies have shown a

Table 1 *Factors evaluated for increased risk of cerebral palsy in multifetal gestations*

Factor	Increased risk
Plurality	in triplets > twins > singletons
Low birth weight	invariably, excess risk for twins > singletons apparent in > 2500 g
Prematurity	invariably, excess risk for twins > singletons apparent after 37 weeks
Monozygosity	when associated with anomalies or twin–twin transfusion syndrome ± fetal death
Twin–twin transfusion syndrome	alone or in combination with fetal death; amnioreduction?
Single fetal death	invariably
Birth weight discordance	probably not associated
Mode of delivery	retrospective study only
'Vanishing twin'	hypothetical stage

similarly increased prevalence of cerebral palsy in twins as compared to singletons: 7.4 vs. 1 in 1000 survivors to 1 year[3] and 6.7 vs. 1.1 in 1000 survivors to 3 years[4]. This trend was also true for higher-order multiples: Petterson and co-workers[5] showed that the prevalence of cerebral palsy in triplets exceeded that of twins and singletons (28 vs. 7.3 vs. 1.6 per 1000 survivors to 1 year) and Pharoah and Cooke reported a crude prevalence of 44.8 vs. 12.6 vs. 2.3 per 1000 survivors in triplets, twins and singletons, respectively[6]. Data from Japan confirmed this tendency also in quadruplets: 0.9% vs. 3.1% vs. 11.1% for twins, triplets and quadruplets, respectively[7]. Therefore, the higher the number of fetuses, the greater the prevalence of cerebral palsy.

The increased prevalence of cerebral palsy related to plurality immediately raises the possibility of over-representation of multiples among LBW infants. Although there are no data related to higher-order multiples, several series stratified the prevalence of cerebral palsy in twins and singletons according to birth weight. Williams and associates[3] found that the relative risk of cerebral palsy was greatest (4.5-fold) among twins weighing more than 2499 g. Grether and colleagues[4] showed that the risk for cerebral palsy among very LBW twins was comparable to that of singletons, whereas twins weighing 2500 g or more had a cerebral palsy risk 3.6 times that of singletons of similar weight. Similarly, Pharoah and Cooke[6] found that, among infants weighing ≥ 2500 g, there was a significantly higher risk in multiple than in singleton births, whereas the birth weight-specific prevalence of cerebral palsy among those weighing < 2500 g was not significantly different. Therefore, although LBW remains an important risk factor for cerebral palsy, the disadvantage of twins as compared to singletons is only apparent in infants of normal birth weight.

The increased prevalence of cerebral palsy in twins is not restricted to prematurity. Yokoyama and colleagues[7] evaluated infants of multiple births and found that the risk of cerebral palsy was 20 times higher in births before 32 weeks than in those at or after 36 weeks. Williams and co-workers[3] also found a strong relationship between the risk for cerebral palsy in twins and gestational age at birth, so that every additional week of gestation decreased the risk by a factor of 0.76. The risk was further increased by a factor of 2.8 for infants delivered before 33 weeks. However, when comparing twin to singleton pregnancies, the relative risk of cerebral palsy was greatest, and significant, only for twins delivered at ≥ 37 weeks' gestation. Therefore, although prematurity is probably the most significant risk factor for cerebral palsy, the disadvantage of twins as compared to singletons is only apparent at term.

The data imply that multiple and singleton pregnancies have similar risks for cerebral palsy until term. However, at the same time as the risk for singletons is decreasing with advanced gestational age and increased birth weight, the risk for multifetal pregnancies is increasing. The excess risk for cerebral palsy beyond 37 weeks may suggest that 'term' occurs earlier in twins. This notion is in accordance with the observations that, as compared with singletons, twins experience increased morbidity and associated costs[8] and are at increased risk of death[9] and severe handicap[10] after reaching 38 weeks' gestation.

RISKS OF CEREBRAL PALSY THAT ARE UNIQUE TO MULTIPLE PREGNANCY

In addition to LBW and prematurity, there are some other risks which are unique to multiple pregnancies.

Zygosity and chorionicity

Monozygotic (MZ) twins occur in about one in three spontaneous and one in 10–15 assisted conceptions[11]. Brain damage in the survivor following single fetal demise is specifically seen in monochorionic (MC) twins (2/3 of MZ twins) in which intertwin–transplacental vascular anastomoses are invariably found but produce the twin–twin transfusion syndrome in only 10–15%[12]. It has been postulated that, following the death of one twin, thromboplastin-like material is transfused through the vascular connection into the survivor's circulation, resulting in end-organ damage (the 'embolic' theory). Alternatively, it has been proposed that blood is shunted via an open anastomosis into the low-resistance vascular system of the dead fetus, resulting in acute hypovolemia, ischemia and end-organ injury (the 'ischemic' theory).

As a result of these theories, it has been expected that MZ twins are at greater risk of cerebral palsy as compared to dizygotic (DZ) twins. The risk may be estimated by comparing like-sex (all MZ + 50% of DZ twins) to unlike-sex ('pure' DZ twins) pairs, as well as by direct zygosity assessment. Petterson and colleagues[5] and Nelson and Ellenberg[13] found a similar prevalence of cerebral palsy in like- and unlike-sex pairs, while Javier Laplaza and associates[2] cited results of two other studies to support the higher number of same-sex twins found among their cerebral palsy series. These authors also cited an MZ : DZ ratio of 1:1.3, which was higher than previously reported figures[2]. Recently, Nelson and Ellenberg[13] found a similar risk of cerebral palsy in MZ and DZ pairs, confirming other observations[14], while Koterazawa and co-workers[15] reported that the risk of cerebral palsy in twins (12.7 times that of singletons) was particularly high in MZ twins. The results of these few comparative studies are obviously conflicting, and the data must be interpreted with caution, since zygosity assessment may not be reliable. Nonetheless, it seems that MZ twinning *per se* does not increase the risk of cerebral palsy, unless associated with fetal anomalies and the twin–twin transfusion syndrome, with or without single fetal demise.

Twin–twin transfusion syndrome

The vascular communications in MC placentas seem to provide the explanation for neurological handicap in cases of single fetal death. However, the risk of cerebral palsy in the twin–twin transfusion syndrome may be unrelated to fetal death. For example, several authors have claimed that amnioreduction to alleviate polyhydramnios associated with the syndrome may be implicated in the genesis of cerebral palsy. Reisner and associates[15] reported a rate of 18% of suspected or confirmed cerebral palsy cases which was not different from a 20% rate in preterm singletons. On the other hand, Ville and colleagues[17] in reply to criticism of their article which described treatment for twin–twin transfusion syndrome with laser coagulation of placental vessels, reported that four of the 16 survivors (25%) of therapeutic amnio-reduction had cerebral palsy. Although it was not stated whether these infants had co-twins who died *in utero*, the authors concluded that laser coagulation was associated with a substantially reduced risk of cerebral palsy, as compared with serial amniocentesis. It is therefore possible that different hemodynamic changes, occurring at different stages of an MZ pregnancy, or severity of the twin–twin transfusion syndrome may cause different patterns of brain damage[18].

Single fetal demise

Although the reported figures vary, all studies have unanimously shown that single fetal death significantly increases the risk of cerebral palsy in the survivor. Two studies have quoted similar risks of 95–96 per 1000 pairs with one survivor vs. 18–12 per 1000 pairs in which both twins survived[2,5], while Grether and colleagues[4] found that cerebral palsy was 108 times more prevalent in children who survived the fetal death of a co-twin. At 8 years of age or more, 4.8% of survivors of single fetal demise of a co-twin were handicapped[19]. Regrettably, no study has yet correlated these figures with chorionicity of the affected twin gestation. Therefore, it is unknown whether or not this formidable risk is restricted to MC placentation only. Yoshida and Matayoshi[20] studied 33 cases of single fetal demise occurring among 133 MC pairs (24.8%). Eight babies (24.2%) were handicapped, but a more favorable prognosis could be recognized when the co-twin died in the early as compared to later stages of gestation.

The observed prevalence of cerebral palsy in triplets with a co-triplet who died *in utero* was 154 per 1000 survivors to 1 year, as compared to 29 per 1000 triplet sets of which all were born alive[5].

Birth weight discordance

The lighter twin in a pair with significant inter-twin birth weight differences is considered to be either absolutely or relatively growth restricted. The association of cerebral palsy with this frequently encountered clinical entity was studied by Rydhstroem in a subgroup of LBW twins[21]. No difference in the distribution of birth weight discordance was found among the 115 disabled twins, as compared to that in the general population. Rydhstroem concluded that birth weight discordance seems not to be related to disability.

Mode of delivery

The only study that examined the risk of cerebral palsy in twins as related to the mode of delivery did not find a reduced risk of cerebral palsy with Cesarean delivery as compared with vaginal birth[22]. Without minimizing the importance of this population-based observation, one should acknowledge its retrospective nature. In addition, Rydhstroem found that abdominal delivery seemed to have little impact on either short or long-term neurological outcome for twins discordant in birth weight by 1000 g or more[23]. It is interesting to note that most studies relating risk of cerebral palsy to the mode of delivery in singletons focused on extremely premature, very LBW infants and on breech presentation. The risk of cerebral palsy as related to the mode of delivery (i.e. vaginal vs. abdominal birth) is not precisely known.

CEREBRAL PALSY AND THE 'VANISHING TWIN' SYNDROME

The proportion of polyembryonic conceptions is higher than the proportion of multiple births. The phenomenon of embryonic demise in a multiple gestation is currently diagnosed by:

(1) Sonographic evidence of more than one embryo with disappearance of one embryo on a subsequent scan ('vanishing twin syndrome');

(2) Histological evidence of embryonic tissue incorporated in the placenta or membranes of a singleton pregnancy;

(3) Cytogenetic evidence of two different cell lines in an otherwise singleton pregnancy (seen in about 4/1000 chorionic villus samplings)[24].

Recently, Pharoah and Cooke[25] hypothesized that cerebral palsy of unknown etiology is the result of embryonic death, in a similar mechanism to that in which death of an MC co-twin may impair the neurological development of the survivor. Despite the ongoing controversy about which of the above-mentioned theories is correct, both the 'embolic' and the 'ischmic' mechanisms require the opening of an existing vascular communication. Therefore, the major objection to this exciting theory is that, in all probability, the sonographic image of the vanishing twin has been exclusively observed in DC placentas, which rarely have anastomoses[26]. Nevertheless, one should not discard this hypothesis, for several reasons. First, there is cytogenetic and hematological evidence of chimerism in MZ twins (all DC), suggesting that inter-twin transport through an open vascular communication occurs in an early embryonic stage[26]. Second, as mentioned above, anastomoses do occur in DC placentas, albeit very rarely. Since our knowledge on placental vascular communications in twin–twin transfusion syndrome comes from the examination of second- and third-trimester placentas, it is possible that a functioning anastomosis disappears and cannot be traced any longer concomitant to or following early embryonic demise. Finally, since sonography is unable to distinguish between DC placentation of MZ and DZ twins, and since most sonographic accounts on the vanishing twin syndrome do not regularly consider chorionicity, it is possible that some vanished twins were MC (all MZ) or that some DC placentas of MZ twins have vascular anastomoses during early pregnancy.

Taken together, it may be proposed that some singletons are, in fact, the survivors of an unknown or a pre- 'vanishing twin' syndrome, that is, embryonic demise occurred before the first sonographic scan. Thus, the plea of Pharoah and Cooke[27] for registering all *fetus papyraceus* cases is justified, and might be extended to registering also vanished twins, not only for scientific reasons but also for counselling patients in whom single embryonic or fetal demise has occurred.

It is believed that in the near future we shall witness increasing interest in the 'vanishing twin' syndrome, as its nature shifts from a simple sonographic curiosity to an important clinical entity.

CONCLUSION

There is an increased risk of cerebral palsy in multifetal pregnancies as compared to singletons. It has been shown that the excessive risk is not only a result of over-representation of multiples among premature and low birth weight infants, but may result from factors related to the twinning process itself. The risk of cerebral palsy should be acknowledged not only when a multifetal pregnancy has been diagnosed, but also when counselling infertility patients in whom an iatrogenic multifetal pregnancy is a calculated risk.

References

1. Blair E, Stanley F, Hockey A. Intrapartum asphyxia and cerebral palsy. *J Pediatr* 1992;121: 170–1
2. Javier Laplaza F, Root L, Tassanawipas A, Cervera P. Cerebral palsy in twins. *Dev Med Child Neurol* 1992;34:1053–63
3. Williams K, Hennessy E, Alberman B. Cerebral palsy: effects of twinning, birthweight, and gestational age. *Arch Dis Child* 1996;75:F178–82
4. Grether JK, Nelson KB, Cummins SK. Twinning and cerebral palsy: experience in four northern California counties, births 1983 through 1985. *Pediatrics* 1993;92:854–8
5. Petterson B, Nelson KB, Watson L, Stanley F. Twins, triplets, and cerebral palsy in births in Western Australia in the 1980s. *Br Med J* 1993; 307:1239–43
6. Pharoah POD, Cooke T. Cerebral palsy and multiple births. *Arch Dis Child* 1996;75:F174–7
7. Yokoyama Y, Shimizu T, Hayakawa K. Prevalence of cerebral palsy in twins, triplets and quadruplets. *Int J Epidemiol* 1995;24:943–8
8. Luke B, Bigger HR, Leurgans S, Sietsema D. The cost of prematurity: a case-control study of twins vs singletons. *Am J Public Health* 1996;86: 809–14
9. Minakami H, Sato I. Reestimating date of delivery in multifetal pregnancies. *J Am Med Assoc* 1996; 275:1432-4
10. Luke B, Keith LG. The contribution of singletons, twins, and triplets to low birth weight, infant mortality, and handicap in the United States. *J Reprod Med* 1992;37:661–6
11. Blickstein I. The new dimensions of multiple pregnancy [Editorial]. *Isr J Obstet Gynecol* 1998;9: 64–6
12. Blickstein I. The twin-twin transfusion syndrome. *Obstet Gynecol* 1990;76:714–22
13. Nelson KB, Ellenberg JH. Childhood neurological disorders in twins. *Paediatr Perinat Epidemiol* 1995;9:135–45
14. Petterson B, Stanley F, Henderson D. Cerebral palsy in multiple births in Western Australia: genetic aspects. *Am J Med Genet* 1990;37:346–51
15. Koterazawa K, Shimgaki K, Nabetani M, Miyata H, Kodama S, Nakamura H. A study on the incidence of cerebral palsy among twins in Himeji City. *No To Aattatsu* 1998;30:20–3
16. Reisner DP, Mahony BS, Petty CN, Nyberg DA, Porter TF, Zingheim RW, Williams MA, Luthy DA. Stuck twin syndrome: outcome in thirty-seven consecutive cases. *Am J Obstet Gynecol* 1993;169: 991–5
17. Ville Y, Hyett J, Nicolaides K. Twin-twin transfusion syndrome. *N Engl J Med* 1995;333: 388–9
18. Sugama S, Kusano K, Akatsuka A, Ochiai Y, Tsuzura S, Maekawa K. Pattern of brain damage

and its developmental mechanisms in mono-zygotic twins. *No To Aattatsu* 1995;27:216–23

19. Rydhstrom H, Ingemarsson I. Prognosis and long-term follow-up of a twin after antenatal death of the co-twin. *J Reprod Med* 1993;38: 142–6

20. Yoshida K, Matayoshi K. A study on prognosis of surviving co-twin. *Acta Genet Med Gemellol* 1990;39: 383–8

21. Rydhstrom H. The relationship of birth weight and birth weight discordance to cerebral palsy or mental retardation later in life for twins weighing less than 2500 grams. *Am J Obstet Gynecol* 1995;173:680–6

22. Rydhstrom H. Twin pregnancies and mode of delivery – too many cesarean sections? *J Perinat Med* 1991;19:220–8

23. Rydhstrom H. Prognosis for twins discordant in birth weight of 1.0 kg or more: the impact of cesarean section. *J Perinat Med* 1990;18:31–7

24. Cytogenetic analysis of chorionic villi for prenatal diagnosis: an ACC collaborative study of U.K. data. Association of Clinical Cytogeneticists Working Party on Chorionic Villi in Prenatal Diagnosis. *Prenat Diagn* 1994;14:363–79

25. Pharoah POD, Cooke RWI. A hypothesis for the aetiology of spastic cerebral palsy – the vanishing twin. *Dev Med Child Neurol* 1997;39:292–6

26. Blickstein I. Reflections on the hypothesis for the aetiology of spastic cerebral palsy caused by the 'vanishing twin' syndrome. *Dev Med Child Neurol* 1998;44:358

27. Pharoah POD, Cooke RWI. Registering a fetus papyraceus. *Br Med J* 1997;314:441–2

Perinatal asphyxia

51

D. J. Evans and M. I. Levene

TERMINOLOGY

Asphyxia is a condition of impaired gas exchange. If persistent, asphyxia leads to progressive hypoxemia and ischemia with resultant hypercarbia and acidosis. The terms hypoxic–ischemic insult and hypoxia–ischemia are also used to describe this process. The insult may occur in the antenatal, perinatal or postnatal periods. A hypoxic–ischemic insult may not necessarily lead to an injury. This depends upon the severity, nature, timing and duration of the insult, which need to overwhelm the ability of the fetus to adapt and survive. The clinical manifestation of any hypoxic–ischemic injury is also variable and probably depends upon a similar interaction between the insult and the fetus.

The terms birth asphyxia, intrapartum asphyxia and intrapartum hypoxic–ischemic injury are widely used and denote a hypoxic–ischemic injury resulting from an insult in the intrapartum period. The terms are also widely misused; they should not be used unless there is specific evidence pointing to an intrapartum hypoxic–ischemic injury. Hypoxic–ischemic encephalopathy refers to the clinical features of central nervous system (CNS) dysfunction following a hypoxic–ischemic insult.

PATHOPHYSIOLOGY OF FETAL HYPOXIA–ISCHEMIA

Fetal adaptation to hypoxia–ischemia

Many newborn infants recover from apparently severe hypoxic–ischemic insults. This reflects the relative resistance of the fetus and neonate to such insults and the adaptive ability of the fetus in response to intrauterine stress. Normal labor is a stressful time for the fetus. As the intrauterine pressure exceeds 30 mmHg during contractions, the perfusion of the intervillous space is impaired, transiently interrupting placental gas exchange. The healthy fetoplacental unit can accommodate this, provided the contractions are of less then 60 s in duration with sufficient respite (2–3 min) in between[1].

The fetus has a wide variety of circulatory and metabolic adaptive mechanisms that can act to minimize the consequences of hypoxia–ischemia:

(1) There is an initial sympathetic response. The elevated catecholamine levels increase peripheral vascular resistance and myocardial contractility, maintaining cerebral perfusion despite fetal bradycardia. Cerebrovascular resistance falls in response to hypoxemia and hypercarbia, maintaining cerebral perfusion[2].

(2) The maternofetal circulation represents a high-output oxygen supply such that almost twice the amount of oxygen can be extracted by fetal hemoglobin before cardiac output needs to increase[3]. Erythropoietin concentrations are increased, stimulating fetal erythrocyte production[4].

(3) There is a redistribution of blood supply to the CNS, myocardium and adrenals at the expense of the kidneys, gastrointestinal tract, liver and muscle[5]. Within the brain, preferential oxygenation is maintained by diverting blood flow to the brainstem, midbrain and cerebellum[6].

(4) Gross body movements, breathing movements and rapid eye movement

(REM) sleep are reduced, thus reducing energy consumption and oxygen demand[7].

(5) The immature CNS can more readily utilize the lactate, pyruvate and ketones generated by anaerobic glycolysis as an alternative to glucose[8]. The sympathetic stimulus also accelerates anaerobic glycolysis with mobilization of liver glycogen stores, thus maintaining the CNS and myocardial energy substrate. Infants with hyperinsulinemia (e.g. those born to mothers with diabetes) are less able to generate these alternative energy sources and are therefore at greater risk from hypoxic–ischemic injury.

A hypoxic–ischemic injury occurs when these adaptive mechanisms are overwhelmed. This can either occur when the stress of labor is compounded by additional pathological stresses such as cord prolapse, placental abruption and placental insufficiency, or occur when the fetus has sustained an earlier, antenatal injury that compromises its adaptive ability.

Mechanisms of hypoxic–ischemic injury

During hypoxia–ischemia, neurons are unable to produce sufficient quantities of adenosine triphosphate (ATP) and have to rely on intracellular stores to maintain activity. The most vulnerable cells will exhaust these stores, undergoing osmotic lysis and cell death because of membrane pump failure. This results in cytotoxic cerebral edema. Resuscitation of the newborn restores oxygenation and perfusion to cells but does not prevent further injury. It appears that the following cascade-like processes are initiated following resuscitation, resulting in delayed or secondary neuronal injury.

Cerebrovascular injury

Autoregulation of cerebral perfusion appears to be impaired: both high cerebral blood flow states, characterized by a reduced vascular reactivity to changes in arterial p_{CO_2}[9], and

states of reduced cerebral blood flow have been reported[10]. Free radicals, activated neutrophils, platelet activating factor (PAF) and eicosanoids may promote vasogenic cerebral edema that further compromises perfusion.

Glutamate release

Hypoxia–ischemia results in the release, and impairment of re-uptake, of glutamate. Glutamate acts upon the N-methyl-D-aspartate (NMDA) receptor, permitting calcium entry into the neuron. High intracellular calcium concentrations activate enzymes responsible for DNA fragmentation and free radical formation, also uncoupling oxidative phosphorylation and resulting in futile ATP consumption[11].

Free radicals

The formation of free radicals results from the action of oxygen upon free fatty acid, prostaglandin and hypoxanthine metabolism. In addition, activation of the NMDA receptor leads to the production of nitric oxide, which can diffuse through membranes and act as a retrograde messenger, further stimulating glutamate release[12]. Nitric oxide can also react with molecular oxygen to form superoxide, peroxide and peroxynitrite radicals. Free radicals cause DNA damage and membrane lipid oxidation, and are potent inducers of apoptosis[13].

Apoptosis

This is a form of programmed cell death, distinct from necrosis in that cells undergoing apoptosis have a characteristic morphology and the process requires energy. Inappropriate activation of the apoptotic program may account for at least part of the delayed cell death observed after hypoxia–ischemia[14]. Suggested mechanisms by which apoptosis is induced include DNA damage, intracellular calcium entry, interruption of intercellular signalling and the actions of free radicals.

Pathological patterns of hypoxic–ischemic injury

The first pattern to be observed following hypoxia–ischemia is the development of cerebral edema within 24–48 h of the insult. This is recognized on imaging or postmortem as marked flattening and widening of the gyri plus obliteration of the sulci. The appearance of cerebral edema has little prognostic significance. With resolution of edema, other patterns emerge and are more indicative of a significant insult.

Selective neuronal necrosis

This is the most commonly observed pathology in term infants, affecting neurons in a scattered fashion and often widely distributed throughout the gray matter. Light microscopy changes are apparent 24–36 h following the insult with cytoplasmic eosinophilia and nuclear fragmentation. Overt necrosis follows within a few days.

Injury to the basal ganglia and brain stem

This is thought to represent the consequence of acute total asphyxia, rather than chronic partial asphyxia. Basal ganglion injury is though to be responsible for the dyskinetic type of cerebral palsy seen in survivors of hypoxia-ischemia, and abnormal signal intensity in the basal ganglia is a common finding on magnetic resonance imaging (MRI). If the infant survives for several months, an abnormal myelination pattern occurs which is detectable on the MRI scan. This is responsible for the marble-like appearance of the basal ganglia seen at postmortem, known as status marmoratus. Hemorrhage and hemorrhagic infarction affecting the thalami following hypoxia-ischemia are also well-recognized phenomena.

Parasagittal injury

Parasagittal injury is an ischemic injury affecting the cerebral cortex and subcortical white matter in vascular watersheds between the anterior, middle and posterior cerebral arteries, giving rise to a parasagittal distribution that is often symmetrical.

White matter injury

White matter injury in the form of periventricular leukomalacia is seen following ischemia in preterm infants. Subcortical white matter abnormalities on MRI are a common finding following hypoxic–ischemic insults at term. If the injury is severe, cystic degeneration is observed, referred to as subcortical leukomalacia. The survivors of the most severe insults usually show a mixed pattern of injury, referred to as multicystic leukoencephalopathy.

Focal cerebral infarction

Focal cerebral infarction, most commonly in the middle cerebral artery, has also been reported in asphyxiated infants. The etiology of focal cerebral infarction is unknown in the majority of cases; hypoxia–ischemia represents the single largest etiological factor, although this does not prove a causative link.

CLINICAL MANIFESTATIONS OF HYPOXIC–ISCHEMIC INJURY

The clinical manifestation of a hypoxic–ischemic injury depends upon the nature and timing of the insult. Insults occurring before the 20th week of gestation tend to result in neuronal migration disorders; those occurring between the 24th and 34th weeks result in periventricular leukomalacia. In the majority of such antepartum injuries, labor progresses to term and the intrapartum and neonatal course is uncomplicated. Presentation may be delayed until later in childhood, usually with signs of neuro-developmental impairment, such as cerebral palsy or generalized developmental delay. In some cases of antepartum injury, however, the fetal adaptive ability has been compromised by the injury and the fetus is unable to cope with the demands of normal labor. The presentation is one of fetal distress and the subsequent brain injury may be incorrectly attributed to an intrapartum hypoxic–ischemic injury. Any intervention undertaken, in response to the fetal distress detected, is unlikely to alter the prognosis in such cases.

There are no uniformly accepted diagnostic criteria for intrapartum hypoxic–ischemic injury. The definition rests upon the weight of evidence that can be accumulated pointing to an intrapartum hypoxic–ischemic insult causing a recognized pattern of neurological injury. The suggestive clinical features are outlined in the following sections. The presence of hypoxic–ischemic encephalopathy is mandatory for the diagnosis, and therefore it is extremely important to exclude the other likely causes of such a disturbance in conscious level.

Intrapartum monitoring

Electronic fetal monitoring was introduced in the 1970s with the aim of being able to detect fetal distress during labor. It is thought that abnormalities in fetal heart rate patterns indicate fetal hypoxia during labor. Fetal blood sampling can be used as an adjunct. Studies have shown that multiple late decelerations and decreased variability in fetal heart rate patterns are associated with an increased risk of intrapartum death and cerebral palsy, but the predictive value is poor[15,16]. Moreover, data from meta-analysis of randomized controlled trials comparing electronic fetal monitoring with or without fetal blood sampling versus intermittent auscultation do not show a therapeutic benefit, despite increases in obstetric intervention rates. It appears that abnormal fetal heart rate patterns are unreliable markers of intrapartum antecedents of neurological damage.

Clinical features at birth

An intrapartum hypoxic–ischemic insult can cause depression of the Apgar score and delay in establishing spontaneous respiration, although this is not invariable. Many other factors can also cause depression of the infant at birth, for example prematurity, maternal analgesia or anesthetic. Nevertheless, the longer the time taken to recover to an Apgar score of above 3, the greater the risk of death and cerebral palsy in term infants (Table 1)[17]. Umbilical arterial acidemia at birth has been widely used as retrospective evidence of tissue hypoxia and fetal distress. In isolation, however, it is only loosely associated with subsequent poor outcome[18], possibly because the acidosis may simply be a consequence of redistribution of blood supply to vital organs in a compensated fetus.

Clinical features after birth

Infants often show a predictable progression of neurological symptoms following intrapartum hypoxia–ischemia, termed hypoxic–ischemic encephalopathy. Initially there is a period of near normality, followed by the onset of seizures and a gradual deterioration in their conscious level. The maximal level of neurological abnormality can be graded and is predictive of outcome (Table 2)[19,20]. It is important to remember that other conditions can produce encephalopathic features, such as metabolic and drug encephalopathies, CNS malformations and CNS infections. During hypoxia–ischemia, blood flow is redistributed in order to preserve circulation to the most vital organs, namely the brain, heart and adrenals, at the expense of the kidneys, liver and gastrointestinal tract. Damage to the latter organs is an additional marker of a hypoxic–ischemic insult. The classic forms of neurological impairment suffered by children who survive intrapartum hypoxia–ischemia at term are spastic quadriplegia and dyskinetic cerebral palsy. There may be associated intellectual impairment, blindness or epilepsy. Mental retardation alone is not a recognized sequela.

INVESTIGATIONS

Due to the difficulties in making a certain diagnosis of intrapartum hypoxic–ischemic injury based upon the clinical features described above, further investigation of the newborn infant is advisable. This enables a

Table 1 *Outcome associated with latest* very low Apgar score (0–3) in infants of birth weight > 2500 g. Adapted from reference 17*

Time (min)	Number liveborn	Death by 1 year (%)	Number known to 7 years	Cerebral palsy (%)	Predictive value[†] (%)	Likelihood ratio[†]	95% CI
1	1729	3.1	1330	0.7	3.6	2.5	1.9–3.1
5	286	7.7	217	0.9	8.4	6.0	3.6–8.6
10	66	18.2	43	4.7	21.2	18.0	8.4–30
15	23	47.8	11	9.1	52.2	72.0	31–170
20	39	59.0	14	57.1	79.5	250.0	130–770

Overall prevalence of death and cerebral palsy = 1.5%; *counts at each time include only those children with very low Apgar scores at that time and no later very low Apgar score; [†]predictive value and likelihood ratio are for poor outcome (death or cerebral palsy)

Table 2 *A clinical grading system for hypoxic–ischemic encephalopathy[19], with associated risk of death and handicap[20]*

	Grade I (mild)	Grade II (moderate)	Grade III (severe)
Conscious level	irritability; 'hyperalert'	lethargy	comatose
Tone	mild hypotonia	marked abnormalities in tone	severe hypotonia
Feeding	poor sucking	requires tube feeds	failure to maintain spontaneous respiration
Seizure activity	no seizures	seizures	prolonged seizures
Predictive value (%)			
death	1.3	5.6	61
death and handicap	1.6	24	78
Likelihood ratio (95% CI in parentheses)			
death	0.09 (0.03–0.30)	0.39 (0.21–0.71)	11.0 (7.56–15.9)
death and handicap	0.05 (0.02–0.15)	0.94 (0.71–1.23)	10.7 (6.71–17.1)

more precise diagnosis for medicolegal purposes and can be helpful in enabling the clinician to counsel parents with regard to prognosis. The investigations reviewed below are those that are commonly performed and produce the information of most value.

Cerebral ultrasound

Cerebral ultrasound is a readily available technique, and sequential examinations provide useful information. The initial phase of cerebral edema produces a generalized increase in echodensity, indistinct sulci and compression of the ventricles. Such findings are of little prognostic significance. Later findings associated with a poor outcome are echogenic thalami and multifocal cystic changes in the subcortical and periventricular white matter.

The blood flow velocities in the major cerebral arteries can be measured using pulsed wave duplex Doppler techniques. When assessed at 24 h of age, a resistance index (RI) of less than 0.55 in the anterior cerebral artery is associated with a likelihood ratio of 5.0 for a poor prognosis[21], reflecting injury to the cerebral vasculature.

Magnetic resonance imaging

By the end of the first week of life, MRI is predictive and findings associated with poor outcomes include an abnormal signal in the basal ganglia, disruption of the posterior limb of the internal capsule and an abnormal signal in the white matter (likelihood ratio = 12.3)[22,23]. Later abnormalities include white matter gliosis, generalized atrophy and delayed myelination.

Electroencephalography

The background (interictal) electro-encephalography (EEG) activity within the first 6 h is more predictive of an adverse outcome than the presence or frequency of seizures. Discontinuous (burst-suppression) and persisting low-voltage states are abnormalities associated with the greatest risk of adverse outcome (likelihood ratio = 7.6)[24]. Experience is required when assessing EEGs of preterm infants, as these normally show discontinuous activity with long interburst intervals.

Other investigations

Magnetic resonance spectroscopy can provide information about the energy state within the brain following hypoxia–ischemia. Near-infrared spectroscopy gives further information about cerebral blood volume and various biochemical markers of tissue injury (e.g. CK-BB, the brain-specific isoenzyme of creatine kinase) have predictive value. These investigations have yet to become established in clinical practice.

PROGNOSIS

Infants with mild hypoxic–ischemic encephalopathy (grade I) are not at increased risk of developing adverse neurological sequelae and, unless complicated by other factors, do not warrant further study. Investigations are useful to aid determination of the prognosis in those infants with moderate (grade II) hypoxic–ischemic encephalopathy, and in confirming the poor prognosis of infants with the severe (grade III) condition at an early enough stage in order that consideration may be given to discontinuing ventilatory support. The best early predictors of poor outcome are

sustained low-voltage states and discontinuous activity on continuous EEG or cerebral function monitoring, appearing by 6 h, and abnormal Doppler cerebral blood flow velocities, appearing by 24 h. If the results of these investigations are unequivocal on two separate occasions after the first 24 h, consideration should be given to withdrawing ventilatory support. In equivocal cases, further imaging (MRI) towards the end of the first week and continued assessment of the neurological state of the infant are recommended. Follow-up outside the neonatal period needs to be for at least 1 year in term infants, 2–3 years in preterm infants. Clinical assessment and, if necessary, further neuroimaging should enable the clinician to detect developing neurological impairments, enabling early referral to the relevant child development specialists. The impairments suffered by children who survive intrapartum hypoxia–ischemia at term are spastic quadriplegia and dyskinetic cerebral palsy.

The hypothesis that intrapartum complications, particularly hypoxia–ischemia, were a major cause of cerebral palsy was proposed over a century ago. This resulted in undue emphasis being placed on the causative role of intrapartum events by the medical profession, lawyers and lay people. However, epidemiological evidence from studies conducted over the past 15 years suggest that less than 10% of cerebral palsy is a result of intrapartum hypoxia–ischemia[25]. The alternative hypothesis is that adverse fetal and genetic events earlier in fetal development cause cerebral palsy and, in some cases, these events are responsible for intrapartum complications and thus fetal distress.

CONCLUSION

Intrapartum hypoxia–ischemia is responsible for significant numbers of neurologically damaged children throughout the world and remains a significant problem for perinatologists. Greater precision in antenatal and intrapartum neurological assessment of the fetus is needed, as well as more accurate prediction of neurological disability, based upon neonatal examination and investigations. A greater accuracy in the detection of potentially damaging fetal compromise should lead to more specific and effective perinatal intervention.

References

1. Peebles DM, Spencer JA, Edwards AD, *et al.* Relation between frequency of uterine contractions and human fetal cerebral oxygen saturation studied during labour by near infrared spectroscopy. *Br J Obstet Gynaecol* 1994;101:44–8

2. Ashwal S, Dale PS, Longo ID. Regional cerebral blood flow studies in the fetal lamb during hypoxia, hypercapnia, acidosis and hypotension. *Pediatr Res* 1984;18:1309–16

3. Bocking AD, White SE, Homan J, Richardson BS. Oxygen consumption is maintained in fetal sheep during prolonged hypoxaemia and hypercapnia in sheep. *J Dev Physiol* 1992;17:169–74

4. Ruth V, Autti-Ramo I, Granstrom M-L, Korkman M, Raivio KO. Prediction of perinatal brain damage by cord plasma vasopressin, erythropoietin, and hypoxanthine values. *J Pediatr* 1988;113:800–15

5. Cohn HE, Sachs EJ, Heyman MA, Rudolph AM. Cardiovascular responses to hypoxemia and acidemia in fetal lambs. *Am J Obstet Gynecol* 1974;120:817–24

6. Richardson BS, Rurak D, Patrick JE, Homan J. Cerebral oxidative metabolism during sustained hypoxaemia in fetal sheep. *J Dev Physiol* 1989;11:37–43

7. Richardson BS, Carmichael L, Homan J, Patrick JE. Electrocortical activity and breathing movements in fetal sheep with prolonged and graded hypoxemia. *Am J Obstet Gynecol* 1992;167:553–8

8. Yager JY, Heitjan DF, Towfighi J, Vannucci RC. Effect of insulin induced and fasting hypoglycaemia on perinatal hypoxic–ischemic brain damage. *Pediatr Res* 1991;31:138–42

9. Pryds O, Greisen G, Lou H, Friis-Hansen B. Vasoparalysis associated with brain damage in asphyxiated term infants. *J Pediatr* 1990;117:119–25

10. van Bel F, Dorrepaal CA, Benders MJ, Zeeuwe PE, van deBor M, Berger HM. Changes in cerebral haemodynamics and oxygenation in the first 24 hours after birth asphyxia. *Pediatrics* 1993;92:365–72

11. Siesjo BK. Pathophysiology and treatment of focal cerebral ischaemia. Part II: Mechanisms of damage and treatment. *J Neurosurg* 1992;77:337–54

12. Lawrence AJ, Jarrott B. Nitric oxide increases interstitial excitatory amino acid release in the rat dorsomedial medulla oblongata. *Neurosci Lett* 1993;151:126–9

13. Buttke TM, Sandstrom PA. Oxidative stress as a mediator of apoptosis. *Immunol Today* 1994;15:7–10

14. Mehmet H, Yue X, Squier MV, *et al.* Increased apoptosis in the cingulate sulcus of newborn piglets following transient hypoxia–ischaemia is related to the degree of high energy phosphate depletion during the insult. *Neurosci Lett* 1994;181:121–5

15. Neilson JP. EFM + scalp sampling vs intermittent auscultation in labour: In Enkin MW, Keirse MJNC, Renfew MJ, Neilson JP, eds. *Pregnancy and Childbirth Module.* Cochrane Database of Systematic Reviews, Review No. 03297, 4 May 1994, Disk Issue 1. Published through *Cochrane Updates on Disk.* Oxford: Update Software, 1994

16. Nelson KB, Dambrosia JM, Ting TY, Grether JK. Uncertain value of electronic fetal monitoring in predicting cerebral palsy. *N Engl J Med* 1996;334:613–18

17. Nelson KB, Ellenberg JH. Apgar scores as predictors of chronic neurologic disability. *Pediatrics* 1981;68:36–44

18. Ruth VJ, Raivio KO. Perinatal brain damage: predictive value of metabolic acidosis and the Apgar score. *Br Med J* 1988;297:24–7

19. Levene MI, Kornberg J, Williams THC. The incidence and severity of post-asphyxial encephalopathy in full-term infants. *Early Hum Dev* 1985;11:21–6

20. Peliowski A, Finer NN. Birth asphyxia in the term infant. In Sinclair JC, Bracken MB, eds. *Effective Care of the Newborn Infant.* Oxford: Oxford University Press 1992:249–79

21. Archer LNJ, Levene MI, Evans DH. Cerebral artery Doppler ultrasonography for prediction of outcome after perinatal asphyxia. *Lancet* 1989;2:1116–18

22. Rutherford M, Pennock J, Schwieso J, Cowan F, Dubowitz L. Hypoxic–ischaemic encephalopathy: early and late magnetic resonance imaging findings in relation to outcome. *Arch Dis Child* 1996;75:F145–51

23. Kuenzle C, Baenziger O, Martin E, *et al.* Prognostic value of early MR imaging in term

infants with severe perinatal asphyxia. *Neuropediatrics* 1994;25:191–200

24. Hellstrom-Westas L, Rosen I, Svenningsen NW. Predictive value of early continuous amplitude integrated EEG recordings on outcome after severe birth asphyxia in full term infants. *Arch Dis Child* 1995;72:F34–8

25. Blair E, Stanley FJ. Intrapartum asphyxia: a rare cause of cerebral palsy. *J Pediatr* 1988;112:515–19

Ultrasound screening policies in the newborn period

52

V. Váradi

INTRODUCTION

Ultrasonographic imaging has achieved widespread use in neonatal units for diagnostic and screening purposes. This is because it is a non-invasive and convenient method for bedside examination. There are, however, some restrictions, which must be considered before advising routine use of ultrasound imaging. First, it is subject to misinterpretation (for example, over-estimation of grade I periventricular bleeding); and second, it can involve excessive handling, especially if performed by inexperienced personnel[1].

One must distinguish between the use of sonography for diagnostic or screening purposes, and whether the screening is carried out among healthy newborn infants or in neonatal intensive care. Ultrasonographic imaging in each site has a different significance.

In their series of 3396 clinically healthy newborn infants, Leonardi and Reither[2] found 4.2% anomalous brain scans, 4.4% renal scans that needed to be followed by further diagnostic and therapeutic steps and 7.4% right-sided and 9.7% left-sided hip dysplasias.

Labádi and co-workers[3] examined 8230 newborns and young infants by abdominal and cranial ultrasound screening. Their results also demonstrated that, in spite of prenatal routine ultrasound screening, a relatively high number of anomalies was revealed, especially in the genitourinary system. The overall incidence of developmental anomalies was 4%, and one-third of these concerned the genitourinary system (0.2–2% of the population). The most frequently seen anomaly was pelvic dilatation

of various severity. Among the 151 intracranial malformations found, the most common were subependymal hemorrhage, choroid plexus hemorrhage, ventriculomegaly and porencephalic cysts.

Most newborn units agree, in terms of healthy newborn care, that the value of ultrasound brain screening is still under discussion, but that the introduction of general ultrasound screening of the urinary system and the hips is mandatory. In neonatal intensive care and in preterm infants under 32 weeks of gestation, it is most important to screen the brain. The heart, kidney and abdomen follow in importance. In preterm (under 32 gestational weeks) and term babies, brain imaging after asphyxia has prognostic value.

ULTRASOUND SCREENING OF THE NEONATAL BRAIN

In healthy neonatal care, cranial sonographic screening is still in dispute. However, apart from a few extreme opinions[4], cranial ultrasonography for preterm infants and term infants after perinatal asphyxia is strongly advised[1].

Among healthy neonates the incidence of brain anomalies is 3–4%. In a recent study, Berger and colleagues[5] screened 5286 babies at 5–8 days postpartum to examine the incidence and severity of brain damage in neonates and to relate these to various obstetric factors. The most frequent abnormality was periventricular–intraventricular hemorrhage (3.6%) of various degrees (grades I–III). Periventricular leukomalacia, porencephaly,

382

subarachnoid hemorrhage and hydrocephalus were rare (less than 2%). The incidence of periventricular–intraventricular hemorrhage increased progressively with decreasing gestational age. It ranged between 1.6% at 38–43 weeks and 50% at 24–30 weeks. A large percentage of babies with periventricular-intraventricular hemorrhage were clinically normal. In immature neonates there was a close relationship between Apgar scores at 1, 5 and 10 min and both the incidence and severity of periventricular–intraventricular hemorrhage. The incidence of periventricular–intraventricular hemorrhage was larger in growth-restricted newborn infants.

Most of what is seen by ultrasound is of no clinical significance (e.g. grade I periventricular–intraventricular hemorrhage, choroid plexus hemorrhage, subependymal pseudocysts, ventricular asymmetry) and only a few anomalies (0.7%) carry prognostic relevance (grade II periventricular-intraventricular hemorrhage, ventriculomegaly, porencephaly). The neurosonographic findings are significantly dependent on mode of delivery. Vacuum extraction, breech presentation and prolonged labor carry a significantly higher risk[2,5].

Most of these cerebral lesions, typical for immature infants, can be reliably screened by ultrasound.

(1) Periventricular–intraventricular hemorrhage: 5–10% of premature babies born before 32 weeks of gestation develop periventricular–intraventricular hemorrhage during the first postnatal week. The hemorrhage itself and the sequelae of grade III–IV intraventricular hemorrhage (i.e. posthemorrhagic hydrocephalus or porencephaly) are also readily diagnosed by sonographic scans around 3–4 weeks postpartum. Later, the dynamics of hydrocephalus can be followed sonographically.

(2) Hypoxic–ischemic lesions in premature infants: periventricular leukomalacia is less frequent than hemorrhage, but carries a more serious neurological outcome. In the acute state (1 week after

birth), increased echogenicity is seen around the lateral ventricle. In the chronic case (3–4 weeks after birth), periventricular cavitation appears (periventricular cystic leukomalacia). At the morphological end-stages, atrophia cerebri can also be clearly vizualised.

As far as postasphyxic mature infants are concerned, only the focal or multifocal hypoxic–ischemic lesions (infarction, subcortical cystic leukomalacia) can be reliably detected in the early postnatal period. In cases of diffuse hypoxic–ischemic brain injury (selective neuron necrosis and edema cerebri) cranial ultrasonography has no diagnostic value. Weeks after the insult, ultrasound can give a reliable diagnosis of morphological sequelae of hypoxic–ischemic brain damage (atrophia cerebri). However, the late sonographic picture in both hemorrhagic and hypoxic–ischemic infants also carries prognostic value.

It is worth screening premature and mature infants as well as babies born after chronic fetal distress (prolonged intrauterine hypoxia) or after massive maternal third-trimester bleeding. In the first cases we can find the sequelae of *in utero* periventricular hemorrhage (i.e. subependymal pseudocysts) in some babies. In the case of maternal blood loss, the consequence of serious intrauterine fetal cerebral hypoperfusion (ischemia) may be seen as connatal periventricular leukomalacia.

The optimal timing for detecting the acute changes by cranial ultrasonography is at the end of the first week of life. For premature infants and postasphyxial mature infants a second investigation, when the infant is 3–4 weeks old, is suggested in order to follow the morphological changes in the brain.

ULTRASOUND SCREENING OF THE URINARY TRACT

There is general agreement that sonographic screening of the urinary system in newborn infants is mandatory, despite widespread prenatal sonographic screening. Among clinically healthy newborn infants the incidence of congenital anomalies of the urinary tract with the need for further investigation or follow-up was found to be 4–5% and the incidence of severe kidney malformation was 1%[3]. The incidence of the prenatally diagnosed severe genitourinary tract anomalies was found to be only 0.2–0.5% in the same population.

Although abnormalities of the urinary tract can be easily recognized, because they are invariably accompanied by fluid-filled masses in the fetal abdomen, only 60–70% of hydronephrotic cases become known prenatally. On the other hand, dilatation of the renal pelvis can be more prominent *in utero* than in the first postnatal days. This is due to the increased amniotic fluid circulation at 27–28 weeks of gestation and the physiological oliguria during of the first days of life. The most common postnatally screened urinary abnormalities are:

(1) Renal pelvis dilatation;

(2) Unilateral renal agenesis;

(3) Renal dysgenesis: unilateral multicystic kidney, polycystic adult kidney disease and congenital hydronephrosis;

(4) Bladder outlet obstruction: posterior urethral valves and urethral stenosis.

The prenatal ultrasound diagnosis significantly influences obstetric management. Antenatal diagnosis of congenital pelvic dilatation and hydronephrosis allows early postnatal intervention and the preservation of renal function. The postnatal screening allows a more precise diagnosis.

Pyelectasis or dilatation of the renal pelvis may occur secondary to any anomaly of the urinary tract located below the level of the pelvis. Its severity is gauged by the size of the renal pelvis in the anteroposterior diameter.

Many studies deal with the diagnostic value of the renal pelvis diameter in pre- and postnatal sonographic screening[6]. One of the conclusions is that the renal pelvis dilatation on prenatal and postnatal sonograms is linked to obstructive uropathies rather than to vesicoureteral reflux. Prenatal sonography seems to be less sensitive than postnatal sonography in revealing obstructive uropathies. The cut-off level for a normal neonatal renal pelvis seems to be 10 mm. A renal pelvis smaller than 10 mm shows no pathological significance, because these renal collecting systems normalize spontaneously within 1 year. If the postnatal ultrasound scan shows an isolated pelvic diameter below this level, a clinical follow-up is advised and the parents are informed of the possibility of vesicoureteral reflux and of the necessity of performing cytobacteriological urine examination in case of unexplained fever[7].

The differentiation between hydronephrotic and multicystic kidney is very important, because of their different significance, although in classic cases differentiation will not cause a problem. In hydronephrosis all kidney tissues are recognizable and the cystic pelvis is connected by similar-looking calyces. The presence or absence of obstruction in hydronephrosis needs further examination[3].

The variables associated with a higher risk of urinary tract obstruction are increased echogenicity, parenchymal rims of 5 mm or less, contralateral hypertrophy, a resistance index with diuresis of 70% or greater, ureter diameter of 10 mm or greater, or aperistaltic ureter. These features help to differentiate between obstructive and non-obstructive hydronephrosis[8].

Vesicoureteral reflux (VUR) affects approximately 1% of newborn infants. The risk is even higher if the patient's family history involves more than one member with VUR or more than one generation affected with VUR. The condition has been associated with urinary tract infection and renal damage and is responsible for approximately 10% of cases of end-stage renal failure in young adults. The renal injury that results from VUR is related to infection, and reflux may be prevented by the early administration of antibiotics or corrective surgery. Ultrasound may not be able to differentiate primary VUR from lower obstructive uropathy with or without reflux in neonates with sonographic evidence of hydronephrosis and/or hydroureter.

The general use of obstetric ultrasound has resulted in an increased frequency of diagnosis of fetal uropathies. Subsequently, various studies have focused on proper postnatal management. It has been debated whether a voiding cystoureterography should be performed in every neonate with antenatal diagnosis of uropathy, or whether a postnatal ultrasound examination should be used to select the neonates needing voiding cystoureterography.

The supporters of performing voiding cystoureterography in every neonate claim that ultrasound is a poor indicator of VUR. In their series, 25–60% of VUR were missed by ultrasound and the urinary tract appeared normal on the scan, even in cases with reflux of grades III–V[9–14]. In the series by Avni and colleagues[15], only 50.9% of the patients presented a significant dilatation of the renal pelvis. Using this criterion alone, we would miss 49% of cases of VUR. Scott and colleagues[12] stated that routine renal ultrasound scanning of newborn babies was of no value in detecting those who may have ureteral reflux, and that the number of other renal abnormalities likely to be detected was small.

The advocates of more selective use of voiding cystoureterography stress that it is ethically and economically impossible to perform this on every neonate with antenatal diagnosis of uropathy. Therefore, after birth, ultrasound should select the neonates subsequently needing voiding cystoureterography.

It appears that pelvic dilatation alone is a poor indicator of the presence of VUR; it underestimates the presence and degree of VUR. Therefore, associated sonographic signs have been sought[11,15]. The detection of calyceal or ureteral dilatation is an important supplemental finding. The lack of corticomedullar dilatation differentiation is the single most common ultrasound finding[15]. Avni and colleagues[15], in their recent study,

sought to determine whether a urinary tract appearing normal by meticulous ultrasound examination may coexist with vesicoureteric reflux and whether a normal ultrasound scan can be used to exclude VUR, thereby avoiding unnecessary voiding cystoureterography. They found that careful ultrasound examination of the neonatal urinary tract allowed the detection of over 87% of cases of VUR by showing at least one sonographic abnormality. They concluded that a normal-appearing urinary tract does not usually coexist with VUR and that in such cases voiding cystoureterography is not necessary. Ultrasound criteria of changes that could result from or be associated with vesicoureteral reflux[11,15] are:

(1) Pelvic dilatation;

(2) Calyceal dilatation (isolated or with pelvic dilatation);

(3) Ureteral dilatation (isolated or with pelvic dilatation);

(4) Pelvic or ureteral wall thickening;

(5) Lack of corticomedullary differentiation;

(6) Signs of dysplasia (cortical thinning, small kidney, cortical hyperechogenicity);

(7) Ballooning of the pelvis during voiding.

The sensitivity of ultrasound evaluation of the urinary tract in the neonate can be increased by lowering the cut-off level for normal fetal pelvic diameter from 10 to 4 mm[16]. In using this cut-off level for renal pelvic dilatation and searching for other anomalies besides pelvic dilatation potentially associated with VUR, a normal careful ultrasound study may be used to exclude VUR in the neonate and thus avoid the use of screening voiding cystoureterography. Although occasional cases of VUR could be missed by this approach, it seems reasonable to consider that the risk of missing low-grade reflux would be outweighed by the benefit of avoiding unnecessary examination in healthy babies.

A new method for the diagnosis of VUR is percutaneous vesicoinfusion. By this method the bladder is slowly expanded with saline solution gently injected through a needle. A progressive dilatation of the renal pelvis indicates VUR[17].

The sequelae of perinatal hypoxia and trauma and tumors of the kidney and adrenal glands can also be screened by ultrasound.

Sequelae of perinatal hypoxia and trauma

Transient neonatal renal medullary hyperechogenicity

This is a common ultrasound finding in healthy neonates in the first few days of life. It usually disappears within the first week of life. Its etiology is unclear, although it may be related to protein cast deposits in the renal tubules. Renal medullary hyperechogenicity may rarely be associated with renal hypoperfusion and transient renal dysfunction, but in healthy neonates it should be recognized as a normal variant[18,19].

Adrenal gland hemorrhage

The incidence of this is 1% and it very often occurs without clinical features. Since adrenal neuroblastoma can imitate the sonographic and clinical pictures of adrenal gland hemorrhage, it is important to follow up all neonates with adrenal hemorrhage until this disappears[20].

Neonatal renal venous thrombosis

This is a serious complication in the newborn infant. Perivascular streaks are first seen at 3 days of age with diffusely enlarged and echogenic kidney. Echolucency then gradually disappears over the medulla, accompanied by shrinking of renal size. Since pathognomic perivascular streaks are present for only a few days, early ultrasound scanning should be performed for every newborn suspected of having renal venous thrombosis[21].

Tumors of the kidney and adrenal gland

Tumors of the kidneys are rare. In the kidney, the similar-looking congenital mesoblastic nephroma and Wilms' tumor can be detected. Congenital adrenal neuroblastoma is the most common abdominal tumor found in newborns, representing 12.3% of all perinatal neoplasms.

Neonatal ultrasound screening has good sensitivity and specificity in the detection of urinary tract malformations. However, a negative ultrasound diagnosis soon after birth does not exclude hydronephrosis, pyelectasis or vesicoureteral reflux. In cases of positive fetal sonographic findings, therefore, the ultrasound examination should be repeated in 7–10 days.

ULTRASOUND SCREENING FOR CONGENITAL HIP DYSPLASIA

Screening for congenital hip dysplasia in newborn infants, mostly by Ortolani's test, is widely performed. Nevertheless, most of the dysplasias (the incidence of dysplasias is 7–9%) are still discovered late[22,23]. The prevalence of subluxated/luxated hips in later infancy is still reported to be as high as 1–3 per 1000 infants. Using ultrasound, it is possible to evaluate both hip morphology and hip stability. Ultrasonographic screening allows early diagnosis, and early start of therapy results in a high success rate and reduces the length of therapy[24].

Clinically hip stability is described as stable, borderline, unstable, dislocatable or dislocated and the morphology on ultrasound as normal, immature or dysplastic. Sonograpic hip screening has proved to be effective in detecting true instability of the hip joint as well as dysplasia. The optimal time for sonographic screening does not seem to be immediately after birth, but at an age between 4 and 6 weeks, when the hip has already shown its true nature[25].

Universal primary ultrasound screening of the hip has been adopted in some European countries[23]. The subsequent increases in treatment and follow-up of screened infants have tempered enthusiasm in many other countries, such as the UK[26]. A general screening of newborns in Austria since 1992 has demonstrated that the rate of treatment can be decreased by about 50% and that sonography used correctly can avoid overtreatment[27].

On the other hand, selective ultrasound screening of the hip to assess and manage infants with clinically detected hip instability and those at high risk (positive family history, breech presentation, twins)[28] did not reduce the incidence of late-presenting congenital hip dysplasia. There are clinically silent dysplastic hips for which early detection is possible only with sonographic screening.

Sonographically, approximately 85% of infants have morphologically normal hips, while 12% have immature hips and 3% have dysplastic hips. About 80–90% of infants with

dysplastic acetabula show only minor changes and many hips may normalize without reducing the occurrence of late-diagnosed congenital hip dislocation. It is known that only babies whose dysplasia is recognized within the first few weeks will recover completely. Restitution after 3 months of age is only 70–80%, and after 6 months only 50%.

Since immature hips recover by themselves, hip screening is advisable at the age of 6–8 weeks. At that time the control examination of immature hips is avoidable and the treatment of dysplastic hips can be started during the best period of hip development[29,30].

References

1. Jorch G. Ultrasound imaging. *J Perinat Med* 1994;22:571–4
2. Leonardi A, Reither M. Ultrasound screening of newborn infants. Uses and role in routine diagnosis. *Klin Pediatr* 1993;205:383–8
3. Labádi L, Tuksa Á, Tekulics P. Routine ultrasound screening in the newborn period. *Gyermekgyógyászat* 1998;44:482–7
4. Harding D, Kuschel C, Evans N. Should preterm infants born after 29 weeks of gestation be screened for intraventricular hemorrhage? *J Pediatr Child Health* 1998;34:57–9
5. Berger R, Bender S, Sefkow S, Klingmuller V, Kunzel W, Jensen A. Peri/intraventricular haemorrhage: a cranial ultrasound study on 5286 neonates. *Eur J Obstet Gynecol Reprod Biol* 1997;75: 191–203
6. Dremsek PA, Gindl K, Voitl P, *et al.* Renal pyelectasis in fetuses and neonates: diagnostic value of renal pelvic diameter in pre- and postnatal sonographic screening. *Am J Roentgenol* 1997;168:1017–19
7. Podevin G, Levard G, Marechaud M, Gurault F, Barret D. Postnatal diagnostic strategy of urinary tract malformations detected by prenatal screening. *Arch Pediatr* 1997;4:411–15
8. Garcia-Pena BM, Keller MS, Schwartz DS, Korsvik HE, Weiss RM. The ultrasonographic differentiation of obstructive versus non-obstructive hydronephrosis in children: a multivariable scoring system. *J Urol* 1997;158: 560–5
9. Blane CE, DiPietro MA, Zerin JM, Sedman AB, Bloom DA. Renal sonography is not a reliable screening examination for vesicoureteral reflux. *J Urol* 1993;150:752–5
10. Kis E, Verebély T, Kövi R, Várkonyi I, Máttyus I. Usefulness of ultrasound in diagnosis of primary vesicoureteralis reflux in neonates and infants. *Orv Hetil* 1998;139:1785–8
11. Masahiro H, Kasuga K, Hori C, Sudo M. Ultrasonic indicators of ureteric reflux in the newborn. *Lancet* 1994;434:519–20
12. Scott JES, Lee REJ, Hunter EW, Coulthard MG, Matthews JNS. Ultrasound screening of the urinary tract. *Lancet* 1991;338:1571–3
13. Tibbals JM, deBruyn R. Primary vesico-ureteric reflux – how useful is US? *Arch Dis Child* 1996;75: 444–7
14. Zerin JM, Ritchey ML, Chang ACH. Incidental vesico-ureteral reflux in neonates with antenatally detected hydronephrosis and other renal abnormalities. *Radiology* 1993;187:157–60
15. Avni EF, Ayadi K, Rypens F, Hall M, Schulman CC. Can careful ultrasound examination of the urinary tract exclude vesicoureteric reflux in the neonate? *Br J Radiol* 1997;70:977–82
16. Anderson NG, Abbot GD, Mogridge N, Allan RB, Maling TM, Wells JE. Vesicoureteric reflux in the newborn: relationship to fetal renal pelvic diameter. *Pediatr Nephrol* 1997;11:610–16
17. Quintero RA, Johnson MP, Arias F, *et al. In utero* sonographic diagnosis of vesicoureteral reflux by percutaneous vesicoinfusion. *Ultrasound Obstet Gynecol* 1995;6:386–9
18. Howlett DC, Greenwood KL, Jarosz JM, MacDonald LM, Saunders AJ. The incidence of transient renal medullary hyperechogenicity in

neonatal ultrasound examination. *Br J Radiol* 1997;70:140–3

19. Riebel TW, Abraham K, Warter R, Muller R. Transient renal medullary hyperechogenicity in ultrasound studies of neonates: is it a normal phenomenon and what are the causes? *J Clin Ultrasound* 1993;21:25–31

20. Jojart G, Bodanszky H. Neonatal neuroblastoma detected by ultrasonic screening. *Orv Hetil* 1993;134:971–4

21. Lin GJ, Yang PH, Wang ML. Neonatal renal venous thrombosis. A case report describing serial sonographic changes. *Pediatr Nephrol* 1994; 8:589–91

22. Geitung JT, Rosendahl K, Sudmann E. Cost-effectiveness of ultrasonographic screening for congenital hip dysplasia in newborns. *Skeletal Radiol* 1996;25:251–4

23. Rosendahl K, Markestad T, Lie RT. Developmental dysplasia of the hip. A population-based comparison of ultrasound and clinical findings. *Acta Paediatr* 1996;85:64–9

24. Rosendahl K, Éie RT, Markestad T. Congenital hip dislocation. Ultrasonic screening of newborn infants. *Tidskr Nor Laegeforen* 1997;117:346–52

25. Grill F, Muller D. Results of ultrasonographic screening in Austria. *Orthopädie* 1997;26:25–32

26. Dezateux C, Godward S. A national survey of screening for congenital dislocation of the hip. *Arch Dis Child* 1996;74:445–8

27. Graf R. Hip ultrasonography. Basic principles and current aspects. *Orthopädie* 1997;26:14–24

28. Chan A, McCaul KA, Cundy PJ, Haan EA, Byron-Scott R. Perinatal risk factors for developmental dysplasia of the hip. *Arch Dis Child* 1997;76;F94–F100

29. Daoud S, Várady M, Kis ZS. Ultrasound examination of the hip in the newborn infant. *Gyermekgyógyászat* 1996;5:1146–54

30. Franke J, Lazovic D, Overhoff HM, von Jan U, Ruhmann O. New approaches to 3D ultrasonographic imaging of infant hips. *Orthopädie* 1997; 26:210–14

Computers and fetal medicine 53

I. E. Zador, L. Chik and R. J. Sokol

INTRODUCTION

It seems that every time we open a newspaper, watch the news or listen to the radio, there is an announcement of some 'breakthrough technology' that will dramatically improve the way we interact with computers. It is also very likely that from the time this book goes to press until its appearance in print the computer industry will undergo another 'technology cycle'. This term refers to the 12–18-month period during which computer processing power doubles and the cost halves. This rapid and unprecedented change puts enormous strain on all the users of computers. Whether an individual is zigzagging through the hardware maze or a manager is looking for a software solution to keep competitive in the rapidly changing health-care environment, this person will face the unenviable task of making the 'right' decision. The best that one can hope is that a current commitment will get one through several technology cycles. The shortness of the technology cycle is straining the classical system life cycle which requires planning, vendor selection, development, implementation and maintenance.

Keeping this rapid pace in mind, we will try to optimize the information presented in this chapter. It is hoped that the material presented here will remain relevant at least until the next edition of this book. The chapter starts with an overview of computer fundamentals. The main focus is on some emerging innovative ideas that might impact on our specialty. The main emphasis is on the application of the Internet. We postulate that Internet-based technologies may profoundly affect the way we will care for the fetus in the new millennium.

OVERVIEW OF COMPUTERS

Hardware

Since the introduction of the personal computer (PC) in the late 1970s, computer use has approximately doubled each year. Today it is estimated that there are 50 million PCs worldwide; 80% of these PCs are used in the industrial world. The most popular 'information appliance', the television set, is about ten times more popular. In the USA the average cost of a moderately equipped desktop computing setup is around $1500. Add around $500 to this price for a comparable notebook computer. To upgrade to a top-of-the-line PC would require an additional $1000. What is amazing in these prices is that, during the past several years, this cost structure has remained remarkably steady. There are no indications to suspect that this trend will not continue in the foreseeable future, despite a major push from large computer manufacturers to market a PC below $1000. The good news is that, as we sail through the 'technology cycle', the same investment buys more computing power, larger storage capacity, improved display resolution – in short, an improvement across the entire spectrum of computer hardware.

There is still a significant debate over the desktop computer platform. The two remaining platforms are what are referred to as the IBM-compatible PC and the Apple-based computer. The former is manufactured by a large number of companies (IBM, Hewlett Packard, Dell, Compaq, Toshiba and many more) while the latter are produced almost exclusively by the Apple Corporation. The passion over the debate of which platform to use can reach the intensity of a religious war. Unfortunately, the market share of Apple-based computers is rapidly slipping. Overall, Apple's market share is below 10%, although among educational institutions and most notably in the video editing industry it is higher.

The central processing unit (CPU) remains the essential component of the computer. It is the heart and the brain of its functionality; it represents around 25% of the total cost of a personal computer. The best known and the largest CPU maker is Intel Corporation. The company, based in Santa Clara, California, supplies microprocessors for about 85% of the world's personal computers. The 1990s could be labelled as the decade of the Intel Pentium CPU chip. Currently, the Pentium II 450-MHz 32-bit CPU chip represents the top of the line. The Intel architecture 64-bit CPU code named Merced is anticipated to be on the market by the end of the decade. The chip should debut at 500 MHz and will be scalable to more than 4 GHz. Other major CPU makers include Motorola, Digital Equipment Corporation, Cyrix and AMD, which are mostly based on the East Asian side of the Pacific basin.

What are some anticipated trends in the computer arena for the next several years? They will occur, either by predictable elements driven by such factors as higher processing power or greater storage space, or by less predictable elements, which may change the nature of the computer in an even more dramatic way. In just these past 2 years, the dramatic drop in the price of computer memory (RAM) has had a major effect on how people think of creating applications. We should expect the impact of emerging innovative screen design. We will have low-cost, high-resolution flat-screen technology. The idea of being able to cover your desk or walls with screens that can actively display information will become very common. Eventually, we will have a portable, tablet-sized device that will provide enough resolution so that actually reading off that device would make sense. The idea of another recent hardware initiative, the NetPC, is that you take all the richness and software capabilities of a Windows PC and put it in a package that minimizes the number of hardware changes during the PC's life. In most cases, the only additional thing you would do is add more RAM. This creates an easy-to-use Internet device that is compatible with existing Windows applications. They will have a browser built into them but, because of the smaller screen and limited resources, they will not have the richness of the full PC. We can also anticipate devices that use the TV set, filling in as an information appliance. The term 'PC' will probably be reserved for things that you sit fairly close to and on which you can edit information easily with a full-screen type of display. However, PC technology will be used in all information appliances, so that we can get the greatest possible sharing of applications and information.

Operating systems and software

Health-care institutions of today are faced with the bewildering task of administering a vast array of computing architectures. It is surely daunting to support the mainframes in which crucial data are stored, as well as a wide variety of smaller computers, including Windows machines of differing powers and flavors (Windows 3.1, Windows 95 and 98, Windows NT, on 386s, 486s and Pentiums); Macintoshes; OS/2-based machines; and Unix boxes, not to mention various palmtops. Although most medical institutions have learned to cope with their collection of diverse computers, it is not difficult to imagine how much they are straining under the extra load of supporting different applications on different computers.

Applications of computers in fetal medicine

The areas of fetal medicine most closely associated with computers are obstetric data management systems, electronic fetal monitoring and ultrasound fetal imaging[1-3].

Obstetric data management systems (OBDMS) are computer systems designed to interface with fetal and maternal monitors[4-6]. This allows monitoring and charting records to be created and maintained electronically and to be viewed from centralized workstations. In theory, these systems could eliminate paper record keeping altogether, although currently at least some paper documentation is being kept. These systems have been almost exclusively developed by large companies such as Hewlett Packard, Marquette Medical Systems and SpaceLabs, to mention a few. The products offered by all of these companies are very similar. The majority of these systems have been developed around Microsoft's Windows NT technology and can be relatively easily interfaced with other departmental computer systems. They also remain very costly. A typical OBDMS system for a department with 3000 deliveries per year might cost in excess of $500 000.

Electronic fetal monitoring is an area that, from its inception in the early 1970s, was closely related to computers[7-12]. The acquisition of a large amount of information and online real-time signal processing generated a vast literature related to computerized antepartum and intrapartum fetal heart rate assessment. Additional computer algorithms were developed to study fetal behavioral states, fetal movements and effects of vibroacoustic stimulation, and various computer models were developed for the interpretation and teaching of fetal monitoring. After a relatively short pause, there is currently a renewed interest in the topic. Among the most promising reports are those of the research related to the processing and interpretation of the abdominal fetal electrocardiogram (FECG). The increased computing power and sophisticated signal processing technique might enable practitioners to analyze the various components of the FECG in real time. An interesting concept is the use of abdominal FECG at around 18 weeks as a screening tool for fetal cardiac anomalies.

Ultrasound fetal imaging remains among the most explosive areas of growth in fetal medicine[13-21]. Its contribution to our understanding of the developing fetus and the ever-increasing worldwide utilization of this modality is propelled by advances in computer technologies. The increase in the computer's processing power lends itself to the design of cost-effective real-time three-dimensional ultrasound hardware. Ultrasound scanners with three-dimensional capabilities are offered today as an option by most of the leading ultrasound manufacturers. Although the clinical usefulness of three-dimensional ultrasound in fetal imaging is still hotly debated, it is just a matter of time till its incorporation into our day-to-day practice. The initial experiences with three-dimensional ultrasound come from reports originating from some selected research institutions. The early articles seem to indicate that three-dimensional imaging is superior in the detection of fetal face and spine anomalies[16-20].

An emerging buzzword in ultrasound imaging that might enhance our ability to detect fetal anomalies is a signal processing technique referred to as 'harmonic tissue imaging'. Introduced almost simultaneously by several major ultrasound hardware manufacturers (including ATL and Acuson), this technology has the potential to alter profoundly the diagnostic course for the most challenging patients – those who are defined as difficult-to-image. Tissue harmonic imaging considerably improves image quality in difficult-to-image patients who are often overweight or have disease conditions that make it difficult, and sometimes impossible, to obtain images of diagnostic quality. This computer power-hungry signal-processing scheme enhances images obtained from patients with large body habitus to the level usually obtained from patients in the normal weight range.

Another interesting innovation in fetal imaging is the development of tools for real-time detection of inner and outer skull boundaries of a fetal head, abdominal circumference and the fetal long bones. It can be speculated that the sonographer of the future will not have to spend a significant portion of scanning time on fetal biometry but rather will be able to focus his/her attention on assessment of fetal morphology. This will be further enhanced by the numerous fetal ultrasound software packages for ultrasound data acquisition and reporting.

The ultrasound information that cannot be directly downloaded will be input, utilizing speech-recognition packages.

THE INTERNET AND THE WORLD WIDE WEB

Brief history

The Internet (also known as ARPANET) started during the cold war in the late 1960s[22-25]. It was conceived and developed by the United States Department of Defense in conjunction with a number of universities to explore the possibility of a communications network that could survive a nuclear attack. After the cold war was over, it continued simply because all the end users found that it provided a very convenient way to communicate. The early applications of the Internet included electronic mail (e-mail), online discussion support groups and the transfer of files among government agencies, companies and universities. During the early 1980s, all the interconnected research networks were converted to a standard protocol (TCP/IP) which enabled all of the networks of the Internet to send data back and forth. In 1990, HTML, a hypertext protocol that could communicate graphic information on the Internet, was introduced. Utilizing HTML, one could create graphic pages (a web site) which would then become a part of the huge, virtual hypertext network called the World Wide Web (WWW). The enhanced Internet was informally renamed the Web and a huge additional user base emerged.

At the moment, the term 'Internet' refers to the physical structure of the Net, including client and server computers and the lines that connect everything. The term 'Web' refers to the collection of sites and the information that can be accessed when one is using the Internet. A number of different services have developed over the years to facilitate the sharing of information among the many sites on the Internet. Because the Internet was originally research-oriented, many of these services were hard to use and poorly documented. Now that the Internet has been opened to commercial and private sites, new services are being developed that are easier to use. Currently, the Internet Society, the group that controls the Internet, is trying to form new protocols in order to have millions of addresses rather than the limited system of today. The problem of how both the old and the new addressing systems will be able to work at the same time during a transition period has not yet been worked out.

Telemedicine

Telemedicine will be the next big wave to inundate the practice of medicine[26-30]. The combined synergy of low-cost computing power, improving telecommunications facilities (including the Internet) and advances in clinical information science will transform the ways in which medicine is practiced.

Trends in telemedicine are being watched closely because of technology's immense promise to connect a large segment of the population living in rural areas with specialists located in distant hospitals for diagnosis and treatment recommendations. Telemedicine can be defined as anything more sophisticated than a telephone and fax machine through interactive video consultations. In general, telemedicine refers to the use of electronic communication networks for the transmission of information and data related to the diagnosis and treatment of medical conditions. The emerging telemedicine headlines include teleradiology, telesonography, telepathology, teleconsultation in psychiatry/mental health, ophthalmology, dermatology, cardiology, oncology, pediatrics, orthopedics, gynecology, neurology, teletriage and telenursing, multimedia obstetrics and teledentistry. The major areas for applications of telemedicine include home health, health triage, electronic house calls, emergency and trauma medicine, battlefield medicine, rural health, van-based telemedicine, prison health, HIV outreach, space medicine and medicine in developing nations. Digital instruments suitable for remote examination now available include the digital stethoscope, otoscope, endoscope, proctoscope, ophthalmoscope, dermascope and microscope.

While the use of telemedicine is experiencing tremendous growth, work is being done on defining policies relating to medical, legal, psychological and reimbursement issues. Late in 1996, California became the first state to pass a bill (the Telemedicine Development Act of 1996 – Senate Bill 1665) which recognized the practice of telemedicine as a legitimate means by which an individual may receive medical services from a health-care provider without person-to-person contact with the provider. The application of telemedicine in the USA may be enhanced by the late 1997 decision of the US Congress to include reimbursement for telemedical consultations for rural areas. Acting on legislation introduced by Senator Ken Conrad of North Dakota, members of the House and Senate agreed that telemedicine consultation reimbursement will be established for all eligible part B Medicare services at normal co-pay rates. No facility fees or transmission costs will be eligible for reimbursement. It is estimated that this will yield $100 million to $200 million per year for telemedicine reimbursement, starting in 1999.

People are spending significant resources trying to resolve the wide array of complex issues that are associated with remote computing. In fact, end-user demand for remote access is likely to increase dramatically as many more people obtain access to a browser. The anticipated demand for telemedicine and other streaming video applications could easily choke the existing network infrastructure. In the next several years, the demand for remote access computing may well eclipse the Internet phenomenon as we struggle to apply existing technologies to solutions of new social and work-related needs.

Online information search

It is now common among medical professionals to seek medical information on a given topic by accessing the Internet and initiating a MEDLINE search[31]. This can be done from the home, office or any location around the world with an access to the Internet. It is obviously a much more efficient method of searching the literature than visiting a library with its limited service hours and looking through the journals. A MEDLINE search does not require any specific training or knowledge. The search engine attached to MEDLINE translates key words or free text entries (e.g. premature labor and ultrasound) to a vocabulary called MESH (Medical Subject Headings) and matches these terms to the article title or subject headings in all publications in the collection of the National Library of Medicine. Currently, there is approximately a 4-week delay between the time of publication and the appearance on MEDLINE. An abstract with all the pertinent information about the authors, language, journal, etc., is usually provided for each such article found. The information obtained from the MEDLINE search can be downloaded into each computer and can be easily incorporated into any application.

A related emerging trend relates to the change in the nature of medical publishing. The leading medical journals, such as the *New England Journal of Medicine*, the *British Journal of Medicine*, the *Journal of the American Medical Association* and *The Lancet*, are now online, as are several leading journals in our specialty. The leading scientific publishers are making their entire journal collections available over the Internet. For example, John Wiley & Sons has recently announced the launch of its Interscience project which will provide online access to nearly all of its more than 400 scientific journals. Interscience will feature searchable content listings, abstracts and, by the end of 1998, access to full-text electronic files for all articles published in its journal (JCU in the Online Era, 26:1, 1997). Other publishers are implementing similar strategies. Consequently, some publishers of scientific journals are concluding that the publication of annual subject and author indices in the respective journals would be of limited, if any, value to their readers and have decided to abandon the practice.

Continuing medical education

Advances in educational software provide new electronic options for earning continuing medical education (CME) credits. Physicians and other health-care providers have the option of obtaining CME credits out of the computers they already use at the office and at home. The American College of Obstetricians and Gynecologists (ACOG) and other organizations are developing computer software that a physician can use to get CME credit. One of the first programs developed by ACOG is an interactive CD-ROM for colposcopy. The multimedia program includes a tutorial, video clips and color images, some of which can be digitally stained to detect pathology. Other multimedia programs on endometriosis, urogynecology, laparoscopic hysterectomy and pelvic anatomy are available from various other sources. Such programs are generally priced at about $50 per credit.

CONCLUSION

In medicine, the availability and immediacy of information on the Web can be a mixed blessing. On one hand, the intimate, uncensored, egalitarian nature of the Web, the idea of cutting out the middleman and the ease with which people can hook up with each other for information and support are indisputable benefits of this technology. On the other hand, and this mostly applies to a novice user who needs information about symptoms, drugs and alternative treatments, there are two important risks. One is the obvious risk of obtaining inaccurate information; the missing middleman in this case is the medical expert. The other, which is harder to assess, is the risk of being scared, overwhelmed and depressed by a personal account of someone with first-hand knowledge of a frightening and mysterious disease. What is so compelling about the Web – the way we can search for a random topic – can be disorienting and even frightening when it comes to searching for medical information on life-altering diseases that affect you or someone close to you.

As with any other medium, the Internet has great possibilities as a tool for human communication. It is the first communication infrastructure to combine features of both mass media and interpersonal communication. It can only be truly useful, however, if we are prepared to face both its strengths and its weaknesses, dealing with each. We often speak of the Internet as our future but, in reality, it is just an important part of our future. Technology can supplant only so much. The Internet is not necessarily a better way of communicating, just a different one.

References

1. Sokol RJ, Chik L, Zador IE. Approaching the millennium: perinatal problems and software solutions. *Early Hum Dev* 1992;29:51-6
2. Zador IE. Computers in obstetrics and gynecology. *Contrib Gynecol Obstet* 1989;17:86-95
3. Dalton KJ, Chard T. *Computers in Obstetrics and Gynecology*. Amsterdam: Elsevier Science Publishers, 1990
4. Amini SB, Catalano PM, Mann LI. Effect of prenatal care on obstetrical outcome. *J Matern Fetal Med* 1996;5:142-50
5. McGhee TD. Observations on database design for improving clinical care. *Int J Clin Monit Comput* 1996;13:143-5
6. Holubkov R, Holt VL, Connell FA, LoGerfo JP. Analysis, assessment, and presentation of risk-adjusted statewide obstetrical care data: the StORQS II study in Washington State. Statewide Obstetrics Review and Quality System. *Health Serv Res* 1998;33:531-48
7. van Wijngaarden WJ, Sahota DS, James DK, *et al.* Improved intrapartum surveillance with PR

interval analysis of the fetal electrocardiogram: a randomized trial showing a reduction in fetal blood sampling. *Am J Obstet Gynecol* 1996;174: 1295–9

8. Birnie E, Monincx WM, Zondervan HA, Bossuyt PM, Bonsel GJ. Cost-minimization analysis of domiciliary antenatal fetal monitoring in high-risk pregnancies. *Obstet Gynecol* 1997;89:925–9

9. Murray ML, Higgins P. Computer versus lecture: strategies for teaching fetal monitoring. *J Perinatol* 1996;16:15–19

10. Weiner Z, Farmakides G, Schulman H, Lopresti S, Schneider E. Surveillance of growth-retarded fetuses with computerized fetal heart rate monitoring combined with Doppler velocimetry of the umbilical and uterine arteries. *J Reprod Med* 1996;41:112–18

11. Martin CB Jr. Electronic fetal monitoring: a brief summary of its development, problems and prospects. *Eur J Obstet Gynecol Reprod Biol* 1998; 78:133–40

12. Devoe LD. Computerized fetal heart rate analysis and neural networks in antepartum fetal surveillance. *Curr Opin Obstet Gynecol* 1996;8:119–22

13. Zador IE. Computers in obstetrical and gynecological imaging. *Ultrasound Obstet Gynecol* 1992;2:309–11

14. Zador IE, Salari V, Chik L, Sokol RJ. Ultrasound measurement of the fetal head: computer versus operator. *Ultrasound Obstet Gynecol* 1991;1:208–11

15. Zador IE, Salari V, Sokol RJ. Computer application in ultrasound imaging. *Ultrasound Q* 1994;12:205–15

16. Hata T, Manabe A, Aoki S, Miyazaki K, Yoshino K, Yamamoto K. Three-dimensional intrauterine sonography in the early first-trimester of human pregnancy: preliminary study. *Hum Reprod* 1998;13:740–3

17. Chang FM, Hsu KF, Ko HC, *et al.* Three-dimensional ultrasound assessment of fetal liver volume in normal pregnancy: a comparison of reproducibility with two-dimensional ultrasound and a search for a volume constant. *Ultrasound Med Biol* 1997;23:381–9

18. Sklansky MS, Nelson TR, Pretorius DH. Three-dimensional fetal echocardiography: gated versus nongated techniques. *J Ultrasound Med* 1998;17: 451–7

19. Levental M, Pretorius DH, Sklansky MS, Budorick NE, Nelson TR, Lou K. Three-dimensional ultrasonography of normal fetal heart: comparison with two-dimensional imaging. *J Ultrasound Med* 1998;17:341–8

20. Riccabona M, Johnson D, Pretorius DH, Nelson TR. Three dimensional ultrasound: display modalities in the fetal spine and thorax. *Eur J Radiol* 1996;22:141–5

21. Laudy JA, Janssen MM, Struyk PC, Stijnen T, Wallenburg HC, Wladimiroff JW. Fetal liver volume measurement by three-dimensional ultrasonography: a preliminary study. *Ultrasound Obstet Gynecol* 1998;12:93–6

22. McKeown MJ. Use of the Internet for obstetricians and gynecologists. *Am J Obstet Gynecol* 1997;176: 271–4

23. Larkin M. Interactive pregnancy, parenting, and ob/gyn websites. *Lancet* 1998;352:916

24. Feingold M, Kewalramani R, Kaufmann GE. Internet and obstetrics and gynecology. *Acta Obstet Gynecol Scand* 1997;76:718–24

25. Smith RP. Internet update. *MD Comput* 1998;15: 10–13,15–27

26. Warner I. Telemedicine applications for home health care. *J Telemed Telecare* 1997;3(Suppl 1): 65–6

27. Malone FD, Nores JA, Athanassiou A, *et al.* Validation of fetal telemedicine as a new obstetric imaging technique. *Am J Obstet Gynecol* 1997;177: 626–31

28. Jones MG. Telemedicine and the national information infrastructure: are the realities of health care being ignored? *J Am Med Inform Assoc* 1997;4:399–412

29. Macedonia CR. Telemedicine and ultrasonography: making waves. *Ultrasound Obstet Gynecol* 1998;12:84–5

30. Landwehr JB, Zador IE, Wolfe HM, Dombrowski MP, Treadwell MC. Telemedicine and fetal ultrasonography: assessment of technical performance and clinical feasibility. *Am J Obstet Gynecol* 1997;177:846–8

31. Satya-Murti S. Medical journals on line. *J Am Med Assoc* 1997;277:673–7

Index

abdomen, B-mode studies of, 47
abortion (spontaneous), intervillous circulation and, 31
absent or reversed end-diastolic blood flow, 89
absent or reversed end-diastolic flow,
    fetal heart rate variability and, 157
    outcome and, 159
acardiac twin, umbilical cord ligation in, 192
achondrogenesis type II, B-mode studies of, 48
acidemia, intrapartum surveillance for, 245
acrania,
    B-mode studies of, 46
    three-dimensional ultrasound of, 104, 105
adenosine deaminase deficiency, hematopoietic stem cell
    transplantation *in utero* for, 199
AIDS (acquired immune deficiency syndrome), gender
    differences in, 317
allantoid cyst, 68
amnionicity, three-dimensional ultrasound of, 107
anemia in fetomaternal transfusion, 214
anencephaly,
    B-mode studies of, 46
    three-dimensional ultrasound of, 20, 104
aneuploidy,
    hyperechogenicity in, 13
    prediction by increased resistance index in umbilical
        circulation, 11
anophthalmia, three-dimensional ultrasound of, 104
anti-coagulants in pre-eclampsia, 352
antiphospholipid, 291
antithrombin III, thrombophilia and, 288
antithrombin III deficiency, 288
Apgar score, 238
Arnold–Chiari malformation, 256
arthrogryposis (congenital), 48
aspirin, role in pre-eclampsia, 350
atrioventricular septal defect, B-mode studies of, 47

banana sign, 256
bilateral renal agenesis, B-mode studies of, 47
biochemistry, maternal serum, 40
biophysical profile of fetus, 9–15
β-blockers in hypertension in pregnancy, 312
blood flow, *see* specific circulations
brain, ultrasound screening of, 382
bronchogenic cysts, 73

calcium supplements in pre-eclampsia, 353
calcium-channel-blocking agents in hypertension in
    pregnancy, 313
Campylobacter, 224
captopril in hypertension in pregnancy, 314
carbon monoxide poisoning, 306
cardiac defects, B-mode studies of, 47
cardiotocography, 251
cerebral circulation,
    hemodynamic changes in, 82, 83
    IUGR and, 81–85
cerebral palsy,
    in multiple pregnancy, 368–373
    risk factors for, 369
    vanishing twin syndrome and, 371
cervix, determination of ripening, 355
Cesarean section,
    after maternal death, 338
    principal indications for, 364
Chiari-II malformation,

development of, 257
etiology of, 257
prevention of by prenatal myelomeningocele coverage, 258
prevention of in fetal lambs, 259
cholestasis of pregnancy, 274–278
    complications of,
        fetal, 275
        maternal, 275
    definition of, 274
    management of, 277
    physiopathology of, 275
    surveillance of, 276
chorioangioma of placenta, 73
chorionic villus sampling, 117–123
    anatomy of chorionic villus and, 117
    complications, 121
    contraindications for, 120
    in twin pregnancy, 119
    indications for, 119
    limb abnormalities after, 121
    safety and efficacy, 120
    techniques of, 118, 119
    transabdominal, 118
    transcervical, 118
    transvaginal, 119
chorionicity,
    as a risk factor for cerebral palsy, 369
    three-dimensional ultrasound of, 107
chromosome abnormalities,
    biometrical markers of, 12
    biophysical profile of, 10
    indirect signs of, 11
    maternal serum biochemistry measures and, 40
    nuchal translucency as a sign of, 11
    nuchal translucency in, 38, 39
    pregnancy dating and, 37
    prevalence, 37
    pyelectasis as a marker of, 60
    screening for, 37
    theoretical risk of, 10
cleft lip, three-dimensional ultrasound of, 104
clonidine in hypertension in pregnancy, 312
clubfoot,
    three-dimensional ultrasound of, 105, 106
combined electronic–biochemical surveillance, 251
computers, use in fetal medicine, 389–395
congenital adrenal hyperplasia, medical therapy *in utero* for, 193
congenital cystic adenomatoid malformation, open *in utero*
    surgery for, 188
congenital diaphragmatic hernia, open *in utero* surgery for,
    188
congenital heart defects,
    diagnosis, 52
    fetal venous return and, 88
    four-chamber view of, 55
    frequency, 53
    prenatal diagnosis, 54
    screening for, 52–57
    severity, 53
congenital hip dysplasia, 386
contraction stress test, 151
corticosteroids in pre-eclampsia, 352
craniopharyngioma, 70
crown–rump length,
    as a sign of IUGR, 13
    importance of, 10

in trisomy, 18 37
cystic adenomatoid malformation, 73
cystoscopy, 191
cysts of umbilical cord, 68
cytomegalovirus,
    cholestasis and, 274
    congenital infection, 219
    diagnosis, 219
    epidemiology of perinatal infection, 217
    infection in pregnancy, 218
    outcome, 220
    pathogenesis of perinatal infection, 218
    prevention, 221
    screening for, 42
    therapy, 221

Dandy–Walker malformation, B-mode studies of, 47
diabetes mellitus,
    fetal lung maturity and, 229
    nucleated red blood cell counts in, 241
diazoxide in hypertension in pregnancy, 313
disseminated intravascular coagulopathy after fetal reduction
    in multiple pregnancy, 137
ductus venosus, developmental anatomy of, 86
dysplastic ear, three-dimensional ultrasound of, 104

ear,
    shape and fetal anomalies, 104
    three-dimensional ultrasound of normal, 105
echocardiography,
    clinical indications for, 54
    ultrasound indications for, 54
embryo,
    anatomy of chorionic villus and, 117
    heart rate anomalies, 10
    kinetics of, 9
    three-dimensional ultrasound of,
        at six weeks, 17
        at seven weeks, 17
        at eight weeks, 17
    umbilical Doppler of, 10
enalapril in hypertension in pregnancy, 314
encephalocele, B-mode studies of, 46
end-diastolic velocity, changes in during gestation, 33
epignathus, 72
Escherichia coli, 225
ethics,
    fetus–family relationship after maternal death, 341
    first codes of in medicine, 3
    HIV infection in pregnancy and, 331–335
    loss of maternal autonomy after brain death, 340
    management of maternal death during pregnancy, 336–342
    of fetal reduction in multiple pregnancy, 146
    virtues needed by doctor, 3
ethnicity,
    fetal distress and, 270
    fetal mortality and, 270
    hyaline membrane disease and, 268
    pre-eclampsia and, 344
    preterm delivery and, 267, 267–273
    variations of gestational age with maturity in, 267–273
ex utero intrapartum treatment (EXIT), 189
exencephaly, B-mode studies of, 46

factor V Leiden mutation, 291
Fas–Fas ligand interactions and fetomaternal tolerance, 111
fetal cells in maternal blood, 130–135
    optimization strategies, 130
    role in disease, 133
fetal heart rate,
    in fetomaternal transfusion, 212
    variability of, 157–164, 165
    variations with fetal behavior, 184
fetal malformation, diagnosis of, 12
fetal reduction in multiple pregnancy, 136–150
    advances in, 141

embryo selection for, 139
ethics of, 146
genetic testing and, 143
history of, 137
management of pregnancy after, 144
outcomes, 143
risk of anomalies after, 145
timing of, 139
fetomaternal tolerance, 111–116
    Fas–Fas ligand interactions in, 111
    HLA and natural killer cells in, 112
    indoleamine 2, 3-dioxygenase, 114
    mechanisms of, 113
    T helper cells in, 113
fetomaternal transfusion, 211–216
    diagnosis, 214
    etiology of, 211
    incidence, 211
    recognition of, 211
α-fetoprotein in fetomaternal transfusion, 214
fetus,
    acid–base status of, 238
    adaptation of to hypoxia–ischemia, 374
    arterial circulation in abnormal, 49
    behavior of,
        and brainstem integrity, 165–170
        fetal heart rate variations and, 184
        hemodynamics and, 181–185
    biophysical profile of, 153
    development of senses in, 171–180
    developmental anatomy of, 86
    distress in and ethnicity, 270
    hearing in, 174–177
    hemodynamic changes in,
        advanced redistribution stage, 82
        decompensatory phase, 83
        Doppler silent stage, 82
        early redistribution stage, 82
    intrapartum blood analysis, 252
    intrapartum surveillance of, 245–253
    medical therapies for, 192–196
    mortality and ethnicity, 270
    movement of,
        basic rest–activity cycle, 167
        eyes, 165
        in anencephaly, 166
        in fetomaternal transfusion, 212
        non-rapid eye movement sleep, 166
            hemodynamics in, 181
        patterns of, 165
        rapid eye movement sleep, 166
            hemodynamics in, 181
        stomach, 165
    olfaction in, 177
    open surgery on, 186–190
    oxygenation of, 301–309
    pain responses in, 173
    perinatal asphyxia in, 374–381
    pulmonary flow in, 76–80
    taste in, 177
    three-dimensional ultrasound of,
        at nine to ten weeks, 18
        at eleven weeks, 19
    tumors in, 70–75
    venous circulation in abnormal, 50
    venous return in, 86–92
    viability of after cardiorespiratory maternal death, 337
    vision in, 178
        damage to pre- and postnatally, 179
    visualization rate of parts in first trimester, 19
    well-being, acoustic responsiveneess as a measure of, 176
    well-being of,
        activity assessment and, 152
        antepartum testing of, 151–156
        contraction stress test, 151
        maternal assessment of fetal activity, 152

non-stress test, 152
umbilical artery Doppler velocimetry, 153
fiduciary role of doctor, 3

galactosemia, medical therapy *in utero* for, 195
Gardnerella vaginalis, 225
gastroschisis, B-mode studies of, 47
Gaucher's disease, hematopoietic stem cell transplantation *in utero* for, 200
genetic testing, fetal reduction in multiple pregnancy after, 143
gestational age,
cf. maturation and ethnicity, 267–273
estimation of in post-term pregnancy, 363
goiter, fetal, 72
gray-level histogram width, 93–101
group A streptococci, 224

hamartoma, renal, 73
hearing in the fetus, 174–177
loss in cytomegalovirus infection, 220
heart rate, embryonic, 10
HELLP syndrome (hemolysis,
elevated liver enzymes,
low platelets),
in the Netherlands, 343–346
role of fetal cells in, 134
hemangioendothelioma, 73
hematopoietic stem cell transplantation, 196–201
hemodynamics, fetal behavior and, 181–185
hemoglobinopathies,
hematopoietic stem cell transplantation *in utero* for, 198
prenatal diagnosis of, 124–129
screening in pregnancy, 127
hemolytic disease,
perinatal, 279–287
see also Rhesus incompatibility
hemorrhage,
adrenal and neuroblastoma, 386
in neonatal brain, 382
hepatitis, cholestasis and, 274
hepatitis B in pregnancy, 44
hip dysplasia (congenital), 386
HIV (human immunodeficiency virus),
antiretroviral therapy in pregnancy, 318
choice of drugs for, 319–322
assessment in pregnancy, 323
ethics of infection in pregnancy,
clinical ethics, 331
contraception, 332
partner notification, 333
patient disclosure to health workers, 333
pregnancy termination, 332
public ethics, 331
vertical transmission prevention, 334
gender differences in infection, 317
guidelines for zidovudine monotherapy in pregnancy, 327
in pregnancy, 44
management of in pregnancy, 317–330
peripartum management, 322
postpartum management, 322
protocol for management of in pregnancy, 324
vertical transmission prevention, 334
holoprosencephaly, B-mode studies of, 47
human leukocyte antigen (HLA), in fetomaternal tolerance, 112
Hurler's syndrome,
first use of fetal reduction in multiple pregnancy for, 137
hematopoietic stem cell transplantation *in utero* for, 200
hyaline membrane disease, ethnicity and, 268
hydralazine in hypertension in pregnancy, 312
hydranencephaly in congenital toxoplasmosis, 43
hydrocephalus, 383
hydronephrosis, 73
hydrops,

arterial circulation in, 49
in fetomaternal transfusion, 212
three-dimensional ultrasound of, 20
hyperhomocysteinemia, 290
hypertension in pregnancy,
angiotensin II receptor agonist in, 314
antihypertensive drugs for, 311
β-blockers in, 312
calcium-channel-blocking agents in, 313
clonidine in, 312
converting enzyme inhibitors in, 314
diazoxide in, 313
hydralazine in, 312
α-methyldopa, 311
nifedipine in, 313
nitrates in, 313
pharmacological management of, 310
see also pre-eclampsia
when to treat, 311
why treat, 311
hyperthyroidism, medical therapy *in utero* for, 194
hypoplasia, lung, 78
hypospadias, 61
hypothyroidism, medical therapy *in utero* for, 194
hypoxemia,
hemodynamic changes during, 81
pathophysiology of, 81
hypoxia, 301–309, 374–381
causes of, 304
intrapartum surveillance for, 245
maternal, 306
maternal oxygen administration in, 307
nucleated red blood cell counts as an index of, 238–244
pathophysiology of, 374
stages of progressive, 246
vasoactive agents for, 307
hypoxia–ischemia,
clinical manifestations of injury by, 376
mechanisms of injury in, 375
pathophysiology of, 374
patterns of injury, 376
prognosis after, 379
hysteroscopic metroplasty, 294–300

immune privilege, 111–116
immunodeficiency diseases, hematopoietic stem cell transplantation *in utero* for, 199
immunoglobulin G, use in perinatal hemolytic disease, 283
indoleamine 2,3-dioxygenase, fetomaternal tolerance and, 114
infections,
after chorionic villus sampling, 121
causative agents, 224, 225
clinical diagnosis, 223–228
cytomegalovirus, 217–222
definitions, 223
diagnosis of, 225
fetal morbidity from, 224
laboratory diagnosis, 223–228
maternal morbidity from, 224
pathogenesis, 224
prevalence, 223
screening for fetal, 41
inferior vena cava, developmental anatomy of, 86
infertility,
multiple pregnancy and treatments for, 136, 144
iniencephaly, B-mode studies of, 46
intermittent auscultation, 251
Internet, 392
intervillous circulation,
continuous flow and spontaneous abortion, 31
evaluation of, 28–36
flow changes during gestation, 33
in late pregnancy, 32
in pre-eclamptic pregnancy, 34

intraplacental circulation, color Doppler evaluation of, 29
intrauterine growth restriction (IUGR),
    ARED and, 157
    as a marker of chromosome abnormalities, 12
    cerebral circulation in, 81–85
    gray-level histogram width studies of, 96
    pre-eclampsia and, 347–354
    Wharton's jelly and, 64
iodine deficiency and fetal goiter, 72
itching, cholestasis of pregnancy and, 274

kidneys,
    B-mode studies of, 47
    multicystic, 73
    polycystic, 73
    pyelectasis in, 58–63
Kleihauer–Betke test, 213, 280

labor induction, 355–361, 366
lambda sign, measure for chorionicity, 40
lemon sign, 47, 256
leukomalacia, 382
limb abmormalities, after chorionic villus sampling, 121
lipoma, intracranial, 70
Listeria monocytogenes, 224
liver, gray-level histogram width studies of, 96
losartan in hypertension in pregnancy, 314
lower obstructive uropathy, endoscopic in utero surgery for, 190
lower urinary tract obstruction, endoscopic in utero surgery for, 190
lung, gray-level histogram width studies of, 96
lung circulation, normal, 76
lung hypoplasia, 78
lung maturity,
    assessment by ultrasound, 93
    assessment of, 229–237
        foam test, 231
        lamellar body count, 234
        lecithin/sphingomyelin ratio, 231
        optical density of amniotic fluid, 234
        phosphatidylglycerol, 231
        surfactant/albumin ratio, 231
        ultrasound, 234

Maroteaux–Lamy syndrome, hematopoietic stem cell
    transplantation in utero for, 200
maternal–fetal blood flow, 302
maturity, cf. gestational age and ethnicity, 267–273
meconium, fetal distress and, 242
MEDLINE, 393
megacystis, B-mode studies of, 47
meningomyelocele, 73
metabolic diseases, hematopoietic stem cell transplantation in
    utero for, 200
metachromatic leukodystrophy, hematopoietic stem cell
    transplantation in utero for, 200
methemoglobinemia, 306
α-methyldopa in hypertension in pregnancy, 311
methylmalonic acidemia, medical therapy in utero for, 195
microcephaly in cytomegalovirus infection, 220
midgut herniation, three-dimensional ultrasound of, 104
mifepristone (RU486), use in labor induction, 357
misoprostol, use in labor induction, 359
monitoring,
    cardiotocography, 251
    combined electronic–biochemical surveillance, 251
    hypoxia–ischemia and, 377
    in cholestasis of pregnancy, 276
    intermittent auscultation, 251
    intrapartum surveillance, 245–253
    judgement of, 247
    of post-term pregnancies, 365
mortality (maternal),
    brain death, 338–340
    cardiorespiratory, 337

Cesarean section during and after, 338
    definition of, 336
    fetus–family relationship after, 341
    incidence, 336
    management of during pregnancy, 336–342
multicystic dysplastic kidney disease, B-mode studies of, 47
multiple carboxylase deficiency, medical therapy in utero for, 195
multiple pregnancy,
    cerebral palsy in, 368–373
    chorionic villus sampling in, 119
    fetal reduction in, 136–150
    first-trimester scans of, 40
    study of cutaneous stimulation reactions in, 172
    three-dimensional ultrasound of, 107
    treatments for infertility as a cause of, 136
myelomeningocele,
    artificial creation of, 259
    B-mode studies of, 47
    Chiari-II malformation prevention by prenatal coverage, 258
    experimental repair of in fetal lambs, 259
    natural history of, 255
    postnatal management of, 255
    prenatal repair of, 254–264
    see also spina bifida
myoblastoma, 72

natural killer cells, in fetomaternal tolerance, 112
nephroblastoma, 73
neural tube defects,
    medical therapy in utero for, 196
    see also specific defects
neuroblastoma, 386
nifedipine in hypertension in pregnancy, 313
nitrates in hypertension in pregnancy, 313
nitric oxide in pre-eclampsia, 351
non-reactive non-stress test, 226
non-stress test, 152
nuchal translucency,
    as a sign of subsequent twin–twin transfusion syndrome, 40
    B-mode studies of, 48
    fetal venous return and, 88
    in chromosome abnormalities, 11, 13, 37
    measurement of, 38
    prognostic value of, 10
nucleated red blood cell counts,
    as an index of hypoxia, 238–244
    calculation from white blood cell counts, 239
    mechanism of production, 241

olfaction in the fetus, 177
oligodendroma, 70
omphalocele,
    B-mode studies of, 47
    three-dimensional ultrasound of, 104
omphalomesenteric duct cyst, 68
osteogenesis imperfecta type II, B-mode studies of, 48
oxygenation of fetus, 301–309
oxyhemoglobin in fetus cf. adult, 303
oxytocin, use in labor induction, 356

pain,
    development of senses and, 171
    fetal responses to, 173
patient, –doctor relationship, 3
peak systolic velicity, changes in during gestation, 33
placenta, gray-level histogram width studies of, 96
placentation, physiopathological aspects of, 347
polydactyly, three-dimensional ultrasound of, 106
polymerase chain reaction, use on fetal cells in maternal
    blood, 131
polyploidy, signs of, 11
porencephaly, 382
Potter syndrome, see bilateral renal agenesis
pre-eclampsia, 310–316
    anti-coagulants, 352

aspirin and, 350
calcium supplements in, 353
corticosteroids in, 352
epidemiology of in the Netherlands, 343–346
intervillous circulation and, 34
nitric oxide in, 351
physiopathology of, 347–354
role of fetal cells in, 133
pregnancy,
anembryonic cf. normal, 30
B-mode studies in first trimester, 46–49
cholestasis of, 274–278
Doppler studies in first trimester, 49–51
fetomaternal tolerance in, 111–116
intervillous circulation in late, 32
management of maternal death during, 336–342
multiple, *see* multiple pregnancy
placentation during, 348
post-term, 362–367
impact of, 363
incidence of, 363
surveillance methods for, 365
screening procedures in first trimester, 37–45
prenatal diagnosis, techniques of, 144
prostaglandins, use in labor induction, 358
protein C deficiency, 288, 289
protein C resistance, 289
protein S deficiency, 288, 289
pruritus, cholestasis of pregnancy and, 274
pulmonary artery flow velocity waveforms, 76
pulmonary venous flow velocity waveforms, 78
pulsatility index, changes in during gestation, 33
pyelectasis, 58–63
as a marker of chromosome abnormalities, 60
definition, 58
outcome in, 61
perinatal management of, 58

resistance index,
changes in during gestation, 33
in spiral artery, 30
of arterial intervillous flow, 30
respiratory distress syndrome, 229
retinopathy, 179
rhabdomyoma, congenital, 72
Rhesus incompatibility, 279–287
biochemistry amd molecular genetics of, 279
etiology of, 280
high-dose intravenous immunoglobulin G for, 283
intrauterine fetal transfusion, 281
pathogenesis of, 280
patient management in, 282
prophylaxis for, 286
risks of, 286
sensitization mechanism for, 280
treatment of, 281
RU486, *see* mifepristone
rubella in pregnancy, 43

sacrococcygeal teratoma, 73
open *in utero* surgery for, 188
sarcoma, intracranial, 70
scleroderma, role of fetal cells in, 133
screening,
for chromosome abnormalities, 37
for congenital heart defects, 52–57
for fetal infections, 41
for hemoglobinopathies, 127
for Rhesus incompatibility, 279–287
of neonate by ultrasound, 382–388
sensitivity, study of cutaneous stimulation reactions in
multiple pregnancy, 172
septate uterus,
diagnosis and treatment of, 295
intervention in, 299

obstetric complications in, 297
prediction of pregnancy outcome in by ultrasound, 298
pregnancy outcome in, 294–300
severe combined immunodeficiency syndrome,
hematopoietic stem cell transplantation *in utero* for, 199
sickle cell disorders,
hematopoietic stem cell transplantation *in utero* for, 198
prenatal diagnosis of, 124
single umbilical artery syndrome, *see* umbilical artery, single
skeletal dysplasias, B-mode studies of, 48
skelton, B-mode studies of, 47
spina bifida,
B-mode studies of, 46
Chiari-II malformation in, 257
prenatal diagnosis of, 256
prenatal repair of, 254–264
see also myelomeningocele; neural tube defects
spiral artery,
flow changes in during gestation, 33
resistance index in, 30
surfactant,
function of, 230
production of, 230
role of, 229
surgery,
hysteroscopic metroplasty, 294–300
intrapartum, 189
surgery (*in utero*),
endoscopic,
laser ablation in twin–twin transfusion, 192
lower obstructive uropathy, 190
myelomeningocele repair in lambs by, 261
umbilical cord ligation by, 192
for myelomeningocele, 254–264
open,
closing of the uterus after, 189
fetal homeostasis during, 187
for congenital cystic adenomatoid malformation, 188
for congenital diaphragmatic hernia, 188
for sacrococcygeal teratoma, 188
monitoring during, 187
timing of, 186
risk and benefit assessments, 254
use in non-lethal defects, 255
syphilis in pregnancy, 44

taste in the fetus, 177
telemedicine, 392
temporal averaged maximum velocity, changes in during
gestation, 33
teratoma,
cervical, 71
gastric, 73
intracranial, 70
nasopharyngeal, 72
sacrococcygeal, 73
open *in utero* surgery for, 188
α-thalassemia, prenatal diagnosis of, 125
β-thalassemia, prenatal diagnosis of, 125
thalassemias, hematopoietic stem cell transplantation *in utero*
for, 198
thanatophoric dwarfism, B-mode studies of, 48
thrombophilia, 288–293
acquired causes, 288
diagnosis, 291
inherited causes of, 288
therapy, 291
toxoplasmosis,
hydranencephaly in neonate with, 43
screening for, 42
tracheal ligation, 189
transfusion,
intrauterine fetal for perinatal hemolytic disease, 281
see also fetomaternal; twin–twin
transplantation *in utero*, 196–201

tricuspoid atresia, 42
trisomy 13, umbilical cord pseudocyst in, 11
trisomy 18,
    crown–rump length in, 37
    umbilical cord pseudocyst in, 11
trisomy 21,
    bilateral ectasia of renal pelvis as a sign of, 13
    nuchal translucency in, 38
    pyelectasis as a marker of, 60
tuberous sclerosis complex,
    congenital rhabdomyomas and, 72
    intracranial tumors and, 70
tumors,
    abdominal, 73
    adrenal gland, 386
    cervical, 71
    diagnosis of, 70–75
    intracranial, 70
    kidney, 386
    management of, 70–75
    mediastinal, 73
    oronasopharyngeal, 72
    placental, 73
    see also specific tumors
    thoracic, 72
twin–twin transfusion syndrome, 205–210
    as a risk factor for cerebral palsy, 370
    diagnosis of, 206
    laser ablation in, 192
    nuchal translucency as a sign of subsequent, 40
    outcome, 208
    pathophysiology of, 205
    treatment of, 207
twins, see multiple pregnancy

ultrasound,
    B-mode studies in first trimester pregnancies, 46–49
    biophysical profile of fetus by, 9–15
    brain screening in neonate, 382
    color Doppler,
        of intervillous circulation, 28
        of yolk sac, 24
    congenital hip dysplasia, 386
    diagnosis and treatment of septate uterus using, 295
    Doppler, 10
        fetal venous return in abnormal fetuses, 88
        fetal venous return in normal fetuses, 87
        fetal venous return in second and third trimesters, 89
        in abnormal fetus, 49
        in first trimester pregnancies, 49–51
        pulmonary flow waveforms, 76–80
        umbilical artery Doppler velocimetry for fetal well-
            being measurement, 153
    fetal lung maturity assessment by, 93
    gray-level histogram width,
        base length measurement in, 95
        comparisons of, 94
        determination of, 94
        development of technique, 93
        of fetal liver, 96   of fetal lung, 96
        of placenta, 96
    in hypoxia–ischemia, 378
    lung maturity assessment by, 234
    markers for chromosome abnormalities, 12
    of umbilical cord, 64–69
    prediction of pregnancy outcome in septate uterus, 298
    role in chorionic villus sampling, 118
    screening for tumors, 386
    screening policies in neonate, 382–388
    three-dimensional,
        advanced sonoembryology by, 16–23

        fetal anomaly identification by, 20
        history of, 21
        in first trimester, 103
        in second trimester, 103
        in third trimester, 103
        methods used, 16
        of embryo, 17
        of fetus, 18, 19
        use in prenatal diagnosis, 102–108
    timing of screening, 48
    tissue characterization by, 93–101
    twin–twin transfusion syndrome diagnosis by, 206
    urinary tract screening in neonate, 384
umbilical artery,
    color Doppler evaluation of flow in, 29
    compression of, 305
    discordant, 65
    single,
        as a sign of chromosome abnormalities, 11
        implications of, 66
        incidence, 66
        three-dimensional ultrasound of, 107
umbilical circulation,
    Doppler studies of, 10
    increased resistance index in and chromosome
        abnormalities, 11
umbilical cord,
    blood flow in and oxygenation of fetus, 302
    cystic lesions of, 68
    maternal–fetal blood flow and, 302
    measurement of by ultrasound, 64
    nucleated red cell count and hypoxia, 238–244
    ultrasound of, 64–69
umbilical cord pseudocyst, 11
ureteropelvic junction obstruction, 59
uterine circulation, fetal hypoxia and, 305
uteroplacental circulation,
    color Doppler evaluation of, 29
    in cynomolgus monkeys, 31

vanishing twin syndrome and cerebral palsy, 371
vasoactive agents for hypoxia, 307
venous return, evaluation in fetus, 86–92
ventricular septal defect, B-mode studies of, 47
vision in the fetus, 178
    damage to, 179
vitamin C in pre-eclampsia, 353
vitamin E in pre-eclampsia, 353
voiding cystourethrography, 59

well-being of fetus, antepartum testing of, 151–156
Wharton's jelly and IUGR, 64
Wilms' tumor, 73, 386

X-linked recessive inheritance, hematopoietic stem cell
    transplantation in utero for, 199

yolk sac,
    echogenicity of, 13
    in abnormal pregnancy, 25
    in normal pregnancy, 24
    size as a marker of chromosome abnormalities, 12
    vascularization of, 24–27
    volume of, 24–27

zidovudine,
    guidelines for monotherapy in pregnancy, 327
    use in HIV infection, 317
zygosity, as a risk factor for cerebral palsy, 369